Ancient and Traditional Foods, Plants, Herbs and Spices used in Cardiovascular Health and Disease

The use of different foods, herbs and spices to treat or prevent disease has been recorded for thousands of years. Egyptian papyrus, hieroglyphics and ancient texts from the Middle East have described the cultivation and preparations of herbs and botanicals to "cure the sick." There are even older records from China and India. Some ancient scripts describe the use of medicinal plants which have never been seen within European cultures. Indeed, all ancient civilizations have pictorial records of different foods, herbs and spices being used for medical purposes. However, there are fundamental questions pertaining to the scientific evidence for the use of these agents or their extracts in modern medicine.

There have been considerable advances in scientific techniques over the last few decades. These have been used to examine the composition and applications of traditional cures. Modern science has also seen the investigation of herbs, spices and botanicals beyond their traditional usage. For example, plants which have been used for "digestion" or "medical ills" since time immemorial are now being investigated for anti-cancer properties or their toxicity, using high throughput screening. Techniques also include molecular biology, cellular biochemistry, physiology, endocrinology and even medical imaging. However, much of the material relating to the scientific basis or applications of traditional foods, herbs, spices and botanicals is scattered among various sources. The widespread applicability of foods or botanicals are rarely described and cautionary notes on toxicity are often ignored. This is addressed in *Ancient and Traditional Foods, Plants, Herbs and Spices used in Cardiovascular Health and Disease*.

Ancient and Traditional Foods, Plants, Herbs and Spices in Human Health

Series Editors

Vinood B. Patel *University of Westminster, London*

Victor R. Preedy *King's College, London*

Rajkumar Rajendram *King Abdulaziz Medical City, Riyadh*

Each volume in the series provides an evidenced-based ethos describing the usage and applications of traditional foods and botanicals in human health. The content provides a platform upon which other scientific studies can be based. These may include the extraction or synthesis of active agents, *in vitro* studies, pre-clinical investigations in animals, and clinical trials.

The key benefits of each volume:

- Chapters provide a historical background on the usage of food and plant-based therapies.
- Chapters are based on the results of studies using scientific techniques and methods.
- Presents wide references to other foods, herbs and botanicals reported to have curative properties.
- Chapters are self-contained, focused toward specific conditions.

Ancient and Traditional Foods, Plants, Herbs and Spices used in Cardiovascular Health and Disease
Edited by Rajkumar Rajendram, Victor R. Preedy, and Vinood B. Patel

For more information about this series, please visit https://www.routledge.com/Ancient-and-Traditional-Foods-Plants-Herbs-and-Spices-in-Human-Health/book-series/ATFHSH

Ancient and Traditional Foods, Plants, Herbs and Spices used in Cardiovascular Health and Disease

Edited by
Rajkumar Rajendram, Victor R. Preedy,
and Vinood B. Patel

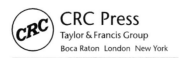

CRC Press is an imprint of the
Taylor & Francis Group, an **informa** business

First edition published 2023
by CRC Press
6000 Broken Sound Parkway NW, Suite 300, Boca Raton, FL 33487–2742

and by CRC Press
4 Park Square, Milton Park, Abingdon, Oxon, OX14 4RN

CRC Press is an imprint of Taylor & Francis Group, LLC

© 2024 selection and editorial matter, Victor R. Preedy, Vinood B. Patel, and Rajkumar Rajendram; individual chapters, the contributors

Reasonable efforts have been made to publish reliable data and information, but the author and publisher cannot assume responsibility for the validity of all materials or the consequences of their use. The authors and publishers have attempted to trace the copyright holders of all material reproduced in this publication and apologize to copyright holders if permission to publish in this form has not been obtained. If any copyright material has not been acknowledged please write and let us know so we may rectify in any future reprint.

Except as permitted under U.S. Copyright Law, no part of this book may be reprinted, reproduced, transmitted, or utilized in any form by any electronic, mechanical, or other means, now known or hereafter invented, including photocopying, microfilming, and recording, or in any information storage or retrieval system, without written permission from the publishers.

For permission to photocopy or use material electronically from this work, access www.copyright.com or contact the Copyright Clearance Center, Inc. (CCC), 222 Rosewood Drive, Danvers, MA 01923, 978–750–8400. For works that are not available on CCC please contact mpkbookspermissions@tandf.co.uk

Trademark notice: Product or corporate names may be trademarks or registered trademarks and are used only for identification and explanation without intent to infringe.

Library of Congress Cataloging-in-Publication Data
Names: Patel, Vinood B., editor. | Preedy, Victor R., editor. | Rajendram, Rajkumar, editor.
Title: Ancient and traditional foods, plants, herbs and spices used in cardiovascular health and disease / edited by Vinood B. Patel, Victor R. Preedy, and Rajkumar Rajendram.
Description: First edition. | Boca Raton : CRC Press, 2023. | Includes bibliographical references. | Summary: "The use of different foods, herbs and spices to treat or prevent disease has been recorded for thousands of years, however, there are fundamental questions pertaining to the scientific evidence for the use of these agents in modern medicine. This book investigates the use of foods, herbs, plants and spices for properties which may be beneficial in the treatment of cardiovascular disease. It provides information on diets; specific agents, items, and extracts; resources; and each chapter focuses on a plant-derived material providing a historical background, uses, toxicity and cautionary notes and summary points"— Provided by publisher.
Identifiers: LCCN 2022060969 (print) | LCCN 2022060970 (ebook) | ISBN 9781032108582 (hardback) | ISBN 9781032115344 (paperback) | ISBN 9781003220329 (ebook)
Subjects: LCSH: Cardiovascular system—Diseases—Diet therapy. | Cardiovascular system—Diseases—Alternative treatment. | Cardiovascular system—Diseases—Prevention. | Heart—Diseases—Diet therapy. | Heart—Diseases—Alternative treatment. | Heart—Diseases–Prevention.
Classification: LCC RC684.D5 A53 2023 (print) | LCC RC684.D5 (ebook) | DDC 616.1/0654–dc23/eng/20230406
LC record available at https://lccn.loc.gov/2022060969
LC ebook record available at https://lccn.loc.gov/2022060970

ISBN: 978-1-032-10858-2 (hbk)
ISBN: 978-1-032-11534-4 (pbk)
ISBN: 978-1-003-22032-9 (ebk)

DOI: 10.1201/9781003220329

Typeset in Times
by Apex CoVantage, LLC

Contents

Editors ix
Contributors xi

SECTION I   Overviews and Dietary Components

Chapter 1   Connecting the Link between Oxidative Stress, Dietary Antioxidants and Hypertension 3

Sukhchain Kaur, Tushar Midha, Oyndril Dutta, Om Prakash Saini, Rasmi Ranjan Muduli, Anil K. Mantha and Monisha Dhiman

Chapter 2   Domestic and International Research on the Relationship between Japanese Diet and Ischemic Heart Disease 19

Tomoko Imai and Hiroshi Shimokata

Chapter 3   Olive Oil and Other Oils as a Part of Traditional Diets and Bioactive Compounds for Cardioprotection 35

Estefanía Sánchez Rodríguez, Laura Alejandra Vázquez Aguilar and María Dolores Mesa García

Chapter 4   Herbs and Molecular Basis of Cardiovascular Protection 49

Shubhang Joshi, Vinay M. Paliwal, Vikram Vamsi Priya and Bidya Dhar Sahu

Chapter 5   Seaweed in Traditional Diets and Relationship with Cardiovascular Disease Incidence and Mortality...65

Kazumasa Yamagishi, Wanlu Sun and Hiroyasu Iso

SECTION II   Specific Agents, Items and Extracts

Chapter 6   Asiatic Pennywort (*Centella asiatica*) and Cardiovascular Protection: A New Narrative 77

Chin Theng Ng, Siau Hui Mah and Lai Yen Fong

Chapter 7   *Terminalia arjuna* and Cardiovascular Protection: A Comprehensive Overview 93

Aashis Dutta and Manas Das

v

Chapter 8 Baicalein Extract from Chinese Herbal Medicine to Use in Cardiovascular Diseases: Focus on Myocardial Ischemia/Reperfusion Injury 111

Ramona D'Amico, Salvatore Cuzzocrea and Rosanna Di Paola

Chapter 9 Balloon Vine (*Cardiospermum halicacabum* L.) and Cardiovascular Protection: Cellular, Molecular and Metabolic Aspects 125

A. Rajasekaran, R. Arivukkarasu and G. Venkatesh

Chapter 10 Black Cumin (*Nigella sativa*): Biological Activities and Molecular Aspects in Relation to Cardiovascular Disease.. 145

Maryam Moradi Binabaj and Fereshteh Asgharzadeh

Chapter 11 Date Palm (*Phoenix dactylifera*) and Cardiovascular Protection: Molecular, Cellular and Physiological Aspects.. 161

Heba Abd Elghany Sahyon

Chapter 12 The Beneficial Action of *Artemisia* Genus on the Cardiovascular System.............. 177

Smail Amtaghri and Mohamed Eddouks

Chapter 13 Kalmegh (*Andrographis paniculata*) and Cardioprotective Mechanisms.............. 193

Vuanghao Lim, Jun Jie Tan and Yoke Keong Yong

Chapter 14 Ka'á Jaguá (*Aloysia polystachya* (Griseb.) Moldenke (Verbenaceae)): From Traditional Use to Pharmacological Investigations in Relation to Cardiovascular Disease 215

Jane Manfron, Karyne Garcia Tafarelo Moreno, Vanessa Samudio Santos Zanuncio, Denise Brentan Silva and Arquimedes Gasparotto Junior

Chapter 15 *Bridelia ferruginea* and Myocardial Protection in Mitochondrial Membrane Permeability 231

Oluwatoyin O. Ojo

Chapter 16 Lingzhi (*Ganoderma lucidum*) and Cardiovascular Disease.................................. 247

Brian Tomlinson, Sze Wa Chan and Paul Chan

Chapter 17 Mexican Orchid (*Prosthechea karwinskii*) and Use in Cardiovascular Protection: Cellular and Physiological Aspects 259

Luicita Lagunez Rivera, Gabriela Soledad Barragan Zarate, Rodolfo Solano, Alfonso Alexander Aguilera and Aracely E. Chavez Piña

Contents   **vii**

Chapter 18 Mushrooms and Cardiovascular Protection: Molecular, Cellular, and Physiological Aspects 281

    Rachel B. Wilson and Nica M. Borradaile

Chapter 19 Pomegranate (*Punica granatum*) and Cardiovascular Protection: Molecular, Cellular, and Metabolic Aspects 297

    María del Rocío Thompson Bonilla and María Eugenia Jaramillo Flores

Chapter 20 Review on Phytochemistry and Pharmacological Properties of *Momordica dioica* Roxb.: Special Emphasis on Cardioprotective Activity 313

    Seema Mehdi, Tamsheel Fatima Roohi, Suman P., M. S. Srikanth and K. L. Krishna

Chapter 21 Saptrees (Genus *Garcinia*) and Cardioprotection: Molecular, Cellular, and Metabolic Aspects 331

    Elvine Pami Nguelefack-Mbuyo and Télesphore Benoît Nguelefack

Chapter 22 Watermelon (*Citrullus lanatus*) and Cardiovascular Protection: A Focus on the Effects of Citrulline 345

    Bilgehan Ozcan, Christophe Moinard and Elise Belaïdi

SECTION III   Resources

Chapter 23 Recommended Resources on Cardiovascular Health and Disease in Relation to Foods, Plants, Herbs and Spices in Human Health 361

    Rajkumar Rajendram, Daniel Gyamfi, Vinood B. Patel and Victor R. Preedy

Index 371

Editors

Dr. Rajkumar Rajendram, AKC, BSc (Hons), MBBS (Dist), MRCP (UK), FRCA, EDIC, FFICM, is a clinician scientist with a focus on internal medicine, anesthesia, intensive care and peri-operative medicine. Dr Rajendram's interest in traditional medicines began at medical school when he attended the Society of Apothecaries' history of medicine course. He subsequently graduated with distinctions from Guy's, King's and St. Thomas Medical School, King's College London in 2001. As an undergraduate he was awarded several prizes, merits and distinctions in pre-clinical and clinical subjects. Dr. Rajendram completed his specialist training in acute and general medicine in Oxford in 2010 and then practiced as a Consultant in Acute General Medicine at the John Radcliffe Hospital, Oxford. Dr. Rajendram also trained in anesthesia and intensive care in London and was awarded fellowships of the Royal College of Anaesthetists (FRCA) and the Faculty of Intensive Care Medicine (FFICM) in 2009 and 2013 respectively. He then moved to the Royal Free London Hospitals as a Consultant in Intensive Care, Anesthesia and Peri-operative Medicine. He has been a fellow of the Royal College of Physicians of Edinburgh (FRCP Edin) and the Royal College of Physicians of London (FRCP Lond) since 2017 and 2019 respectively. He is currently a Consultant in Internal Medicine at King Abdulaziz Medical City, National Guard Health Affairs, Riyadh, Saudi Arabia. Dr. Rajendram recognizes that integration of traditional medicines into modern paradigms for healthcare can significantly benefit patients. As a clinician scientist he has therefore devoted significant time and effort to nutritional science research and education. He is an affiliated member of the Nutritional Sciences Research Division of King's College London and has published more than 300 textbook chapters, review articles, peer-reviewed papers and abstracts.

Victor R. Preedy, BSc, PhD, DSc, FRSB, FRSPH, FRCPath, FRSC, is a staff member of the Faculty of Life Sciences and Medicine within King's College London. Professor Preedy is also a member of the Department of Nutrition and Dietetics (teaching), Director of the Genomics Centre of King's College London and Professor of Clinical Biochemistry (Hon) at Kings College Hospital. Professor Preedy graduated in 1974 with an Honours Degree in Biology and Physiology with Pharmacology. He gained his University of London PhD in 1981. In 1992, he received his Membership of the Royal College of Pathologists and in 1993 he gained his second doctorate (DSc), for his outstanding contribution to protein metabolism in health and disease. Professor Preedy was elected as a Fellow to the Institute of Biology in 1995 and to the Royal College of Pathologists in 2000. Since then he has been elected as a Fellow to the Royal Society for the Promotion of Health (2004) and The Royal Institute of Public Health (2004). In 2009, Professor Preedy became a Fellow of the Royal Society for Public Health and in 2012 a Fellow of the Royal Society of Chemistry. Professor Preedy has carried out research when attached to Imperial College London, The School of Pharmacy (now part of University College London) and the MRC Centre at Northwick Park Hospital. He has collaborated with research groups in Finland, Japan, Australia, USA and Germany. Professor Preedy is a leading expert on the science of health and has a long-standing interest in dietary and plant-based components. He has lectured nationally and internationally. To his credit, Professor Preedy has published more than 700 articles, which include peer-reviewed manuscripts based on original research, abstracts and symposium presentations, reviews and numerous books and volumes.

Vinood B. Patel, BSc, PhD, FRSC, is currently Reader in Clinical Biochemistry at the University of Westminster and honorary fellow at King's College London. He presently directs studies on metabolic pathways involved in liver disease, particularly related to mitochondrial energy regulation and cell death. Research is being undertaken to study the role of nutrients, antioxidants, phytochemicals, iron, alcohol and fatty acids in the pathophysiology of liver disease. Other areas of interest are identifying new biomarkers that can be used for the diagnosis and prognosis of liver disease and understanding mitochondrial oxidative stress in Alzheimer's disease and gastrointestinal dysfunction in autism. Dr Patel graduated from the University of Portsmouth with a degree in Pharmacology and completed his PhD in protein metabolism from King's College London in 1997. His postdoctoral work was carried out at Wake Forest University Baptist Medical School studying structural-functional alterations to mitochondrial ribosomes, where he developed novel techniques to characterize their biophysical properties. Dr Patel is a nationally and internationally recognized researcher and has several edited biomedical books related to the use or investigation of active agents or components. These books include *The Handbook of Nutrition, Diet, and Epigenetics; Branched Chain Amino Acids in Clinical Nutrition; Cancer: Oxidative Stress and Dietary Antioxidants and Diet Quality: An Evidence-Based Approach; Toxicology: Oxidative Stress and Dietary Antioxidants,* and *Molecular Nutrition: Vitamins.* In 2014 Dr Patel was elected as a Fellow to The Royal Society of Chemistry.

Contributors

Laura Alejandra Vázquez Aguilar
Department of Biochemistry and Molecular
Biology II
Institute of Nutrition and Food Technology
"José Mataix," Biomedical Research
Centre University of Granada
Spain

Alfonso Alexander Aguilera
Facultad de Bioanálisis
Universidad Veracruzana
Mexico

Smail Amtaghri
Faculty of Sciences and Techniques
Errachidia
Moulay Ismail University of Meknes
Morocco

R. Arivukkarasu
Department of Pharmacognosy
KMCH College of Pharmacy
Tamil Nadu, India

Fereshteh Asgharzadeh
Department of Physiology
Faculty of Medicine
Mashhad University of Medical Sciences
Iran

Elise Belaïdi
HP2 Laboratory
Univ. Grenoble Alpes
CHU Grenoble Alpes
France

Maryam Moradi Binabaj
Cellular and Molecular Research Center
Sabzevar University of Medical Sciences
Iran

María del Rocío Thompson Bonilla
Laboratorio de Medicina Genómica
Investigación Biomédica y
Traslacional
ISSSTE, Hospital Regional
Mexico

Nica M. Borradaile
Department of Physiology and Pharmacology
Western University
Canada

Paul Chan
Division of Cardiology
Department of Internal Medicine
Wan Fang Hospital
Taipei Medical University
Taiwan

Sze Wa Chan
School of Health Sciences
Caritas Institute of Higher Education
Hong Kong SAR
China

Salvatore Cuzzocrea
Department of Chemical, Biological,
Pharmaceutical and Environmental Sciences
University of Messina
Italy

Ramona D'Amico
Department of Chemical, Biological,
Pharmaceutical and Environmental Sciences
University of Messina
Italy

Manas Das
Animal Physiology and Biochemistry
Laboratory
Department of Zoology
Gauhati University
India

Monisha Dhiman
Department of Microbiology
School of Basic and Applied Sciences
Central University of Punjab
India

Aashis Dutta
Animal Physiology and Biochemistry
Laboratory
Department of Zoology
Gauhati University
India

Oyndril Dutta
Department of Microbiology
School of Basic and Applied Sciences
Central University of Punjab
India

Mohamed Eddouks
Faculty of Sciences and Techniques Errachidia
Moulay Ismail University of Meknes
Morocco

María Eugenia Jaramillo Flores
Department of Biochemical Engineering
School of Biological Sciences
Instituto Politécnico Nacional
Mexico

Lai Yen Fong
Department of Preclinical Sciences
Faculty of Medicine and Health Sciences
Universiti of Tunku Abdul Rahman
Malaysia

María Dolores Mesa García
Department of Biochemistry and Molecular
    Biology II
Institute of Nutrition and Food Technology
    "José Mataix," Biomedical Research Centre
University of Granada
Spain

Arquimedes Gasparotto Junior
Laboratory of Electrophysiology and
    Cardiovascular Pharmacology
Faculty of Health Sciences
Federal University of Grande Dourados
Brazil

Daniel Gyamfi
The Doctors Laboratory Ltd
London, United Kingdom

Tomoko Imai
Department of Food Science and Nutrition
Faculty of Human Life and Science
Doshisha Women's College of Liberal Arts
Japan

Hiroyasu Iso
Department of Social Medicine
Osaka University
Japan

Shubhang Joshi
National Institute of Pharmaceutical Education
    and Research (NIPER)-Guwahati
Assam, India

Sukhchain Kaur
Department of Microbiology
School of Basic and Applied Sciences
Central University of Punjab
India

K. L. Krishna
Department of Pharmacology
JSS College of Pharmacy
JSS Academy of Higher Education & Research
India

Vuanghao Lim
Integrative Medicine Cluster
Advanced Medical and Dental Institute
Universiti Sains Malaysia
Malaysia

Siau Hui Mah
School of Biosciences
Centre for Drug Discovery and Molecular
    Pharmacology
Faculty of Health and Medical Sciences
Taylor's University
Malaysia

Jane Manfron
Department of Pharmaceutical Sciences
State University of Ponta Grossa
Brazil

Anil K. Mantha
Department of Zoology
School of Basic and Applied Sciences
Central University of Punjab
India

Seema Mehdi
Department of Pharmacology
JSS College of Pharmacy
JSS Academy of Higher Education & Research
India

Tushar Midha
Department of Microbiology
School of Basic and Applied Sciences
Central University of Punjab
India

Contributors

Christophe Moinard
LBFA
Univ. Grenoble Alpes
France

Karyne Garcia Tafarelo Moreno
Laboratory of Electrophysiology and
Cardiovascular Pharmacology
Faculty of Health Sciences
Federal University of Grande Dourados
Brazil

Rasmi Ranjan Muduli
Department of Microbiology
School of Basic and Applied Sciences
Central University of Punjab
India

Chin Theng Ng
Faculty of Medicine
AIMST University
Kedah, Malaysia

Télesphore Benoît Nguelefack
Research Unit of Animal Physiology and
Phytopharmacology
Department of Animal Biology
Faculty of Science
University of Dschang
Cameroon

Elvine Pami Nguelefack-Mbuyo
Research Unit of Animal Physiology and
Phytopharmacology
Department of Animal Biology
Faculty of Science
University of Dschang
Cameroon

Oluwatoyin O. Ojo
Department of Chemical Sciences,
Faculty of Natural and Applied Sciences
Anchor University Lagos
Nigeria

Bilgehan Ozcan
HP2 Laboratory
Univ. Grenoble Alpes
CHU Grenoble Alpes
France

Dr. Suman P.
Department of Dravyaguna
Govt. Ayurvedic Medical College & Hospital
India

Vinay M. Paliwal
National Institute of Pharmaceutical Education
and Research (NIPER)-Guwahati
Assam, India

Rosanna Di Paola
Department of Chemical, Biological,
Pharmaceutical and Environmental
Sciences
University of Messina
Italy

Vinood B. Patel
School of Life Sciences
University of Westminster
London, United Kingdom

Aracely E. Chavez Piña
Laboratorio de Farmacología
Escuela Nacional de Medicina y Homeopatía
Instituto Politécnico Nacional
Mexico

Victor R. Preedy
School of Life Course and Population Sciences
King's College London
London, United Kingdom

Vikram Vamsi Priya
National Institute of Pharmaceutical Education
and Research (NIPER)-Guwahati
Assam, India

A. Rajasekaran
Department of Pharmaceutical Analysis
KMCH College of Pharmacy
Tamil Nadu, India

Rajkumar Rajendram
College of Medicine
King Saud bin Abdulaziz University for Health
Sciences
Riyadh, Saudi Arabia

Luicita Lagunez Rivera
Laboratorio de Extracción y Análisis de
Productos Naturales Vegetales

Centro Interdisciplinario de Investigación para
el Desarrollo Integral Regional
Unidad Oaxaca
Instituto Politécnico Nacional
Mexico

Estefanía Sánchez Rodríguez
Department of Biochemistry and Molecular
Biology II
Institute of Nutrition and Food Technology
"José Mataix," Biomedical Research Centre
University of Granada
Spain

Tamsheel Fatima Roohi
Department of Pharmacology
JSS College of Pharmacy
JSS Academy of Higher Education & Research
India

Bidya Dhar Sahu
Department of Pharmacology & Toxicology
National Institute of Pharmaceutical Education
and Research (NIPER)-Guwahati
Assam, India

Heba Abd Elghany Sahyon
Department of Chemistry
Faculty of Science
Kafrelsheikh University
Egypt

Om Prakash Saini
Department of Microbiology
School of Basic and Applied Sciences
Central University of Punjab
India

Hiroshi Shimokata
Institute of Health and Nutrition
Nagoya University of Arts and Sciences
Japan

Denise Brentan Silva
Laboratory of Natural Products and Mass
Spectrometry
Faculty of Pharmaceutical Sciences, Food, and
Nutrition
Federal University of Mato Grosso do Sul
Brazil

Rodolfo Solano
Centro Interdisciplinario de Investigación para
el Desarrollo Integral Regional Unidad
Oaxaca
Instituto Politécnico Nacional
Mexico

M. S. Srikanth
Department of Pharmacy Practice
JSS College of Pharmacy
JSS Academy of Higher Education &
Research
India

Wanlu Sun
Department of Public Health Medicine
Faculty of Medicine and Health
Services Research and Development
Center
University of Tsukuba
Japan

Jun Jie Tan
Advanced Medical and Dental Institute
Universiti Sains Malaysia
Malaysia

Brian Tomlinson
Faculty of Medicine
Macau University of Science and Technology
China

G. Venkatesh
Department of Pharmacology
KMCH College of Pharmacy
Coimbatore, India

Rachel B. Wilson
Department of Physiology and
Pharmacology
Western University
Canada

Kazumasa Yamagishi
Department of Public Health Medicine
Faculty of Medicine and Health
Services Research and Development
Center
University of Tsukuba
Japan

Yoke Keong Yong
Department of Human Anatomy
Faculty of Medicine and Health Sciences
Universiti Putra Malaysia
Malaysia

Vanessa Samudio Santos Zanuncio
Laboratory of Natural Products and
  Mass Spectrometry
Faculty of Pharmaceutical Sciences, Food,
  and Nutrition
Federal University of Mato Grosso do Sul
Brazil

Gabriela Soledad Barragan Zarate
Laboratorio de Extracción y Análisis de
  Productos Naturales Vegetales
Centro Interdisciplinario de Investigación para
  el Desarrollo Integral Regional Unidad
  Oaxaca
Instituto Politécnico Nacional
Mexico

Section I

Overviews and Dietary Components

1 Connecting the Link between Oxidative Stress, Dietary Antioxidants and Hypertension

Sukhchain Kaur, Tushar Midha, Oyndril Dutta,
Om Prakash Saini, Rasmi Ranjan Muduli,
Anil K. Mantha and Monisha Dhiman

CONTENTS

1.1	Introduction	4
1.2	Hypertension	4
1.3	Oxidative Stress	6
1.4	Protein Oxidation (PO)	7
1.5	Lipid Peroxidation (LPO)	7
1.6	DNA/RNA or Nucleic Acid Oxidation	7
1.7	Antioxidants and CVDs	8
1.8	Natural Antioxidants as Anti-Hypertensive Agents	8
1.9	Vitamin A	8
1.10	Ascorbic Acid or Vitamin C	9
1.11	Vitamin E	10
1.12	Coenzyme Q10	10
1.13	Sirtuins	11
1.14	Flavonoids	11
1.15	Plants with Antioxidant Properties	12
1.16	Toxicity and Cautionary Notes	13
1.17	Summary Points	13
References		14

LIST OF ABBREVIATIONS

8-oxodG	8-Oxo-7,8-Dihydro-2'-Deoxyguanosine
8-oxoG	8-Oxo-7,8-Dihydroguanosine
AA	Ascorbic Acid
ACE	Angiotensin-Converting Enzyme
AGE	Advanced Glycation End Product
AOPPs	Advanced Oxidation Protein Products
ASCVD	Atherosclerotic Cardiovascular Diseases
CAD	Coronary Artery Disease
CHD	Coronary Heart Disease
CKD	Chronic Kidney Disease
CoQ	Coenzyme Q10
CVD	Cardiovascular Disease
DBP	Diastolic Blood Pressure
DNA	Deoxyribonucleic Acid

DOI: 10.1201/9781003220329-2

DPPH	2,2-Diphenyl-1-Picrylhydrazyl
EGC	Epigallocatechin
EGCG	Epigallocatechin Gallate
Hg	Mercury
HT	Hypertension
IMA	Ischemia Modified Albumin
LDL	Low-Density Lipoprotein
LPO	Lipid Peroxidation
MAP	Mitogen-Activated Protein
MDA	Malondialdehyde
mm	Millimetre
mtDNA	Mitochondrial DNA
NADPH	Nicotinamide Adenine Dinucleotide Phosphate
NCDs	Non-Communicable Diseases
NO	Nitric Oxide
NOS	Nitric Oxide Synthase
NOX	NADP Oxidase
Nrf	Nuclear Transcription Factor
OH	Hydroxyl
PCO	Protein Carbonyl
PO	Protein Oxidation
RAAS	Renin Angiotensin Aldosterone System
RBC	Red Blood Corpuscles
RNA	Ribonucleic Acid
ROS	Reactive Oxygen Species
SBP	Systolic Blood Pressure
SHR	Spontaneously Hypertensive Rats
SIRT	Sirtuins
SOD	Superoxide Dismutase
T-SH	Total Thiol
WYK	Wistar Kyoto Rats

1.1 INTRODUCTION

Cardiovascular disease (CVD) is used as umbrella terminology for various interlinked ailments that may affect the heart and the blood vessels and includes hypertension, coronary heart disease (CHD), cerebrovascular disease, heart failure, cardiomyopathies, atherosclerosis, rheumatic/congenital heart disease and chronic kidney disease (CKD) (WHO 2021; Escobar 2002). CVDs are responsible for approximately 18 million deaths per annum which contribute to 31% of mortality worldwide and a majority of premature deaths occurs due to CHD and cerebrovascular mishaps (Stewart et al. 2017). In India, the occurrence rate of non-communicable diseases (NCDs) is more than 54% of total deaths and surprisingly, out of which 25% is shared by CVDs (Chopra and Ram 2019). The association between CVDs, oxidative stress and antioxidants are multifaceted. Oxidative stress plays a crucial role in the pathophysiology of CVD linked disorders such as hypertension, atherosclerosis, ischemic heart disease, cardiomyopathies and congestive heart failure by causing cardiac and vascular abnormalities (García et al. 2017).

1.2 HYPERTENSION

Hypertension is one of the important CVDs which is characterized by an abnormal increase in blood pressure such as systolic blood pressure (SBP) > 130 mmHg or diastolic blood pressure

(DBP) > 80 mmHg. Hypertension is accountable for 7.5 billion deaths annually worldwide (Delacroix and Chokka 2014). Hypertension is a crucial predisposing factor for heart failure, stroke, peripheral arterial disease, and is a reason for chronic kidney disease. Hypertension is frequently connected with metabolic disorders such as diabetes and dyslipidaemia, and the occurrence rate of these diseases is very high nowadays (Václavík 2018). According to the American Heart Association, blood pressure less than 120/80 mm Hg is considered within the normal limits whereas the blood pressure range from 120–129 systolic and greater than 80 mm Hg diastolic, is said to be elevated pressure, and persons with elevated blood pressure are more prone to develop high blood pressure (Arnett et al. 2019). Stage I hypertension is when systolic blood pressure ranges from 130–139 mm Hg or diastolic blood pressure ranges from 80–89 mm Hg. Stage I hypertension is involved with a greater risk of developing atherosclerotic cardiovascular diseases (ASCVD), such as heart attack or stroke. When blood pressure steadily ranges at 140/90 mm Hg or higher, the condition is known to be stage II hypertension. A hypertensive crisis occurs when the blood pressure unexpectedly outstrips 180/120 mm Hg (Arnett et al. 2019).

The association between hypertension and Renin Angiotensin Aldosterone System (RAAS) is very multifarious. The up-regulated activation of the RAAS plays a crucial role in the occurrence of endothelial dysfunction and hypertension. Up-regulation of RAAS induces insulin resistance and increases ROS production in cardiovascular tissues (Yagi et al. 2013). Aliskiren was the first oral renin inhibitor approved to be used as an anti-hypertensive agent and is also reported to lower the increase in ROS produced by RAAS (Alshahrani 2020); hence the pathophysiology of hypertension is greatly affected by oxidative stress (Figure 1.1). The production of excessive ROS and a limited supply of antioxidants in the living system are known as oxidative stress.

TABLE 1.1
Classification of Blood Pressure Based upon Various Stages of Hypertension

Blood Pressure Classification	Normal	Elevated	Hypertension (Stage I)	Hypertension (Stage II)	Hypertension Emergency
Systolic (mm Hg)	< 120	120–129	130–139	140 or > 140	> 180
Systolic (mm Hg)	< 80	> 80	80–89	90 or > 90	> 120

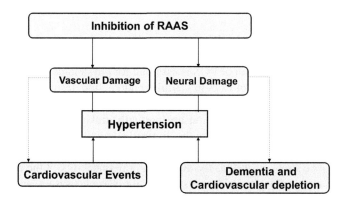

FIGURE 1.1 Role of Renin Angiotensin pathway in the implication of hypertension.

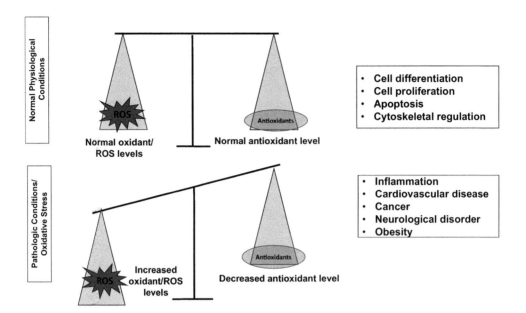

FIGURE 1.2 Excessive ROS production leads to pathological conditions, while moderate levels of ROS are required for normal physiological functions in the cells.

The reduced levels of various antioxidants such as superoxide dismutase and glutathione peroxidase activity are associated with hypertension in newly diagnosed and untreated hypertensive patients and these reduced levels of antioxidants are inversely interrelated with blood pressure. The increased levels of hydrogen peroxide production also seem to be associated with hypertensive patients (Baradaran et al. 2014). Moreover, higher lipid hydroperoxide and protein carbonyls production has been seen in hypertensive subjects. The hypertensive patients with renal abnormalities showed a significant increase in oxidative stress suggesting antioxidant therapy can be proven as a beneficial remedy to control the effects of hypertension and to reduce the oxidative damage which ultimately can control blood pressure. While dietary antioxidants have positive effects on hypertension and cardiovascular risk factors, these effects are not very consistent for effective and improved results for high-risk hypertension. So, it is required to set up such strategies which enhance the action of single or combined antioxidants in the treatment of hypertension and hypertension linked ailments (Figure 1.2).

1.3 OXIDATIVE STRESS

Oxidative stress is known to be involved in numerous diseases. It is a condition of abnormal production of reactive oxygen species (ROS) and an insufficient supply of antioxidants in the body. On other hand, the normal production of ROS is essential for physiological processes in the human body. But the increased production of ROS in vascular endothelium results in endothelial dysfunction that further aids the occurrence of atherosclerosis and CKD.

Endothelial dysfunction and inflammation are mutually linked to each other during CVDs. The hallmarks of endothelial dysfunction are the diminished nitric oxide (NO) bioavailability, low endothelium-based vasorelaxation, and increased expression of inflammatory genes, extreme ROS generation and oxidative stress, as well as the alteration in permeability of the cell layer. A number of ROS sources are responsible for oxidative stress in the vascular system such as NADPH oxidase, NO synthase and xanthine oxidase. NADPH oxidases (NOXs) (e.g. NOX1 and NOX2) are the class of enzymes that produce ROS and imperative sponsors of endothelial dysfunction as well as inflammation in vascular ailments for instance in hypertension, diabetes and ageing, etc. (Chen et al. 2018). The increased expression of vascular NOX1 has been observed in ethanol induced hypertension which is further associated with the expression of different proteins involved in abnormal vascular contraction and ROS production (Marchi et al. 2016).

1.4 PROTEIN OXIDATION (PO)

Protein oxidation is demarcated as any covalent modification of a protein prompted by interaction with reactive oxygen species (ROS) or with by-products of oxidative stress. ROS targets and oxidizes both amino acid chains and protein-protein backbones that results in protein fragmentation and the normal functioning of protein get altered. The major targeted amino acids are cysteine and methionine due to the presence of the sulfur group in those amino acids. Oxidative-stress-induced alterations in proteins induce structural and conformational changes and affect the solubility of the proteins. These alterations make proteins more susceptible to proteolysis and further upsets their enzymatic properties (Davies 2016). Protein carbonyls and advanced glycation end products (AGEs) are the main imprints of protein oxidation in the cells. A group of 30 hypertensive patients and 30 normotensive individuals were demonstrated to check the association between hypertension and protein oxidation and the study revealed that Plasma total thiol (T-SH), protein carbonyl (PCO), advanced oxidation protein products (AOPPs), ischemia modified albumin (IMA) were significantly increased in hypertensive patients in comparison to healthy individuals. This finding shows that oxidative stress or ROS generated in cells act as a leading cause in the progression of hypertension as well as ageing events (S. Yavuzer et al. 2016). The high levels of MDA and protein carbonyls, as well as low antioxidant levels, were found to be associated with the pathophysiology of Coronary artery disease (CAD) (Tejaswi et al. 2017).

1.5 LIPID PEROXIDATION (LPO)

Lipid peroxidation is a stamp of oxidative stress in CVDs that indicates the exposure of membrane lipids of cells to excessive ROS production. LPO results in the altered membrane permeability and oxidation of lipids present in the cellular membranes. Stimulated inflammatory cells produce ROS and enzymes such as myeloperoxidase which initiate lipid peroxidation. When the process of LPO continues in cells, then the 8-isoprostane and malondialdehyde (MDA), 8-isoprostane, 8-ISO; 4-hydroxy-2-nonenal, 4-HNE have often reported by-products of this process. Altered lipid peroxidation might be implicated in vascular mild cognitive impairment and also lead to redox imbalance with neuronal mitochondrial damage which further accelerates the cognitive consequences of vascular disease (Suridjan et al. 2017). LPO events also demonstrated in hypertension due to a weakened oxidant/antioxidant status. Peroxidative damage decreases the antioxidants with an increase in blood pressure and age progression (Yavuzer et al. 2016).

1.6 DNA/RNA OR NUCLEIC ACID OXIDATION

The oxidative-stress-induced DNA/RNA oxidation shows a strong link between the pathophysiology of various diseases. Nucleic acid oxidation mainly involves base substitution, addition, deletion and other mutations. Nucleic acid oxidation results in the formation of by-products (e.g. 8-Oxo-7,8-dihydro-2'-deoxyguanosine (8-oxodG) and 8-oxo-7,8-dihydroguanosine (8-oxoG)); these by-products are identified to be associated with CAD and heart failure. Accumulation of oxidized DNA and DNA damage response elements such as atherosclerotic plaques of human samples and animal models is evidence of ROS-induced destruction that further fuels apoptosis and ageing, which are conceivable outcomes of the DNA damage response. Mitochondrial DNA (mtDNA) is more prone to oxidative damage as compared to nuclear DNA because of continuous exposure to ROS in the inner mitochondrial membrane through the electron transport chain. Mitochondrial DNA oxidative

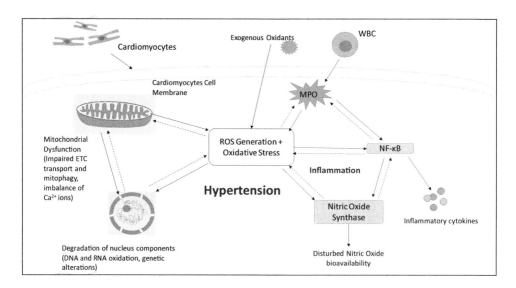

FIGURE 1.3 Role of ROS/oxidative stress in hypertension.

damage interferes with cellular respiration and promotes lethal concerns for the cell. High levels of 8-oxodG were demonstrated in serum and urine samples of hypertension and CAD patients with an increased rate of heart failure (Guo et al. 2017; Yavuzer et al. 2016) (Figure 1.3).

1.7 ANTIOXIDANTS AND CVDS

During the normal physiological function, the body's antioxidant defense systems are proficient in scavenging the ROS generated in the body due to oxidative stress to sustain the oxidant-antioxidant balance (Siti et al. 2015). This antioxidant defense system comprises enzymatic antioxidants such as superoxide dismutase, glutathione peroxidase and catalase. The non-enzymatic ones include glutathione, albumin and bilirubin (Figure 1.4).

1.8 NATURAL ANTIOXIDANTS AS ANTI-HYPERTENSIVE AGENTS

Vitamins are indispensable nutrients that are prerequisites for several physio-chemical processes in the human body. The fact is universally acknowledged that appurtenance of some vitamins is required as these vitamins are not manufactured in the body. The categorization of vitamins is done based upon their solubility in water (B complexes and C) and fat (A, D, E and K) (Uribe et al. 2017).

Various antioxidants such as vitamin A precursors and derivatives, ascorbic acid (vitamin C), α-Tocopherol (vitamin E), L-Arginine, flavonoids, some mitochondrial-specific antioxidants (Coenzyme Q10, Acetyl-L-Carnitine and α-Lipoic Acid) and garlic, glutamate, N-acetylcysteine, sour milk and vitamin D all have shown anti-hypertensive effects through antioxidant mechanisms that may involve inhibition of sources of excessive ROS (Siti et al. 2015).

1.9 VITAMIN A

Retinoids are the precursor and derivatives of vitamin A which comprises a beta-carotene ring with an isoprenoid carbon chain (Craft and Furr 2019). The main sources of vitamin A are liver, sweet potato, carrot, pumpkin, and broccoli leaf, etc. Beta-carotene, a compound related to vitamin A, is known for its cardio-protective roles but the participation of vitamin A as an anti-hypertensive agent is a bit contradictory because some reports showed the contribution of vitamin A as a pro-oxidative factor in hypertension complications (Figure 1.5) (Petiz et al. 2017).

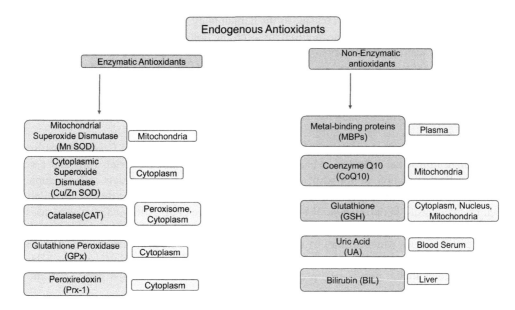

FIGURE 1.4 Various endogenous enzymatic and non-enzymatic antioxidants present in the cells.

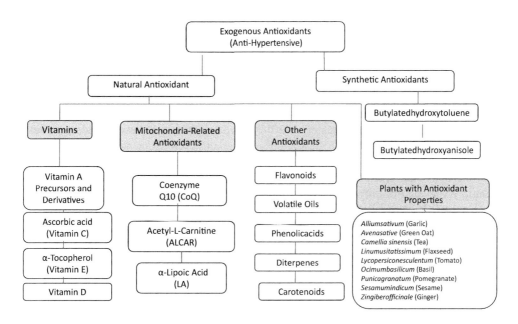

FIGURE 1.5 Classification of some exogenous antioxidants having anti-hypertensive properties.

1.10 ASCORBIC ACID OR VITAMIN C

Vitamin C, also known as ascorbic acid (AA), occurs in two biologically active forms: reduced form – ascorbate and oxidized form – dehydroascorbic acid. It consists of six-carbon lactone and is an important nutrient in humans (Linowiecka et al. 2020). The potential role of ascorbic acid supplementation is the scavenging of free radicals that contains a single pair electron (Kaźmierczak-Barańska et al. 2020). The plasma concentrations of ascorbate may efficiently contend for superoxide and decrease thiols. Ascorbic acid has the potential to suppress the NADPH oxidase activity and it shows limited pro-oxidant capacity (Baradaran et al. 2014).

Vitamin C is supplemented from outside as the human body is unable to synthesize this vitamin due to the deficiency of a key enzyme required for its production (i.e. enzyme gulonolactoneoxidase) (Ma et al. 2020). Whereas the majority of plant species have a tremendous capacity to fabricate vitamin C, and these plant sources contain a high amount of this vitamin (i.e. up to 5,000 mg/100 g). The main dietary sources of vitamin C are citrus fruits, strawberries, tomatoes, green and red peppers, broccoli, Indian gooseberry and other green vegetables. Vitamin C usually gets absorbed by passive diffusion/active diffusion in the buccal cavity/gastrointestinal tract respectively (Devaki and Raveendran 2017).

Existing studies demonstrate how the antioxidant capability of vitamin C contributes to cardiovascular health. Atherosclerosis is characterized as the ailment of arterial walls and a series of events of lipid oxidation, and modification, which further leads to persistent inflammation and plaque formation. Vitamin C reduces the risk of atherosclerosis by precluding the oxidative damage caused by low-density lipoprotein (LDL)-cholesterol (Salvayre et al. 2016) and also condenses the adhesion of monocytes. The apoptosis episodes in vascular smooth muscle increase the stability of atherosclerotic plaques which further exaggerate the pathophysiology of atherosclerosis, and vitamin C stops apoptosis, which makes plaques unstable. Furthermore, vitamin C aids the balanced production of endothelial nitric oxide production which is directly associated with a reduction in increased blood pressure.

The anti-hypertensive efficacy of ascorbic acid has been estimated in a number of trials. Some studies showed modest discounts in blood pressure in both normal and hypertensive subjects. Studies based upon meta-analysis divulged the significant role of vitamin C in the reduction of blood pressure in hypertensive groups (Guan et al. 2020).

1.11 VITAMIN E

It is a group of compounds such as tocopherols and tocotrienols (Szewczyk et al. 2021). The main dietary sources enriched in vitamin E include avocados, asparagus, nuts, leafy green vegetables and vegetable oils (Shahidi and de Camargo 2016). Vitamin E is a powerful antioxidant that hinders LDL and lipid peroxidation (Galmés et al. 2018). Further, vitamin E lowers oxidative stress by inhibiting the actions of NADPH oxidase, lipoxygenase and cyclo-oxygenase. Still, some studies represent vitamin E's pro-oxidant capacity under certain cellular conditions. Combined antioxidant therapy (e.g. combination of vitamin E with vitamin C or A) significantly improves the proficiency of vitamin E and significantly decreases the blood pressure. The decreased antioxidant capacity and increased ROS production have been observed in patients with essential hypertension. The SOD activity in erythrocytes and vitamin E levels is decreased in essential hypertensive subjects. The hypertensive patients with uncontrolled blood pressure showed increased superoxide ions and H_2O_2 levels; also a significant increase in concentrations of lipid peroxides in plasma was observed (Manning et al. 2005).

Since the positive results of antioxidant treatment have been observed in animal experimental studies, so many clinical trials have been executed to determine if antioxidant treatment can improve cardiovascular disease. Several antioxidant treatments such as vitamins C and E decreases O^{2-} production in renal tissue, thus preventing renal damage, and also improving renal function and decreasing blood pressure.

1.12 COENZYME Q10

CoQ (2, 3 dimethoxy-5 meth-6-decaprenyl benzoquinone) is a derivative of mevalonic acid and phenylalanine. This complex is a key factor of the electron transport chain that accepts electrons from Complexes I and II and the glyceraldehyde-3-phosphate shuttle (Linkner and Humphreys 2018). The lower CoQ levels are found to be associated with a greater risk of hypertension in older adults. CoQ reduces the production of superoxide ions in mitochondria by increasing the productivity of electron transfer from Complexes I and II down the mitochondrial electron transport chain (Alcázar-Fabra et al. 2016). Coenzyme Q is also known for its antioxidant effect by dropping lipid peroxidation in the plasma membrane. The CoQ supplementation is found to be associated with reductions in blood pressure in hypertensive subjects (Sood and Keenaghan 2021). In animal models of hypertension such as in spontaneously hypertensive rats (SHR), the increased urinary excretion of NO metabolites and marked up-regulation of renal, vascular and cardiac NOS isotype expression were observed. Whereas the administration of the effective antioxidant compound desmethyltirilazad improved hypertension, dropped excretion of urinary NO metabolite and decreased the compensatory up-regulation of NOS isotypes in SHR. This study showed the role of oxidative stress and chaotic NO metabolism in the pathogenesis of hypertension, and antioxidant therapy altered the deleterious effects of oxidative stress in SHR.

1.13 SIRTUINS

The sirtuins are the nicotinamide adenine dinuclcotide dependent deacetylases and are grouped based on their subcellular location. The nuclear sirtuins include SIRT1, SIRT6 and SIRT7 while the mitochondrial sirtuins include SIRT3, SIRT4 and SIRT5 (Miller 2020). The potential of SIRT3 as a therapeutic target in hypertension was proved by Dikalova et al. (Dikalova et al. 2020), where restoring the SIRT3 levels in hypertensive mice lead to a decrease in blood pressure and normalization of vascular superoxide levels. SIRT 3 increases the activity of mitochondrial superoxide dismutase 2 by de-acetylating the lysine residues. The depletion of SIRT3 in hypertension promotes vascular inflammation, hypertrophy and endothelial dysfunction.

1.14 FLAVONOIDS

Flavonoids are the group of naturally occurring polyphenolic compounds with a specialized structure of benzo-γ-pyrone ring (Feng et al. 2017). Flavonoids are universally found in most plants and are manufactured by the phenylpropanoid pathway. Fruits, vegetables, grains, bark, roots, stems, flowers, tea and wine are the main sources of flavonoids. Flavonoids are being used in various pharmaceutical, medicinal and nutraceutical sectors because these compounds act as excellent antioxidants against oxidative stress, also play a role as anti-inflammatory and anti-carcinogenic agents. Flavonoids are also known to modify the activities of crucial enzymes to maintain cellular homeostasis (Panche et al. 2016). The flavonoids prevent the cells from oxidative damage by inhibiting the activities of oxidant enzymes such as glutathione S-transferase, NADH oxidase, monooxygcnase, etc. as these enzymes are associated with ROS production (Kumar and Pandcy 2013).

An existing study demonstrated that the antioxidant properties of quercetin (a flavonoid) lower the blood pressure and heart rate in spontaneously hypertensive (SHR) as compared to normotensive Wistar Kyoto rats (WKY) when quercetin is administrated orally to these rats. Quercetin also showed a positive effect on cardiac and renal hypertrophy in SHR, whereas in the case of WKY, no effect was seen (Duarte et al. 2001) and it suggested the anti-hypertensive effect of flavonoids.

Regular consumption of other flavonoids such as dietary catechins (e.g. epigallocatechin (EGC) and epigallocatechin gallate (EGCG) etc.) maintains healthy systolic blood pressure and blood glucose levels that ultimately lower the risk of hypertension as well as diabetes. Further, these catechins show a protective role against oxidative stress responses in rat models.

Another flavonoid, myricetin, shows anti-hypertensive and antioxidant properties by reversing the augmented levels of lipid peroxidation in the heart tissue of the hypertensive rat model. Myricetin also increased the diminished antioxidant status (superoxide dismutase, catalase and glutathione) in hypertensive rat models (Borde et al. 2011). Flavonoids increase the bioavailability of nitric oxide (NO) and improve endothelial functioning, suggesting their anti-hypertensive role against hypertension pathophysiology (Maaliki et al. 2019; Wang et al. 2021).

1.15 PLANTS WITH ANTIOXIDANT PROPERTIES

The anti-hypertensive effect of dietary black sesame meal was checked in pre-hypertensive patients and it was observed that black sesame seeds showed positive effects on oxidative stress by targeting increased levels of lipid peroxidation and by lowering the blood pressure in hypertensive subjects (Wichitsranoi et al. 2011).

In a double-blind, placebo-controlled pilot study, the 31 subjects suffering from grade-1 HT, without any associated ailments, who were not taking any anti-hypertensive drug therapy, were complemented with tomato extract for four weeks. Tomato extract is loaded with plenty of carotenoids and lycopene is a major carotenoid that is known for its antioxidant and free-radical scavenging properties. This short-term treatment of tomato extract decreased the systolic and diastolic pressures, as well as lowered the production of the maker of lipid peroxidation (i.e. thiobarbituric-acid-reactive substances) (Engelhard et al. 2006).

An investigation showed that the supplementation of Resveratrol, a key ingredient of red wine enriched with polyphenols, positively affects the blood pressure and endothelial dysfunction biomarkers such as F_2-isoprostanes, malondialdehyde and protein carbonyls in the model of essential hypertension (Upadhyay et al. 2018). The four-week administration of red wine in male spontaneously hypertensive rats (SHRs) gradually declined blood pressure significantly; also this administration further lowered the oxidation of proteins and lipids with increased production of nitric oxide (Del Pino-García et al. 2017). So, these studies proved that various antioxidants act as anti-hypertensive agents against hypertension and various CVDs. The antioxidant extracts of blueberry are reported to throttle oxidative stress by quelling ROS production and also by choking off lipid peroxidation in hypertensive animal models. Nrf2 inhibition has been shown to aggravate oxidative stress and inflammation (Farooqui et al. 2021). Blueberry extract re-establishes the antioxidant protection shield by equipping antioxidants at transcriptional (Nrf-2) and translational levels (SOD). Simultaneously, the blueberry extract wards off the levels of oxidant enzymes in pulmonary hypertension (Türck et al. 2020).

Black cumin (*Nigella sativa* L.) is a herb with nutraceutical values and is famous for its spicy nature, culinary uses, and medicinal properties. It is widely found in the Indian subcontinent along with southwest Asia, northeastern Africa and the eastern Mediterranean. Thymoquinone is the primary bioactive component present in black cumin and it acts majorly to reduce oxidative stress and inflammation. The compound thymoquinone and its derivatives are the major chemical groups in black cumin. It is an important natural antioxidant, and it helps in lowering the reactive oxygen species and up-regulates superoxide dismutase, catalase, and glutathione (Hannan et al. 2021).

Ginseng (*Panax ginseng*) is a pharmaceutically important plant with medicinal properties that are widely used in Asian countries to treat a variety of diseases including hypertension. Fermented ginseng root extract is rich in ginsenosides Rg3 and Rh2, which largely suppress the ROS production that reduces the damage to the RBC membranes. Fermented and non-fermented ginseng root extracts decrease the nitrite levels inside macrophages, enhancing the anti-inflammatory activity. Antioxidants like superoxide dismutase and glutathione peroxidase can be greatly increased by the administration of ginseng (Lee and Kim 2014).

Celery (*Apium graveolens* L.) is an ancient plant from India with numerous health benefits including anti-hypertensive properties. It is widely used in Indian traditional medicines, due to the presence of compounds like limonene, selinene, frocoumarin glycosides, flavonoids and vitamin A. The flavonoids, phenolic acids and tansipropanoids compounds have antioxidant properties. These compounds act as an antioxidant, which prevents peroxidation and free radicals. Polyphenols neutralize free radicals by utilizing their phenolic groups to accept hydrogen from the hydrogen donors. The roots of the plant can successfully remove OH groups and DPPH (2,2-diphenyl-1-picrylhydrazyl) radicals (Kooti and Daraei 2017).

Mango (*Mangifera indica*) is one of the famous fruits from the Indian subcontinent and is the second most famous tropical fruit crop in the world. Its leaves are a rich source of antioxidants and are used to treat hypertension. The dichloromethanic fraction of the *M. indica* leaves are exceptionally good antioxidants and its effect is similar when compared to that of enalapril, an anti-hypertensive drug. The main components of the dichloromethanic fraction are flavonoids that promote the antioxidant properties. The fraction also has an inhibitory role in ACE and reduction of MAP activity leading to its anti-hypertensive property, and hence decreased risks of cardiovascular diseases and strokes (Ronchi et al. 2015).

The leaf of *Piper betel* (betel vine) is best known for its anti-cancer, antimicrobial and antioxidant properties. The antioxidant property of *P. betel* leaf is due to high phenolic and flavonoid content. Quercetin and eugenol are two major constituents of *P. betel* that promote the antioxidant properties, by modulating glutathione levels (Yasin et al. 2018).

Cocoa products are also polyphenol rich and have been reported to improve blood pressure and NO bioavailability. Feeding cocoa powder in hypertensive uninephrectomized rats showed reduction of inflammation and oxidative stress (Jayeola et al. 2020).

Garlic (*Allium sativum*) is an ancient plant with numerous medicinal uses due to its safe consumption. Allicin, a major active component of garlic, promotes vasodilating effects by targeting angiotensin II. Further, this active ingredient also improves the NO bioavailability and lowers the blood pressure in hypertension (Matsutomo 2020).

In vitro studies verified that licorice (*Glycyrrhiza glabra*) root extract protects the cardiomyocytes against anti-cancer drugs such as doxorubicin and maintains a healthy microenvironment for cardiac health. This study indicated that plant-based formulations can be potential treatment strategies in therapeutic linked cardio-toxicity (Upadhyay et al. 2020).

Watermelon (*Citrullus lanatus*) contains citrulline, α-amino acid and is a precursor of nitrogen oxide and argentine. Citrulline is known to enhance nitric oxide bioavailability and regulate glycaemic status, and inflammation (Azizi et al. 2020). A spiny herb Lepidagathis is used as traditional medicine due to the presence of a high concentration of its flavonoids and phenolic compounds which make it a remarkable antioxidant. *L. pungent* extract can be used in the treatment of free-radical-mediated diseases because of its antioxidant and anti-cancerous constituents (Dhanalakshmi and Thangadurai 2021). So, plant-based antioxidants also have great potential to act as anti-hypertensive agents by quenching effects associated with oxidative stress.

1.16 TOXICITY AND CAUTIONARY NOTES

Despite the benefits of plant-based phytochemicals, reports show toxic effects in *in vivo* and *in vitro* studies. The high doses of phytochemical resveratrol is reported to inhibit P450 cytochrome (Shaito et al. 2020). Further, this phytochemical attenuates the effect of various drugs upon interaction. The persistent consumption of thymoquinone causes liver toxicity (Ong et al. 2016) and γ-tocopherol, a natural substitute of vitamin E, promotes airway hyper-reactivity during eosinophilic allergic lung inflammation in mice (Moreno-Macias and Romieu 2014). Flavonoid intake more than the recommended limits is toxic and carcinogenic. Flavonoids bind to non-heme iron which increases the risk of iron deficiency in the elderly population (Birt and Jeffery 2013). Flavonoid drug interaction may lead to liver failure and aids cancer progression and reproductive abnormalities (Galati and O'Brien 2004; Tang and Zhang 2021).

So, it is suggested that some dietary phytochemicals could be harmful, allergic and silent carcinogens. The appropriate evaluation of synergistic and antagonistic actions of phytochemicals is required to improve their bioavailability and therapeutic potential to treat various disorders.

1.17 SUMMARY POINTS

- Hypertension is affiliated with enhanced cardiovascular oxidative stress and compromised endothelial function, which is the result of imbalanced levels of intracellular oxidants and nitric oxide bioavailability.
- Numerous diseases have been allied with oxidative stress suggesting that this can trigger disease pathophysiology and the use of antioxidant therapy could be effective treatment to quench the deleterious effects of oxidative stress.

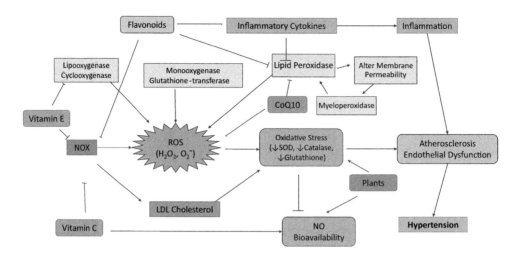

FIGURE 1.6 Possible mode of action of natural antioxidants as anti-hypertensive agents.

- The consumption of anti-hypertensive antioxidants appears to be the most effective treatment in the managing of hypertension since they can reduce increased blood pressure by affecting molecular mechanisms which are involved in the regulation of both vascular function and oxidative state (Figure 1.6).
- More studies need to be conducted to better understand the causes and targets of ROS/RNS and their harmful or beneficial roles, the specific molecular mechanisms, and their cross-talks between antioxidants.
- With the lack of side effects and economical preparation, the regular ingestion of dietary antioxidants may be beneficial for CVD prevention in individuals with pre-hypertension, or even those with hypertension with combined therapy.

REFERENCES

Alcázar-Fabra, María, Plácido Navas, and Gloria Brea-Calvo. 2016. "Coenzyme Q Biosynthesis and Its Role in the Respiratory Chain Structure." *Biochimica et Biophysica Acta (BBA): Bioenergetics* 1857 (8): 1073–1078. https://doi.org/10.1016/j.bbabio.2016.03.010.

Alshahrani, Saeed. 2020. "Aliskiren: A Promising Antioxidant Agent beyond Hypertension Reduction." *Chemico-Biological Interactions* 326: 109145. https://doi.org/10.1016/j.cbi.2020.109145.

Arnett, Donna K., Roger S. Blumenthal, Michelle A. Albert, Andrew B. Buroker, Zachary D. Goldberger, Ellen J. Hahn, Cheryl Dennison Himmelfarb. 2019. "ACC/AHA Guideline on the Primary Prevention of Cardiovascular Disease: A Report of the American College of Cardiology/American Heart Association Task Force on Clinical Practice Guidelines." *Circulation* 140 (11). American Heart Association: e596–646. doi:10.1161/CIR.0000000000000678.

Azizi, Samaneh, Reza Mahdavi, Elnaz Vaghef-Mehrabany, Vahid Maleki, Nahid Karamzad, and Mehrangiz Ebrahimi-Mameghani. 2019. "Potential Roles of Citrulline and Watermelon Extract on Metabolic and Inflammatory Variables in Diabetes Mellitus, Current Evidence and Future Directions: A Systematic Review." *Clinical and Experimental Pharmacology and Physiology* 47 (October). doi:10.1111/1440-1681.13190.

Baradaran, Azar, Hamid Nasri, and Mahmoud Rafieian-Kopaei. 2014. "Oxidative Stress and Hypertension: Possibility of Hypertension Therapy with Antioxidants." *Journal of Research in Medical Sciences: The Official Journal of Isfahan University of Medical Sciences* 19 (4): 358–367.

Birt, Diane F., and Elizabeth Jeffery. 2013. "Flavonoids." *Advances in Nutrition (Bethesda, Md.)* 4 (5). American Society for Nutrition: 576–577. doi:10.3945/an.113.004465.

Borde, Pravin, Mahalaxmi Mohan, and Sanjay Kasture. 2011. "Effect of Myricetin on Deoxycorticosterone Acetate (DOCA)-Salt-Hypertensive Rats." *Natural Product Research* 25 (16). England: 1549–1559. doi:10.1080/14786410903335190.

Oxidative Stress, Dietary Antioxidant and Hypertension

Chen, Qishan, Qiwen Wang, Jianhua Zhu, Qingzhong Xiao, and Li Zhang. 2018. "Reactive Oxygen Species: Key Regulators in Vascular Health and Diseases." *British Journal of Pharmacology* 175 (8): 1279–1292. doi:10.1111/bph.13828.

Chopra, H. K., and C. Venkata S. Ram. 2019. "Recent Guidelines for Hypertension." *Circulation Research* 124 (7). American Heart Association: 984–986. doi:10.1161/CIRCRESAHA.119.314789.

Craft, Neal E., and Harold C. Furr. 2019. "Chapter 2: Methods for Assessment of Vitamin a (Retinoids) and Carotenoids." In *Laboratory Assessment of Vitamin Status Harrington*, edited by B. T. Dominic, 21–47. Academic Press. https://doi.org/10.1016/B978-0-12-813050-6.00002-4.

Davies, Michael J. 2016. "Protein Oxidation and Peroxidation." *The Biochemical Journal* 473 (7). Department of Biomedical Sciences, Panum Institute, University of Copenhagen, Blegdamsvej 3, Copenhagen 2200, Denmark davies@sund.ku.dk: 805–825. doi:10.1042/bj20151227.

Delacroix, Sinny, and Ramesh G. Chokka. 2014. "Hypertension: Pathophysiology and Treatment." *Journal of Neurology & Neurophysiology* 5 (6). doi:10.4172/2155-9562.1000250.

Devaki, Sudha J., and Reshma Lali Raveendran. 2017. "Vitamin C: Sources, Functions, Sensing and Analysis." In *Vitamin C*. InTech. doi:10.5772/intechopen.70162.

Dhanalakshmi, Manoharan, and Subramaniam Ananda Thangadurai. 2021. "Antioxidant and Anticancer Activities of Whole Plant Extracts of Lepidagathis Pungens Nees: In Vitro Evaluation." *Pharmacognosy Magazine* 17 (5). India: 63. doi:10.4103/pm.pm_356_20.

Dikalova, Anna E., Arvind Pandey, Liang Xiao, Liaisan Arslanbaeva, Tatiana Sidorova, Marcos G. Lopez, Frederic T. Billings, et al. 2020. "Mitochondrial Deacetylase Sirt3 Reduces Vascular Dysfunction and Hypertension While Sirt3 Depletion in Essential Hypertension Is Linked to Vascular Inflammation and Oxidative Stress." *Circulation Research* 126 (4). American Heart Association: 439–452. doi:10.1161/CIRCRESAHA.119.315767.

Duarte, Juan, Raquel Pérez-Palencia, Felix Vargas, Maria Angeles Ocete, Francisco Pérez-Vizcaino, Antonio Zarzuelo, and Juan Tamargo. 2001. "Antihypertensive Effects of the Flavonoid Quercetin in Spontaneously Hypertensive Rats." *British Journal of Pharmacology* 133 (1): 117–124. doi:10.1038/sj.bjp.0704064.

Engelhard, Yechiel N., Benny Gazer, and Esther Paran. 2006. "Natural Antioxidants from Tomato Extract Reduce Blood Pressure in Patients with Grade-1 Hypertension: A Double-Blind, Placebo-Controlled Pilot Study." *American Heart Journal* 151 (1). United States: 100. doi:10.1016/j.ahj.2005.05.008.

Escobar, E. 2002. "Hypertension and Coronary Heart Disease." *Journal of Human Hypertension* 16 (Suppl 1) (March). England: S61–63. doi:10.1038/sj.jhh.1001345.

Farooqui, Zeba, Razia Sultana Mohammad, Mustafa F. Lokhandwala, and Anees Ahmad Banday. 2021. "Nrf2 Inhibition Induces Oxidative Stress, Renal Inflammation and Hypertension in Mice." *Clinical and Experimental Hypertension* 43 (2). Taylor & Francis: 175–180. doi:10.1080/10641963.2020.1836191.

Feng, Weisheng, Zhiyou Hao, and Meng Li. 2017. "Isolation and Structure Identification of Flavonoids." In *Flavonoids: From Biosynthesis to Human Health*. InTech. doi:10.5772/67810.

Galati, Giuseppe, and Peter J. O'Brien. 2004. "Potential Toxicity of Flavonoids and Other Dietary Phenolics: Significance for Their Chemopreventive and Anticancer Properties." *Free Radical Biology & Medicine* 37 (3). United States: 287–303. doi:10.1016/j.freeradbiomed.2004.04.034.

Galmés, Sebastià, Francisca Serra, and Andreu Palou. 2018. "Vitamin E Metabolic Effects and Genetic Variants: A Challenge for Precision Nutrition in Obesity and Associated Disturbances." *Nutrients* 10 (12). doi:10.3390/nu10121919.

García, Noemí, Cecilia Zazueta, and Leopoldo Aguilera-Aguirre. 2017. "Oxidative Stress and Inflammation in Cardiovascular Disease." In *Oxidative Medicine and Cellular Longevity* 2017. Hindawi: 5853238. doi:10.1155/2017/5853238.

Guan, Yuanyuan, Pengju Dai, and Hongwu Wang. 2020. "Effects of Vitamin C Supplementation on Essential Hypertension: A Systematic Review and Meta-Analysis." *Medicine* 99 (8).

Guo, Cheng, Peili Ding, Cong Xie, Chenyang Ye, Minfeng Ye, Chi Pan, Xiaoji Cao, Suzhan Zhang, and Shu Zheng. 2017. "Potential Application of the Oxidative Nucleic Acid Damage Biomarkers in Detection of Diseases." *Oncotarget*. doi:10.18632/oncotarget.20801.

Hannan, Md. Abdul, Md. Ataur Rahman, Abdullah Al Mamun Sohag, Md. Jamal Uddin, Raju Dash, Mahmudul Hasan Sikder, Md. Saidur Rahman, et al. 2021. "Black Cumin (*Nigella sativa* L.): A Comprehensive Review on Phytochemistry, Health Benefits, Molecular Pharmacology, and Safety." *Nutrients* 13 (6): 1784. doi:10.3390/nu13061784.

Jayeola, Olayinka Christianah, Ademola Adetokunbo Oyagbemi, Omolara Ibiwunmi Okunlola, Olayiwola Olubamiwa, Temidayo Olutayo Omobowale, Temitayo Olabisi Ajibade, Foluso Bolawaye Bolaji-Alabi, et al. 2020. "Effect o-f Cocoa Powder on Hypertension and Antioxidant Status in Uninephrectomized Hypertensive Rats." *Veterinary World* 13 (4). Veterinary World: 695–705. doi:10.14202/vetworld.2020.695-705.

Kaźmierczak-Barańska, Julia, Karolina Boguszewska, Angelika Adamus-Grabicka, and Bolesław T. Karwowski. 2020. "Two Faces of Vitamin C: Antioxidative and Pro-Oxidative Agent." *Nutrients* 12 (5): 1501. doi:10.3390/nu12051501.

Kooti, Wesam, and Nahid Daraei. 2017. "A Review of the Antioxidant Activity of Celery (*Apium graveolens* L)." *Journal of Evidence-Based Complementary & Alternative Medicine* 22 (4). SAGE Publications Inc STM: 1029–1034. doi:10.1177/2156587217717415.

Kumar, Shashank, and Abhay K. Pandey. 2013. "Chemistry and Biological Activities of Flavonoids: An Overview." In *The Scientific World Journal*, edited by K. P. Lu and J. Sastre. Hindawi Publishing Corporation: 162750. doi:10.1155/2013/162750.

Lee, Chang Ho, and Jong-Hoon Kim. 2014. "A Review on the Medicinal Potentials of Ginseng and Ginsenosides on Cardiovascular Diseases." *Journal of Ginseng Research* 38 (3): 161–166. doi:10.1016/j.jgr.2014.03.001.

Linkner, Edward (Lev), and Corene Humphreys. 2018. "Chapter 32: Insulin Resistance and the Metabolic Syndrome." In *Integrative Medicine* (Fourth Edition), edited by B. T. David. Rakel, 320–333.e5. Elsevier. https://doi.org/10.1016/B978-0-323-35868-2.00032-3.

Linowiecka, Kinga, Marek Foksinski, and Anna A. Brożyna. 2020. "Vitamin c Transporters and Their Implications in Carcinogenesis." *Nutrients* 12 (12): 1–19. doi:10.3390/nu12123869.

Ma, Gang, Lancui Zhang, Minoru Sugiura, and Masaya Kato. 2020. "Citrus and Health." In *The Genus Citrus: The Genus Citrus Gmitter*, edited by Manuel Talon, Marco Caruso, and G. B. T. Fred, 495–511. Elsevier. doi:10.1016/B978-0-12-812163-4.00024-3.

Maaliki, Dina, Abdullah A. Shaito, Gianfranco Pintus, Ahmed El-Yazbi, and Ali H. Eid. 2019. "Flavonoids in Hypertension: A Brief Review of the Underlying Mechanisms." *Current Opinion in Pharmacology* 45: 57–65. https://doi.org/10.1016/j.coph.2019.04.014.

Manning, R. Davis, Jr., Niu Tian, and Shumei Meng. 2005. "Oxidative Stress and Antioxidant Treatment in Hypertension and the Associated Renal Damage." *American Journal of Nephrology* 25 (4). Switzerland: 311–317. doi:10.1159/000086411.

Marchi, Katia Colombo, Carla Speroni Ceron, Jaqueline J. Muniz, Bruno S. De Martinis, José E. Tanus-Santos, and Carlos Renato Tirapelli. 2016. "NADPH Oxidase Plays a Role on Ethanol-Induced Hypertension and Reactive Oxygen Species Generation in the Vasculature." *Alcohol and Alcoholism* 51 (5): 522–534. doi:10.1093/alcalc/agw043.

Matsutomo, Toshiaki. 2020. "Potential Benefits of Garlic and Other Dietary Supplements for the Management of Hypertension." *Experimental and Therapeutic Medicine* 19 (2): 1479–1484. doi:10.3892/etm.2019.8375.

Miller, Francis J. 2020. "Hypertension and Mitochondrial Oxidative Stress Revisited." *Circulation Research* 126 (4). American Heart Association: 453–455. doi:10.1161/CIRCRESAHA.120.316567.

Moreno-Macias, Hortensia, and Isabelle Romieu. 2014. "Effects of Antioxidant Supplements and Nutrients on Patients with Asthma and Allergies." *Journal of Allergy and Clinical Immunology* 133 (5): 1237–1244. https://doi.org/10.1016/j.jaci.2014.03.020.

Ong, Yong Sze, Latifah Saiful Yazan, Wei Keat Ng, Mustapha M. Noordin, Sarah Sapuan, Jhi Biau Foo, and Yin Sim Tor. 2016. "Acute and Subacute Toxicity Profiles of Thymoquinone-Loaded Nanostructured Lipid Carrier in BALB/c Mice." *International Journal of Nanomedicine* 11: 5905–5915. doi:10.2147/IJN.S114205.

Panche, A. N., A. D. Diwan, and S. R. Chandra. 2016. "Flavonoids: An Overview." *Journal of Nutritional Science* 5: e47. doi:10.1017/jns.2016.41.

Petiz, Lyvia Lintzmaier, Carolina Saibro Girardi, Rafael Calixto Bortolin, Alice Kunzler, Juciano Gasparotto, Thallita Kelly Rabelo, Cristiane Matté, José Claudio Fonseca Moreira, and Daniel Pens Gelain. 2017. "Vitamin A Oral Supplementation Induces Oxidative Stress and Suppresses IL-10 and HSP70 in Skeletal Muscle of Trained Rats." *Nutrients*. doi:10.3390/nu9040353.

Pino-García, Raquel Del, María D. Rivero-Pérez, María L. González-San José, Kevin D. Croft, and Pilar Muñiz. 2017. "Antihypertensive and Antioxidant Effects of Supplementation with Red Wine Pomace in Spontaneously Hypertensive Rats." *Food & Function* 8 (7): 2444–2454. doi:10.1039/C7FO00390K.

Ronchi, Silas Nascimento, Girlandia Alexandre Brasil, Andrews Marques do Nascimento, Ewelyne Miranda de Lima, Rodrigo Scherer, Helber B. Costa, Wanderson Romão, et al. 2015. "Phytochemical and in Vitro and in Vivo Biological Investigation on the Antihypertensive Activity of Mango Leaves (*Mangifera Indica* L.)." *Therapeutic Advances in Cardiovascular Disease* 9 (5). SAGE Publications: 244–256. doi:10.1177/1753944715572958.

Salvayre, R., A. Negre-Salvayre, and C. Camaré. 2016. "Oxidative Theory of Atherosclerosis and Antioxidants." *Biochimie* 125 (June). France: 281–296. doi:10.1016/j.biochi.2015.12.014.

Shahidi, Fereidoon, and Adriano Costa de Camargo. 2016. "Tocopherols and Tocotrienols in Common and Emerging Dietary Sources: Occurrence, Applications, and Health Benefits." *International Journal of Molecular Sciences* 17 (10). doi:10.3390/ijms17101745.

Shaito, Abdullah, Anna M. Posadino, Nadin Younes, Hiba Hasan, Sarah Halabi, Dalal Alhababi, Anjud Al-Mohannadi, et al. 2020. "Potential Adverse Effects of Resveratrol: A Literature Review." *International Journal of Molecular Sciences.* doi:10.3390/ijms21062084.

Siti, Hawa N., Y. Kamisah, and J. Kamsiah. 2015. "The Role of Oxidative Stress, Antioxidants and Vascular Inflammation in Cardiovascular Disease (a Review)." *Vascular Pharmacology* 71 (August). United States: 40–56. doi:10.1016/j.vph.2015.03.005.

Sood, Brittany, and Michael Keenaghan. 2021. "Coenzyme Q10." In Treasure Island (FL).

Stewart, Jack, Gavin Manmathan, and Peter Wilkinson. 2017. "Primary Prevention of Cardiovascular Disease: A Review of Contemporary Guidance and Literature." *JRSM Cardiovascular Disease* 6: 2048004016687211. doi:10.1177/2048004016687211.

Suridjan, Ivonne, Nathan Herrmann, Alex Adibfar, Mahwesh Saleem, Ana Andreazza, Paul I. Oh, and Krista L. Lanctôt. 2017. "Lipid Peroxidation Markers in Coronary Artery Disease Patients with Possible Vascular Mild Cognitive Impairment." Edited by Ignacio Casado Naranjo. *Journal of Alzheimer's Disease* 58 (3): 885–896. doi:10.3233/JAD-161248.

Szewczyk, Kacper, Aleksandra Chojnacka, and Magdalena Górnicka. 2021. "Tocopherols and Tocotrienols: Bioactive Dietary Compounds; What Is Certain, What Is Doubt?" *International Journal of Molecular Sciences* 22 (12). MDPI: 6222. doi:10.3390/ijms22126222.

Tang, Zhimei, and Qiang Zhang. 2021. "The Potential Toxic Side Effects of Flavonoids." *BIOCELL.* doi:10.32604/biocell.2021.015958.

Tejaswi, G., M. M. Suchitra, D. Rajasekhar, V. S. Kiranmayi, and P. V. L. N. Srinivasa Rao. 2017. "Myeloperoxidase, Protein Carbonyls and Oxidative Stress in Coronary Artery Disease." *Journal of Indian College of Cardiology* 7 (4): 149–152. doi:https://doi.org/10.1016/j.jicc.2017.10.004.

Türck, Patrick, Schauana Fraga, Isadora Salvador, Cristina Campos-Carraro, Denise Lacerda, Alan Bahr, Vanessa Ortiz, et al. 2020. "Blueberry Extract Decreases Oxidative Stress and Improves Functional Parameters in Lungs from Rats with Pulmonary Arterial Hypertension." *Nutrition (Burbank, Los Angeles County, Calif.)* 70 (February). United States: 110579. doi:10.1016/j.nut.2019.110579.

Upadhyay, Shishir, Kunj Bihari Gupta, Sukhchain Kaur, Rubal, Sandeep Kumar, Anil K. Mantha, and Monisha Dhiman. 2018. "Resveratrol: A Miracle Drug for Vascular Pathologies." In *Functional Food and Human Health*, 119–142. Singapore: Springer Singapore. doi:10.1007/978-981-13-1123-9_7.

Upadhyay, Shishir, Anil Kumar Mantha, and Monisha Dhiman. 2020. "Glycyrrhiza Glabra (Licorice) Root Extract Attenuates Doxorubicin-Induced Cardiotoxicity via Alleviating Oxidative Stress and Stabilising the Cardiac Health in H9c2 Cardiomyocytes." *Journal of Ethnopharmacology* 258: 112690. https://doi.org/10.1016/j.jep.2020.112690.

Uribe, Noclia García, Manuel Reig García-Galbis, and Rosa María Martínez Espinosa. 2017. "New Advances about the Effect of Vitamins on Human Health: Vitamins Supplements and Nutritional Aspects." In *Functional Food: Improve Health through Adequate Food*. InTech. doi:10.5772/intechopen.69122.

Václavík, Jan. 2018. "Dyslipidemia and Hypertension: What to Worry about More?" *Vnitrni lekarstvi* 64 (4). Czech Republic: 395–401.

Wang, Jialing, Hailong Li, Tian Xia, Jun Feng, and Ru Zhou. 2021. "Pulmonary Arterial Hypertension and Flavonoids: A Role in Treatment." *The Chinese Journal of Physiology* 64 (3). India: 115–124. doi:10.4103/cjp.cjp_25_21.

WHO. 2021. "Cardiovascular Diseases (CVDs)."

Wichitsranoi, Jatuporn, Natthida Weerapreeyakul, Patcharee Boonsiri, Chatri Settasatian, Nongnuch Settasatian, Nantarat Komanasin, Suchart Sirijaichingkul, Yaovalak Teerajetgul, Nuchanart Rangkadilok, and Naruemon Leelayuwat. 2011. "Antihypertensive and Antioxidant Effects of Dietary Black Sesame Meal in Pre-Hypertensive Humans." *Nutrition Journal* 10 (1): 82. doi:10.1186/1475-2891-10-82.

Yagi, Shusuke, Masashi Akaike, Takayuki Ise, Yuka Ueda, Takashi Iwase, and Masataka Sata. 2013. "Renin-Angiotensin-Aldosterone System Has a Pivotal Role in Cognitive Impairment." *Hypertension Research* 36 (9): 753–758. doi:10.1038/hr.2013.51.

Yasin, Z. A. Mat, Ahmad Suhail Khazali, Firas Khalil Ibrahim, Nurshamimi Nor Rashid, and Rohana Yusof. 2018. "Antioxidant and Enzyme Inhibitory Activities of Areca Catechu, Boesenbergia Rotunda,

Piper Betle and Orthosiphon Aristatus for Potential Skin Anti-Aging Properties." *Current Topics in Nutraceutical Research* 17 (3): 229–235. doi:10.37290/ctnr2641-452X.17:229-235.

Yavuzer, Hakan, Serap Yavuzer, Mahir Cengiz, Hayriye Erman, Alper Doventas, Huriye Balci, Deniz Suna Erdincler, and Hafize Uzun. 2016. "Biomarkers of Lipid Peroxidation Related to Hypertension in Aging." *Hypertension Research: Official Journal of the Japanese Society of Hypertension* 39 (5).

Yavuzer, Serap, Hakan Yavuzer, Mahir Cengiz, Hayriye Erman, Filiz Demirdag, Alper Doventas, Huriye Balci, Deniz Suna Erdincler, and Hafize Uzun. 2016. "The Role of Protein Oxidation and DNA Damage in Elderly Hypertension." *Aging Clinical and Experimental Research* 28 (4).

2 Domestic and International Research on the Relationship between Japanese Diet and Ischemic Heart Disease

Tomoko Imai and Hiroshi Shimokata

CONTENTS

2.1 Introduction: What Is a Japanese Diet? 19
2.2 Background: Japanese Diet and Ischemic Heart Disease 20
2.3 Usefulness of Japanese Diet Patterns According to Statistical Studies 22
2.4 Japanese Diet Patterning Score Generated from DASH, HEI, and MED 24
2.5 Japanese Diet's Unique Dietary Score 25
2.6 Japanese Diet Intervention Trial 27
2.7 International Research on the Relationship between Japanese
Diet and Ischemic Heart Disease 28
2.8 Future of Japanese Diet, an Ecological Study with Open Data 29
2.9 Summary Points 31
References 31

LIST OF ABBREVIATIONS

CVDs   cardiovascular disease
CDs   cerebrovascular diseases
HDL   high-density lipoprotein cholesterol
IHD   ischemic heart disease
LDL   low-density lipoprotein cholesterol

2.1 INTRODUCTION: WHAT IS A JAPANESE DIET?

In December 2013, the Japanese diet was inscribed in the United Nations Educational, Scientific and Cultural Organization Intangible Cultural Heritage List. It is the fifth diet to be inscribed in this list. The reasons for the inclusion of Japanese diets on the list are as follows: the use of a variety of fresh ingredients and the development of cooking techniques and utensils that are used in making most of these ingredients; the ideal nutritional balance of a diet based on three kinds of dishes, which promotes healthy eating habits and longevity and prevents obesity; and the enjoyment of nature and the sense of the seasons, such as the use of seasonal furniture and dishes. It is closely related to the traditional annual events such as the New Year. The Japanese diet is one of the main attractions in Japan.

DOI: 10.1201/9781003220329-3

2.2 BACKGROUND: JAPANESE DIET AND ISCHEMIC HEART DISEASE

According to the Global Burden of Disease (GBD) database 2019, the incidence of ischemic heart disease (IHD) per 100,000 people in Japan is 126.3, the prevalence of IHD is 1084.0, and the mortality rate from IHD is 29.9, which is the lowest among those reported in developed countries; moreover, Japan has the second highest healthy life expectancy rate (73.8 years) among the countries worldwide. According to the World Bank, Japan also has the highest average life expectancy (84.4 years) among the countries worldwide. It is not surprising that the Japanese diet is gaining attention as a healthy food worldwide.

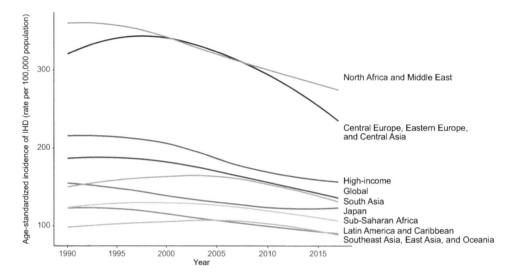

FIGURE 2.1 Global and regional changes in IHD incidence from 1990 to 2017.

Note: This figure shows the age-standardized incidence of IHD per 100,000 people, covering the period from 1990 to 2017, which was derived from the GBD 2017.

Source: From Sezaki et al. (2021) with permission. Added Japanese lines.

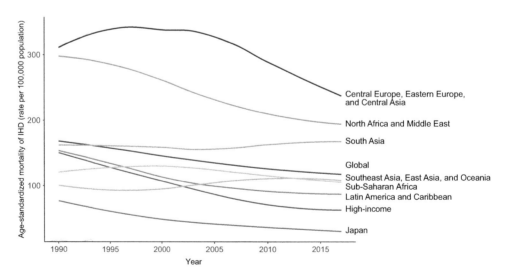

FIGURE 2.2 Global and regional changes in IHD mortality from 1990 to 2017.

Note: This figure shows the age-standardized mortality of IHD per 100,000 people, covering the period from 1990 to 2017, which was derived from the GBD 2017.

Source: From Sezaki et al. (2021) with permission. Added Japanese lines.

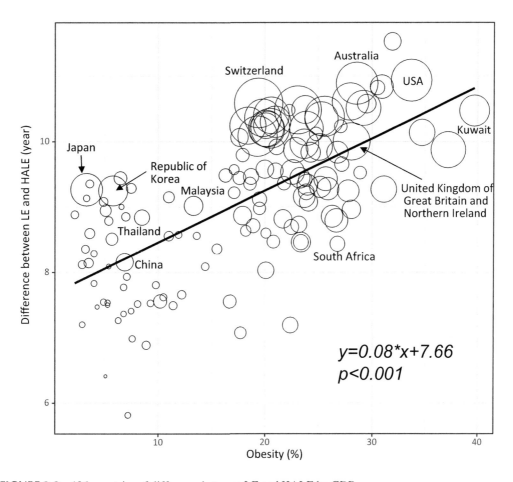

FIGURE 2.3 136 countries of difference between LE and HALE by GDP.

Note: This figure shows the 136 countries of difference between LE and HALE by GDP, which was derived from the GBD 2015. HALE, healthy life expectancy; LE.

Source: From Miyamoto et al. (2018) with permission. Translated into English, with some corrections.

The Japanese diet is based on three kinds of dishes: one staple food (shu-shoku), one main dish (shu-sai), and two side dishes (fuku-sai). The main staple food is rice, while the main dish is only composed of a single serving of meat or seafood. The side dishes mainly consist of vegetables, seaweed, or soybean products. This may be accompanied by soup (shiru-mono) or Japanese pickled vegetables (tsuke-mono). Some dishes, such as sushi and sukiyaki (cooked meat and vegetables, etc., in one pot), are a combination of main and side dishes.

Tsugane (2020) introduced the food and nutrients that characterize the Japanese diet, based on the results of the Japan Public Health Center-based prospective (JPHC) study and other studies, and explained that the Japanese diet is associated with a longer healthy life span among the Japanese individuals. In the 1960s, Japan's average life expectancy was lower than that of other developed countries because of the relatively high mortality rate associated with cerebrovascular diseases (CDs). In the last half-century, the average Japanese life expectancy was the longest in the world.

Japan has the lowest obesity rates worldwide because Japanese individuals consume less red meat, which contains saturated fatty acids, and more fish, which contains n-3 polyunsaturated fatty acids; plant foods such as soybeans; and non-sweetened beverages such as green tea. In addition, a moderate increase in the consumption of animal foods, milk, and dairy products, and a decreased

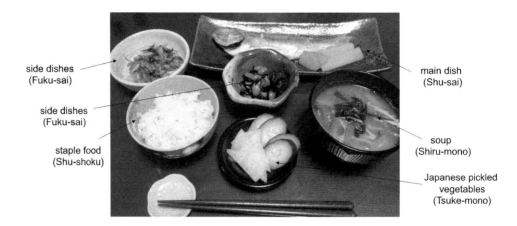

PHOTO 2.1 The basic principles of the Japanese diet.

Note: This photo shows the basic principles of Japanese diet of "one soup and three dishes", taken by the author.

salt intake have contributed to a longer life span and a healthier lifestyle. These foods can be consumed as part of the Japanese diet without difficulty. Yamori et al. (2008) reported that Japanese diets, especially Okinawan diets consumed at the time of the survey, were effective against the prevention of cardiovascular diseases (CVDs) based on the World Health Organization (WHO)-Coordinated Cardiovascular Diseases and Alimentary Comparison study of 60 communities in 25 countries, and other studies reported the characteristics of the Japanese diet (Seidelmann et al. 2018; Koga et al. 2017; Murakami et al. 2018; Sproesser et al. 2018; Suzuki et al. 2018; Toda et al. 2011).

2.3 USEFULNESS OF JAPANESE DIET PATTERNS ACCORDING TO STATISTICAL STUDIES

Htun et al. (2017) identified three food intake patterns (traditional Japanese, Westernized, and meat and fat patterns) by conducting a principal component analysis using the de-identified data from the 2012 Japan National Health and Nutrition Survey (NHNS) conducted in 11,365 individuals aged 20–84 years. A "traditional Japanese" food intake pattern was defined as a high consumption of miso (Japanese fermented soybean paste), soy sauce, fresh vegetables and fruits, beans, and potatoes. A "Westernized" food intake pattern was defined as higher consumption of bread, dairy products, butter and margarine, and jam, but less consumption of rice and miso. The "meat and fat" food intake pattern was defined as higher consumption of meat, fat, sauces, mayonnaise, wheat, and wheat products. The "traditional Japanese" food intake pattern showed protective effects against hypertension in men. The multivariate-adjusted odds ratios (OR) and 95% confidence interval (CI) were estimated for the highest quartile and compared with those of the lowest quartile of hypertension (0.67, 0.53–0.84, p for trend = 0.003) in men. The Westernized food intake pattern was positively associated with hypercholesterolemia (1.80, 1.41–2.29, $p < 0.001$) and higher low-density lipoprotein (LDL) (1.75, 1.30–2.35, $p < 0.001$) in women, while the "meat and fat" food intake pattern was associated with hypertension (1.41, 1.11–1.79, $p = 0.008$), diabetes (1.38, 0.98–1.95, $p = 0.021$), and hypercholesterolemia (1.64, 1.17–2.29, $p = 0.036$) in men.

Sadakane et al. (2008) surveyed 6,886 (2,742 men and 4,144 women, for the analysis of blood pressure) and 7,641 (2,992 men and 4,649 women, for the analysis of serum lipids) individuals aged 40–69 years in 12 regions of Japan from 1992 to 1995 in a cross-sectional study using the food frequency questionnaire (FFQ). Three dietary patterns were determined by a factor analysis:

vegetarian pattern, which involved the high intake of vegetables, potatoes, tofu, fermented soybeans, fruits, seaweed, citrus fruits, legumes, and dried fish; meat pattern, which involved the high intake of processed meat, meats, fish products, fatty foods, and butter; and Western dietary pattern, which involved the high intake of bread, butter, and yogurt, and a low intake of rice, salted foods, and miso soup. The participants' dietary pattern scores were calculated and compared across quartiles. The highest meat pattern score was significantly associated with higher levels of high-density lipoprotein (HDL) and LDL in men (p for trend < 0.05, all), while the highest vegetarian pattern score was significantly associated with lower blood pressure levels and higher HDL levels in women (p for trend < 0.05).

In the 1994 Ohsaki National Health Insurance Cohort study in Miyagi, Shimazu et al. (2007) conducted a survey using the FFQ in 40,547 men and women aged 40–79 years, divided their dietary patterns by factor analysis, and followed them for seven years. Three patterns were scored and compared in quartiles: Japanese pattern, which involved high consumption of soy products, fish, seaweed, vegetables, fruits, and green tea; meat pattern, which involved high consumption of meat, coffee, and alcohol; and dairy, vegetable, and fruit patterns, which involved high consumption of dairy products and low consumption of alcohol. Participants with the highest Japanese pattern score consumed more salt than the other groups and had a significantly higher incidence of hypertension. Participants with the highest Japanese pattern score had a significantly lower risk of death from CDs; the hazard ratio (HR) of the highest quartile group was 0.73 (95% CI: 0.59–0.90, p for trend = 0.003) compared with that of the lowest quartile group; meanwhile, the group with the highest meat pattern score had a higher risk of death (HR: 1.49, 95% CI: 0.94–2.34, 0.06).

Morimoto et al. (2012) conducted an FFQ survey of 1,995 men and 3,670 women aged 40–69 years living in Nagano from 1990 to 1992, and divided the participants' dietary pattern into the following three groups by conducting a principal component analysis: healthy pattern, which involved the high intake of vegetables, potatoes, seaweed, fruits, and soybean products, and the other two patterns. The participants were followed up until the end of 2006. Participants with the highest healthy pattern score had a lower risk of developing diabetes (multivariable-adjusted HR for highest vs. lowest quartiles: 0.78, 95% CI: 0.61–0.95, p for trend = 0.008). In particular, those who ate regular meals (HR: 0.76, 95% CI: 0.58–0.96, 0.012), performed exercise (HR: 0.65, 95% CI: 0.44–0.96, 0.018), and were classified as non-smokers or former smokers (HR: 0.72, 95% CI: 0.53–0.96, 0.001) had a lower risk of developing diabetes.

Iwasaki et al. (2019) studied the association between nutrient patterns and metabolic syndrome (MetS) using the baseline data of 30,108 individuals aged 35–69 years who participated in the Japan Multi-Institutional Collaborative Cohort Study, which was conducted in the seven study areas in Japan. MetS was diagnosed based on the body mass index. The three nutrient patterns were determined using a factor analysis. Factor 1 scores (fiber, potassium, and vitamin pattern) were associated with a reduced OR of MetS (OR: 0.69, 95% CI: 0.63–0.77, p for trend < 0.001), obesity (OR: 0.75, 95% CI: 0.69–0.82, < 0.001), high blood pressure (OR: 0.78, 95% CI: 0.72–0.85, < 0.001), high serum triglyceride levels (OR: 0.77, 95% CI: 0.70–0.85, < 0.001), low HDL levels (OR: 0.87, 95% CI: 0.76–0.99, < 0.09), and high blood glucose levels (OR: 0.82, 95% CI: 0.76–0.90, < 0.001). Factor 2 scores (fats and fat-soluble vitamin pattern) were associated with an increased prevalence of MetS (OR: 1.27, 95% CI: 1.17–1.38, < 0.001), obesity (OR: 1.27, 95% CI: 1.18–1.38, < 0.001), and high blood pressure (OR: 1.15, 95% CI: 1.07–1.24, < 0.001). Factor 3 scores (saturated fatty acid, calcium, and vitamin B_2 pattern) were associated with a lower OR of MetS (OR: 0.87, 95% CI: 0.79–0.95, < 0.001), high blood pressure (OR: 0.84, 95% CI: 0.78–0.90, < 0.001), high serum triglyceride levels (OR: 0.90, 95% CI: 0.83–0.98, < 0.002), and low HDL levels (OR, 0.79; 95% CI: 0.70–0.90, < 0.001).

Other studies have investigated the relationship between Japanese dietary patterns and CVDs, which was calculated using statistical methods. However, the names of the patterns and the foods included in the patterns vary from report to report. The number of food groups that comprise a Japanese diet varies from five to nine and includes miso and soy sauce, dried fish, citrus fruits, green tea, etc. The other disadvantage of the statistical method is that it cannot be widely used to obtain a score that represents the Japanese diet in general as it depends on the population.

Zhang, Tomata et al. (2019) developed a nine-component weighted Japanese Diet Index (JDI) by conducting a factor analysis and a confirmatory factor analysis of the daily consumption of 39 food items from the FFQ in 1,129 Japanese individuals aged ≥70 years included in the Ohsaki Cohort study (Tomata et al. 2019). Afterward, the 12-component modified JDI (mJDI12) was defined in the cross-sectional data of another cohort study (fifth wave: 2006 to 2008) conducted by the National Institute for Longevity Sciences-Longitudinal Study of Aging. Among the mJDI12 items, rice, fish and shellfish, green and yellow vegetables, seaweed, green tea, beef and pork, soybeans and soybean products, fruits, and mushrooms were significantly associated with the nutrient density (ND) score. These nine components were chosen from the mJDI12, and a new weighted JDI (wJDI9) was developed. The JDI, mJDI12, and wJDI9 scores were positively correlated with the ND score (JDI; Spearman's $\rho = 0.34$, 95% CI: 0.31–0.38, $p < 0.05$, mJDI12; $\rho = 0.44$, 95% CI: 0.41–0.48, < 0.05, wJDI9; $\rho = 0.61$, 95% CI: 0.58–0.64, < 0.05).

This study suggested that when using dietary patterns from statistical studies conducted in another population, the validity of the scores for each population must be considered, and a modified scoring system must be developed. This indicates that the development of a general Japanese diet scoring system that can be used worldwide is still in progress.

2.4 JAPANESE DIET PATTERNING SCORE GENERATED FROM DASH, HEI, AND MED

Dietary Approaches to Stop Hypertension (DASH), Health Eating Index (HEI), and Mediterranean diet (MED) are dietary scoring systems that are recognized worldwide as useful for promoting health and preventing CVDs. All of these scoring systems are equally useful for assessing an individual's health, regardless of the region or ethnicity (Baxter et al. 2006; Liese et al. 2015), but some have been modified based on the Japanese diet pattern.

Kawamura et al. (2018) developed a washoku-modified DASH diet called DASH-JUMP. The DASH-JUMP diet is rich in green and yellow vegetables, seaweed, milk, and mushrooms, while it has low contents of meat, eggs, confectionery, oils and fats, Japanese pickled vegetables, shellfish boiled in sweetened soy sauce, and fruits. The participants (28 men and 27 women; mean age: 54.2 ± 8.0 years) were placed on a DASH-JUMP diet for two months. Four months after the intervention, they were allowed to consume their usual diets. A nutritional survey was conducted using the FFQ at baseline and after one, two, three, and six months. The participants who exhibited an increase in blood pressure one month after discontinuing the intervention developed an eating habit that broadly imitated the DASH-JUMP diet four months after cessation of the said intervention. The systolic and diastolic blood pressure values at four months after cessation of the intervention decreased significantly compared with those at baseline. A strong hypotensive effect was associated with the DASH-JUMP diet, which is based on the traditional Japanese foods with a tailored nutritional composition of the DASH diet, including reduced salt.

Murakami et al. (2020) assessed the overall diet quality of Japanese individuals using the Healthy Eating Index-2015 (HEI-2015) and Nutrient-Rich Food Index 9.3 (NRF9.3), and compared the diet quality scores between Japanese and American adults. The HEI-2015 is a composite measure of compliance with the 2015–2020 Dietary Guidelines for Americans. NRF9.3 is a validated, composite measure of the nutrient density of the total diet, calculated using the reference daily values of nine qualifying nutrients. They used one-day dietary record data from 19,719 adults (aged ≥20 years) in the NHNS 2012 and the first 24-h dietary recall data from 4,614 adults in the US National Health and Nutrition Examination Survey 2011–2012. A higher total score in the HEI-2015 and NRF9.3 was associated with favorable patterns of overall diet in the Japanese population. The mean total scores of HEI-2015 and NRF9.3 were similar between the Japanese and US populations (HEI-2015, Japan: 51.9, US: 52.8; NRF9.3: Japan: 448, US: 435, respectively). However, the component scores of the two populations were considerably different. For HEI-2015, the Japanese population had higher scores for whole fruits, total vegetables, green and beans, total protein foods, seafood and plant proteins, fatty acids, added sugars, and saturated fats, but lower scores for total fruits, whole grains, dairy, refined grains, and sodium.

Kanauchi and Kanauchi (2015) investigated the association between dietary quality and the prevalence of untreated hypertension in 433 Japanese male workers in a cross-sectional study. Dietary quality was assessed using four adherence indices: the WHO-based Healthy Diet Indicator (HDI), the American Heart Association 2006 Diet and Lifestyle Recommendations (AI-84), the DASH diet, and the MED. Patients with untreated hypertension had significantly lower HDI and AI-84 scores than those without hypertension. The DASH and MED scores across the three hypertension classes were comparable. Low adherence to HDI and the lowest quartile of AI-84 score were associated with a significantly higher prevalence of untreated hypertension (OR: 3.33, 95% CI: 1.39–7.94, $p = 0.007$, OR: 2.23, 95% CI: 1.09–4.53, 0.027), respectively. However, the DASH score was not associated with hypertension.

The Japanese diet might be similar to the DASH diet, except that it has a high salt content. The HEI and MED scores are obtained based on the eating patterns of the US and the Mediterranean populations, respectively, and it remains unclear whether they represent the characteristics of the Japanese diet. A few studies have utilized these dietary scoring system in Japan (Migliaccio et al. 2020). However, whether these dietary scores can prove the effectiveness of the Japanese diet needs further investigation.

2.5 JAPANESE DIET'S UNIQUE DIETARY SCORE

Are there any useful dietary scores that have been created independently in Japan?

Zhang, Otsuka et al. (2019) investigated the association between the Japanese dietary pattern and disability-free survival (DFS) time in the older Japanese population to analyze the ten-year follow-up data of 9,456 older Japanese individuals aged ≥65 years who participated in a community-based prospective cohort study. Dietary habits were assessed using the FFQ, and nine food items were used to calculate the JDI score: rice, miso soup, fish and shellfish, green and yellow vegetables, seaweed, Japanese pickled vegetables, green tea (1 point for each item if the consumption value was more than or equal to the median, and 0 otherwise), beef and pork, and coffee (0 points for each item if the consumption value was more than or equal to the median, and 1 point otherwise). JDI was developed based on the results of a previous study that reported the Japanese dietary patterns using statistical methods. During the follow-up period, 4,233 (44.8%) incident disability or death events occurred. In addition, a higher JDI score was significantly associated with longer DFS time, and the multivariate-adjusted 50% differences and 95% CI was 7.1 (1.8–12.4) longer for the highest quartile. Each 1-standard deviation increase of the JDI score was associated with 3.7 (1.7–5.7) additional months of life without disability (p trend < 0.01). No differences were observed in sex or chronic condition (no or ≥1 chronic condition) at baseline.

Matsuyama et al. (2021) examined the association between adherence to the eight-item Japanese Diet Index (JDI8) score and the subsequent risk of all-cause and cause-specific mortality in 92,969 Japanese adults aged 45–74 years, in JPHC study. Adherence to the Japanese diet consisting of eight components was assessed using JDI8, with scores ranging from 0 to 8. This score was based on the score reported by Zhang et al., in which coffee was removed from the items in order to make an eight-item score. During a median follow-up of 18.9 years, a higher JDI8 score was significantly associated with a lower risk of all-cause and CVD mortality. The multivariable-adjusted HR of all-cause and CVD mortality for the highest JDI8 score group (score: 6–8) and the lowest JDI8 score group (score: 0–2) were 0.86 (95% CI: 0.81–0.90, p trend < 0.001) and 0.89 (95% CI 0.80–0.99, 0.007), respectively. These scores may be useful for calculating the original Japanese diet score. However, all of these scores were examined only in the Japanese cohort.

In 2005, the Ministry of Health, Labour and Welfare is promoting and educating about Japanese diet at the national level; the Japan Ministry of Agriculture, Forestry and Fisheries established the

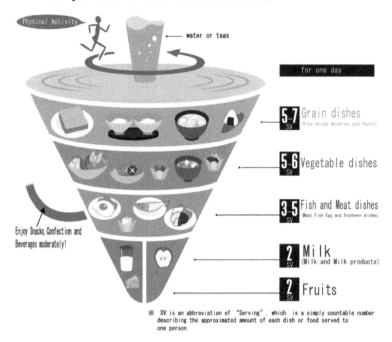

FIGURE 2.4 Japanese Food Guide Spinning Top.

Source: Japanese diet scores according to Japanese food-based dietary guidelines, from HP of MAFF (www.maff.go.jp/j/balance_guide/b_use/pdf/eng_reiari.pdf) (Japanese food guide).

Japanese Food Guide Spinning Top, which shows in a framed illustration the approximate serving (SV) of "what" and "how much" to eat each day. It was created using the data of 100 typical Japanese dishes obtained from the NHNS. The nutritional standards were consistent with the Dietary Reference Intakes for Japanese 2010. One of the three is best for each individual (1,400–2,000 kcal, basic; 2,200 ± 200 kcal; and 2,400–3,000 kcal) depending on sex, age, and physical activity level. It consists of five categories. The daily serving (SV) for each category of basic are as follows: 5–7 SV for "grain dishes (staple food)", 5–6 SV for "vegetable dishes (side dishes)", 3–5 SV for "fish and meat dishes (main dish)", 2 SV for "milk and dairy products" and "fruits". The standard one SV for each category is as follows: "grain dishes" contain 40 g of carbohydrates derived from grains; vegetable dishes" contain 70 g of vegetables, mushrooms, potatoes, beans, and seaweeds (dried foods are rehydrated); "fish and meat dishes" contain 6 g of protein derived from fish, meat, soybeans, and soybean products; "milk and dairy products" contain 100 mg of calcium derived from milk and dairy products; and "fruits" contain 100 g of fruit as the main ingredients. "Snack, confection, and beverages" are represented as the string that turns the top and should be consumed in an enjoyable and moderate amount (200 kcal a day). One regular rice ball is equivalent to 1 SV; one bowl of udon (Japanese noodles), 2 SV of "grain dish"; a hamburger steak for one person, 3 SV; a fish dish for one person, 2 SV of "fish and meat dish"; and a bottle of milk (about 200 ml), 2 SV of "milk and dairy products".

Some Japanese diet scores, obtained using the Japanese Food Guide Spinning Top, are used as indicators of the Japanese diet. For example, 13,355 men and 15,724 women from the Takayama Cohort study, which was initiated in 1992, performed a dietary survey using the FFQ. Adherence to Japanese food guide was rated from 0 to 70 based on the intake of the recommended number of SV of "grains dishes", "vegetable dishes", "fish and meat dishes", "milk and dairy products", and "fruits", as well as the total energy intake and intake of energy from "snacks, confection, and beverages"; higher scores indicated better adherence to the recommendations. The association between the score and mortality risk was evaluated until 1999. The adherence score was associated with a lower risk of mortality from all causes (comparing the highest and lowest quartiles of the score (hazard ratios [HR]: 0.78, 95% CI: 0.65–0.94, p for trend 0.01), non-cardiovascular and non-cancer causes (HR: 0.69, 95% CI: 0.50–0.96, 0.04), and cardiovascular disease (HR: 0.76, 95% CI: 0.56–1.04, 0.05) in women) (Oba et al. 2009).

Kurotani et al. (2016) examined the association between adherence to the modified Japanese food guide score and total and cause specific mortality in the JPHC study. They administered the FFQ at baseline (1990/1993); the diets of 36,624 men and 42,970 women aged 45–75 were investigated using a new score created by the previous 70-point scale. Compliance of the Japanese food guide was calculated by adding the ratio of white meat to red meat to give a score of 80 points, and the subjects were divided into quartiles, with follow-up for a median of 15 years. The highest compliance score had a 0.85 lower risk of total mortality than with the lowest compliance score (95% CI: 0.79–0.91, p for trend < 0.001), and an increase of 10 points in the score resulted in a 0.93 lower risk of total mortality (95% CI: 0.91–0.95, < 0.001). Highest compliance had lower risk of death from CVD (HR: 0.93, 0.89–0.98, 0.005), and CDs (HR: 0.89, 0.82–0.95, 0.002). There was a significant decrease in the risk of CVDs in the group with higher compliance scores for "vegetable dishes" and "fruits", especially.

Furthermore, there was a significant decrease in the risk of CVDs in the group with higher compliance scores for "vegetable dishes" and "fruits". Nishimura et al. (2015) examined whether adherence to the Japanese food guide was associated with the metabolic risk factors in 1,083 Japanese female college students aged 18–22 years in the dietitian training department of 15 universities included in the cross-sectional study conducted in 2006–2007. Adherence to the Japanese food guide was assessed using the dietary information on the consumed SVs of "grain dishes", "vegetable dishes", "fish and meat dishes", "milk and dairy products", and "fruits", and energy intake from "snack, confection, and beverages", during the preceding month, which were derived using a comprehensive diet history questionnaire. Higher dietary adherence was associated with higher intake of protein, carbohydrate, dietary fiber, Na, K, and vitamin C, and lower intakes of total and saturated fats. An inverse association was also observed between dietary adherence and dietary energy density. Dietary adherence was inversely associated with waist circumference (p for trend = 0.002). It also showed an inverse association with LDL (p for trend = 0.04).

2.6 JAPANESE DIET INTERVENTION TRIAL

Inoue et al. (2014) conducted a non-randomized controlled trial by offering a Japanese-style healthy lunch menu to 35 middle-aged men (control: seven men, intervention: 28 men; mean age: 47.2 ± 7.9 years) in a workplace cafeteria, which was designed to prevent and reduce MetS. The participants were assigned to either the control group or intervention group. The control group consumed habitual lunches. The intervention group was provided with a Japanese-style healthy lunch at a workplace cafeteria for three months. The control group did not show significant differences in the anthropometric data at baseline and after three months. However, a healthy lunch menu intake frequency of ≥ 50 percentile in the intervention group decreased the body fat percentage ($p = 0.019$), systolic blood pressure ($p = 0.023$), diastolic blood pressure ($p = 0.001$), total cholesterol level ($p = 0.006$), and LDL level ($p = 0.010$), but increased the plasma ghrelin levels ($p = 0.008$) after the intervention.

Yamauchi et al. (2014) randomized overweight and obese diabetic individuals (n = 19, 10 women) in an intervention group (n = 10) and included educational classes on lifestyle modification using a healthy plate or a waiting-list control group (n = 9). The intervention period was three months, and the educational classes using the healthy plate were conducted every month as a group session for the intervention group. The healthy plate measured 21 cm long, 27.4 cm wide, and 2.5 cm deep, which was divided into five sections. The staple food comprised 1/6 of the plate, the main dish comprised 2/6 of the plate, and the two side dishes each comprised 1/4 of the plate so that the participants would not only eat a healthy menu, but also determine the proper amount of food and the proportion of food that could help maintain health. The intervention group lost an average of 3.7 kg, while the control group lost an average of 0.1 kg.

In addition, Maruyama et al. (2017) reported that more than 90% of middle-aged men (n = 33, 30–49 years) with MetS who were provided with a Japanese diet for six weeks as part of a clinical trial reported that their weight and one or more of the risk factors for CVDs, such as serum lipids (before/after comparison, $p < 0.001$), decreased. However, only a few intervention studies were conducted in Japan. In any case, it is impossible to use food scores from Japanese food guides in countries other than Japan, where there is no concept of staple food, main dishes, and side dishes, or where rice is not considered a staple food. Therefore, it is necessary to develop a Japanese food score that can be used internationally. Some studies on the Japanese diet have developed an indicator based on the nutrients rather than dishes from the Japanese food guide.

Yoneoka et al. (2019) performed a critical appraisal of the Japanese food guide. They used the data of the 2016 NHNS conducted in 3,861 Japanese individuals aged ≥20 years, with low risks of diabetes, hypertension, hyperlipidemia, and obesity. The indicator was developed to reflect the adherence to the recommended intake of seven nutrients defined by the Japanese food guide, including proteins, fat, saturated fatty acids, carbohydrates, dietary fiber, sodium, and potassium. Only 0.3% of the participants adhered to the Japanese food guide (adherence rate) for all seven nutrients. There was considerable variation in the rate of adherence to the different nutrients (24.2%–61.8%). For most health outcomes, regardless of age category and quartile, no clear association was observed between the Japanese food guide adherence indicator and outcomes. Therefore, the impact of nutrients on health may not necessarily depend on the amount of each nutrient in the diet.

These domestic studies used Japanese data. In order to prove the usefulness of Japanese diet internationally, research on the usefulness of the Japanese diet conducted in countries other than Japan is necessary.

2.7 INTERNATIONAL RESEARCH ON THE RELATIONSHIP BETWEEN JAPANESE DIET AND ISCHEMIC HEART DISEASE

Since no indicators have a high level of evidence, such as the HEI produced by the US Department of Agriculture and the DASH produced by the National Institutes of Health, which are managed by public institutions, research on Japanese diet has not been conducted overseas. However, countries where rice is a staple food are conducting their own studies to determine the relationship between dietary patterns and CVDs.

Li and Shi (2017) reported the association of dietary pattern in 1991–2011 and metabolic risk in China based on the eight waves of annual data obtained from the China Health and Nutrition Survey (≥18 years, n = 9,499) conducted in a longitudinal study. Three-day food consumption was collected by 24-h recall. The anthropometric measures, blood pressure, fasting blood glucose level, and lipid levels were obtained in 2009. The dietary pattern was determined using a principal component analysis. The "traditional" pattern was characterized by high intakes of rice, meat, and vegetables, while the "modern" pattern was characterized by high intakes of fast food, milk, and deep-fried food. The "traditional" pattern was inversely associated with cardiometabolic risks, with linear slopes ranging from −0.15 (95% CI: −0.18 to −0.12) for hypertension to −0.67 (−0.73 to −0.60) for impaired glucose control. The "modern" pattern was positively associated with those factors, with slopes ranging from 0.10 (0.04–0.17) for high cholesterol to 0.42 (0.35–0.49) for impaired glucose control.

In Korea, the "rice and kimchi" pattern was associated with low prevalence of hypercholesterolemia and high prevalence of hypertriglyceridemia based on the 24-h dietary recall data from a cross-sectional survey conducted by the Korea National Health and Nutrition Examination Survey 2007–2012 (Kim et al. 2019).

As for dietary patterns of the Multi-Ethnic Cohort study of Chinese, Malay, and Indian populations (8,433 Singapore residents, aged 21–94 years) from cross-sectional data, a "healthy" dietary pattern, similar across ethnic groups and characterized by high intakes of whole grains, fruit, dairy, vegetables, and unsaturated cooking oil and low intakes of Western fast foods, sugar-sweetened beverages, poultry, processed meat, and flavored rice, was inversely associated with body mass index (−0.26 per 1 SD of the pattern score; 95% CI: −0.36 to −0.16), waist circumference (−0.57 cm; 95% CI: −0.82 to −0.32), total cholesterol (−0.070 mmol/L; 95% CI: −0.091 to −0.048), LDL (−0.054 mmol/L; 95% CI: −0.074 to −0.035), and fasting triglyceride levels (−0.22 mmol/L; 95% CI: −0.04 to −0.004) and directly associated with HDL (0.013 mmol/L; 95% CI: 0.006–0.021).

It may be necessary to examine the health benefits of Asian dietary styles, not limited to Japan, in which rice is a staple food (Gadgil et al. 2015).

2.8 FUTURE OF JAPANESE DIET, AN ECOLOGICAL STUDY WITH OPEN DATA

In recent years, open data from the Food and Agriculture Organization of the United Nations Statistics Division database (FAOSTAT), GBD, WHO, and other sources have been used for research. Figures 2.5–2.7 show the 132 countries of obesity (Figure 2.5), age-standardized incidence of IHD (Figure 2.6), and HALE (Figure 2.7) per 100,000 people and TJDS by GDP, which

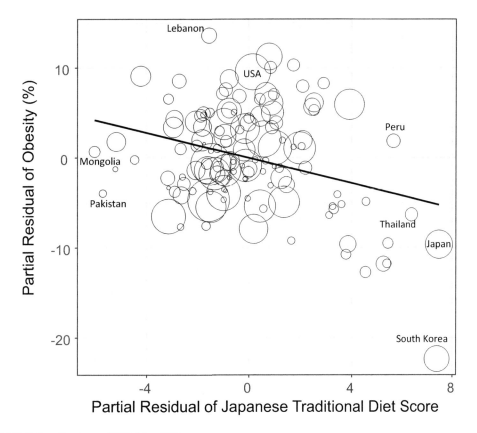

FIGURE 2.5 Obesity and TJDS by GDP.

Source: From Imai et al. (2019) with permission.

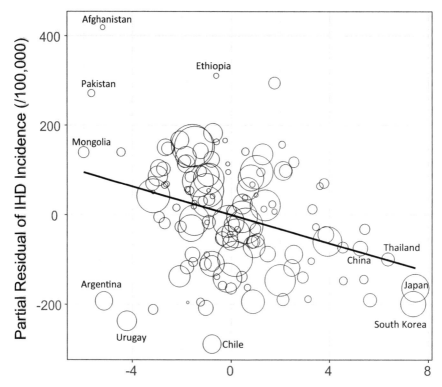

FIGURE 2.6 IHD and TJDS by GDP.

Source: From Imai et al. (2019) with permission.

were derived from the WHO database 2014, the GBD 2015, and the FAOSTAT 2013. Obesity is defined as a BMI $\geq$30.

Imai et al. (2019) created a traditional Japanese diet score (TJDS) and clarified the relationship between TJDS and obesity, IHD, and healthy life expectancy (HALE) using an ecological study. Food (g/day/capita) and energy supply (kcal/day/capita) were determined using the FAOSTAT 2013. The characteristic traditional Japanese foods (beneficial food components in the Japanese diet: rice, fish, soybeans, vegetables, eggs, and seaweeds; food components rarely used in the Japanese diet: wheat, milk, and red meat) were divided into tertiles (beneficial food components: −1, 0, and 1; rarely used food components: 1, 0, and −1). The obesity rate was determined using the WHO 2014 data. The incidence of IHD, HALE were determined using the GBD 2015; the other confounders were obtained from open data in the same way. The associations between TJDS and obesity, IHD, and HALE were examined in 132 countries, using the most current data (since 2010). The TJDS ranged from −6 to 7. TJDS was inversely correlated with obesity ($\beta \pm$ SE; −0.70 $\pm$ 0.19, p <0.001) and IHD (−19.4 $\pm$ 4.3, < 0.001), and positively correlated with HALE (0.40 $\pm$ 0.14, < 0.01). They collected the longitudinal open data (from 1990–1991 to 2017) using the same scoring system and reported that it was also negatively associated with breast cancer, depression, and suicide (Abe et al. 2021; Sanada et al. 2021).

However, no panel data analyses, cohort studies, or intervention studies were conducted using this score. It will take some time to develop a Japanese diet scoring system that can be used internationally with a high level of evidence.

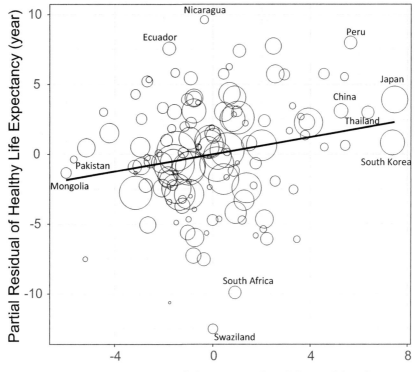

FIGURE 2.7 HALE and TJDS by GDP.

Source: From Imai et al. (2019) with permission.

Willett et al. (2019) announced a sustainable healthy diet called the EAT-Lancet Commission in 2019. The Japanese diet is essentially a meal made from locally grown ingredients, cooked in a way that makes the most of the ingredients. Scientific research has been conducted to determine the health benefits and sustainability of the Japanese diet and to develop a Japanese diet indicator that can describe it scientifically.

2.9 SUMMARY POINTS

- The Japanese diet, consisting of rice, fish, and soybean products, is nutritionally balanced.
- The Japanese diet consists of a staple dish, a main dish, and two side dishes.
- Healthy Japanese diet patterns have been studied using statistical methods, reviews, and Japanese food guides.
- There is no official Japanese diet scoring system established yet.
- Several useful Japanese diet scoring systems have been developed.

REFERENCES

Abe C, Imai T, Sezaki A, Miyamoto K, Kawase F, Shirai Y, Sanada M, et al. 2021. A longitudinal association between the traditional Japanese diet score and incidence and mortality of breast cancer: An ecological study. European Journal of Clinical Nutrition 75:929–936.

Baxter A, Coyne T, and McClintock C. 2006. Dietary patterns and metabolic syndrome: A review of epidemiologic evidence. Asia Pacific Journal of Clinical Nutrition 15:134–142.

Gadgil MD, Anderson CAM, Kandula NR, and Kanaya AM. 2015. Dietary patterns are associated with metabolic risk factors in South Asians living in the United States. The Journal of Nutrition 145:1211–1217.

Htun NC, Suga H, Imai S, Shimizu W, and Takimoto H. 2017. Food intake patterns and cardiovascular risk factors in Japanese adults: Analyses from the 2012 National Health and nutrition survey, Japan. Nutr J. Sep 19;16(1):61. doi: 10.1186/s12937-017-0284-z.

Imai T, Miyamoto K, Sezaki A, Kawase F, Shirai Y, Abe C, Fukaya A, Kato T, Sanada M, and Shimokata H. 2019. Traditional Japanese diet score: Association with obesity, incidence of ischemic heart disease, and healthy life expectancy in a global comparative study. The Journal of Nutrition Health and Aging 23:717–724.

Inoue H, Sasaki R, Aiso I, and Kuwano T. 2014. Short-term intake of a Japanese-style healthy lunch menu contributes to prevention and/or improvement in metabolic syndrome among middle-aged men: A non-randomized controlled trial. Lipids Health Dis. Mar 27;13:57. doi: 10.1186/1476-511X-13-57.

Iwasaki Y, Arisawa K, Katsuura-Kamano S, Uemura H, Tsukamoto M, Kadomatsu Y, Okada R, et al. 2019. Associations of nutrient patterns with the prevalence of metabolic syndrome: Results from the baseline data of the Japan multi-institutional collaborative cohort study. Nutrients. Apr 30;11(5):990. doi: 10.3390/nu11050990.

Japan Ministry Agriculture, Forestry and Fisheries. The Washoku Way-Japan's Nuanced Approach to Food-. www.maff.go.jp/j/shokusan/gaisyoku/pamphlet/

Kanauchi M, and Kanauchi K. 2015. Diet quality and adherence to a healthy diet in Japanese male workers with untreated hypertension. BMJ Open. Jul 10;5(7):e008404. doi: 10.1136/bmjopen-2015-008404.

Kawamura A, Kajiya K, Kishi H, Inagaki J, Mitarai M, Oda H, Umemoto S, and Kobayashi S. 2018. The nutritional characteristics of the hypotensive WASHOKU-modified DASH Diet: A sub-analysis of the DASH-JUMP study. Current Hypertension Reviews 14:56–65.

Kim S, Joung H, and Shin S. 2019. Dietary pattern, dietary total antioxidant capacity, and dyslipidemia in Korean adults. Nutr J. Jul 13;18(1):37. doi: 10.1186/s12937-019-0459-x.

Koga M, Toyomaki A, Miyazaki A, Nakai Y, Yamaguchi A, Kubo C, Suzuki J et al. 2017. Mediators of the effects of rice intake on health in individuals consuming a traditional Japanese diet centered on rice. PLoS One. Oct 2;12(10):e0185816. doi: 10.1371/journal.pone.0185816. eCollection 2017.

Kurotani K, Akter S, Kashino I, Goto A, Mizoue T, Noda M, Sasazuki S, Sawada N, and Tsugane S. 2016. Quality of diet and mortality among Japanese men and women: Japan Public Health Center based prospective study. BMJ. Mar 22;352:i1209. doi: 10.1136/bmj.i1209.

Li M, and Shi Z. 2017. Dietary pattern during 1991–2011 and its association with cardio metabolic risks in Chinese adults: The China health and nutrition survey. Nutrients. Nov 6;9(11):1218. doi: 10.3390/nu9111218.

Liese AD, Krebs-Smith SM, Subar AF, George SM, Harmon BE, Neuhouser ML, Boushey CJ, Schap TE, and Reedy J. 2015. The dietary patterns methods project: Synthesis of findings across cohorts and relevance to dietary guidance. J Nutr. Mar;145(3):393–402. doi: 10.3945/jn.114.205336. Epub 2015 Jan 21.

Maruyama C, Nakano R, Shima M, Mae A, Shijo Y, Nakamura E, Okabe Y, et al. 2017. Effects of a Japan Diet Intake Program on metabolic parameters in middle-aged men. J Atheroscler Thromb 24:393–401.

Matsuyama S, Sawada N, Tomata Y, Zhang S, Goto A, Yamaji T, Iwasaki M, Inoue M, Tsuji I, and Tsugane S. 2021. Association between adherence to the Japanese diet and all-cause and cause-specific mortality: The Japan Public Health Center-based prospective study. European Journal of Nutrition 60:1327–1336.

Migliaccio S, Brasacchio C, Pivari F, Salzano C, Barrea L, Muscogiuri G, Savastano S, and Colao A. 2020. What is the best diet for cardiovascular wellness? A comparison of different nutritional models international. Journal of Obesity Supplements 10:50–61.

Miyamoto K, lmai T, SezAki A, Kawase F, and Shimokata H. 2018. International comparative study on the difference between life expectancy and healthy life expectancy. Nagoya Journal of Nutritional Sciences 4:1–7.

Morimoto A, Ohno Y, Tatsumi Y, Mizuno S, and Watanabe S. 2012. Effects of healthy dietary pattern and other lifestyle factors on incidence of diabetes in a rural Japanese population. Asia Pacific Journal of Clinical Nutrition 21:601–608.

Murakami K, Livingstone MBE, and Sasaki S. 2018. Thirteen-year trends in dietary patterns among Japanese Adults in the National Health and Nutrition Survey 2003–2015: Continuous westernization of the Japanese. Nutrients. Jul 30;10(8):994. doi: 10.3390/nu10080994.

Murakami K, Livingstone MBE, Fujiwara A, and Sasaki S. 2020. Application of the healthy eating index-2015 and the nutrient-rich food index 9.3 for assessing overall diet quality in the Japanese context: Different nutritional concerns from the US. PLoS One 15(1):e0228318. https://doi.org/10.1371/journal.pone.0228318

Nishimura T, Murakami K, Livingstone MBE, Sasaki S, and Uenishi K. 2015. Adherence to the food-based Japanese dietary guidelines in relation to metabolic risk factors in young Japanese women. British Journal of Nutrition 114:645–653.

Oba S, Nagata C, Nakamura K, Fujii K, Kawashi T, Takathuka N, and Shimizu H. 2009. Diet based on the Japanese food guide spinning top and subsequent mortality among men and women in a general Japanese population. Journal of the American Dietetic Association 109:1540–1547.

Sadakane A, Tsutsumi A, Gotoh T, Ishikawa S, Ojima T, Kario K, Nakamura Y, and Kayaba K. 2008. Dietary patterns and levels of blood pressure and serum lipids in a Japanese population. Journal of Epidemiology 18:58–67.

Sanada M, Imai T, Sezaki A, Miyamoto K, Kawase F, Shirai Y, Abe C, et al. 2021. Changes in the association between the traditional Japanese diet score and suicide rates over 26 years: A global comparative study. Journal of Affective Disorders 294:382–390.

Seidelmann SB, Claggett B, Cheng S, Henglin M, Shah A, Steffen LM, Folsom AR, Rimm EB, Willett WC, and Solomon SD. 2018. Dietary carbohydrate intake and mortality: A prospective cohort study and meta-analysis. Lancet Public Health. Sep;3(9):e419–e428.

Sezaki A, Imai T, Miyamoto K, Kawase F, Shirai Y, Abe C, Sanada M, et al. 2021. Global relationship between Mediterranean diet and the incidence and mortality of ischaemic heart disease. European Journal of Public Health 31:608–612.

Shimazu T, Kuriyama S, Hozawa A, Ohmori K, Sato Y, Nakaya N, Nishino Y, Tsubono Y, and Tsuji I. 2007. Dietary patterns and cardiovascular disease mortality in Japan: A prospective cohort study. International Journal of Epidemiology 36:600–609.

Sproesser G, Imada S, Furumitsu I, Rozin P, Ruby MB, Arbit N, Fischler C, Schupp HT, and Renner B. 2018. What constitutes traditional and modern eating? The case of Japan. Nutrients 10(2):118. doi: 10.3390/nu10020118

Suzuki N, Goto Y, Ota H, Kito K, Mano F, Joo E, Ikeda K, Inagaki N, and Nakayaka T. 2018. Characteristics of the Japanese diet described in epidemiologic publications: A qualitative systematic review. Journal of Nutritional Science and Vitaminology. 64:129–137.

Toda N, Mayuyama C, Koba S, Tanaka H, Birou S, Teramoto T, and Sasaki J. 2011. Japanese dietary lifestyle and cardiovascular disease. Journal of Atherosclerosis and Thrombosis 18:723–734.

Tomata Y, Zhang S, Kaiho Y, Tanji F, Sugawara Y, and Tsuji I. 2019. Nutritional characteristics of the Japanese diet: A cross-sectional study of the correlation between Japanese diet index and nutrient intake among community-based elderly Japanese. Nutrition. Jan;57:115–121. doi: 10.1016/j.nut.2018.06.011. Epub 2018 Jul 11.

Tsugane S. 2020. Why has Japan become the world's most long-lived country: Insights from a food and nutrition perspective. European Journal of Clinical Nutrition 75:921–928.

Yamauchi K, Katayama T, Yamauchi T, Kotani K, Tsuzaki K, Takahashi T, and Sakane N. 2014. Efficacy of a 3-month lifestyle intervention program using a Japanese-style healthy plate on body weight in overweight and obese diabetic Japanese subjects: A randomized controlled trial. Nutr J. Nov 24;13:108. doi: 10.1186/1475-2891-13-108.

Yamori Y, Miura A, and Taire K. 2008. Implications from and for food cultures for cardiovascular diseases: Japanese food, particularly Okinawan diets. Asia Pacific Journal of Clinical Nutrition 10:144–145.

Yoneoka D, Nomura S, Kurotani K, Tanaka S, Nakamura K, Uneyama H, Hayashi N, and Shibuya K. 2019. Does Japan's national nutrient-based dietary guideline improve lifestyle-related disease outcomes? A retrospective observational cross-sectional study. PLoS One. Oct 17;14(10):e0224042. doi: 10.1371/journal.pone.0224042. eCollection 2019.

Willett W, Rockström J, Loken B, Springmann M, Lang T, Vermeulen S, Garnett T, et al. 2019. Food in the Anthropocene: The EAT-lancet commission on healthy diets from sustainable food systems. Lancet. 393:447–492.

Zhang S, Otsuka R, Tomata Y, Shimokata H, Tange C, Tomida M, Nishita Y, Matsuyama S, and Tsuji I. 2019. A cross-sectional study of the associations between the traditional Japanese diet and nutrient intakes: The NILS-LSA project. Nutrition Journal Jul 30;18(1):43. doi: 10.1186/s12937-019-0468-9.

Zhang S, Tomata Y, Sugawara Y, Tsuduki T, and Tsuji I. 2019. The Japanese dietary pattern is associated with longer disability-free survival time in the general elderly population in the Ohsaki Cohort 2006 study. J Nutr. Jul 1;149(7):1245–1251. doi: 10.1093/jn/nxz051.

3 Olive Oil and Other Oils as a Part of Traditional Diets and Bioactive Compounds for Cardioprotection

Estefanía Sánchez Rodríguez, Laura Alejandra Vázquez Aguilar and María Dolores Mesa García

CONTENTS

3.1 Introduction 36
3.2 Background 36
3.3 Virgin Olive Oil Composition: Oleic Acid and Minor Bioactive Compounds 37
3.4 Protective Activity of VOO against Cardiovascular Diseases 38
    3.4.1 Cardioprotective Effects of Oleic Acid from Olive Oil 40
    3.4.2 Cardioprotective Effects of Phenolic Compounds from Olive Oil 41
    3.4.3 Cardioprotective Effects of Triterpenes Derivatives from Olive Oil 42
3.5 Bioavailability and Toxicity of Bioactive and Minor Compounds 42
3.6 Other Foods, Herbs, Spices, and Botanicals Used in Cardiovascular
    Health and Disease 43
3.7 Toxicity and Cautionary Notes 43
3.8 Summary Points 44
References 44

LIST OF ABBREVIATIONS

CVD	Cardiovascular disease
DHA	Docosahexaenoic acid
EFSA	European Food Safety Authority
EPA	Eicosapentaenoic acid
EVOO	Extra virgin olive oil
FDA	Food and Drug Administration
HDLc	High-density lipoprotein cholesterol
LDLc	Low-density lipoprotein cholesterol
MUFA	Monounsaturated fatty acid
NF-κB	Nuclear factor kappa B
PREDIMED	Prevention with Mediterranean Diet
PUFA	Polyunsaturated fatty acids
SFA	Saturated fatty acids
sICAM-1	Soluble intercellular adhesion molecule-1
sVCAM-1	Soluble vascular adhesion molecule-1
VOO	Virgin olive oil

DOI: 10.1201/9781003220329-4

3.1 INTRODUCTION

Cardiovascular diseases (CVD) are the leading causes of mortality and disability worldwide. These are non-communicable chronic diseases usually associated with a build-up of fatty deposits inside the arteries wall (atherosclerosis), that activate oxidative, inflammatory and immune system response, smooth muscle cell proliferation, and thrombotic processes. In addition, they can also be associated with hypertension and metabolic complications.

CVD can often be prevented and co-treated by leading a healthy lifestyle, including healthy diets and physical activity; aiming to reduce weight and plasma lipids, as low-density lipoprotein cholesterol (LDLc) and triacylglycerides; while increasing high-density lipoprotein cholesterol (HDLc). Food components may reduce oxidative and inflammatory biomarkers offering cardioprotection. On the other hand, antihypertensive and metabolic healthy tools may also contribute to these benefits against CVD.

In this regard, dietary oils play a key role in many of these conditions, not only because of the influence of fats on blood lipids but also because of the presence of bioactive compounds (Bester et al. 2010). It is important to pay attention not only to the quantity but also to the quality of dietary fat. In general, vegetable unsaturated oils have demonstrated to be healthier than saturated fats; specifically saturated fats from animals or plants offer less cardioprotection. Indeed, diets high in saturated fatty acids (SFA) or *trans* fatty acids increase plasma LDLc and have been associated with increased risk of CVD (Siri-Tarino et al. 2010). In addition, the European Food Safety Authority (EFSA) has concluded that replacement of dietary SFA by unsaturated fatty acids reduces the risk of CVD (EFSA Journal 2011a). In fact, the substitution of SFA by polyunsaturated fatty acids (PUFA) and to a lesser extent by monounsaturated fatty acids (MUFA), decreases LDLc plasma concentration and the total cholesterol:HDLc ratio. Apart from the fatty acid profile, oils obtained from fruits and seed contain different minor compounds exerting antioxidant, anti-inflammatory, antihypertensive, or anti-thrombotic activities, contributing to their cardioprotective functional properties.

In general, virgin olive oil (VOO) and sunflower oil are known to reduce serum cholesterol; VOO and coconut oil increase the HDLc; VOO contains antioxidant, anti-inflammatory and cardiovascular protective molecules; and fish oil exerts anti-inflammatory activities and reduces potentially fatal cardiac arrhythmias. In this chapter we summarize the main cardioprotective effects of VOO and other edible oils, describing the main components responsible for these actions and their mechanisms of action.

3.2 BACKGROUND

The Mediterranean diet is characterized by high intake of extra virgin olive oil (EVOO), vegetables, nuts, legumes, whole grains, moderate consumption of fish, dairy products, eggs and poultry, and alcohol – especially red wine – and low intake of red and processed meats (Willett et al. 1995). The Mediterranean diet is recognized as a healthy dietary pattern for CVD, in part due to the high consumption of VOO, which is the main fatty source. The interest in the Mediterranean diet began in the 1950s when a decrease of heart disease incidence in Mediterranean countries was observed. Since then, numerous studies have confirmed that the Mediterranean diet helps to prevent heart disease and stroke (Mozaffarian 2016).

Dietary fats and oils are edible food components providing nutritional, technological, and organoleptic characteristics, but also, they may exert some health benefits and contribute to cardioprotection. The main edible oil exerting cardioprotective properties is undoubtedly VOO. This is a vegetable oil obtained from the fruit of *Olea europaea*, a tree native from the Syrian-Palestinian region. The cultivation of the olive tree to obtain oil began in Crete in the 6th century BC, from where it spread throughout the Mediterranean Basin, and has been extended to different areas all over the world nowadays (Castellano-Orozco 2017).

The composition of olive oils varies depending on the variety of the tree, the cultivar characteristics, the type of the soil, the altitude and climate conditions, the time of harvesting (from October

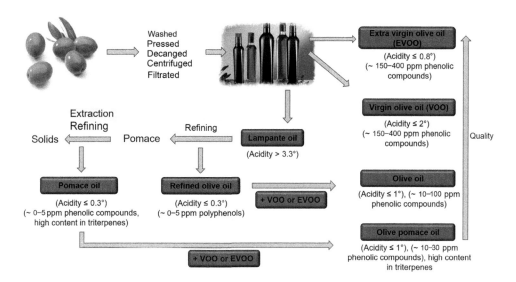

FIGURE 3.1 Types of olive oil.

Note: Elaboration and physicochemical characteristics of different types of olive oils.

to February), and the extraction process. These differences on olive oil composition may explain the diversity of healthy properties attributed to them.

Olive oil is extracted from ripe olives between six and eight months old, when they contain their maximum amount of oil, which usually occurs in late autumn. Figure 3.1 shows the different types and characteristics of olive oils described by the International Olive Council (2021). Note that VOOs are those obtained from the fruit of the olive tree solely by controlled cool mechanical or other physical procedures that do not lead to alterations in the oil composition, and which have not undergone any treatment other than washing, decantation, centrifugation, and filtration. Within them, EVOO has specific organoleptic characteristics established by a specialized panel of experts, while ordinary VOO does not reach those specific high-quality characteristics of EVOO. Physicochemical and organoleptic characteristics depend on the presence of different minor compounds that also provide healthy properties. Refining processes extract phenolic compounds, and therefore the healthy properties of refined olive oils are minimized. In addition, olive pomace oil, obtained by treating olive waste pomace, is rich in triterpenic acids extracted from the skin and the seeds of the fruit. These compounds have demonstrated potential cardioprotective properties, but they provide an unpleasant taste to the pomace oil and therefore it is not adequate for human consumption.

Since ancient times, olive oil and olive by-products, such as pomace and leaf extracts, have been used as traditional remedies for the treatment of multiple pathologies thanks to their antioxidant, anti-inflammatory, and antimicrobial properties. Specifically, olive oil was highly prized as a remedy to heal burns, sores, and ulcers, to strengthen the skin and muscles, and to relieve stomach, liver, and headaches. But those antioxidant and anti-inflammatory properties have converted VOOs into a good dietary tool useful for the prevention and treatment of pathologies such as CVD, diabetes, cancer, and neurodegenerative diseases (Sanchez-Rodriguez and Mesa 2018).

3.3 VIRGIN OLIVE OIL COMPOSITION: OLEIC ACID AND MINOR BIOACTIVE COMPOUNDS

VOO is mainly composed of a saponifiable fraction of triacylglycerides (97–99%), of which the main fatty acid is monounsaturated oleic acid (68–81.5%), besides other unsaturated fatty acids such as linoleic and palmitoleic acids, and around 14% of saturated fatty acids (SFA) such as palmitic

TABLE 3.1

Main Bioactive Compounds from Virgin Olive Oils

Phenolic Compounds of Virgin Olive Oil (40–1000 ppm)

Phenolic Acids

Derived from benzoic acid	Derived from cinnamic acid
benzoic, p-hydroxybenzoic, protocatechinic, gallic, vanillic, and syringic acid	cinnamic, p-coumaric, o-coumaric, caffeic, ferulic, and sinapic acids

Phenolic Alcohols

(p-hydroxyphenyl) ethanol or **tyrosol** (3,4-dihydroxyphenyl) ethanol or **hydroxytyrosol**, and the (3,4-dihydroxyphenyl) ethanol-glucoside

Secoiridoids (elenolic acid or its derivatives)

Oleuropein: elenolic acid + hydroxytyrosol and glucose or oleuropein aglycone
Oleocanthal: elenolic acid ester of the tyrosol

Terpenic acids of virgin olive oil (00.5–3%)

Dihydroxyterpenes	Pentacyclic hydroxyterpenic acids
Erytrodiol (homo-olestranol, 5α-olean-12-en-3β, 28-diol)	Oleanolic acid
Uvaol (Δ-12-ursen-3β, 28diol)	Maslinic acid
	Ursolic acid
	Botulinic acid

Note: This table shows the different types of bioactive compounds of virgin olive oils, phenolic compounds, and triterpenes.

and stearic acids. In addition, VOO contains a minor non-saponifiable fraction (2%) which includes more than 230 compounds, such as vitamins and some antioxidants (Ramirez-Tortosa et al. 2006), which are responsible for its organoleptic and functional properties (Mehmood et al. 2020).

Table 3.1 summarizes the main bioactive compounds found in VOOs. Among them, olives contain specific antioxidant phenolic compounds, mainly hydroxytyrosol, tyrosol, and their derivatives oleuropein and oleocanthal, respectively (Ramirez-Tortosa et al. 2006). These molecules have at least one aromatic ring attached to one or more hydroxyl groups and are found as simple forms or forming polymers (Figure 3.2). Oleuropein is responsible for the bitterness of VOO. It accumulates in new extracted oils and hydrolysates during the storage of the VOO releasing hydroxytyrosol. Oleocanthal is implicated in the bitterness and pungency, and is mainly responsible of the pharyngeal astringency properties of olive oils.

In addition to polyphenols, VOO contains other minor components that are also being investigated for their potential health effects. Terpenic derivatives are concentrated in the skin and bone of the fruit, and therefore are mainly found in pomace oils (Ramirez-Tortosa et al. 2006). In this chapter we focus on bioactive components that have been shown to exert beneficial health effects, which are oleic acid, and hydrophilic phenols and terpene derivatives representing the major bioactive fraction of VOO. Figure 3.2 represents chemical structures of these molecules.

3.4 PROTECTIVE ACTIVITY OF VOO AGAINST CARDIOVASCULAR DISEASES

In 1966, an epidemiological study showed a lower mortality rate from coronary heart disease in populations that consumed products derived from the olive tree. This study was preliminary to the "seven countries study" that established the relationship between dietary fat and the incidence of

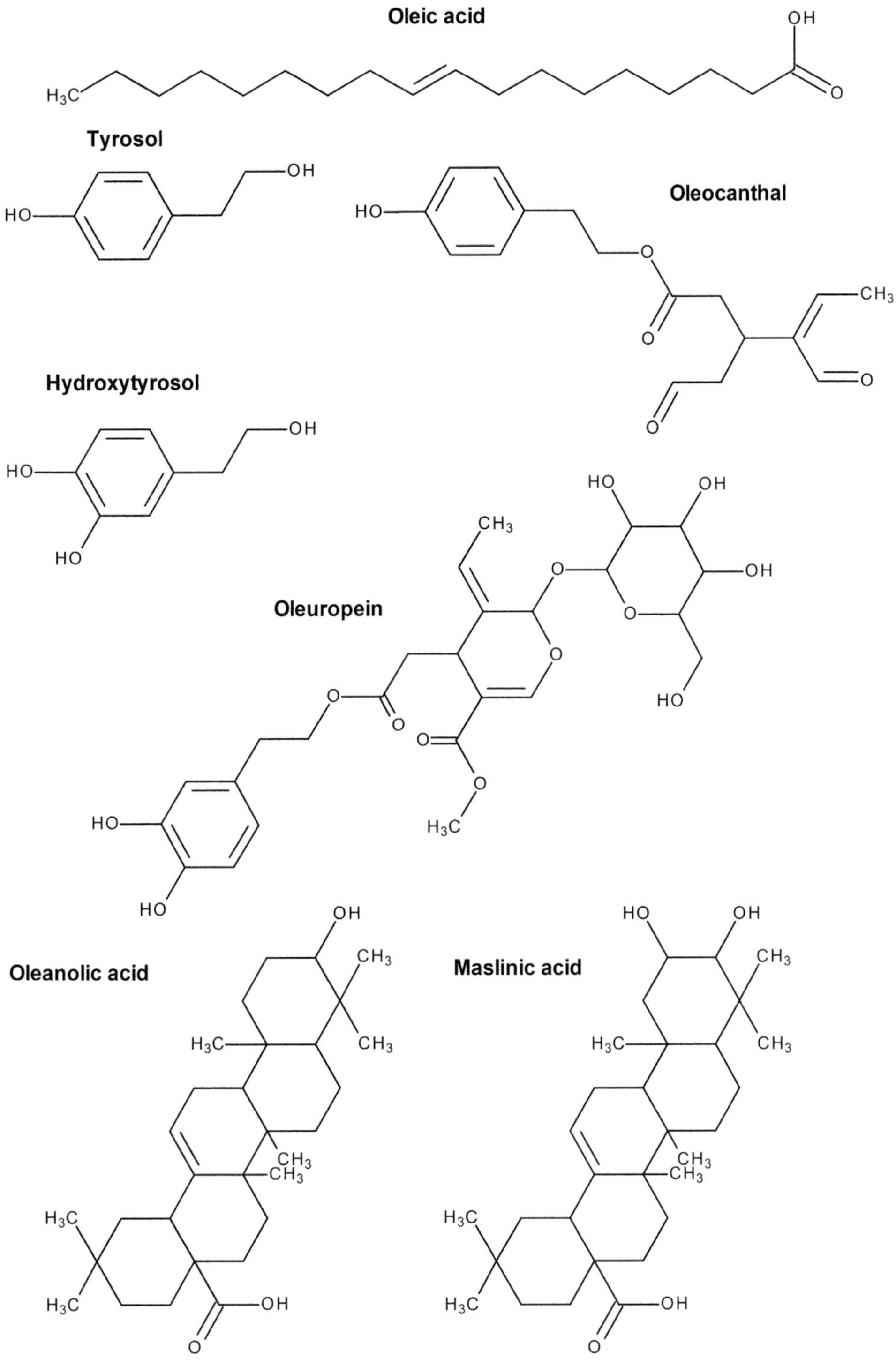

FIGURE 3.2 Chemical structures of the most interesting molecules in the virgin olive oils.

Note: Representative molecules from the virgin olive oil: oleic acid, as the most important fatty acid in the olive oil; tyrosol, hydroxytyrosol, and their derivatives oleocanthal and oleuropein, respectively, as phenolic compounds; and the most important triterpenes in olive oil, oleanolic acid and maslinic acid.

CVD, and highlighted the difference between the Mediterranean diet characterized by the high consumption of fats (15–30% of total dietary energy), mainly as olive oil, and other more saturated-fats diets (Delarue 2021).

The Prevention with Mediterranean Diet (PREDIMED) study was a long intervention clinical trial, designed to determine the effect of prolonged (five years) consumption of a Mediterranean diet enriched with VOO or nuts on the prevention of CVD in individuals at high cardiovascular risk. Indeed, this was the first randomized controlled study demonstrating cardioprotective properties of VOO. The volunteers were divided into three groups: a group consuming Mediterranean diet supplemented with VOO (one liter per week), a group of volunteers consuming a Mediterranean diet and 30 g of nuts daily, and a control group that ate a low-fat diet. The data showed that people having the Mediterranean diet supplemented with walnuts or VOO had a lower rate of major cardiovascular events (myocardial infarction, stroke, and death from cardiovascular causes) than those assigned to a reduced-fat diet by approximately 30% (Estruch et al. 2018). In addition, a Mediterranean diet supplemented with olive oil or nuts improved the plasma glucose, HDLc and C-reactive protein levels, systolic blood pressure (Estruch et al. 2006), and oxidized LDLc (Fito et al. 2007a) in individuals at high cardiovascular risk compared with the low-fat diet, improving endothelial markers in hypertensive population (Storniolo et al. 2017). Figure 3.3 shows the main cardioprotective mechanisms of action of olive oil and their minor compounds.

Many studies and clinical trials have been carried out in this field, and results are not always easy to interpret, due to the variability of the experimental designs and intervention times, the characteristics of the population studied, and the composition of oils or the use of isolated compounds. Therefore, more randomized, well-designed, and controlled studies are needed to demonstrate the functional activities of VOO and its components.

3.4.1 CARDIOPROTECTIVE EFFECTS OF OLEIC ACID FROM OLIVE OIL

Traditionally, the health benefits of olive oil were attributed to the high presence of oleic acid (18:1n-9), a MUFA that provides stability and adequate fluidity to cell membranes, facilitating their functions without increasing instability. The substitution of SFA with oils enriched in MUFA from olive oil decreases plasma concentrations of total cholesterol, LDLc (EFSA Journal 2011a), and increases HDLc being negatively associated with cardiovascular risk. This effect has not been confirmed with other types of oleic acid-rich oils with a lower content of phenolic compounds (Covas et al. 2006).

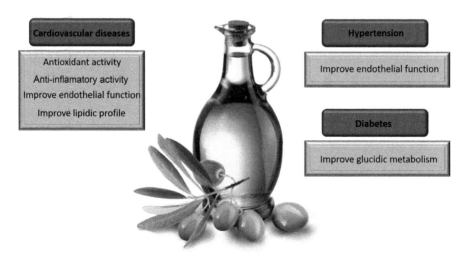

FIGURE 3.3 Beneficial effects of virgin olive oil on cardiovascular risk factors.

In addition, most studies have shown that MUFA-rich diets reduce susceptibility to LDL oxidation, an independent risk factor associated with the development of coronary heart disease in the general population, since it contributes to oxidative stability of the particles.

Oleic acid can also be found naturally in numerous food sources, including edible oils, meat (pork, beef, chicken), cheese, nuts, sunflower seeds, eggs, pasta, milk, olives, and avocados. A systematic review and meta-analysis of cohort studies has indicated an overall risk reduction of all-cause mortality (11%), cardiovascular mortality (12%), cardiovascular events (9%), and stroke (17%) independently of the source and the origin of MUFA within a specific diet (Schwingshackl and Hoffmann 2014). However, the same study showed that, concretely, only the consumption of olive oil was associated with a significant risk reduction for several outcomes. Later in 2018, the U.S. Food and Drug Administration (FDA) determined that there is strong evidence to support a qualified health claim that consuming oleic acid in edible oils (containing at least 70% of oleic acid per serving), such as olive oil, sunflower oil, or canola oil, in replacement of SFA may reduce the risk of coronary heart disease (FDA 2018).

3.4.2 Cardioprotective Effects of Phenolic Compounds from Olive Oil

In 2015, a meta-analysis concluded that olive oils with a high content of polyphenols (150–800 mg/kg) exert a moderate effect on systolic blood pressure without affecting diastolic blood pressure (Hohmann et al. 2015). In 2019, a meta-analysis compared the effects of olive oils with different amounts of phenolic compounds on cardiovascular risk factors, and concluded that high-polyphenol EVOO may improve plasma LDLc, oxidized-LDL levels, and systolic blood pressure, although evidences were low or moderate (Schwingshackl et al. 2019).

Hydroxytyrosol and oleuropein share an orthodiphenolic structure that provides antioxidant activity that helps the control of the blood and cellular oxidative state (Gorzynik et al. 2018). Clinical studies have shown an increase in the postprandial serum antioxidant capacity after the ingestion of VOO compared to ordinary olive oil and corn oil, as well as a decrease in lipid oxidation (Fito et al. 2007b). The EUROLIVE (Effect of Olive Oil Consumption on Oxidative Damage in European Populations) study described a dose-dependent beneficial effect of olive oils on lipid oxidative damage and blood HDLc levels, at doses comparable to usual daily intakes during three weeks (Covas et al. 2006). Taking into accounts these results, in 2011 the EFSA gave a positive scientific opinion on the substantiation of health claims related to polyphenols in olive oils and the protection of LDL particles from oxidative damage. They concluded that 5 mg of hydroxytyrosol and its derivatives (oleuropein and tyrosol) in 20 mL of olive oil should be consumed daily in the context of a balanced diet (EFSA Journal 2011b).

Phenolic compounds of EVOO exert positive effects on plasma lipids, improving HDLc functionality, by increasing their size and cholesterol efflux capacity, stability, and antioxidant activity, and therefore their antiatherogenic capacity (Stadler and Marsche 2021). They also increase the expression of genes involved in the elimination of cellular cholesterol by HDL (Farras et al. 2013). In addition, supplementation with olive oil rich in minor compounds can decrease the number and size of postprandial triacylglycerides-rich particles that constitute a cardiovascular risk factor, while other studies showed a decrease in postprandial hyperlipidemia and hyperglycemia after ingestion of VOO (Pacheco et al. 2007).

Hydroxytyrosol, tyrosol, and oleuropein exert anti-inflammatory activity (Robles-Almazan et al. 2018). Experimental and clinical trials have shown that high phenolic VOOs may reduce pro-inflammatory mediators (Casas et al. 2016) (Souza et al. 2017). In addition, oleuropein can inhibit smooth muscle cells proliferation (Abe et al. 2011). Oleocanthal inhibits cyclooxygenase 1 and 2 *in vitro* exerting strong anti-inflammatory activity (Lucas et al. 2011), and reduces collagen-stimulated platelet aggregation in healthy men (Agrawal et al. 2017) (Segura and Curiel 2018). These anti-inflammatory effects are mediated by the modification of the nuclear factor kappa B (NF-κB) signaling cascade, and consequently by the reduction of pro-inflammatory mediators and adhesion molecules that mediate endothelial dysfunction (Tangney and Rasmussen 2013).

Daily consumption of phenolic compounds-rich VOO may improve endothelial function in humans, although results are not conclusive (Perona et al. 2006). A meta-analysis found a significant reduction of plasma soluble intercellular adhesion molecule-1 (sICAM-1) but not of soluble vascular adhesion molecule-1 (sVCAM-1) concentration after the intervention with VOO for at least four weeks (Papageorgiou et al. 2011), by modulating the expression of several genes related to the renin-angiotensin-aldosterone system (Martin-Pelaez et al. 2017). In addition, supplementation with a VOO with different extract from the olive fruit during eight weeks benefits endothelial function and decreases blood pressure in spontaneously hypertensive rats (Vazquez et al. 2019).

3.4.3 Cardioprotective Effects of Triterpenes Derivatives from Olive Oil

Olive-derived triterpenic acids have demonstrated antioxidant and anti-inflammatory activities (Sanchez-Quesada et al. 2013), as well as capacity to restore vascular disorders associated with cardiovascular risk, showing a potential therapeutic strategy to prevent vascular dysfunction (Rodriguez-Rodriguez 2015). In animal models, a triterpene-enriched pomace oil improved endothelium relaxation in spontaneously hypertensive rats (Valero-Muñoz et al. 2014).

The NUTRAOLEUM study was a randomized, double-blind, crossover, controlled clinical trial, aimed to evaluate the effect of the intake of 30 mL/d of three olive oils with different amounts of bioactive compounds: 1) a control VOO with a low content of phenolic compounds and triterpenes, 2) an optimized VOO with a high phenolic content and low triterpenic acids; and 3) a functional VOO rich in phenolic and triterpenic acids from the olive fruit. That study provided for the first time evidence of the bioavailability (de la Torre et al. 2020) and cardioprotective benefits of olive oil-derived triterpenes (oleanolic and maslinic acid) in healthy humans (Biel et al. 2016). This study reported benefits of VOO rich in polyphenols and triterpenic acids on endothelial function, HDL plasma levels (Sanchez-Rodriguez et al. 2018), oxidative and inflammatory biomarkers (Sanchez-Rodriguez et al. 2019), and on the postprandial insulin release and peripheral tissue sensitivity (Sanchez-Rodriguez et al. 2021). In addition, a beneficial effect of these compounds on endothelial function and blood pressure has been described in animal models (Valero-Muñoz et al. 2014).

3.5 BIOAVAILABILITY AND TOXICITY OF BIOACTIVE AND MINOR COMPOUNDS

Bioavailability of phenolic compounds has been studied in humans and it varies depending on the specific compound and the food matrix. Human hydroxytyrosol excretion is higher after its administration as a natural component of olive oil (44.2% of hydroxytyrosol administered) than as an isolated component added into other foods (Visioli et al. 2003).

Once absorbed, phenolic compounds are metabolized in the intestine and liver and eliminated in the urine as conjugated derivatives. Considering that, some authors have proposed that the biological activity of hydroxytyrosol and tyrosol could be also attributed to their metabolites. This rapid metabolism avoids its accumulation in the body and its toxicity (Robles-Almazan et al. 2018). The pharmacokinetics of maslinic and oleanolic acids present in olive oils has been demonstrated in humans (de la Torre et al. 2020). Maslinic bioavailability was seven-fold higher than that of oleanolic acid, on the basis of the maximum concentration and area under the curve calculated, despite only a 1.3-fold difference in doses administered. They are metabolized after absorption, and eliminated in the urine. Maslinic and, to a lesser extent, oleanolic acid, accumulate in biological fluids in a dose-dependent manner. Maslinic and oleanolic acids plasma concentrations showed progressive accumulation after 24 h and three weeks of ingestion of daily doses (30 mL) of an olive oil enriched with these compounds. Maslinic acid plasma concentrations ranged from 1.8 ng/mL at baseline to

Olive Oil and Other Oils as a Part of Traditional Diets

6.7 ng/mL at 24 h after and up to 21.5 ng/mL after three weeks of ingestion. Oleanolic acid plasma concentrations ranged from 0.31 ng/mL at baseline to 0.49 ng/mL at 24 h and up to 2.5 ng/mL three weeks later. These results agree with other studies in rats, suggesting a low oleanolic acid oral bio-availability due to poor gastrointestinal absorption (de la Torre et al. 2020).

3.6 OTHER FOODS, HERBS, SPICES, AND BOTANICALS USED IN CARDIOVASCULAR HEALTH AND DISEASE

In addition to olive oil, other oils may benefit cardiovascular risk, such as sunflower oil, coconut oil, and fish oil. Sunflower oil is produced by refining sunflower seeds. This oil is rich in linoleic acid (60–70%), the major n-6 PUFA, but also contains oleic and stearic acid. Scientific evidence has shown that the main cardioprotective effect of sunflower oil is the modulation of the serum lipid profile, decreasing total cholesterol and LDLc, due to those PUFA. Despite this, sunflower oil has a neutral effect since the extraction process eliminates minor compounds (Bester et al. 2010). It only contains appreciable amounts of vitamin E, the main lipidic antioxidant that stabilizes the high amount of n-6 PUFA in this oil, and therefore no antioxidant benefits have been observed after ingestion (Eder et al. 2006).

Coconut oil is rich in medium-chain SFA, in particular lauric (48%) and myristic acids (19%) that have been claimed to have numerous health benefits (Teng et al. 2020). This SFA-rich oil raises total cholesterol and LDLc to a greater extent than unsaturated plant oils, but to a lesser extent than butter (Eyres et al. 2016). Virgin coconut oil, extracted from the fresh coconut kernel, is rich in polyphenols with antioxidant and anti-inflammatory activities. When compared with animal oils, coconut oil may increase HDLc and decrease LDLc, whereas when compared with other PUFA-rich plant oils it increases LDLc but had no significant effect on HDLc (Teng et al. 2020). Therefore, it is not a good choice for the prevention of CVD.

Fish and commercially available fish oil preparations are sources of omega-3 long-chain (LC)-PUFAs, eicosapentaenoic acid (EPA, 20:5) and docosahexaenoic acid (DHA, 22:6), and vitamins B12 and D. Early epidemiologic studies show an inverse relationship between fish consumption and the risk of coronary heart disease, due to the presence of these omega-3 LC-PUFAs (Whelton et al. 2004). Many experimental studies and some clinical trials have documented the benefits of fish oil supplementation in decreasing the incidence and progression of atherosclerosis, myocardial infarction, heart failure, arrhythmias, and stroke (Kris-Etherton et al. 2002), by reducing plasma triacylglycerides, improving membrane fluidity and cardiac ion channels, and because of their anti-inflammatory, anti-thrombotic, and anti-arrhythmic effects. However, large-scale studies have failed to demonstrate any benefit of fish oil supplements on cardiovascular outcomes and mortality (Goel et al. 2018) (Risk and Prevention Study Collaborative Group 2013) (Galan et al. 2010), maybe because the higher oxidizability of these LC-PUFA. Therefore, more studies are needed to reach final conclusion.

3.7 TOXICITY AND CAUTIONARY NOTES

The high intake of any type of oil provides energy disbalance that induces body weight gain and obesity that is an independent CVD risk factor. Apart from this fact, no adverse effects have been reported after the intake VOO with different amounts of phenolic compounds (Rodriguez-Lara et al. 2019) or in experimental *in vitro* and animal models (Mehmood et al. 2020). To our best knowledge, no studies have reported any toxic effects derived from the consumption of sunflower or coconut oil.

Finally, fish oil supplements are generally safe, and the risk of toxicity with methylmercury, an environmental toxin, is minimal. However, it is advisable to consume no more than 1 g of omega-3 LC-PUFA per day in adults to avoid possible anticoagulant pathological situation (Goel et al. 2018).

3.8 SUMMARY POINTS

- This chapter mainly focuses on cardioprotective effects of VOO.
- The replacement of SFA with MUFA or PUFA reduces plasma LDLc concentrations.
- The cardioprotective effect of VOO is due to oleic acid and other minor bioactive compounds.
- VOO phenolic compounds and triterpenes can exert beneficial health effects through different mechanisms of action: lipid lowering, antioxidant, anti-inflammatory, antihypertensive, and anti-thrombotic.
- EFSA recommends the daily consumption of 20 g of olive oil containing at least 5 mg of hydroxytyrosol and its derivatives for LDL oxidative protection.
- The main cardioprotective effect of sunflower oil is the modulation of the serum lipid profile, decreasing total cholesterol and LDLc.
- To our best knowledge, virgin coconut oil does not provide a positive cardiovascular effect.
- The cardioprotective effect of omega-3 LC-PUFA from fish oil is related to its triacylglycerides-lowering properties, the modulation of membrane fluidity and cardiac ion channels, and anti-inflammatory, anti-thrombotic, and anti-arrhythmic effects.

REFERENCES

Abe, R., J. Beckett, R. Abe, A. Nixon, A. Rochier, N. Yamashita, and B. Sumpio. 2011. "Olive oil polyphenol oleuropein inhibits smooth muscle cell proliferation."*European Journal of Vascular and Endovascular Surgery* 41 (6): 814–820. doi:10.1016/J.EJVS.2010.12.021.

Agrawal, Karan, Eleni Melliou, Xueqi Li, Theresa L. Pedersen, Selina C. Wang, Prokopios Magiatis, John W. Newman, and Roberta R. Holt. 2017. "Oleocanthal-rich extra virgin olive oil demonstrates acute anti-platelet effects in healthy men in a randomized trial."*Journal of Functional Foods* 36: 84–93. doi:10.1016/j.jff.2017.06.046.

Bester, D., A.J. Esterhuyse, E.J. Truter, and J. Van Rooyen. 2010. "Cardiovascular effects of edible oils: A comparison between four popular edible oils."*Nutrition Research Reviews* 23 (2): 334–348. doi:10.1017/S0954422410000223.

Biel, Sara, Maria-Dolores Mesa, Rafael de la Torre, Juan-Antonio Espejo, Jose-Ramon Fernandez-Navarro, Montserrat Fito, Estefania Sanchez-Rodriguez, et al. 2016. "The NUTRAOLEOUM study, a randomized controlled trial, for achieving nutritional added value for olive oils."*BMC Complementary and Alternative Medicine* 16 (1): 404. doi:10.1186/s12906-016-1376-6.

Casas, Rosa, Emilio Sacanella, Mireia Urpi-Sarda, Dolores Corella, Olga Castañer, Rosa-Maria Lamuela-Raventos, Jordi Salas-Salvado, Miguel-Angel Martinez-Gonzalez, Emilio Ros, and Ramon Estruch. 2016. "Long-term immunomodulatory effects of a Mediterranean diet in adults at high risk of cardiovascular disease in the prevención con dieta mediterránea (PREDIMED) randomized controlled trial."*The Journal of Nutrition* 146 (9): 1684–1693. doi:10.3945/jn.115.229476.

Castellano Orozco, J.M. 2017. "Grasas y Aceites."In *Tratado de Nutricion, Tomo III*, ed. A. Gil, 3rd Edition, 279–308. Madrid: Editorial Médica Panamericana.

Covas, Maria-Isabel, Kristiina Nyyssönen, Henrik E. Poulsen, Jari Kaikkonen, Hans-Joachim F. Zunft, Holger Kiesewetter, Antonio Gaddi, et al. 2006. "The effect of polyphenols in olive oil on heart disease risk factors."*Annals of Internal Medicine* 145 (5): 333. doi:10.7326/0003-4819-145-5-200609050-00006.

Delarue, Jacques. 2021. "Mediterranean diet and cardiovascular health: An historical perspective."*British Journal of Nutrition*, 1–14. doi:10.1017/S0007114521002105.

De la Torre, Rafael, Marceli Carbo, Mitona Pujadas, Sarah Biel, Maria Dolores Mesa, Maria Isabel Covas, Manuela Exposito, et al. 2020. "Pharmacokinetics of maslinic and oleanolic acids from olive oil-effects on endothelial function in healthy adults: A randomized, controlled, dose-response study."*Food Chemistry* 322: 126676. doi:10.1016/j.foodchem.2020.126676.

Eder E., M. Wacker, U. Lutz, J. Nair, X. Fang, H. Bartsch, F.A. Beland, J. Schlatter and W.K. Lutz. 2006. "Oxidative stress related DNA adducts in the liver of female rats fed with sunflower-, rapeseed-, olive- or coconut oil supplemented diets."*Chemico-Biological Interactions* 159(2): 81–89. doi:10.1016/j.cbi.2005.09.004

EFSA Panel on Dietetic Products. 2011a. "Scientific Opinion on the substantiation of a Health claim related to low fat and low trans spreadable fat rich in unsaturated and omega-3 fatty acids and reduction of

LDL-cholesterol concentrations pursuant to Article 14 of Regulation (EC) nº 1924/2006." *EFSA Journal* 9(5):2168. doi:10.2903/j.efsa.2011.2168

EFSA Panel on Dietetic Products. 2011b. "Scientific opinion on the substantiation of health claims related to polyphenols in olive and protection of LDL particles from oxidative damage (ID 1333, 1638, 1639, 1696, 2865)."*EFSA Journal* 9. doi:10.2903/j.efsa.2011.2033.

Estruch, Ramon. 2006. "Effects of a Mediterranean-style diet on cardiovascular risk factors."*Annals of Internal Medicine* 145 (1): 1. doi:10.7326/0003-4819-145-1-200607040-00004.

Estruch, Ramon, Emilio Ros, Jordi Salas-Salvado, Maria-Isabel Covas, Dolores Corella, Fernando Aros, Enrique Gomez-Gracia, et al. 2018. "Primary prevention of cardiovascular disease with a Mediterranean diet supplemented with extra-virgin olive oil or nuts."*New England Journal of Medicine* 378 (25): e34. doi:10.1056/NEJMoa1800389.

Eyres, Laurence, Michael F. Eyres, Alexandra Chisholm, and Rachel C. Brown. 2016. "Coconut oil consumption and cardiovascular risk factors in humans."*Nutrition Reviews* 74 (4): 267–280. doi:10.1093/nutrit/nuw002.

Farras, Marta, Rosa M. Valls, Sara Fernandez-Castillejo, Montserrat Giralt, Rosa Sola, Isaac Subirana, Maria-Jose Motilva, Valentini Konstantinidou, Maria-Isabel Covas, and Montserrat Fito. 2013. "Olive oil polyphenols enhance the expression of cholesterol efflux related genes in vivo in humans: A randomized controlled trial."*The Journal of Nutritional Biochemistry* 24 (7): 1334–1339. doi:10.1016/j.jnutbio.2012.10.008.

FDA. 2018. "FDA completes review of qualified health claim petition for oleic acid and the risk of coronary heart disease." November 19. www.fda.gov/food/cfsan-constituent-updates/fda-completes-review-qualified-health-claim-petition-oleic-acid-and-risk-coronary-heart-disease#:~:text=The%20U.S.%20Food%20and%20Drug,risk%20of%20coronary%20heart%20disease (accessed January 29, 2022).

Fito, Montserrat, Monica Guxens, Dolores Corella, Guillermo Saez, Ramon Estruch, Rafael de la Torre, Francesc Frances, et al. 2007a. "Effect of a traditional Mediterranean diet on lipoprotein oxidation: A randomized controlled trial."*Archives of Internal Medicine* 167 (11): 1195–1203. doi:10.1001/archinte.167.11.1195.

Fito, Montserrat, Rafael de la Torre, and Maria Isabel Covas. 2007b. "Olive oil and oxidative stress."*Molecular Nutrition Food Research* 51(10):1215–1224. doi:10.1002/mnfr.200600308

Galan, Pilar, Emmanuelle Kesse-Guyot, Sebastien Czernichow, Serge Briancon, Jacques Blacher, and Serge Hercberg. 2010. "Effects of b vitamins and omega 3 fatty acids on cardiovascular diseases: A randomised placebo controlled trial."*British Medical Journal* 341: c6273–c6273. doi:10.1136/bmj.c6273.

Goel, Akshay, Naga Pothineni, Mayank Singhal, Hakan Paydak, Tom Saldeen, and Jawahar Mehta. 2018. "Fish, fish oils and cardioprotection: Promise or fish tale?"*International Journal of Molecular Sciences* 19 (12): 3703. doi:10.3390/ijms19123703.

Gorzynik-Debicka, Monika, Paulina Przychodzen, Francesco Cappello, Alicja Kuban-Jankowska, Antonella Marino Gammazza, Narcyz Knap, Michal Wozniak, and Magdalena Gorska-Ponikowska. 2018. "Potential health benefits of olive oil and plant polyphenols."*International Journal of Molecular Sciences* 19 (3): 686. https://doi.org/10.3390/ijms19030686.

Hohmann, C.D., H. Cramer, A. Michalsen, C. Kessler, N. Steckhan, K. Choi, and G. Dobos. 2015. "Effects of high phenolic olive oil on cardiovascular risk factors: A systematic review and meta-analysis."*Phytomedicine* 22 (6): 631–640. doi:10.1016/j.phymed.2015.03.019.

International Olive Council. 2021. "2020/21 crop year: Production down, consumption up." www.international oliveoil.org/2020-21-crop-year-production-down-consumption-up/ (accessed January 30, 2022).

Kris-Etherton, Penny M., William S. Harris, and Lawrence J. Appel. 2002. "Fish consumption, fish oil, omega-3 fatty acids, and cardiovascular disease."*Circulation* 106 (21): 2747–2757. doi:10.1161/01.CIR. 0000038493.65177.94.

Lucas, Lisa, Aaron Russell, and Russell Keast. 2011. "Molecular mechanisms of inflammation: Anti-inflammatory benefits of virgin olive oil and the phenolic compound oleocanthal."*Current Pharmaceutical Design* 17 (8): 754–768. doi: 10.2174/138161211795428911.

Martin-Pelaez, Sandra, Olga Castañer, Valentini Konstantinidou, Isaac Subirana, Daniel Muñoz-Aguayo, Gemma Blanchart, Sonia Gaixas, et al. 2017. "Effect of olive oil phenolic compounds on the expression of blood pressure-related genes in healthy individuals."*European Journal of Nutrition* 56 (2): 663–670. doi:10.1007/s00394-015-1110-z.

Mehmood, Arshad, Muhammad Usman, Prasanna Patil, Lei Zhao, and Chengtao Wang. 2020. "A review on management of cardiovascular diseases by olive polyphenols."*Food Science and Nutrition* 8: 4639–4655. doi:10.1002/fsn3.1668.

Mozaffarian, Dariush. 2016. "Dietary and policy priorities for cardiovascular disease, diabetes, and obesity."*Circulation* 133(2): 187–225. doi:10.1161/CIRCULATIONAHA.115.018585.

Pacheco, Yolanda M., Beatriz Bermudez, Sergio Lopez, Rocio Abia, Jose Villar, and Francisco J.G. Muriana. 2007. "Minor compounds of olive oil have postprandial anti-inflammatory effects."*British Journal of Nutrition* 98 (2): 260. doi:10.1017/S0007114507701666.

Papageorgiou, N., D. Tousoulis, T. Psaltopoulou, A. Giolis, C. Antoniades, E. Tsiamis, A. Miliou, K. Toutouzas, G. Siasos, and C. Stefanadis. 2011. "Divergent anti-inflammatory effects of different oil acute consumption on healthy individuals."*European Journal of Clinical Nutrition* 65 (4): 514–519. doi:10.1038/ejcn.2011.8.

Perona, Javier, Rosana Cabello Moruno, and Valentina Ruiz Gutierrez. 2006. "The role of virgin olive oil components in the modulation of endothelial function."*The Journal of Nutritional Biochemistry* 17 (7): 429–445. doi:10.1016/j.jnutbio.2005.11.007.

Ramirez-Tortosa, M. C., S. Granados, and J. L. Quiles. 2006. "Chemical composition, types and characteristics of olive oil." In *Olive Oil and Health*, ed. M. C. Ramirez-Tortosa, S. Granados and J. L. Quiles, 45–62. Oxford, UK: CABI Publishing. doi:10.1079/9781845930684.0045.

Risk and Prevention Study Collaborative Group. 2013. "N – 3 fatty acids in patients with multiple cardiovascular risk factors."*New England Journal of Medicine* 368 (19): 1800–1808. https://doi.org/10.1056/NEJMoa1205409.

Robles-Almazan, Maria, Mario Pulido-Moran, Jorge Moreno-Fernandez, Cesar Ramirez-Tortosa, Carmen Rodriguez-Garcia, Jose L. Quiles, and Maria Carmen Ramirez-Tortosa. 2018. "Hydroxytyrosol: Bioavailability, toxicity, and clinical applications."*Food Research International* 105: 654–667. https://doi.org/10.1016/j.foodres.2017.11.053.

Rodriguez-Lara, Avilene, Maria Dolores Mesa, Jeronimo Aragon Vela, Rafael A. Casuso, Cristina Casals Vazquez, Jesus M. Zuñiga, and Jesus Rodriguez Huertas. 2019. "Acute/subacute and sub-chronic oral toxicity of a hidroxytyrosol-rich virgin olive oil extract."*Nutrients* 11 (9): 2133. doi:10.3390/nu11092133.

Rodriguez-Rodriguez, Rosalia. 2015. "Oleanolic acid and related triterpenoids from olives on vascular function: Molecular mechanisms and therapeutic perspectives."*Current Medicinal Chemistry* 22 (11): 1414–1425. doi:10.2174/0929867322666141212122921.

Sanchez-Quesada, Cristina, Alicia Lopez-Biedma, Fernando Warleta, Maria Campos, Gabriel Beltran, and Jose J. Gaforio. 2013. "Bioactive properties of the main triterpenes found in olives, virgin olive oil, and leaves of olea europaea."*Journal of Agricultural and Food Chemistry* 61 (50): 12173–12182. https://doi.org/10.1021/jf403154e.

Sanchez-Rodriguez, Estefania and M. D. Mesa. 2018. "Compuestos bioactivos del aceite de oliva virgen." *Nutrición Clínica en Medicina* 12 (2): 80–94. doi:10.7400/NCM.2018.12.2.5064.

Sanchez-Rodriguez, Estefania, Sara Biel-Glesson, Jose R. Fernandez-Navarro, Miguel A. Calleja, Juan A. Espejo-Calvo, Blas Gil-Extremera, Rafael de La Torre, et al. 2019. "Effects of virgin olive oils differing in their bioactive compound contents on biomarkers of oxidative stress and inflammation in healthy adults: A randomized double-blind controlled trial."*Nutrients* 11 (3): 561. doi:10.3390/nu11030561.

Sanchez-Rodriguez, Estefania, Elena Lima-Cabello, Sara Biel-Glesson, Jose R. Fernandez-Navarro, Miguel A. Calleja, Maria Roca, Juan A. Espejo-Calvo, et al. 2018. "Effects of virgin olive oils differing in their bioactive compound contents on metabolic syndrome and endothelial functional risk biomarkers in healthy adults: A randomized double-blind controlled trial."*Nutrients* 10 (5):626. doi:10.3390/nu10050626.

Sanchez-Rodriguez, Estefania, Laura Alejandra Vazquez-Aguilar, Sara Biel-Glesson, Jose Ramon Fernandez-Navarro, Juan Antonio Espejo-Calvo, Jose Maria Olmo-Peinado, Rafael de la Torre, et al. 2021. "May bioactive compounds from the olive fruit improve the postprandial insulin response in healthy adults?"*Journal of Functional Foods* 83: 104561. doi:10.1016/j.jff.2021.104561.

Schwingshackl, Lukas, and Georg Hoffmann. 2014. "Monounsaturated fatty acids, olive oil and health status: A systematic review and meta-analysis of cohort studies."*Lipids in Health and Disease* 13:154. doi:10.1186/1476-511X-13-154.

Schwingshackl, Lukas, Marc Krause, Christine Schmucker, Georg Hoffmann, Gerta Rücker, and Joerg J. Meerpohl. 2019. "Impact of different types of olive oil on cardiovascular risk factors: A systematic review and network meta-analysis."*Nutrition, Metabolism and Cardiovascular Diseases* 29 (10): 1030–1039. doi:10.1016/j.numecd.2019.07.001.

Segura-Carretero, Antonio, and Jose Curiel. 2018. "Current disease-targets for oleocanthal as promising natural therapeutic agent."*International Journal of Molecular Sciences* 19 (10): 2899. https://doi.org/10.3390/ijms19102899.

Siri-Tarino, Patty W., Qi Sun, Frank B. Hu and Ronald M. Krauss. 2010. "Saturated fat, carbohydrate, and cardiovascular disease."*American Journal of Clinical Nutrition* 91 (3): 502–509. doi: 10.3945/ajcn.2008.26285

Souza, Priscilla, Aline Marcadenti, and Vera Portal. 2017. "Effects of olive oil phenolic compounds on inflammation in the prevention and treatment of coronary artery disease."*Nutrients* 9 (10): 1087. doi:10.3390/nu9101087.

Stadler, Julia T., and Gunther Marsche. 2021. "Dietary strategies to improve cardiovascular health: Focus on increasing high-density lipoprotein functionality."*Frontiers in Nutrition* 8 8:761170. doi:10.3389/fnut.2021.761170.

Storniolo, C. E., R. Casillas, M. Bullo, O. Castañer, E. Ros, G. T. Saez, E. Toledo, et al. 2017. "A Mediterranean diet supplemented with extra virgin olive oil or nuts improves endothelial markers involved in blood pressure control in hypertensive women."*European Journal of Nutrition* 56 (1): 89–97. doi:10.1007/s00394-015-1060-5.

Tangney, Christy C., and Heather E. Rasmussen. 2013. "Polyphenols, inflammation, and cardiovascular disease."*Current Atherosclerosis Reports* 15 (5): 324. doi:10.1007/s11883-013-0324-x.

Teng, Monica, Ying Jiao Zhao, Ai Leng Khoo, Tiong Cheng Yeo, Quek Wei Yong, and Boon Peng Lim. 2020. "Impact of coconut oil consumption on cardiovascular health: A systematic review and meta-analysis."*Nutrition Reviews* 78 (3): 249–259. doi:10.1093/nutrit/nuz074.

Valero-Muñoz, Maria, Beatriz Martin-Fernandez, Sandra Ballesteros, Esther de la Fuente, Jose Carlos Quintela, Vicente Lahera, and Natalia de las Heras. 2014. "Protective effect of a pomace olive oil concentrated in triterpenic acids in alterations related to hypertension in rats: Mechanisms involved."*Molecular Nutrition & Food Research* 58 (2): 376–383. doi:10.1002/mnfr.201300256.

Vazquez, Alejandra, Estefania Sanchez-Rodriguez, Felix Vargas, Sebastian Montoro-Molina, Miguel Romero, Juan Antonio Espejo-Calvo, Pedro Vilchez, et al. 2019. "Cardioprotective effect of a virgin olive oil enriched with bioactive compounds in spontaneously hypertensive rats."*Nutrients* 11 (8). doi:10.3390/nu11081728.

Visioli, Francesco, Claudio Galli, Simona Grande, Katia Colonnelli, Cristian Patelli, and Giovanni Galli. 2003. "Hydroxytyrosol excretion differs between rats and humans and depends on the vehicle of administration."*The Journal of Nutrition* 133 (8): 2612–2615. doi: 10.1093/jn/133.8.2612.

Whelton, Seamus Paul, Jiang He, Paul Kieran Whelton, and Paul Muntner. 2004. "Meta-analysis of observational studies on fish intake and coronary heart disease."*The American Journal of Cardiology* 93 (9): 1119–1123. doi:10.1016/j.amjcard.2004.01.038.

Willett, W. C., F. Sacks, A. Trichopoulou, G. Drescher, A. Ferro-Luzzi, E. Helsing, and D. Trichopoulos. 1995. "Mediterranean diet pyramid: A cultural model for healthy eating." *The American Journal of Clinical Nutrition* 61 (6): 1402S–1406S. doi:10.1093/ajcn/61.6.1402S.

4 Herbs and Molecular Basis of Cardiovascular Protection

Shubhang Joshi, Vinay M. Paliwal,
Vikram Vamsi Priya and Bidya Dhar Sahu

CONTENTS

4.1 Introduction 50
4.2 Cardioprotective Herbs 51
    4.2.1 *Crataegus* spp. (Hawthorn)..51
    4.2.2 *Styphnolobium japonicum* L. 51
    4.2.3 *Vaccinium vitis-idaea* L..52
    4.2.4 *Leonurus cardiaca* L. 53
    4.2.5 *Berberis aristata* DC. 53
    4.2.6 *Melissa officinalis* L. 54
    4.2.7 *Piper longum* L..54
    4.2.8 *Crocus sativus* L. 55
    4.2.9 *Allium sativum* L. 55
    4.2.10 *Andrographis paniculata*..56
    4.2.11 *Amaranthus viridis* L..56
    4.2.12 *Centella asiatica* L. 57
    4.2.13 *Tinospora cordifolia* 57
4.3 Toxicity and Cautionary Notes on the Use of Herbal Formulations 58
4.4 Summary Points 59
4.5 Conflicts of Interest 60
4.6 Acknowledgments..60
References...60

LIST OF ABBREVIATIONS

ACE	Angiotensin-converting enzyme
AMPK	5-Adenosine monophosphate-activated protein kinase
CAD	Coronary artery disease
cAMP	Cyclic adenosine monophosphate
CK-MB	Creatine kinase myocardial band isoenzyme
COX	Cyclooxygenase
CRP	C-reactive protein
CVD	Cardiovascular disease
DHFR	Dihydrofolate reductase
EDHF	Endothelium-derived hyperpolarizing factor
eNOS	Endothelial nitric oxide synthase
ERK	Extracellular regulated kinase
GPx	Glutathione peroxidase
GSH	Reduced glutathione
GST	Glutathione S-transferases
GTPCH1	Guanosine triphosphate cyclohydrolase 1

DOI: 10.1201/9781003220329-5

HDL	High-density lipoprotein
HMG CoA	β-Hydroxy β-methyl glutaryl coenzyme A
IL	Interleukin
iNOS	Inducible nitric oxide synthase
IP3	Inositol 1,4,5-triphosphate
JNK	c-Jun N-terminal kinase
LDH	Lactate dehydrogenase
LDL	Low-density lipoprotein
LOX	Lectin-type oxidized LDL receptor
MAPK	Mitogen-activated protein kinase
MCP	Monocyte chemoattractant protein
NADPH	Nicotinamide adenine dinucleotide phosphate
NF-κB	Nuclear factor kappa light chain enhancer of activated B cells
Nrf2	Nuclear factor erythroid 2 – related factor 2
PAF	Platelet-activating factor
PI3K	Phosphatidylinositol 3-kinase
PKC	Protein kinase C
PPAR	Peroxisome proliferator-activated receptor
ROS	Reactive oxygen species
SOD	Superoxide dismutase
TAC	Transverse aortic constriction
TC	Total cholesterol
TGF-β	Transforming growth factor-β
TNF-α	Tumor necrosis factor-α
VLDL	Very-low-density lipoprotein

4.1 INTRODUCTION

Herbs and spices are frequently used as food and flavoring agents in most recipes worldwide. The great emperor and botanist Charlemagne is quoted as saying "an herb is a friend of physicians and the praise of cooks," which shows their importance and use since ancient times. Due to their medicinal properties, they have great significance in human health. Several researchers have been working on herbs and natural products in recent years, considering chemically synthesized drugs' limitations. Herbs, known as "phytomedicine," have many health benefits in treating various diseases. Plant-based products have higher popularity because they have fewer side effects and are considered food products rather than drugs (Tapsell et al. 2006). The presence of many bioactive compounds like alkaloids, glycosides, tannins, resins, terpenes, volatile oils, and vitamins increases their medicinal value. They are found to have antioxidative, anti-inflammatory, chemopreventive, antimutagenic, and immunomodulatory activities. Many plants present around us show at least some medicinal properties. A total of 21,000 plants were listed by the World Health Organization (WHO) as having health benefits worldwide (Sharma et al. 2017).

Cardiovascular disease (CVD) is the leading cause of global mortality and represents the most significant health burden with a recurring prevalence. CVDs alone cause more deaths than all forms of cancer (Shaito et al. 2020). CVDs include a wide range of diseases, including ischemic heart diseases, stroke, hypertension, myocardial infarction, heart failure, peripheral artery disease, coronary artery disease, congenital heart disease, and rheumatic heart disease. CVDs mainly arise from vascular dysfunction and ultimately cause organ damage. Prevention of vascular endothelium dysfunction can show a lower risk of CVDs by alleviating atherosclerosis, coronary vasoconstriction, and several inflammatory responses. The graph of patients with CVD and mortality is continuously increasing every year. In 2019 a total of 523 million CVD patients were noted, with 18.6 million deaths (Roth et al. 2020). Despite the availability of modern medications, interest is gaining in alternative approaches. Herbs play a crucial role in health care, and many people heavily rely on them for their health needs (Beik et al. 2020). Natural products' structural diversity and biological activity are unrivaled because of their proven efficacy in various diseases, including CVDs. Medicinal plants or herbs produce many bioactive phytochemicals. These bioactive molecules can modulate various physiological events associated with cardiovascular health through multiple mechanisms, such as antioxidant, anti-ischemic, antiproliferative, antihypertensive, antithrombotic, and antihypercholesterolemic agents (Kumar et al. 2021). The plants having a potential cardioprotective activity are discussed next.

4.2 CARDIOPROTECTIVE HERBS

4.2.1 *CRATAEGUS* SPP. (HAWTHORN)

Crataegus spp. contains approximately 300 species from the Rosaceae family found in Asia, Europe, and North America (Tassell et al. 2010; Venskutonis 2018). It has cardiotonic, antispasmodic, antihypertensive, anti-atherosclerotic, antiarrhythmic, anti-ischemic, anti-platelet aggregation, anti-inflammatory, and anti-hypoxic (Beik et al. 2020).

Hawthorn has a vasorelaxant effect due to its ability to induce nitric oxide in the vascular smooth muscle cells. It induces phosphorylation of eNOS via the PI3-kinase/Src/Akt pathway. An increase in intracellular calcium concentration by the inositol 1,4,5-triphosphate (IP3) pathway is also one of the causes of vasorelaxant activity (Zorniak et al. 2017). This ability is due to the oligomeric procyanidins present in hawthorn. It also has a weak angiotensin-converting enzyme (ACE) inhibition activity which could be of importance in hypertension. The vasorelaxant property of hawthorn precontracted by catecholamine is helpful in most cardiovascular diseases because of a reduction in peripheral vascular resistance and an increase in coronary blood flow without involving beta receptors (Tassell et al. 2010). Apart from vasorelaxant action, hawthorn has outstanding antioxidant activity. The antioxidant action is responsible for scavenging reactive oxygen species and enhancing superoxide dismutase (SOD) and catalase activities. This results from inhibiting human neutrophil elastase inhibition (Zorniak et al. 2017). All of it leads to increasing the viability of cells and cardioprotection. The anti-atherosclerotic activity is due to downregulation in caspase 3, leading to inhibition of apoptosis and lipoprotein lipase expression regulation (Tassell et al. 2010). It reduces very-low-density lipoprotein cholesterol (VLDL), low-density lipoprotein cholesterol (LDL), and total cholesterol (TC) by an increase in excretion of bile acids through cholesterol 7α-hydroxylase upregulation and inhibiting the absorption of cholesterol from the intestine by reducing intestinal acyl CoA cholesterol acyltransferase (Tassell et al. 2010; Venskutonis 2018). It reduces plasma lactate dehydrogenase and creatine kinase isoenzymes. It has been shown to reduce inflammation and oxidative stress through inhibition of the PKCα signaling pathway which may be helpful in cardiomyopathy (Venskutonis 2018). It also possesses positive chronotropic and inotropic effects, possibly due to inhibition of 3', 5'-cyclic adenosine monophosphate phosphodiesterase. There are not many safety issues of hawthorn in humans though it could be a concern if unaware of its mild positive inotropic effect in diseases like heart failure (Tassell et al. 2010). When taken with digitalis, Hawthorn can cause some interaction by increasing digitalis activity and toxicity, so it is advisable to take precautions (Beik et al. 2020).

4.2.2 *STYPHNOLOBIUM JAPONICUM* L.

Styphnolobium japonicum L. or *Sophora japonica* is commonly known as the Japanese pagoda tree or Chinese scholar tree and belongs to the Fabaceae family. It is a medium-sized tree mainly found in tropical areas like China, Korea, Japan, and Vietnam and found in Europe, the United States, and India (He et al. 2016). It has beneficial effects in treating cardiac arrhythmias, hypertension, coronary artery disease, and atherosclerosis with anti-inflammatory and antioxidant properties (He et al. 2016; Hong-li et al. 2008). It contains quercetin, sophoricoside, rutin, oxymatrine, isorhamnetin, kaempferol, and genistein as main constituents (He et al. 2016).

Sophora japonica plant extract has a cardioprotective effect by different mechanisms. The ethanolic flower extracts of *Sophora japonica* inhibit nitric oxide (NO) and tumor necrosis factor (TNF)-α production and show anti-inflammatory action. It blocks the production of various inflammatory mediators, inflammatory factors, and cytokines. The primary inflammatory mediator, interleukin (IL)-5, is inhibited along with IL-3 and IL-6 dose-dependently. Sophoroside has an inhibitory effect on cyclooxygenase (COX)-2 specifically, but it does not stop its synthesis (He et al. 2016). Apart from this, oxymatrine, the primary alkaloid found in the roots of *Sophora japonica*, affects cardiac ischemic arrhythmia by blocking sodium and L-type calcium currents in rat cardiomyocytes. Oxymatrine is metabolized into matrine *in vivo*, which also plays a cardioprotective role (Runtao et al. 2011). It decreases cell apoptosis by activation of Bcl-2, reduction in intracellular calcium overload, and reducing apoptotic mediator-Fas and protects from myocardial injury in ischemic rats (Hong-li et al. 2008). Oxymatrine plays a crucial role in inhibiting myocardial fibrosis. Oxymatrine interferes with the transforming growth factor (TGF)-β1/Smad signaling axis, preventing cardiac fibrosis. The action of inhibiting cardiac fibrosis, reducing infarct size, and ameliorating ventricular remodeling in rats could be helpful in congestive heart failure and cardiac hypertrophy (Shen et al. 2011). Moreover, this plant has remarkable antioxidant and free radical scavenging activity, the highest in methanolic extract due to its high phenolic and flavonoid contents. Along with this, the fruits of *Sophora japonica* decrease triglycerides, total cholesterol, and low-density lipoproteins and prevent weight gain by inhibiting adipocyte dedifferentiation by 5'-Adenosine monophosphate-activated protein kinase (AMPK) and mitogen-activated protein kinases (MAPK) pathways. This plant has few side effects like mild diarrhea, as suggested by the Chinese Food and Drug Administration (He et al. 2016).

4.2.3 *VACCINIUM VITIS-IDAEA* L.

Lingonberry, a small red fruit, is scientifically known as *Vaccinium vitis-idaea* L. and belongs to the Ericaceae family. It is found in North America, Scandinavia, North Asia, Russia, and Central Europe. It is classified as "superfruits" because of its broad range of health benefits and richness in antioxidant contents like vitamin A, C, E, and polyphenols. It has a wide range of activities including anticancer, antioxidant, antimicrobial, anti-inflammatory, antiobesity, neuroprotective, and cardioprotective activities (Isaak et al. 2015; Kowalska 2021). Lingonberry is rich in dietary micronutrients and bioactive compounds such as vitamins, minerals, anthocyanins, procyanidins, triterpenoids, kaempferol, and quercetin. Anthocyanin glycosides are responsible for the red and blue color of berries (Kowalska 2021).

Lingonberries have the highest antioxidant properties compared to other berry fruits like cranberry, strawberry, raspberry, blackberry, and blueberry. Anthocyanins have a magnificent antioxidant and free radical scavenging action, which prevents oxidative cell damage and CVDs. It decreases intracellular ROS production by several mechanisms, including downregulation of NADPH oxidase 4 expressions, upregulation of glutathione peroxidase (GPx), catalase, and superoxide dismutase 2 (SOD2) (Kowalska 2021). ROS can trigger oxidative stress and apoptosis in cardiomyocytes, and it even can progress to heart failure. Oxidative stress also occurs during acute ischemia-reperfusion events like myocardial infarction. Therefore, it is necessary to reduce ROS to stop activating apoptotic mechanisms by activating MAPK, such as c-Jun N-terminal kinase and caspases. Lingonberry anthocyanins have protective activity from this apoptotic activity of cardiomyocytes (Isaak et al. 2017). Lingonberry juice shows relaxation in the mesenteric arteries of spontaneously hypertensive rats due to the production of endothelium NO and endothelium-derived hyperpolarizing factor (EDHF) (Kivimäki et al. 2011). Additionally, lingonberry extract suppresses pro-inflammatory cytokines IL-6, monocyte chemoattractant protein-1 (MCP-1), and IL-1β expression and increases anti-inflammatory cytokines like IL-10 in 3T3-L1 adipocytes (Kowalska et al.

2019). In macrophage cells, it decreases the production of IL-6, IL-1β, TNF-α, MCP-1, and the expression of COX-2 and iNOS, providing its anti-inflammatory effect. Lingonberry reduced the levels of triglycerides and increased HDL to LDL/VLDL ratio in animal models leading to fewer atherosclerotic plaque formations in the aortic root region. These effects of lingonberry suggest that regular consumption of it shows cardioprotective results (Kowalska 2021).

4.2.4 *Leonurus cardiaca* **L.**

The scientific name of motherwort is *Leonurus cardiaca* L., and it belongs to the Lamiaceae family. It is a perennial herb indigenous to Himalayan regions of East Asia, Southern Europe, North Africa, and North America. The plant has historically been used as a cardiotonic and has applications in treating several disorders of the heart and circulatory system (Fierascu et al. 2019; Wojtyniak et al. 2013). Motherwort is rich in furanic diterpenes like labdens, monoterpenes like iridoids, triterpenes like oleanolic acids, alkaloids such as stachydrine, and leonurine, pentacyclic triterpenoid carboxylic acid (i.e., ursolic acid), sterols, tannins minerals, and other compounds (Fierascu et al. 2019; Wojtyniak et al. 2013).

The refined extract acts as an anti-anginal and class-III antiarrhythmic agent through antagonism of L-type calcium current and inward potassium current responsible for depolarization and repolarization, respectively, in isolated rabbit heart resulting in lengthened QT and PQ intervals, increased coronary blood flow, and reduced left ventricular pressure (Ritter et al. 2010). Leonurin, an alkaloid isolated from motherwort, showed anti-apoptotic activity by increasing expression of Bcl-2 and protective activity on myocardium during ischemia by reducing lipid peroxidation and levels of creatinine kinase and lactate dehydrogenase (LDH) in rats (Liu et al. 2010). In a clinical trial involving 100 patients having nervous, cardiovascular conditions, atherosclerosis, hypertension, hyperthyroidism, and heart diseases, the administration of tablets containing motherwort extract showed a significant reduction in heart rate, blood pressure, and decrease in palpitations and sensation of tightness in heart area (Wojtyniak et al. 2013). Ursolic acid from ethanolic extract of aerial parts of *Leonurus cardiaca* exhibited the suppression of H_2O_2 generation in the mitochondrial fraction of the rat heart. Furthermore, it showed uncoupling of mitochondrial oxidative phosphorylation and prevention of mitochondrial respiratory chain inhibition (Bernatoniene et al. 2014). In a clinical trial involving 50 patients with stage 1 and 2 hypertension, the administration of this extract showed a reduction in the systolic and diastolic blood pressure and heart rate (Shikov et al. 2011). Stachydrine, an alkaloid of this plant, has shown protection on endothelium function by Nrf2 dependent upregulation of dihydrofolate reductase (DHFR) and guanosine triphosphate cyclohydrolase 1 (GTPCH1) enzymes and also increase of the NO and tetrahydrobiopterin (BH4) levels (Xie et al. 2018). *Leonurus cardiaca* L. is responsible for some bleeding abnormalities, and it should be avoided during pregnancy due to its uterine stimulating property and emmenagogue property (Fierascu et al. 2019).

4.2.5 *Berberis aristata* **DC.**

Berberis aristata DC. is an erect spiny shrub belonging to the Berberidaceae family. It is native to the Himalayan region of India, Sri Lanka, Bhutan, and Nepal. It has traditionally been used in Ayurveda for treating several disorders (Mazumder et al. 2011). The plant root and wood contains a high amount of cardioprotective alkaloid berberine. Other phytochemicals found are oxyberberine, berbamine, oxycanthine, a protoberberine alkaloid karachine, dehydrocaroline, taxilamine, aromoline, palmatine, and other substances like sugar, starch, and tannins (Mazumder et al. 2011).

The fruit shows a tonic effect on the heart. An experiment showed the dose-dependent positive inotropic effect of the n-butanolic fraction of fruit extract from *Berberis aristata* on the heart of guinea pigs. The ionotropic action suggested a novel mechanism modulating the calcium-dependent interaction of actin and myosin binding in skinned myocardial preparation. Apart from this mechanism, it also acted through a cAMP-dependent mechanism (Mazumder et al. 2011). Berberine, a major alkaloid found in *Berberis aristata*, also shows a wide variety of cardioprotective properties (Wang et al. 2015b). Berberine is suggested to protect from severe congestive heart failure by improving cardiac function in patients (Marin-Neto et al. 1988; Zeng et al. 2003). It also helps to prevent doxorubicin-induced cardiomyocyte apoptosis (Lv et al. 2012). In another study, administration of berberine reduces myocardial infarction area, prevents injury of cardiomyocytes by preventing apoptosis, attenuates myocardial dysfunction, and protects the heart from ischemia-reperfusion injury in rats (Wang et al. 2015b). Berberine significantly reduced cardiac troponin, CK-MB, and LDH in serum. It increases mitochondrial membrane potential and prevents cytochrome C release from mitochondria to cytosol, thereby exhibiting anti-apoptosis activity via the mitochondrial pathway. Moreover, it also upregulated Bcl-2 and downregulated Bax expression in the heart (Wang et al. 2015b).

4.2.6 *MELISSA OFFICINALIS* L.

Lemon balm is scientifically known as *Melissa officinalis* L. and belongs to the Lamiaceae (mint) family. *Melissa officinalis* L. is considered a rich source of bioactive compounds. The leaves have a lemon-like taste and smell due to the presence of monoterpenes and sesquiterpene citral. It mainly contains geraniol, β-caryophyllene, citronellal, thymol, and phenolic acids such as rosmarinic acid, caffeic acid, and protocatechuic acid flavonoids such as quercetin, luteolin, and apigenin, triterpenes, and tannins (Draginic et al. 2021).

It is reported that *Melissa officinalis* extract (MOE) has cardioprotective properties like antiarrhythmogenic, vasorelaxant, hypotensive, negative chronotropic and dromotropic, and myocardial infarct size reducing effects. Aqueous MOE showed endothelium-dependent vasorelaxant properties through NO and endothelium-derived hyperpolarizing factor pathways and partly due to blockage of calcium channels in isolated thoracic aortic rings. Furthermore, rosmarinic acid also produced a dose-dependent vasorelaxant effect on the isolated thoracic aorta from rats (Draginic et al. 2021). The MOE has antioxidant action, and it reduces oxidation of LDL and exhibits superoxide scavenging activity (Pearson et al. 1997; Safaeian et al. 2016). Moreover, the active compounds of MOE like quercetin, luteolin, and apigenin showed anti-inflammatory activity by modulating immune response and suppressed cardiac tissue remodeling in animal models of myocarditis (Milenković et al. 2010; Wu et al. 2020; Zhang et al. 2016). Administration of quercetin upregulates IL-10 levels and downregulates pro-inflammatory cytokines like TNF-α and IL-17 in an experimental myocarditis rat model (Milenković et al. 2010). Apigenin also inhibits the production of TNF-α, IL-2, and interferon-γ and upregulates IL-4 and IL-10 levels in experimental autoimmune myocarditis models in Balb/C mice (Zhang et al. 2016). Moreover, luteolin decreases the phosphorylation of p38 and JNK MAPK and nuclear translocation of NF-κB thereby showing a cardioprotective effect (Wu et al. 2020). The MOE also has LDL-lowering effects in hyperlipidemic patients (Jun et al. 2012). *Melissa officinalis* L. has no serious reported side effects and is mostly considered safe, but increased appetite is reported in a recent clinical trial involving patients with heart palpitation (Draginic et al. 2021).

4.2.7 *PIPER LONGUM* L.

Piper longum L. belongs to the family Piperaceae and is commonly called "long pepper." The biological importance of the long pepper is due to the presence of an active constituent known as piperine and some of its derivatives. Zaveri M et al. (2010) reported that an amide derivative of piperine known as dehydropipernonaline has the activity of coronary vasorelaxation. *Piper longum* L. also contains the active components that can inhibit platelet aggregation through antagonism of the thromboxane A2 receptor. Four acidamides, piperine, pipernonaline, piperoctadecalidine, and piperlongumine which are isolated from the fruits of *Piper longum* L., have the dose-dependent

Herbs and Molecular Basis of Cardiovascular Protection

inhibitory activities on platelet aggregation induced via collagen, arachidonic acid, and platelet-activating factor (PAF). It is also reported that piperlongumine has a stronger platelet aggregation inhibitory activity than other acidamides (Zaveri et al. 2010). Wakade et al. (2008) reported the ameliorative effect of *Piper longum* on adriamycin-induced cardiotoxicity in rats. Adriamycin-induced elevation of serum enzymatic biomarkers, namely aspartate transaminase, alanine transaminase, lactate dehydrogenase, and creatine kinase, was significantly decreased in *Piper longum* administered rats. Moreover, *Piper longum* administration also markedly restored the myocardial antioxidant enzymes, for instance, catalase, superoxide dismutase, glutathione peroxidase, glutathione reductase, and reduced glutathione levels compared to the adriamycin per se group. Histopathological evaluation of adriamycin-treated rats revealed cellular infiltration and degenerative changes in the heart, while treatment with *Piper longum* lowered the intensity of those lesions. The results showed that the *Piper longum* administration protects against adriamycin-induced oxidative stress and reduces cardiotoxicity because of its antioxidant activity (Wakade et al. 2008).

4.2.8 *Crocus sativus* L.

Crocus sativus L., commonly known as "saffron," is a stemless perennial herb that belongs to the family Iridaceae. Crocin, anthocyanin, carotene, lycopene, and zeaxanthin are the active constituents of saffron (Lahmass et al. 2021). Evidence suggests that saffron has cardioprotective activity. The protective effects of an active component of *Crocus sativus* (i.e., crocin), on diazinon-induced cardiotoxicity in rats has been reported. Diazinon is a pesticide compound that elevates the lipid peroxides levels and imbalance of myocardial antioxidants causing myocardial oxidative injury. The histopathological evaluation suggests that the sub-chronic exposure of diazinon could induce congestion, infiltration of inflammatory cells, and multifocal necrosis in cardiac tissue. At the same time, the administration of crocin ameliorated these pathological changes owing to its antioxidant potential (Razavi et al. 2013). In a randomized placebo-controlled clinical study on 84 coronary artery disease (CAD) patients, administration of crocin markedly prevented the CAD condition. Atherosclerosis is the primary cause of CAD. Atherosclerosis is the condition in which an uncontrolled entry of ox-LDL into the macrophages by lectin-type oxidized LDL receptor 1 (LOX1) aggravates and progresses the formation of atherosclerotic plaques. Various molecular pathways are involved in the disease's progression and development. 5'-Adenosine monophosphate-activated protein kinase (AMPK) is the crucial regulator of cellular metabolism, which lowers the expression of downstream genes such as NF-κB and LOX1 and therefore subsides the inflammation, macrophage ox-LDL uptake, and formation of atherosclerotic lesions. Administration of the active component of saffron (i.e., crocin), ameliorates atherosclerosis via activating the AMPK pathway and suppressing the activation of LOX1 and NF-κB, which are responsible for myocardial cell injury and ROS generation. The data also suggests that there is a decline in serum ox-LDL and MCP-1 levels in these patients upon supplementation with crocin (Abedimanesh et al. 2020).

4.2.9 *Allium sativum* L.

Allium sativum (garlic) is a bulbous flowering plant belonging to the Alliaceae family. It has both nutritional and medicinal importance due to its health benefits. Garlic is a rich source of sulfur-containing chemical constituents (82%). Dried garlic contains approximately 1% alliin, while crushed garlic contains its most biologically active compound, allicin (Rastogi et al. 2016). Allinase enzyme converts alliin to allicin when garlic is cut and crushed. Other constituents include ajoenes (*E*-ajoene, *Z*-ajoene), vinyldithiins (2-vinyl-(4H)-1,3-dithiin, 3-vinyl-(4H)-1,2-dithiin), sulfides (diallyl disulfide (DADS), diallyl trisulfide (DATS)). The odor of garlic is due to the presence of S-propyl-cysteine-sulfoxide (PCSO), allicin, and S-methyl cysteine-sulfoxide (MCSO) (Chan et al. 2013).

Various research and experiments proved that garlic prevents CVDs. Recent studies suggest that allicin can decrease blood pressure, prevent atherosclerosis, and reduce the serum cholesterol-triglyceride level. The lipid-lowering property is also observed as it inhibits the enzymes involved in lipid synthesis and platelet aggregation (Chan et al. 2013). Also, *ex vivo* and *in vivo* studies proved that allicin shows a vasodilatory effect by increasing nitric oxide levels and blocking Ca^{+2} channels (Mayeux et al. 1988). Another mechanism of garlic may be due to its ability to form hydrogen sulfide (H2S). Erythrocytes convert the organic polysulfides into hydrogen sulfide, which relax smooth muscle, stimulate vasodilation, and decrease blood pressure. It can also lower LDL and total cholesterol and enhance HDL levels by inhibiting the HMG-CoA enzyme (Ashraf et al. 2005). Thiosulphonate obtained from garlic can prevent aggregation of platelets, while diallyl tri-sulfide (DATS) present in garlic oil shows an antithrombotic effect (Hussein et al. 2017). In another study, it has also been demonstrated that garlic can modulate the peroxisome proliferator-activated receptor (PPAR-gamma) pathway and inhibits CD36 expression in macrophages to normalize the uptake of oxidized LDL and prevent atherosclerosis (Khatua et al. 2013).

4.2.10 *Andrographis paniculata*

Andrographis paniculata (Kalmegh/green chiretta) is a well-known herbaceous plant that belongs to the Acanthaceae family. Due to the presence of two bitter compounds, namely andrographolide and kalmeghin, this plant is known as the "king of bitters." The roots are rich in flavonoids, while the aerial part contains four important lactone compounds, namely chuanxinlian A (deoxyandrographolide), B (andrographolide), C (neoandrographolide), and D (14-deoxy-11, 12-didehydroandrographolide) (Akbar 2011).

Andrographis paniculata extract is effective in treating hypertension by decreasing angiotensin-converting enzyme (ACE) activity in rats (Zhang and Tan 1997). Another study on dogs suggests that the extract of the plant effectively treats myocardial infarction. The infarct size and ischemic area were found less harmed in the treatment group compared to the control group. The possible mechanism was reported to be the ability of the extract to decrease the level of Ca^{+2} in the ischemic region to prevent ventricle end-diastolic pressure and maintain average cardiac output (Huayue and Wei-yi 1990). Prophylactic use of andrographolide in rats protected them from hypoxia and reoxygenation injury by upregulating reduced glutathione (GSH) levels (Woo et al. 2008). Andrographolide also inhibits platelet aggregation by decreasing platelet-activating factor (PAF) and serotonin levels in plasma (Akbar 2011).

4.2.11 *Amaranthus viridis* L.

Amaranthus viridis is commonly known as slender amaranth or green amaranth belonging to the Amaranthaceae family. The important phytoconstituents in *Amaranthus viridis* are quercetin and rutin. The leaves contain tannin, resin, phlobatannins, flavonoids, phenols, cardiac glycosides, and saponins, namely pentatriacontane, hexatriacontane, triacontane, and ecdysterone (Reyad-ul-Ferdous et al. 2015).

Amaranthus viridis is found to be effective in the treatment of atherosclerosis by decreasing the level of cholesterol and triglyceride. Prophylactic use of the ethanolic extract of the plant drops the levels of LDL and VLDL and raises the level of HDL in rats (Bisen et al. 2020). In the preclinical isoprenaline-induced myocardial infarction model, plant extract supplementation ameliorated the myocardial damage and restored the histological alterations (Bisen et al. 2020). HMG-CoA reductase inhibition (about 70%) property of *Amaranthus viridis* was also reported, which leads to inhibition of cholesterol biosynthesis (Baskaran et al. 2015). Reduced glutathione, along with GPx and GST, which protects myocardial tissue from ROS, is found to be increased in *Amaranthus viridis* oral treatment in isoproterenol-induced cardiotoxic rats, which confirms the antioxidant property of the plant (Saravanan et al. 2013). C-reactive protein (CRP) is considered a sensitive marker of myocardial infarction, cardiovascular disorders, and tissue damage (Ridker et al. 2000). During systemic inflammation, the liver increases its production by a thousand times more than normal in response to inflammatory stimuli (Cusack et al. 2002). Oral treatment of *Amaranthus viridis* in isoproterenol-induced myocardial infarction in rats showed a decreased level of serum CRP by inhibition of platelet mediated inflammation and the reduced release of pro-inflammatory cytokines (Saravanan and Ponmurugan 2012).

4.2.12 *Centella asiatica* L.

Centella asiatica is a perennial flowering herb belonging to the Apiaceae family. Because of its property of strengthening the nerves and brain cells, it is also known as "brain food" (Seevaratnam et al. 2012). *Centella asiatica* is a rich source of important triterpenes, including asiatic acid, madecassic acid, brahminoside, centelloside, madasiatic acid, thankiniside, isothankunisode, centic acid, cenellic acid, asiaticosside, madecassoside, brahmoside, and brahmic acid. *Centella asiatica* also contains quercetin, rutin, apigenin, kaempferol, catechin, naringin, and volatile oils such as caryophyllene, farnesol, and elemene (Seevaratnam et al. 2012).

Centella asiatica and asiatic acid block TGF-β1-mediated MAPK signaling in cardiomyocytes and protect against cardiac hypertrophy (Si et al. 2014). Moreover, asiatic acid inhibits cardiac hypertrophy in transverse aortic constriction (TAC) induced cardiac hypertrophy experimental model in C57BL/6 mice. The inhibition of IL-1β-activated nuclear factor-κB signaling and inhibition of profibrotic factor TGF-β1 and p38 ERK phosphorylation may be the mechanism through which asiatic acid prevents cardiac hypertrophy (Xu et al. 2015). Aqueous extract of *Centella asiatica* is found to decrease various cardiac marker enzymes like lactate dehydrogenase, glutamate oxaloacetate transaminase, glutamate pyruvate transaminase, and creatine phosphokinase in the adriamycin-induced cardiomyopathy rat model. The restoration of myocardial antioxidants, namely GSH, glutathione-S-transferase, GPx, and SOD in the heart of rats, may account for the cardioprotective effect (Gnanapragasam et al. 2004). In another study, oral administration of 10 and 30 mg/kg of asiatic acid for seven weeks to mice prevented cardiac hypertrophy and fibrosis by inhibiting ERK, mTOR, and activation of AMPKα (Ma et al. 2016). Similarly, four weeks of administration of asiatic acid with a 30 mg/kg dose in renovascular hypertensive rats normalized the mean arterial pressure and heart rate. The mechanism behind this effect was the ability of asiatic acid to diminish the renin-angiotensin system and overproduction of oxidative stress markers, along with inhibition of TNF-α, gp91phox, and NF-κB protein overexpression (Maneesai et al. 2017). Nitric oxide level, which plays a vital role in the progression of hypertension, is increased by plant extract when given in a daily dose of 10 to 20 mg/kg for two weeks (Razali et al. 2019). Another study proved that a 50 mg/kg daily dose of asiaticoside is helpful to treat pulmonary hypertension, cardiac hypertrophy, and pulmonary arterial pressure (Wang et al. 2015a). The molecular mechanism is shown in Figure 4.1.

4.2.13 *Tinospora cordifolia*

Tinospora cordifolia is a popular Indian herb named "Guduchi" in Ayurveda and belongs to the family Menispermaceae (Lugun et al. 2018). The main constituents present in *Tinospora cordifolia* are alkaloids, glycosides, lactones, terpenoids, phenols, aliphatic compounds, steroids, sesquiterpenoids, and polysaccharides. Other chemicals isolated from plant extracts are berberine, tembeterine, columbine, tinospora acid, and tinosporin (Pradhan et al. 2013).

Tinospora cordifolia has significant cardioprotective and hematopoietic activity. Aqueous extract of the plant decreases blood pressure and heart rate in physical stress and cold pressure volunteers when administered for 28 days (Salve et al. 2015). The methanolic extract possesses anti-platelet and anticoagulant activity as it prevents thrombin-induced platelet activation (Lugun et al. 2018). Sharma et al. (2011) in their study found that 150 mg/kg, 250 mg/kg, and 450 mg/kg *Tinospora cordifolia* extract decreases heart rate by 26.3%, 29.16%, 38.29%, respectively, in $CaCl_2$ induced arrhythmic rats and could be the option for atrial fibrillation and ventricular flutter. In

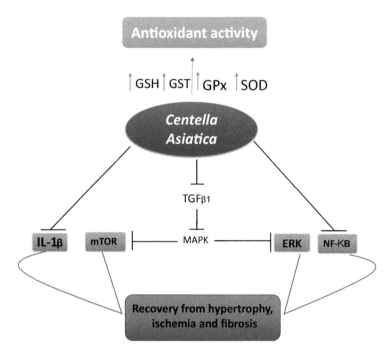

FIGURE 4.1 The proposed cardioprotective mechanism of *Centella asiatica* L.

Note: GSH, reduced glutathione; GST, glutathione S-transferase; GPx, glutathione peroxidase; SOD, superoxide dismutase; TGFβ1, transforming growth factor β1; MAPK, mitogen-activated protein kinases; ERK, extracellular regulated kinase; NF-κB, nuclear factor kappa light chain enhancer of activated B cells; mTOR, mammalian target of rapamycin; IL-1β, interleukin 1beta.

another study, the methanolic extract of the plant showed a cardioprotective effect by strengthening the heart tissue membrane integrity and inhibiting membrane damage in cadmium-induced cardiac injury (Priya et al. 2017). Furthermore, the chloroform extract of *Tinospora cordifolia* has shown to decrease the LPS-induced expression of pro-inflammatory markers like iNOS, COX-2, and TNF-α in the heart tissue of Wistar rats. In addition, this extract also significantly reduced the levels of TNF-α and IL-1β in plasma (Philip et al. 2021). In another study, the alcoholic extract of *Tinospora cordifolia* antagonized the free radical mediated inhibition of sarcolemmal Na$^+$-K$^+$-ATPase in the rat model of ischemia-reperfusion induced myocardial infarction (Rao et al. 2005). The cardioprotective potential of *Tinospora cordifolia* in different experimental models is shown in Figure 4.2.

4.3 TOXICITY AND CAUTIONARY NOTES ON THE USE OF HERBAL FORMULATIONS

Despite the number of health benefits of herbs, plants, and spices, their toxicity has also been a significant concern. Mostly, contaminated soil is responsible for the accumulation of heavy metals and metalloids inside the roots, stems, and leaves of the herbs. Generally, heavy metals like copper, cadmium, iron, lead, and chromium were observed along with arsenic and mercury in different proportions. The estimated health hazards due to the excess consumption of these high metal-containing herbs can include genotoxicity, neurotoxicity, nephrotoxicity, hepatotoxicity, and cardiotoxicity (Charen and Harbord 2020). Moreover, herb-specific toxicity should not be ignored. According to animal studies published on *Crocus sativus*, saffron, safranal, crocin, and crocetin showed embryonic malformation at high doses. A very high dose of saffron leads to an increased miscarriage rate in pregnant females, while safranal has a toxic effect on hematological parameters (Bostan et al.

Herbs and Molecular Basis of Cardiovascular Protection

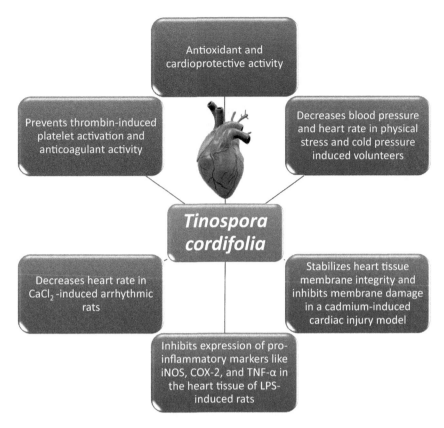

FIGURE 4.2 The cardioprotective mechanism of *Tinospora cordifolia* in different experimental models.

Note: iNOS, inducible nitric oxide synthase; COX-2, cyclooxygenase 2; and TNF-α, tumor necrosis factor alpha.

2017). Similarly, higher doses of *Allium sativum* extract cause depression, partial paralysis, and loss of appetite and may also cause death in rabbits (Mikail 2010). The administration of *Piper longum* in mice at a high dose causes severe hemorrhagic ulcerations and edema in the stomach, urinary bladder, and small intestine (Daware et al. 2000). Hence, all herbal formulations must be examined for their toxicity profiling before their use in research so that possible hazards identification and risk management can be possible.

4.4 SUMMARY POINTS

- The focus of this chapter is to highlight the importance of different herbs and spices in cardiovascular diseases.
- Herbs, considered the "gift of nature," need the world's attention so that the lack of treatment availability can be fulfilled.
- As CVD is reported to cause the highest mortality worldwide, there is a need for reliable and effective treatment options, for which herbs can be the better solution.
- The molecular mechanism of herbs like their antioxidant properties, cardioprotective properties, lipid-lowering effects, and inhibition of disease exacerbation properties along with disease alleviation is discussed in a detailed and mechanistic way.
- Various scientific studies performed on different animal models and human volunteers using plant extract or plant-derived constituents demonstrated their beneficial effect on CVDs.

4.5 CONFLICTS OF INTEREST

The authors report no conflicts of interest.

4.6 ACKNOWLEDGMENTS

The author thanks the Director of NIPER-Guwahati for constant support and encouragement. All authors also acknowledge the Department of Pharmaceuticals, Ministry of Chemicals and Fertilizers, Government of India for financial support.

REFERENCES

Abedimanesh N, Motlagh B, Abedimanesh S, Bathaie SZ, Separham A, Ostadrahimi A (2020) Effects of crocin and saffron aqueous extract on gene expression of SIRT1, AMPK, LOX1, NF-κB, and MCP-1 in patients with coronary artery disease: A randomized placebo-controlled clinical trial. Phytotherapy Research 34(5):1114–1122.

Akbar S (2011) Andrographis paniculata: A review of pharmacological activities and clinical effects. Alternative Medicine Review 16(1):66–77.

Ashraf R, Aamir K, Shaikh AR, Ahmed T (2005) Effects of garlic on dyslipidemia in patients with type 2 diabetes mellitus. J Ayub Med Coll Abbottabad 17(3):60–64.

Baskaran G, SAlvamani S, Ahmad SA, Shaharuddin NA, Pattiram PD, Shukor MY (2015) HMG-CoA reductase inhibitory activity and phytocomponent investigation of Basella alba leaf extract as a treatment for hypercholesterolemia. Drug Design, Development and Therapy 9:509.

Beik A, Joukar S, Najafipour H (2020) A review on plants and herbal components with antiarrhythmic activities and their interaction with current cardiac drugs. Journal of Traditional and Complementary Medicine 10(3):275–287.

Bernatoniene J, Kopustinskiene DM, Jakstas V, et al. (2014) The effect of Leonurus cardiaca herb extract and some of its flavonoids on mitochondrial oxidative phosphorylation in the heart. Planta Medica 80(07):525–532.

Bisen P, ChAturvedi A, Ganeshpurkar A, Dubey N (2020) Cardioprotective effect of ethanolic extract of leaves of amaranthus cruentus in isoprenaline-induced myocardial infarction in rats. Free Radicals and Antioxidants 10(1):24–28.

Bostan HB, Mehri S, Hosseinzadeh H (2017) Toxicology effects of saffron and its constituents: A review. Iranian Journal of Basic Medical Sciences 20(2):110–121.

Chan JYY, Yuen ACY, Chan RYK, Chan SW (2013) A review of the cardiovascular benefits and antioxidant properties of allicin. Phytotherapy Research 27(5):637–646.

Charen E, Harbord N (2020) Toxicity of herbs, vitamins, and supplements. Advances in Chronic Kidney Disease 27(1):67–71.

Cusack MR, Marber MS, Lambiase PD, Bucknall CA, Redwood SR (2002) Systemic inflammation in unstable angina is the result of myocardial necrosis. Journal of the American College of Cardiology 39(12):1917–1923.

Daware MB, Mujumdar AM, Ghaskadbi S (2000) Reproductive toxicity of piperine in Swiss albino mice. Planta Medica 66(03):231–236.

Draginic N, Jakovljevic V, Andjic M, et al. (2021) Melissa officinalis L. as a nutritional strategy for cardioprotection. Frontiers in Physiology 12:661778.

Fierascu RC, Fierascu I, Ortan A, et al. (2019) Leonurus cardiaca L. as a source of bioactive compounds: An update of the European medicines agency assessment report (2010). BioMed Research International 2019:4303215.

Gnanapragasam A, Ebenezar KK, Sathish V, Govindaraju P, Devaki T (2004) Protective effect of Centella asiatica on antioxidant tissue defense system against adriamycin induced cardiomyopathy in rats. Life Sciences 76(5):585–597.

He X, Bai Y, Zhao Z, et al. (2016) Local and traditional uses, phytochemistry, and pharmacology of Sophora japonica L.: A review. Journal of Ethnopharmacology 187:160–182.

Hong-li S, Lei L, Lei S, et al. (2008) Cardioprotective effects and underlying mechanisms of oxymatrine against Ischemic myocardial injuries of rats. Phytotherapy Research 22(7):985–989.

Hua-yue Z, Wei-yi F (1990) Protective effects of Andrographis paniculata Nees on post-infarction myocardium in experimental dogs. Journal of Tongji Medical University 10(4):212–217.

Hussein HJ, Hameed IH, Hadi MY (2017) A review: Anti-microbial, anti-inflammatory effect and cardiovascular effects of garlic: Allium sativum. Research Journal of Pharmacy and Technology 10(11):4069–4078.

Isaak CK, Petkau JC, Blewett H, O K, Siow YL (2017) Lingonberry anthocyanins protect cardiac cells from oxidative-stress-induced apoptosis. Canadian Journal of Physiology and Pharmacology 95(8):904–910.

Isaak CK, PetKau JC, O K, Debnath SC, Siow YL (2015) Manitoba lingonberry (Vaccinium vitis-idaea) bioactivities in ischemia-reperfusion injury. Journal of Agricultural and Food Chemistry 63(23):5660–5669.

Jun H-j, Lee JH, Jia Y, et al. (2012) Melissa officinalis essential oil reduces plasma triglycerides in human apolipoprotein E2 transgenic mice by inhibiting sterol regulatory element-binding protein-1c-dependent fatty acid synthesis. The Journal of nutrition 142(3):432–440.

Khatua TN, Adela R, Banerjee SK (2013) Garlic and cardioprotection: Insights into the molecular mechanisms. Canadian Journal of Physiology and Pharmacology 91(6):448–458.

Kivimäki AS, Ehlers PI, Turpeinen AM, Vapaatalo H, Korpela R (2011) Lingonberry juice improves endothelium-dependent vasodilatation of mesenteric arteries in spontaneously hypertensive rats in a long-term intervention. Journal of Functional Foods 3(4):267–274.

Kowalska K (2021) Lingonberry (Vaccinium vitis-idaea L.) fruit as a source of bioactive compounds with health-promoting effects: A review. International Journal of Molecular Sciences 22(10):5126.

Kowalska K, OleJnik A, Zielińska-Wasielica J, Olkowicz M (2019) Inhibitory effects of lingonberry (Vaccinium vitis-idaea L.) fruit extract on obesity-induced inflammation in 3T3-L1 adipocytes and RAW 264.7 macrophages. Journal of Functional Foods 54:371–380.

Kumar G, Dey SK, Kundu S (2021) Herbs and their bioactive ingredients in cardio-protection: Underlying molecular mechanisms and evidences from clinical studies. Phytomedicine 92:153753.

Lahmass I, El Khoudri M, Ouahhoud S, et al. (2021) Biological effects and pharmacological activities of saffron of Crocus sativus. Arabian Journal of Medicinal and Aromatic Plants 7(2):254–268.

Liu X, Pan L, Chen P, Zhu Y (2010) Leonurine improves ischemia-induced myocardial injury through antioxidative activity. Phytomedicine 17(10):753–759.

Lugun O, Bhoi S, Kujur P, Kumar DV, Surin WR (2018) Evaluation of antithrombotic activities of solanum xanthocarpum and tinospora cordifolia. Pharmacognosy Research 10(1):98–103.

Lv X, Yu X, Wang Y, et al. (2012) Berberine inhibits doxorubicin-triggered cardiomyocyte apoptosis via attenuating mitochondrial dysfunction and increasing Bcl-2 expression. PLoS ONE 7(10):e47351.

Ma Z-G, Dai J, Wei W-Y, et al. (2016) Asiatic acid protects against cardiac hypertrophy through activating AMPKα signalling pathway. International Journal of Biological Sciences 12(7):861–871.

Maneesai P, Bunbupha S, Kukongviriyapan U, et al. (2017) Effect of asiatic acid on the Ang II-AT 1 R-NADPH oxidase-NF-κB pathway in renovascular hypertensive rats. Naunyn-Schmiedeberg's Archives of Pharmacology 390(10):1073–1083.

Marin-Neto J, MAciel B, Secches A, Gallo L (1988) Cardiovascular effects of berberine in patients with severe congestive heart failure. Clinical Cardiology 11(4):253–260.

Mayeux P, Agrawal K, Tou J-S, et al. (1988) The pharmacological effects of allicin, a constituent of garlic oil. Agents and Actions 25(1):182–190.

Mazumder PM, Das S, Das MK (2011) Phyto-pharmacology of Berberis aristata DC: A review. Journal of Drug Delivery and Therapeutics 1(2):46–50.

Mikail HG (2010) Phytochemical screening, elemental analysis and acute toxicity of aqueous extract of Allium sativum L. bulbs in experimental rabbits. Journal of Medicinal Plants Research 4(4):322–326.

Milenković M, Arsenović-Ranin N, Stojić-Vukanić Z, Bufan B, Vučićević D, Jančić I (2010) Quercetin ameliorates experimental autoimmune myocarditis in rats. Journal of Pharmacy and Pharmaceutical Sciences 13(3):311–319.

Pearson DA, FRankel EN, Aeschbach R, German JB (1997) Inhibition of endothelial cell-mediated oxidation of low-density lipoprotein by rosemary and plant phenolics. Journal of Agricultural and Food Chemistry 45(3):578–582.

Philip S, Tom G, Balakrishnan Nair P, Sundaram S, Velikkakathu Vasumathy A (2021) Tinospora cordifolia chloroform extract inhibits LPS-induced inflammation via NF-κB inactivation in THP-1 cells and improves survival in sepsis. BMC Complementary Medicine and Therapies 21(1):1–13.

Pradhan D, Ojha V, Pandey A (2013) Phytochemical analysis of Tinospora cordifolia (Willd.) Miers ex Hook. F. & Thoms stem of varied thickness. International Journal of Pharmaceutical Sciences and Research 4(8):3051–3056.

Priya LB, Baskaran R, Elangovan P, DhiVya V, Huang C-Y, Padma VV (2017) Tinospora cordifolia extract attenuates cadmium-induced biochemical and histological alterations in the heart of male Wistar rats. Biomedicine & Pharmacotherapy 87:280–287.

Rao PR, Kumar VK, Viswanath RK, Subbaraju GV (2005) Cardioprotective activity of alcoholic extract of Tinospora cordifolia in ischemia-reperfusion induced myocardial infarction in rats. Biological and Pharmaceutical Bulletin 28(12):2319–2322.

Rastogi S, Pandey MM, Rawat A (2016) Traditional herbs: A remedy for cardiovascular disorders. Phytomedicine 23(11):1082–1089.

Razali NNM, Ng CT, Fong LY (2019) Cardiovascular protective effects of Centella asiatica and its triterpenes: A review. Planta Medica 85(16):1203–1215.

Razavi BM, Hosseinzadeh H, Movassaghi AR, IMenshahidi M, Abnous K (2013) Protective effect of crocin on diazinon induced cardiotoxicity in rats in subchronic exposure. Chem Biol Interact 203(3):547–555.

Reyad-ul-Ferdous M, Shahjahan DS, Tanvir S, Mukti M (2015) Present biological status of potential medicinal plant of amaranthus viridis: A comprehensive review. Am J Clin Exp Med 3:12–17.

Ridker PM, Hennekens CH, Buring JE, Rifai N (2000) C-reactive protein and other markers of inflammation in the prediction of cardiovascular disease in women. New England Journal of Medicine 342(12):836–843.

Ritter M, Melichar K, Strahler S, et al. (2010) Cardiac and electrophysiological effects of primary and refined extracts from Leonurus cardiaca L. (Ph. Eur.). Planta Medica 76(6):572–582.

Roth GA, Mensah GA, Johnson CO, et al. (2020) Global burden of cardiovascular diseases and risk factors, 1990–2019: Update from the GBD 2019 study. Journal of the American College of Cardiology 76(25):2982–3021.

Runtao G, Guo D, Jiangbo Y, Xu W, Shusen Y (2011) Oxymatrine, the main alkaloid component of Sophora roots, protects heart against arrhythmias in rats. Planta Medica 77(03):226–230.

Safaeian L, Sajjadi SE, Javanmard SH, Montazeri H, Samani F (2016) Protective effect of Melissa officinalis extract against H2O2-induced oxidative stress in human vascular endothelial cells. Research in Pharmaceutical Sciences 11(5):383–389.

Salve BA, Tripathi RK, Petare AU, Raut AA, Rege NN (2015) Effect of Tinospora cordifolia on physical and cardiovascular performance induced by physical stress in healthy human volunteers. Ayu 36(3):265–270.

Saravanan G, Ponmurugan P (2012) Amaranthus viridis Linn., a common spinach, modulates C-reactive protein, protein profile, ceruloplasmin and glycoprotein in experimental induced myocardial infarcted rats. Journal of the Science of Food and Agriculture 92(12):2459–2464.

Saravanan G, PonMurugan P, Sathiyavathi M, Vadivukkarasi S, Sengottuvelu S (2013) Cardioprotective activity of Amaranthus viridis Linn: Effect on serum marker enzymes, cardiac troponin and antioxidant system in experimental myocardial infarcted rats. International Journal of Cardiology 165(3):494–498.

Seevaratnam V, Banumathi P, Premalatha MR, Sundaram SP, Arumugam T (2012) Functional properties of Centella asiatica (L.): A review. International Journal of Pharmacy and Pharmaceutical Sciences 4(5):8–14.

Shaito A, Thuan DTB, Phu HT, et al. (2020) Herbal medicine for cardiovascular diseases: Efficacy, mechanisms, and safety. Frontiers in Pharmacology 11:422.

Sharma AK, Kishore K, Sharma D, et al. (2011) Cardioprotective activity of alcoholic extract of Tinospora cordifolia (Willd.) Miers in calcium chloride-induced cardiac arrhythmia in rats. Journal of Biomedical Research 25(4):280–286.

Sharma M, Gupta A, Prasad R (2017) A review on herbs, spices and functional food used in diseases. International Journal of Research & Review 4(1):103–108.

Shen X-C, Yang Y-P, Xiao T-T, Peng J, Liu X-D (2011) Protective effect of oxymatrine on myocardial fibrosis induced by acute myocardial infarction in rats involved in TGF-β1-Smads signal pathway. Journal of Asian Natural Products Research 13(3):215–224.

Shikov AN, Pozharitskaya ON, Makarov VG, Demchenko DV, Shikh EV (2011) Effect of Leonurus cardiaca oil extract in patients with arterial hypertension accompanied by anxiety and sleep disorders. Phytotherapy Research 25(4):540–543.

Si L, Xu J, Yi C, et al. (2014) Asiatic acid attenuates cardiac hypertrophy by blocking transforming growth factor-β1-mediated hypertrophic signaling in vitro and in vivo. International Journal of Molecular Medicine 34(2):499–506.

Tapsell LC, Hemphill I, Cobiac L, et al. (2006) Health benefits of herbs and spices: The past, the present, the future. Medical Journal of Australia 185(4):S1–S24.

Tassell MC, Kingston R, Gilroy D, Lehane M, Furey A (2010) Hawthorn (Crataegus spp.) in the treatment of cardiovascular disease. Pharmacognosy Reviews 4(7):32–41.

Venskutonis PR (2018) Phytochemical composition and bioactivities of hawthorn (Crataegus spp.): Review of recent research advances. Journal of Food Bioactives 4:69–87.

Wakade A, Shah A, Kulkarni M, Juvekar A (2008) Protective effect of Piper longum L. on oxidative stress induced injury and cellular abnormality in adriamycin induced cardiotoxicity in rats. Indian Journal of Experimental Biology 46:528–533.

Wang X-b, Wang W, Zhu X-C, et al. (2015a) The potential of asiaticoside for TGF-β1/Smad signaling inhibition in prevention and progression of hypoxia-induced pulmonary hypertension. Life Sciences 137:56–64.

Wang Y, Liu J, MA A, Chen Y (2015b) Cardioprotective effect of berberine against myocardial ischemia/reperfusion injury via attenuating mitochondrial dysfunction and apoptosis. International Journal of Clinical and Experimental Medicine 8(8):14513–14519.

Wojtyniak K, Szymański M, Matławska I (2013) Leonurus cardiaca L. (motherwort): A review of its phytochemistry and pharmacology. Phytotherapy Research 27(8):1115–1120.

Woo AY, Waye MM, Tsui SK, Yeung ST, Cheng CH (2008) Andrographolide up-regulates cellular-reduced glutathione level and protects cardiomyocytes against hypoxia/reoxygenation injury. Journal of Pharmacology and Experimental Therapeutics 325(1):226–235.

Wu S, Wang H-Q, Guo T-T, Li Y-H (2020) Luteolin inhibits CVB3 replication through inhibiting inflammation. Journal of Asian Natural Products Research 22(8):762–773.

Xie X, Zhang Z, Wang X, et al. (2018) Stachydrine protects eNOS uncoupling and ameliorates endothelial dysfunction induced by homocysteine. Molecular Medicine 24(1):1–10.

Xu X, Si L, Xu J, et al. (2015) Asiatic acid inhibits cardiac hypertrophy by blocking interleukin-1β-activated nuclear factor-κB signaling in vitro and in vivo. Journal of Thoracic Disease 7(10):1787–1797.

Zaveri M, Khandhar A, Patel S, Patel A (2010) Chemistry and pharmacology of Piper longum L. International Journal of Pharmaceutical Sciences Review and Research 5(1):67–76.

Zeng X-H, Zeng X-J, Li Y-Y (2003) Efficacy and safety of berberine for congestive heart failure secondary to ischemic or idiopathic dilated cardiomyopathy. The American Journal of Cardiology 92(2):173–176.

Zhang C, Tan B (1997) Mechanisms of cardiovascular activity of Andrographis paniculata in the anaesthetized rat. Journal of Ethnopharmacology 56(2):97–101.

Zhang S, Liu X, Sun C, et al. (2016) Apigenin attenuates experimental autoimmune myocarditis by modulating Th1/Th2 cytokine balance in mice. Inflammation 39(2):678–686.

Zorniak M, Szydlo B, Krzeminski T (2017) Review atricle. Journal of Physiology and Pharmacology 68(4):521–526.

5 Seaweed in Traditional Diets and Relationship with Cardiovascular Disease Incidence and Mortality

Kazumasa Yamagishi, Wanlu Sun and Hiroyasu Iso

CONTENTS

5.1 Introduction 65
5.2 Background...65
5.3 Seaweeds Consumed in Asia...66
5.4 JPHC Study..66
5.5 JACC Study..67
5.6 CIRCS..68
5.7 Meta-Analysis of the Existing Evidence 68
5.8 Mechanisms 71
5.9 Other Foods, Herbs, Spices and Botanicals Used in Cardiovascular
      Health and Disease 71
5.10 Toxicity and Cautionary Notes 71
5.11 Summary Points 72
References...72

LIST OF ABBREVIATIONS

CIRCS   Circulatory Risk in Communities Study
JACC   Study Collaborative Cohort Study for Evaluation of Cancer Risk
JPHC   Study Public Health Center-based Prospective Study

5.1 INTRODUCTION

Since seaweed is mainly consumed in East Asia, such as Japan, Korea and China, and is not a familiar food in the West, epidemiological evidence was very limited on a potential effect of seaweed intake on cardiovascular diseases. Since 2019, three large cohort studies in Japan have reported on the association between seaweed and the incidence of mortality from ischemic heart disease and stroke. A review article on this topic was published in 2021 (Murai et al. 2021), and one new original paper has since been published. This paper outlines the findings of the three studies.

5.2 BACKGROUND

Seaweed contains minerals such as potassium, calcium, phosphorus, zinc and iodine, soluble fibers such as fucoidan and alginates, vitamins (A, B, C and E), peptides, and carotenoids including fucoxanthin, which has been thought to be beneficial for cardiovascular health. However, as mentioned earlier, it was not part of the food culture outside of Asia, and the evidence for it has not been clear

DOI: 10.1201/9781003220329-6

for a long time. Basic or epidemiological studies have shown that seaweed has a positive effect on blood pressure, lipids, glucose and body weight (Murai et al. 2021), and therefore it has been vaguely thought that it should be also beneficial for ischemic heart disease and stroke.

In 2019, the results of the world's first cohort study analyzing this association were published from Japan, followed by successive publications of similar associations from two Japanese cohorts in 2020 and 2021. So far, these are the only three cohort studies that have clarified the relationship between seaweed and cardiovascular disease, and therefore this is a new topic in nutritional epidemiology. After introducing each of them, this paper will show the results of its own meta-analysis of the three studies.

5.3 SEAWEEDS CONSUMED IN ASIA

Seaweed is traditionally and broadly consumed in Asia, especially in East Asian countries such as Japan, Korea and parts of China. Major edible seaweed species in Japan are: wakame (brown seaweeds, *Undaria pinnatifida*); kombu (kelp, *Laminaria*); nori (red seaweeds and green seaweeds); and hijiki (*Hizikia fusiformis*).

Wakame is a dark green seaweed which is widely eaten in Japan and Korea, and is rich in mineral and soluble fiber. Edible wakame is harvested from winter to spring and is preserved by drying after being salted. It is often found in miso soup. Fresh wakame can be boiled and then made into cold dishes.

Kombu is a type of edible kelp which is also popularly eaten in China as well as Japan and Korea. There are many ways to eat kombu. In Japan, kombu is usually sun-dried and is used to make soup stock with small pieces of bonito. It can also be chopped into long strips and boiled with soy sauce, sugar and mirin (a type of cooking rice wine). In the coastal cities of China, kombu is usually eaten whole. Stir-fried kombu is the main way to eat it. In some cold northern area in China, people cut kombu into shreds and stew it with tofu and vegetables. It is also considered to have medicinal value such as being effective in dispelling phlegm and softening hardened lesion tissues in China.

Natural nori is found in the sea attached to rocks, but nori in the market is often farmed. In East Asian countries, nori is usually roasted and pressed into dried nori sheets. Japanese and Korean people use nori to wrap rice balls, while Chinese people prefer to tear dried nori to make soup. Nori is also eaten as a snack.

Hijiki is widely eaten in Japan, but not necessarily in China and Korea although it is often farmed in these countries. It is a dark brown, curved stick with a unique shape. In Japan, dried hijiki is often boiled in soy sauce, sugar and vegetables, which is a kind of "nimono" (boiled dish).

Other seaweeds such as tengusa, aosa, mozuku, mekabu and others are also consumed in Japan, but their consumption is considered to be less than the aforementioned four.

There have been no cohort studies that have examined the long-term effects of the intake of these individual seaweeds. The following three studies all analyzed them as total seaweeds.

5.4 JPHC STUDY

The JPHC Study (Japan Public Health Center-based Prospective Study) is a nationwide study that follows approximately 140,000 local residents aged 40–69 years old in 11 public health centers in Japan (Tsugane and Sawada 2014). It consists of two subcohorts. Cohort I started in 1990 in five public health centers and Cohort II started in 1993 in six public health centers. A self-administered questionnaire about lifestyle, including a food frequency questionnaire, was conducted in all eligible study participants at the start of the study.

The JPHC Study, led by the National Cancer Center of Japan, was initially launched to follow up not only cancer but also stroke and ischemic heart disease (myocardial infarction and sudden cardiac death), to identify risk factors for multiple outcomes. It is the largest study in Japan to follow the incidence of ischemic heart disease and stroke with a systematic survey of medical records

Seaweed in Traditional Diets

including electrocardiogram and blood tests and brain images (computed tomography and/or magnetic resonance imaging) in medical institutions.

The food frequency questionnaire in the baseline survey was somewhat different between Cohort I and Cohort II. In Cohort I, seaweed was asked as "seaweed such as nori, wakame, kombu" and four options for frequency were provided. For Cohort II, seaweed was asked as "seaweed (kombu, wakame, mozuku, etc)" and five options for frequency were provided. They combined two cohorts and a total of 86,113 men and women aged 40–69 years without history of cancer or cardiovascular disease at the time of baseline questionnaires were examined (Murai et al. 2019). During a follow-up for 17 years in average, 5,873 incident cases of total cardiovascular diseases were identified. This is the first cohort study that showed the association between the frequency of seaweed intake and incidence of ischemic heart disease and stroke in the world.

The frequency of seaweed intake was inversely associated with incident ischemic heart disease for both men and women. For men, the results showed that the hazard ratios for incident ischemic heart disease were 0.84 (0.69–1.03) for participants who consumed seaweed <1–2 days per month, 0.79 (0.64–0.98) for those who consumed it 3–4 days per month and 0.76 (0.58–0.99) for those who consumed it almost every day compared to those who consumed almost no seaweed, and the trend of the association was significant ($p = 0.04$). For women the respective hazard ratios were 0.75 (0.54–1.05), 0.74 (0.53–1.05), and 0.56 (0.36–0.85), and p for trend = 0.006. In contrast, no such associations for risk of total stroke, ischemic stroke, intraparenchymal hemorrhage and subarachnoid hemorrhage were observed among either men or women in this study.

5.5 JACC STUDY

The JACC Study (the Japan Collaborative Cohort Study for Evaluation of Cancer Risk) was a multicenter collaborative cohort study sponsored by the Japanese Ministry of Education, Culture, Sports, Science and Technology (Tamakoshi et al. 2013). This study has originally conducted by cancer epidemiologists, and the primary objective was to seek the risk factors for cancer. Therefore, they followed up cause-specific death as well as incident cancer which allowed them to examine the risk of mortality from ischemic heart disease and stroke. The JACC and JPHC studies have been recognized as the most large-scaled studies of cardiovascular nutritional epidemiology in Japan.

The JACC Study recruited study participants from 45 districts across Japan. Baseline survey was conducted from 1988 through 1990. Self-administered questionnaires about lifestyle including a food frequency questionnaire and medical histories of cardiovascular disease or cancer was conducted at the beginning of the study. In their questionnaire, seaweed was asked as "seaweed (nori, wakame, kombu, etc)" and five options for frequency were provided. For the study of seaweed, a total of 96,215 men and women aged 40 to 79 years without a history of cardiovascular disease or cancer during the baseline period were involved in the analyses (Kishida et al. 2020). During the follow-up for an average of 16 years, 6,525 deaths from cardiovascular disease occurred. The association between the frequency of seaweed intake and the mortality of ischemic heart disease and stroke was analyzed.

The association of seaweed intake and mortalities were slightly different between men and women, and the associations were generally non-linear. Among men, the hazard ratios for mortality from total stroke were 0.56 (0.38–0.82) for participants who consumed seaweed <1–2 times per month, 0.66 (0.47–0.94) for those consumed it <1–2 times per week, 0.73 (0.51–1.03) for those consumed it 3–4 times per week and 0.70 (0.49–0.99) for those consumed it almost every day, compared to those who never ate seaweed (p for trend = 0.47). Similar associations for mortality from ischemic stroke were observed, of which the hazard ratios were 0.51 (0.28–0.91), 0.55 (0.33–0.94), 0.67 (0.40–1.14) and 0.69 (0.41–1.16), and p for trend = 0.11. Among women, the respective hazard ratios for mortality from total stroke were 0.87 (0.56–1.35), 0.81 (0.54–1.22), 0.74 (0.49–1.12) and 0.70 (0.46–1.06), p for trend = 0.01; and those for mortality from ischemic stroke were 0.49 (0.25–0.97), 0.58 (0.32–1.05), 0.49 (0.27–0.90) and 0.49 (0.27–0.90), p for trend = 0.20. No associations were observed between seaweed intake and risks of intraparenchymal hemorrhage and CHD among either men or women.

5.6 CIRCS

The CIRCS (Circulatory Risk in Communities Study) is a cohort study of lifestyle-related disease involving approximately 12,000 adults from five communities of Japan. It is an ongoing community-based epidemiological dynamic cohort in which health examinations are conducted using the same method every year. This study was originally conducted as preventive measures of stroke in each community. It is one of the oldest large-scale epidemiological studies of cardiovascular diseases in Japan that follows the incidence of ischemic heart disease and stroke with the earliest communities (Akita and Osaka) to start since 1963 (Yamagishi et al. 2019).

A 24-hour recall dietary survey was conducted to collect the dietary data. A total of 6,169 residents aged 40 to 79 years from four communities (Akita, Ibaraki, Osaka and Kochi) who participated in the health check-ups and completed at least one dietary survey between 1984 to 2000 were involved in the study of seaweed. The participants were followed up for an average period of 22 years, and a total of 523 cases of total cardiovascular diseases were confirmed. The relationship between the amount of seaweed intake and the subsequent incidence of ischemic heart disease and stroke was analyzed (Chichibu et al. 2021). The amount of seaweed intake was divided into four groups: no seaweed intake, and tertiles of the amount of seaweed intake on the day before the survey estimated by 24 h recall method. Since this was a face-to-face interview, not self-administrated questionnaire, the participants were asked about their intake of individual seaweeds within a 24-hour period.

The association between seaweed intake and risk of cardiovascular diseases differed between men and women. The hazard ratio for incident total stroke was 0.63 (0.42–0.94) for men who ate the most seaweed (15 g or more the day before the survey) compared to those who ate no seaweed, and the trend of the association was also significant (p for trend = 0.01). Similar association was found for cerebral infarction with hazard ratio of 0.59 (0.36–0.97) (p for trend = 0.03). In women, however, the hazard ratios for total stroke and cerebral infarction were 0.85 (0.55–1.31) and 1.05 (0.59–1.88), respectively. No statistically significant associations were found for hemorrhagic stroke and ischemic heart disease in either sex. Therefore, an inverse association between seaweed and risk of total stroke and cerebral infarction was found among Japanese men in the CIRCS.

5.7 META-ANALYSIS OF THE EXISTING EVIDENCE

The three cohort studies mentioned earlier independently examined the association between seaweed intake and the risk of onset or death of ischemic heart disease and stroke. A part of the findings on sex and outcome differed from each other. These discrepancies were probably due to following reasons: the study population (e.g., the age of the participants, sex-distribution and the communities which the participants were from), the era of the baseline (i.e., 1990–1994 for JPHC Study, 1988–1990 for JACC Study and 1984–2000 for CIRCS), the method in the dietary survey to collect data of seaweed intake (i.e., 24-hour dietary recall methods or food frequency questionnaire methods; and food frequency questionnaire differed across the cohorts) and the method of evaluating the outcomes (i.e., incident cardiovascular disease or mortality from cardiovascular disease). However, in the big picture, there seemed to be an inverse association between seaweed intake and risk of cardiovascular disease. In this context, a meta-analysis integrating these three epidemiological studies were conducted here in this paper. The results are shown in Figure 5.1.

The pooled hazard ratios of ischemic heart disease in the group with the highest seaweed intake compared to the group with no intake were 0.78 (0.61–1.01) for men and 0.91 (0.78–1.06) for women; and the respective hazard ratios of stroke were 0.90 (0.67–1.20) and 0.74 (0.72–1.31). That is, for both men and women, the risk of the incidence of or mortality from both ischemic heart disease

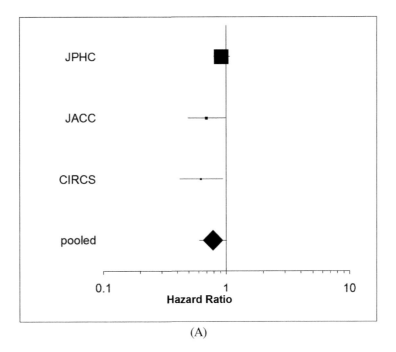

(A)

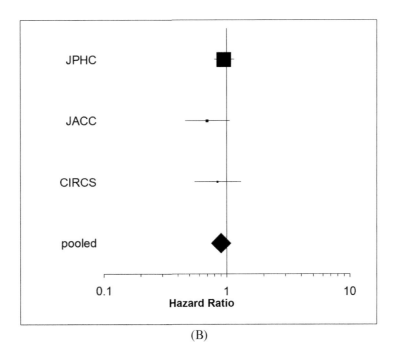

(B)

FIGURE 5.1 Meta-analysis integrating existing three cohort studies examining association between seaweed intake and (A) ischemic heart disease in men; (B) ischemic heart disease in women; (C) stroke in men; (D) stroke in women.

Note: The hazard ratios of individual studies and pooled hazard ratio for the highest vs. lowest categories of seaweed intake were presented. The pooled hazard ratio was (A) 0.78 (0.61–1.01) for stroke in men; (B) 0.91 (0.78–1.06) for stroke in women; (C) 0.90 (0.67–1.20) for ischemic heart disease in men; and (D) 0.74 (0.42–1.31) for ischemic heart disease in women.

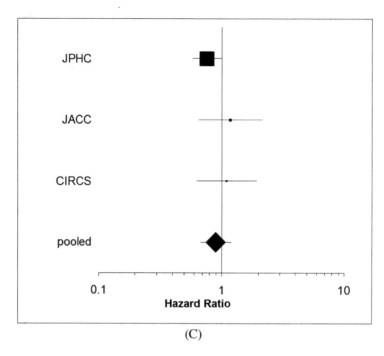

(C)

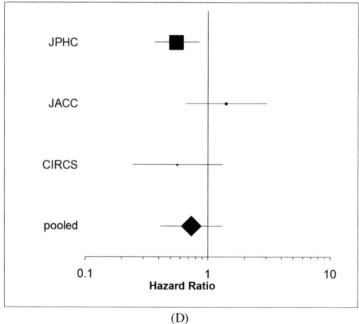

(D)

FIGURE 5.1 (*Continued*)

and stroke tended to be generally lower in the group with the highest seaweed intake than that in the group with no seaweed intake. Although more evidence needs to be accumulated in the future, and the mechanism of metabolic processes of various nutrients contained in the seaweed need to be explored, a high intake of seaweed may contribute to the prevention of cardiovascular diseases, especially for ischemic heart disease and stroke.

5.8 MECHANISMS

There are several possible mechanisms for the association between seaweed and cardiovascular disease.

One possible mechanism is a blood pressure-lowering effect. Some trial studies have showed that the using of seaweed supplement decreased diastolic or mean blood pressure among hypertensive patients (Hata et al. 2001) (Krotkiewski et al. 1991). Seaweeds contain alginate which is a kind of polysaccharide. A study showed that low molecular mass potassium alginate derived from brown algae reduced blood pressure levels in rats with experimentally induced hypertension (Chen et al. 2010). Another way to reduce blood pressure level can be due to peptides included in brown seaweeds. These peptides were reported to show an antihypertensive effect in rats inhibiting angiotensin I-converting enzyme activity (Sato et al. 2002). In addition, potassium and calcium, although they are not specifically contained in seaweeds, lower blood pressure levels.

Another possible mechanism is a lipid-lowering effect. Fucoidan, a sort of polysaccharide, is contained in seaweed and reported to increase lipoprotein lipase activity, reducing serum triglycerides and LDL cholesterol concentrations in apoE-deficient mice (Yokota et al. 2016).

The protective effects of seaweeds against cardiovascular disease also include controlling blood glucose levels (Kim et al. 2008; Yoshinaga and Mitamura 2019), insulin levels (Yoshinaga and Mitamura 2019), postprandial glucose levels (Kato et al. 2018), postprandial insulin sensitivity (Paradis et al. 2011), reducing body weight (Georg Jensen et al. 2012) and waist circumference (Teas et al. 2009).

Other mechanisms are considered as the neuroprotective and antioxidant effects generated by nutritional components such as fucoxanthin (Ikeda et al. 2003), vitamins A, B, C and E (Fabregas and Herrero 1990) contained in seaweeds.

5.9 OTHER FOODS, HERBS, SPICES AND BOTANICALS USED IN CARDIOVASCULAR HEALTH AND DISEASE

Japanese diets or Washoku (Yatsuya and Tsugane 2021) are characterized as high content of rice, fish, soy and green tea as well as seaweed, which is mostly considered to be beneficial for cardiovascular health (Abe and Inoue 2021; Iso et al. 2020; Murai et al. 2021; Nagata 2021; Umesawa et al. 2021). These health benefits of Japanese foods are thought to be the reason why Japan is now one of the world's top countries in terms of longevity (Tsugane 2021). However, one drawback of the Japanese diet is the high sodium content. This is a common nutritional problem in East Asia. In the past, Japan suffered from excessive salt and low nutrition, resulting in a high incidence of stroke and stomach cancer. Even today, the high incidence of stroke and stomach cancer among East Asians can be attributed to the fact that they still consume a large amount of salt compared to the western countries. Therefore, from the standpoint of health, it is recommended to reduce salt intake when adopting the Japanese diet.

5.10 TOXICITY AND CAUTIONARY NOTES

The three studies reported so far have all been conducted on Japanese subjects, and the applicability to non-Japanese populations should be carefully considered. In particular, it is considered that the majority of the seaweeds actually eaten by the Japanese in these studies were wakame. Therefore, one should be cautious when interpretating the results for seaweed in general.

There are several concerns that seaweed has potential adverse effects on health. First, seaweeds contain arsenic and iodine. Feldmann and Krupp categorized arsenic into three species: toxic (inorganic arsenic), nontoxic (arsenobetaine) and potentially toxic (fat-soluble arsenic, arsenosugars, etc.) (Feldmann and Krupp 2011). Most of the arsenic contained in wakame and kombu (kelp) is organic arsenic (arsenosugars), and its adverse effects are thought to be less than those of inorganic arsenic.

Hijiki, another kind of seaweed, contains a large amount of inorganic arsenic. However, at this time, there is no evidence that consuming hijiki is harmful to health although eating it in an extreme manner should be avoided (Ministry of Agriculture, Forestry and Fisheries of Japan 2019). Iodine, which is abundant in seaweeds especially in kombu (kelp), can adversely affect the thyroid function with overdose (Konno et al. 1994). Since kombu is generally used as soup stock in Japanese food, its adverse effects are not considered to be significant, but as with arsenic, extreme consumption of iodine should be avoided. Taken together, to date, there is little evidence that seaweed intake, especially wakame intake, is harmful, and it can be said that it is a food that is recommended to be consumed actively, as long as it is not eaten in an extreme way.

5.11 SUMMARY POINTS

- This chapter focuses on the epidemiological evidence and mechanisms on the association between seaweed intake and risk of cardiovascular disease (ischemic heart disease and stroke).
- There have been three cohort studies on this issue, all of which are from Japan.
- All three studies found an inverse association between seaweed and cardiovascular disease, but there was some inconsistency by sex and outcome.
- Meta-analysis showed a generally inverse association between seaweed and cardiovascular disease for both sexes and outcomes.
- Possible mechanisms for the association between seaweed and cardiovascular diseases may mainly be due to blood pressure-lowering and lipid-lowering effects, and other effects including regulation of glucose tolerance, body weight reduction, neuroprotection and antioxidation.
- Although the toxicity of individual seaweeds should be noted, it can be said that seaweed is a food that is recommended to be consumed actively, as long as it is not eaten in an extreme way.

REFERENCES

Abe, S. K. and Inoue, M. 2021. Green tea and cancer and cardiometabolic diseases: A review of the current epidemiological evidence. European Journal of Clinical Nutrition 75: 877–889.

Chen, Y. et al. 2010. Preventive effects of low molecular mass potassium alginate extracted from brown algae on DOCA salt-induced hypertension in rats. Biomedicine and Pharmacotherapy 64(4): 291–295.

Chichibu, H. et al. 2021. Seaweed intake and risk of cardiovascular disease: The Circulatory Risk in Communities Study (CIRCS). Journal of Atherosclerosis and Thrombosis 28:1298–1306.

Fabregas, J. and Herrero, C. 1990. Vitamin content of four marine microalgae: Potential use as source of vitamins in nutrition. Journal of Industrial Microbiology 5: 259–263.

Feldmann, J. and Krupp, E. M. 2011. Critical review or scientific opinion paper: Arsenosugars – a class of benign arsenic species or justification for developing partly speciated arsenic fractionation in food-stuffs? Analytical and Bioanalytical Chemistry 399: 1735–1741.

Georg Jensen, M. et al. 2012. Effect of alginate supplementation on weight loss in obese subjects completing a 12-wk energy-restricted diet: A randomized controlled trial. The American Journal of Clinical Nutrition 96(1): 5–13.

Hata, Y. et al. 2001. Clinical effects of brown seaweed, *Undaria pinnatifida* (Wakame), on blood pressure in hypertensive subjects. Journal of Clinical Biochemistry and Nutrition 30: 43–53.

Ikeda, K. et al. 2003. Effect of *Undaria pinnatifida* (Wakame) on the development of cerebrovascular diseases in stroke-prone spontaneously hypertensive rats. Clinical and Experimental Pharmacology and Physiology 30: 44–48.

Iso, H. et al. 2020. 11. Chronic diseases and risk factor trends in Japan. In Health in Japan: Social Epidemiology of Japan since the 1964 Tokyo Olympics, ed E. Brunner, N. Cable, and H. Iso, 163–178. Oxford: Oxford University Press.

Kato, T. et al. 2018. Effect of Chinese noodles containing calcium alginate on postprandial blood glucose level: A randomized, double-blind, crossover clinical trial. Japanese Pharmacology and Therapeutics 46(12): 2083–2089.

Kim, M. S. et al. 2008. Effects of seaweed supplementation on blood glucose concentration, lipid profile, and antioxidant enzyme activities in patients with Type 2 diabetes mellitus. Nutrition Research and Practice 2: 62.

Kishida, R. et al. 2020. Frequency of seaweed intake and its association with cardiovascular disease mortality: The JACC study. Journal of Atherosclerosis and Thrombosis 27: 1340–1347.

Konno, N. et al. 1994. Association between dietary iodine intake and prevalence of subclinical hypothyroidism in the coastal regions of Japan. The Journal of Clinical Endocrinology and Metabolism 78(2): 393–397.

Krotkiewski, M. et al. 1991. Effects of a sodium-potassium ion-exchanging seaweed preparation in mild hypertension. American Journal of Hypertension 4: 483–488.

Ministry of Agriculture, Forestry and Fisheries of Japan. 2019. *Shokuhin karano hiso no sesshuryou* (Arsenic intake from food). in Japanese. www.maff.go.jp/j/syouan/nouan/kome/k_as/exposure.html

Murai, U. et al. 2019. Seaweed intake and risk of coronary heart diseases: The Japan Public Health Center-Based Prospective (JPHC) study. American Journal of Clinical Nutrition 110: 1449–1455.

Murai, U. et al. 2021. Impact of seaweed intake on health. European Journal of Clinical Nutrition 75: 877–889.

Nagata, C. 2021. Soy intake and chronic disease risk: Findings from prospective cohort studies in Japan. European Journal of Clinical Nutrition 75: 890–901.

Paradis, M. E. et al. 2011. A randomised crossover placebo-controlled trial investigating the effect of brown seaweed (Ascophyllum nodosum and Fucus vesiculosus) on postchallenge plasma glucose and insulin levels in men and women. Applied Physiology, Nutrition and Metabolism 36: 913–919.

Sato, M. et al. 2002. Angiotensin I-converting enzyme inhibitory peptides derived from Wakame (*Undaria pinnatifida*) and their antihypertensive effect in spontaneously hypertensive rats. Journal of Agricultural and Food Chemistry 50: 6245–6252.

Tamakoshi, A. et al. 2013. Cohort profile of the Japan Collaborative Cohort Study at final follow-up. Journal of Epidemiol 23: 227–232.

Teas, J. et al. 2009. Could dietary seaweed reverse the metabolic syndrome? Asia Pacific Journal of Clinical Nutrition 18: 145–154.

Tsugane, S. 2021. Why has Japan become the world's most long-lived country: Insights from a food and nutrition perspective. Journal of Clinical Nutrition 75: 921–928.

Tsugane, S. and Sawada, N. 2014. The JPHC study: Design and some findings on the typical Japanese diet. Japanese Journal of Clinical Oncology 44: 777–782.

Umesawa, M. et al. 2021. Intake of fish and long-chain n-3 polyunsaturated fatty acids and risk of diseases in a Japanese population: A narrative review. European Journal of Clinical Nutrition 75: 902–920.

Yamagishi, K. et al. 2019. The Circulatory Risk in Communities Study (CIRCS): A long-term epidemiological study for lifestyle-related disease among Japanese men and women living in communities. Journal of Epidemiology 29: 83–91.

Yatsuya, H. and Tsugane, S. 2021. What constitutes healthiness of Washoku or Japanese diet? European Journal of Clinical Nutrition 75: 863–864.

Yokota, T. et al. 2016. Fucoidan alleviates high-fat diet-induced dyslipidemia and atherosclerosis in ApoE[shl] mice deficient in apolipoprotein E expression. Journal of Nutritional Biochemistry 32: 46–54.

Yoshinaga, K. and Mitamura, R. 2019. Effects of *Undaria pinnatifida* (Wakame) on postprandial glycemia and insulin levels in humans: A randomized crossover trial. Plant Foods for Human Nutrition 74: 461–467.

Section II

Specific Agents, Items and Extracts

6 Asiatic Pennywort (*Centella asiatica*) and Cardiovascular Protection
A New Narrative

Chin Theng Ng, Siau Hui Mah and Lai Yen Fong

CONTENTS

6.1 Introduction 78
6.2 Background 79
6.3 Major Beneficial Effects of *C. asiatica* in Cardiovascular Diseases (CVD).......80
6.4 Protection against Myocardial Infarction 80
6.5 Inhibition of Cardiac Hypertrophy 82
6.6 Anti-Hyperlipidaemic and Anti-Obesity Effects...82
6.7 Anti-Hyperglycaemic Effect...83
6.8 Anti-Atherosclerotic Effect...84
6.9 Anti-Hypertensive Effect..85
6.10 Improvement of Venous Insufficiency 85
6.11 Enhancement of Endothelial Barrier Function...86
6.12 Other Foods, Herbs, Spices and Botanicals Used in Cardiovascular
         Health and Disease 86
6.13 Toxicity and Cautionary Notes 87
6.14 Summary Points 88
6.15 Acknowledgements 89
References..89

LIST OF ABBREVIATIONS

Akt   Protein kinase B
AMPK   Adenosine monophosphate-activated protein kinase
AngII   Angiotensin II
AT_1R Angiotensin II receptor type 1
Bcl-2   B-cell lymphoma 2
CVD   Cardiovascular diseases
CYP450   Cytochrome P450
ERK   Extracellular signal-regulated kinase
GLUT4   Glucose transporter type 4
GSH   Glutathione
GSK   Glycogen synthase kinase 3
HIF-1α Hypoxia-inducible factor 1 alpha
HIF-3α1   Hypoxia-inducible factor 3 alpha 1
HK2   Hexokinase II
IRS1   Insulin receptor substrate 1

DOI: 10.1201/9781003220329-8

JNK	c-Jun N-terminal kinase
L-NAME	N$^\omega$-nitro-L-arginine methyl ester hydrochloride
MAPK	Mitogen-activated protein kinase
MI/R	Myocardial ischemic/reperfusion
miR-	MicroRNA
mRNA	Messenger RNA
mTOR	Mammalian target of rapamycin
NADPH	Nicotinamide adenosine dinucleotide phosphate
NF-κB	Nuclear factor kappa B
NO	Nitric oxide
NOS	Nitric oxide synthases
P70S6K	Ribosomal protein S6 kinase
pCO$_2$	Partial pressure of carbon dioxide
PI3K	Phosphoinositide-3-kinase
PIK3R2	PI3K regulatory subunit 2
pO$_2$	Partial pressure of oxygen
PPAR	Peroxisome proliferator-activated receptor
pp-MLC	Diphosphorylated myosin light chain
ROS	Reactive oxygen species
SOD	Superoxide dismutase
SREBP	Sterol regulatory element-binding protein
TNF-α	Tumour necrosis factor-α
VCAM-1	Vascular cell adhesion molecule 1

6.1 INTRODUCTION

Centella asiatica (L.) Urban, previously named as *Hydrocotyle asiatica* L., is a popular medicinal herb that has been utilized around the world since ancient times. It has a widespread application in both traditional and pharmaceutical areas and thus, numerous research studies have been conducted to explore its pharmacological activities including wound-healing, anti-inflammatory, immuno-modulation, anti-diabetic, cardiovascular-protective, anti-cancer, memory enhancement and neuroprotective effects (Sun et al. 2020; Mohd Razali et al. 2019). *C. asiatica* belongs to the Apiaceae family and is well known with the name of *Mandookaparni* in Ayurveda. It is also known as Asiatic pennywort, Indian pennywort, Indian water navelwort, marsh pepperwort, wild violet, tiger herb and *Gotu Kola*. The common names of *C. asiatica* vary depending on the geographical region. For instance, it is called as *pegaga* in Malaysia; *Babassa, Brahmi, Karinga, Karivana, Mandookaparni, Thankuni, Vallarai* and *Vondelaga* in India; *asiatisches Wassernabelkraut* in Germany; *coquelariat* in France; *talapetraka, anamanitra, korokorona* and *silabola* in Madagascar; *bodila-ba-dinku* and *tabao en Amhara* in Africa; *luo de da* and *ji xue cao* in China (Jamil et al. 2007).

C. asiatica is a slender herbaceous plant that grows well on moist, sandy or clayey soils such as tropical or temperate swampy areas. The roots grow vertically downwards with nodes while the stems are smooth with long fleshy leaves in fan-shape, 1–3 arising from each node of the stems. The flowers are umbels with 3–4 white or light pink-to-purple petals and the fruit is dry and long oval to globular in shape (Ramli et al. 2020). Parts of the plant that have been used for medicinal purposes are dried leaves, stems and whole plants. The whole plant of *C. asiatica* is shown in Figure 6.1.

C. asiatica is commonly extracted using alcoholic and aqueous solutions in scientific studies. Many classes of phytochemicals have been identified in this plant including triterpenic acids, steroids, alkaloids, flavonoids, glycosides, fatty acids and volatile oils. Among them, the triterpenic acids – asiatic acid, madecassic acid – and the sugar esters – asiaticoside, asiaticoside A (madecassoside) and asiaticoside B – have the highest therapeutic interest. Thus, these compounds are commonly used in the quantitative profiling of this species (Brinkhaus et al. 2000).

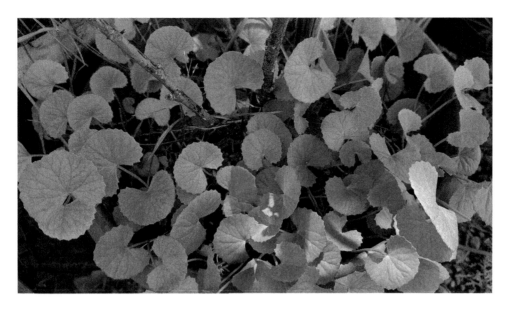

FIGURE 6.1 Whole plant of *C. asiatica*.

6.2 BACKGROUND

C. asiatica is commonly used in cuisine as green salad, curry vegetables, soup vegetables, thin porridge, herbal tea and fresh juices in Asian countries (Cox et al. 1993). It is also used as a medicinal plant in different ancient cultures by natives, including India, China, Sri Lanka, Madagascar, South Africa, Indonesia and Malaysia. The earliest usage of this plant can be traced back at least 3,500 years ago in the Indian Ayurvedic system of medicine. *Unani* system of medicine in India has documented *C. asiatica* as *Brahmi* and showed that the plant was first adopted by the Greeks and was developed by the Arabs in later dates. Besides, this plant has been recorded in the ancient *Shennong* traditional Chinese Herbal system about 2,000 years ago as one of the "miracle elixirs of life" herbs. Although this plant was first mentioned in the French Pharmacopoeia (ed. 1884), but the first plant extract was only reported in 1941, and this was followed by reports on isolation of triterpenoids compounds three years later. The British Herbal Pharmacopoeia also recorded the systemic use of this plant starting from year 1983 for rheumatic conditions and cutaneous affections, as well as topical wound healing, ulcers and cicatrization after surgery (Calapai 2012).

In India, *C. asiatica* has been used in folk medicines for asthma, dropsy, elephantiasis, gastritis, kidney problems, leprosy, urethritis, leucorrhoea and dermatitis while Southeast Asian used it for the treatment of inflammation, rheumatism, syphilis, epilepsy, mental illness, hysteria, dehydration and diarrhoea. Some other traditional usages of *C. asiatica* include memory enhancer, blood purifier, and alleviation of fever, hemorrhoids, high blood pressure, jaundice, keloids, smallpox, toothaches (Biswas et al. 2021). The plant remedy can be applied in the form of leaf powder, ointment, syrup or juices, depending on the illness. The triterpenic fraction of this plant is best studied in scientific research due to the richness of its bioactive components. By using the plant extracts, fractions and isolates, many preclinical studies and clinical trials have been conducted in the forms of topical and systemic therapies to validate the therapeutic claims of folk medicines. Some of the scientifically proven effects are wound healing, and its anti-cancer, anti-inflammatory, antioxidant, gastroprotective, anti-obesity, cardioprotective, hepatoprotective and neuroprotective properties (Sun et al. 2020; Mohd Razali et al. 2019). Pharmacological activities of *C. asiatica* are believed to be mainly attributed to its pentacyclic triterpenoids such as asiatic acid, asiaticoside, madecassic acid and madecassoside. Structures of the major triterpenoids of *C. asiatica* are shown in Figure 6.2.

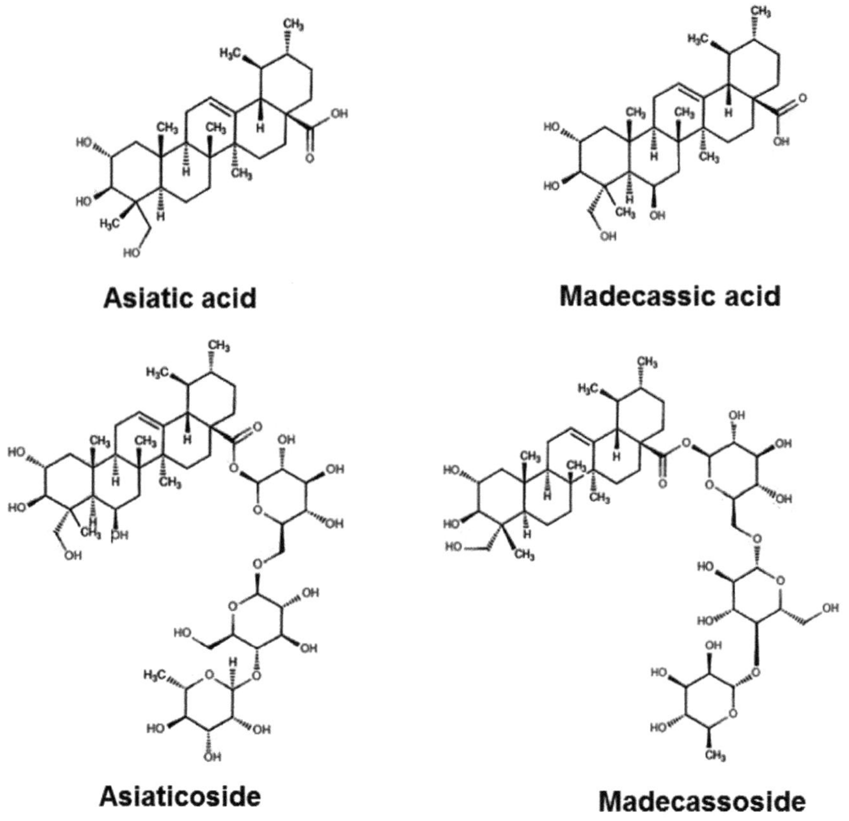

FIGURE 6.2 Structure of major pentacyclic triterpenoids isolated from *C. asiatica*.

Source: Adapted from Mohd Razali et al. (2019).

6.3 MAJOR BENEFICIAL EFFECTS OF *C. ASIATICA* IN CARDIOVASCULAR DISEASES (CVD)

The earliest scientific data about benefits of *C. asiatica* in vascular health was reported in the late 1980s where a highly refined *C. asiatica* extract was demonstrated to improve chronic venous insufficiency in human subjects (Pointel et al. 1987). Emerging evidence in the last two decades has demonstrated that *C. asiatica* exhibits cardiovascular-protective effects such as protection against myocardial infarction, inhibition of cardiac hypertrophy, anti-atherosclerosis, anti-hypertension, alleviation of chronic venous insufficiency and enhancement of endothelial barrier function (Figure 6.3). Besides, *C. asiatica* is also effective in preventing risk factors for cardiovascular diseases (CVD) such as hyperlipidaemia, obesity and hyperglycaemia (Figure 6.3).

6.4 PROTECTION AGAINST MYOCARDIAL INFARCTION

Myocardial ischemia occurs as a result of a decrease in cardiac tissue perfusion, which causes insufficient oxygen supply to the cardiac tissue and eventually progresses to myocardial infarction. Reperfusion of ischemic cardiac tissue also damages the cardiac tissue and results in myocardial ischemic/reperfusion (MI/R) injury. Active constituents of *C. asiatica* have been reported to protect against MI/R in *in vivo* and *in vitro* models. Asiatic acid protects cardiomyocytes

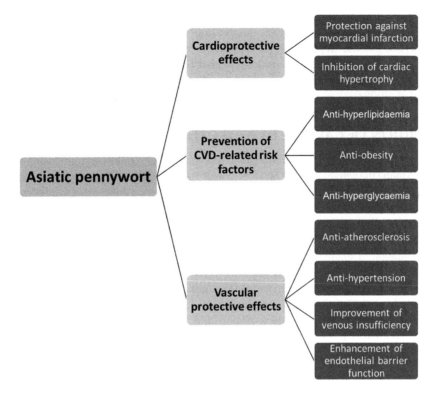

FIGURE 6.3 Pharmacological use of *C. asiatica* in cardiovascular diseases.

from hypoxia-induced cell death by upregulating miR-1290 and hypoxia-inducible factor 1 alpha (HIF-1α) expression while downregulating HIF-3α1 expression (Wu et al. 2017). Dai et al. demonstrated that asiatic acid reduced myocardial infarction size in a dose-dependent manner following MI/R injury. The authors reported that the protective effect of asiatic acid may be associated with regulation of glycometabolism through translocation of glucose transporter type 4 (GLUT4) to membrane and upregulation of peroxisome proliferator-activated receptor (PPAR) (Dai et al. 2018). Besides, asiatic acid has also been shown to protect against cardiac complications induced by doxorubicin by increasing viability, superoxide dismutase (SOD) activity and glutathione (GSH) level of cardiomyocytes and suppressing intracellular reactive oxygen species (ROS) and malondialdehyde levels (Hu, Li, et al. 2020). Moreover, asiatic acid also improved body weight, cardiac output, stroke work and relaxation time in doxorubicin-induced mice. The antioxidant and anti-apoptotic activities of asiatic acid were postulated to be related to protein kinase B (Akt) activation.

In MI/R injury, an increase in ROS production causes an elevation of autophagy activity. Asiatic acid was found to suppress increased autophagy activity in glucose deprivation/reperfusion model, suggesting its potential therapeutic effect in the treatment of MI/R injury (Yi et al. 2020). Furthermore, asiatic acid has been shown to improve myocardial energy metabolism by enhancing cytosolic glycogen autophagy and mitochondrial autophagy, which are accompanied by phosphoinositide-3-kinase/Akt (PI3K/Akt) activation and adenosine monophosphate-activated protein kinase (AMPK) activation, respectively (Qiu et al. 2022). Zhang et al. demonstrated that oxygen-glucose deprivation/reoxygenation impaired glycolysis rate through suppression of hexokinase II (HK2) expression in H9c2 cells. However, asiaticoside treatment at doses of 10 and 20 μM inhibited reduced glucose consumption, lactate production and HK2 expression in oxygen-glucose deprivation/reoxygenation-induced H9c2 cells. These data suggest that asiaticoside exerts beneficial effect in restoration of glycolysis, supporting its use as a potential therapeutic agent in reversing oxygen-glucose deprivation/reoxygenation injury (Zhang et al. 2020). Another active constituent of *C. asiatica*, madecassoside, has also been reported to decrease the infarct size, lactate dehydrogenase, creatine phosphokinase, malondialdehyde and C-reactive protein levels *in vivo* (Bian et al. 2008).

6.5 INHIBITION OF CARDIAC HYPERTROPHY

Cardiac hypertrophy is the pathological enlargement of heart muscles following reperfusion of ischaemic heart tissue. Among the active components of *C. asiatica*, asiatic acid is the most well studied compound in terms of the prevention of cardiac hypertrophy. Histological analysis showed that asiatic acid attenuated cardiac hypertrophy, collagen volume and cardiac fibrosis in chronic pressure overload-induced mice (Ma et al. 2016). The authors also demonstrated that asiatic acid inhibits increased expression of ribosomal protein S6 kinase beta-1 (P70S6K), ribosomal protein S6, extracellular signal-regulated kinase (ERK) and phosphorylation of mammalian target of rapamycin (mTOR) in angiotensin II (AngII)-induced cardiomyocytes, possibly through activation of AMPKα. Besides, asiatic acid has also been reported to attenuate the cell surface area and hypertrophic markers of H9c2 cells following AngII challenge (Li et al. 2021). Li et al. also showed that asiatic acid upregulates miRNA-126 and downregulates both PI3K regulatory subunit 2 (PIK3R2) and activation of PI3K/Akt signalling pathway in myocardium of AngII-treated rats. Other possible signalling pathways which contribute to the anti-hypertropic effect of asiatic acid include p38 mitogen-activated protein kinase (MAPK), c-Jun N-terminal kinase (JNK) and nuclear factor kappa B (NF-κB) pathways (Si et al. 2015; Xu et al. 2015).

To date, clinical data on the cardioprotective effect of *C. asiatica* are widely lacking and thereby hindering the clinical use of this plant for the treatment of cardiac diseases. There is a need to conduct randomized and controlled trials in order to justify the cardioprotective effect of *C. asiatica* reported *in vitro* and *in vivo*.

6.6 ANTI-HYPERLIPIDAEMIC AND ANTI-OBESITY EFFECTS

Increased plasma levels of cholesterols and obesity are the major risk factors for cardiovascular diseases. The main therapeutic approaches for these risk factors include lifestyle modifications and medications. However, there is still an unmet medical need in the development of novel therapeutic agents for cardiovascular diseases, as lipid-lowering drugs including statins, and anti-obesity drugs such as orlistat and sibutramine cause undesirable side effects. Extracts of *C. asiatica* and its triterpenoids have been reported to inhibit hyperlipidaemia and obesity in several preclinical studies. Oral administration of 0.25–1 g/kg of *C. asiatica* water extract for 28 days decreased plasma total cholesterol and triglycerides levels and improved altered SOD and GSH levels in hyperlipidaemic rats (Kumari et al. 2016). In addition, *C. asiatica* water extract also scavenges free radicals including nitric oxide (NO) and hydrogen peroxide *in vitro*. Yan et al. reported that asiatic acid, at doses of 10 and 20 mg/kg/day, reduced total cholesterol and triglycerides levels in plasma and liver tissue of C57BL/6 mice fed with high-fat diet for 7 weeks (Yan et al. 2014). Asiatic acid was also found to prevent fat deposition in hepatocytes by inhibiting increased expression of sterol regulatory element-binding protein (SREBP)-1c and the downstream targets identified include fatty acid synthase and stearoyl CoA desaturase, which are enzymes involved in lipogenesis. Consistent with other studies, Yan et al. postulated that asiatic acid prevents hyperlipidaemia by ameliorating hepatic oxidative stress and decreasing hepatic expressions of NFκB, p38 MAPK and JNK.

In obese Sprague-Dawley rats, asiatic acid improved lipid profiles in serum, liver and kidney tissues as well as reduced fat pad weight and adiposity index (Uddandrao et al. 2020). This protective effect of asiatic acid is associated with reduced expression of PPAR-γ, a nuclear receptor, which regulates adipogenesis and lipid metabolism, and some factors secreted by adipose tissue, including adiponectin, leptin and tumour necrosis factor-α (TNF-α). A similar study also demonstrated anti-obesity effect of asiatic acid in high-fat-diet-fed obese rats and the beneficial effect is attributed to altered expression of markers for fatty acid metabolism and oxidative stress (Rameshreddy et al. 2018). Using a high-carbohydrate, high-fat diet-induced rat models, asiatic acid has also been demonstrated to attenuate development of metabolic syndrome where asiatic acid inhibits hyperlipidaemia, increased blood pressure, increased blood glucose levels, insulin resistance and alteration of haemodynamic parameters (Pakdeechote et al. 2014). Asiatic acid also restored superoxide anion production and protein expression of nitric oxide synthases (NOS) including endothelial NOS (eNOS) and inducible NOS in the aorta of metabolic syndrome rats to basal levels.

Taken together, these *in vivo* data imply that *C. asiatica* and its triterpenoid derivatives exert hypolipidaemic and anti-obesity activities, in which improvement of lipid metabolism, suppression of inflammatory responses and prevention of oxidative stress are the major contributing factors. Although the preclinical data appear to be promising, a huge gap of knowledge still exists on whether *C. asiatica* can demonstrate the similar anti-hyperlipidaemic and anti-obesity potentials clinically. More clinical studies should be conducted to fill these important data gaps.

6.7 ANTI-HYPERGLYCAEMIC EFFECT

In a randomised placebo-controlled clinical trial conducted among 43 diabetic subjects with well-controlled blood glucose levels, daily administration of *C. asiatica* selected triterpenes at escalating doses between 120 mg to 240 mg via oral route for 52 weeks alleviated symptoms of diabetic neuropathy, a complication of diabetic mellitus which affects the microcirculation supplying nervous tissue and results in nerve damage (Lou et al. 2018). Daily treatment with 400 mg/kg of *C. asiatica* ethanol extract for 2 months was reported to alleviate increased blood glucose levels and glomerulosclerosis in streptozotocin-induced diabetic rats (Setyaningsih et al. 2021). Interestingly, the same anti-hyperglycaemic effect was not observed in animals receiving *C. asiatica* treatment for 1 month post-diabetes. This finding highlights the importance of *C. asiatica* in halting early stage of diabetes mellitus. *C. asiatica* ethanol extract not only abrogates vascular dysfunction by upregulating eNOS expression and downregulating endothelin-1 expression, but also inhibits the remodelling of intrarenal arteries in the diabetic animals. Furthermore, anti-hyperglycaemic activity of *C. asiatica* leaf aqueous extract is found concomitantly with augmentation of the insulin signalling pathway and suppression of cerebral inflammation, apoptosis and oxidative stress in diabetic rats (Giribabu et al. 2020). These data suggest that *C. asiatica* may protect against cerebral damage in diabetes mellitus through its anti-inflammatory, anti-apoptotic and antioxidant effects.

Diabetic nephropathy is a common complication of diabetes mellitus and is greatly associated with increased risk of cardiovascular diseases. In a diabetic nephropathy rat model, chronic treatment of asiatic acid for 2 months has been shown to improve morphological abnormality of renal tissues including glomeruli, mesangial cells and foot processes of podocytes (Chen et al. 2018). In addition, asiatic acid also prevents changes in the mRNA level of nephrin and desmin, which are podocyte proteins essential for glomerular filtration barrier. Using a coculture model of RAW 264.7 macrophages and 3T3-L1 mature adipocytes, Kusumastuti et al. demonstrated that 500 μg/ml of standardized *C. asiatica* extract alleviated lipopolysaccharide-induced decreased insulin sensitivity, where this protective effect may be associated with activation of the insulin receptor substrate 1 (IRS1)/GLUT4 pathway and suppression of inflammatory responses (Kusumastuti et al. 2019).

Collectively, various mechanisms of actions including enhancement of insulin signalling, improvement of insulin sensitivity, prevention of vascular dysfunction, restoration of glomerular filtration function, inhibition of cerebral inflammation and oxidative stress, were previously proposed to underlie the anti-hyperglycaemic activity of *C. asiatica* and its active constituents. Identification of a common therapeutic target such as microRNA which controls these mechanisms could further strengthen the role of *C. asiatica* as an anti-hyperglycaemic agent. The signalling pathways and mechanisms involved in cardioprotective effect of *C. asiatica* are summarized in Table 6.1.

TABLE 6.1

Protective Effect of *C. asiatica* and Its Active Constituents on Cardiac Diseases and Cardiovascular Disease-Related Risk Factors

Protective Effect	Extract/Compound	Model	Signalling Pathway/Major Finding	Reference
Inhibition of cardiac hypertrophy	Asiatic acid	*In vivo* and *in vitro*	AMPKα	(Ma et al. 2016)
		In vivo and *in vitro*	miR-126-dependent PI3K/AKT pathway	(Li et al. 2021)
		In vivo	• p38 MAPK • JNK	(Si et al. 2015)
		In vivo and *in vitro*	NF-κB	(Xu et al. 2015)
Protection against myocardial infarction	Asiatic acid	*In vitro*	miR-1290/HIF-3α	(Wu et al. 2017)
		In vivo	Akt/GSK3β	(Dai et al. 2018)
		In vivo and *in vitro*	Akt/GSK3β	(Hu, Li, et al. 2020)
		In vivo and *in vitro*	p38 MAPK/Bcl-2/beclin-1	(Yi et al. 2020)
		In vivo and *in vitro*	• PI3K/Akt • AMPK	(Qiu et al. 2022)
	Asiaticoside	*In vitro*	HK2	(Zhang et al. 2020)
	Madecassoside	*In vivo*	Oxidative stress-related markers	(Bian et al. 2008)
Anti-hyperlipidaemic	*C. asiatica* water extract	*In vivo* and *in vitro*	Oxidative stress-related markers	(Kumari et al. 2016)
	Asiatic acid	*In vivo*	• p38 MAPK • JNK • NF-κB	(Yan et al. 2014)
Anti-obesity	Asiatic acid	*In vivo*	PPAR-γ	(Uddandrao et al. 2020)
		In vivo	lipid metabolism pathway-related markers	(Rameshreddy et al. 2018)
		In vivo	• eNOS • iNOS	(Pakdeechote et al. 2014)
Anti-hyperglycaemic	*C. asiatica* selected triterpenes	Clinical study	Alleviation of diabetic neuropathy	(Lou et al. 2018)
	C. asiatica ethanol extract	*In vivo*	eNOS	(Setyaningsih et al. 2021)
	C. asiatica leaf aqueous extract	*In vivo*	• Insulin signalling pathway (IRS/PI3K/Akt pathway) • MAPK (p38, JNK and ERK) • NF-κB	(Giribabu et al. 2020)
	Asiatic acid	*In vivo*	JNK	(Chen et al. 2018)
	Standardized *C. asiatica* extract	*In vitro*	Insulin signalling pathway (IRS-1/GLUT4)	(Kusumastuti et al. 2019)

6.8 ANTI-ATHEROSCLEROTIC EFFECT

Recent clinical research studied the effect of *C. asiatica* in atherosclerosis by using *C. asiatica* extract which was supplemented with Pycnogenol®, an extract of pine bark (*Pinus pinaster*). Combined treatment of *C. asiatica* (450 mg/day) and Pycnogenol® (150 mg/day) for 6 months improved echogenicity and stabilised plaque structure in asymptomatic and low-risk patients

(Belcaro and Cornelli 2017). After a follow-up of four years, the combined treatment was reported to reduce the progression of asymptomatic arterial plaques to more advanced stages (Belcaro et al. 2017; Belcaro et al. 2015). On top of that, the combined treatment also reduced carotid intima-media thickening and improved oxidative stress status when compared to cardioaspirin-treated group (Belcaro et al. 2020). Noteworthy, the number of coronary calcifications was decreased by the combined supplements (Hu, Belcaro, et al. 2020). Furthermore, the combined supplements also decreased the progression of the stented artery in a 12-month follow-up period, which was in concomitant with a reduction of oxidative stress (Belcaro et al. 2019).

Although the combined treatment of *C. asiatica* with Pycnogenol® shows favourable outcomes, the single effect of *C. asiatica* on atherosclerosis is still lacking. Future clinical studies using *C. asiatica* alone and the effect of long-term intake of *C. asiatica* on atherosclerosis could provide interesting and useful information that support the use of *C. asiatica* as a therapeutic agent for cardiovascular diseases.

6.9 ANTI-HYPERTENSIVE EFFECT

A recent clinical data revealed that consumption of *C. asiatica* tea at a dose of 0.016 g/ml, thrice a day, for 2 weeks decreased both systolic and diastolic blood pressure levels in 60- to 70-year-old hypertensive patients (Astutik et al. 2021). This protective effect of *C. asiatica* tea was observed despite about one-third of the patients involved in the study not consuming *C. asiatica* tea regularly within the study period. Other than clinical data, anti-hypertensive effect of *C. asiatica* and its triterpenes have also been demonstrated in several preclinical studies. Administration of 10 and 20 mg/kg of asiatic acid for 2 weeks attenuated increased blood pressure levels and improved vascular functions including vasodilation and vasoconstriction responses in hypertensive rats stimulated with N^{ω}-nitro-L-arginine methyl ester hydrochloride (L-NAME) (Bunbupha et al. 2014). Asiatic acid also alleviates vascular oxidative stress by enhancing NO release and suppressing production of superoxide anion. In addition, the expression of eNOS and p47phox, a nicotinamide adenosine dinucleotide phosphate (NADPH) oxidase subunit, in L-NAME-induced rats are also restored by asiatic acid.

Asiaticoside has also been shown to normalize mean pulmonary arterial pressure levels in hypoxia-induced rats through both preventive and therapeutic approaches (Wang et al. 2018). The authors suggested that asiatic acid alleviates pulmonary hypertension without affecting the systemic blood pressure levels. The anti-hypertensive effect of asiatic acid is also concomitant with a restoration of basal NO and basal phosphorylated eNOS levels *in vivo* and *in vitro,* a finding which is in agreement with the study reported by Bunbupha et al. Abolishment of the anti-hypertensive effect of asiatic acid by a pharmacological inhibitor of PI3K also suggests the involvement of PI3K-Akt-eNOS pathway.

Several studies also investigated the effect of chronic treatment of *C. asiatica* in hypertensive animals. A recent study showed that intragastric administration of 500 mg/kg of *C. asiatica* ethanolic extract daily for 8 weeks lowered the increased systolic blood pressure and prevented decreased serum NO levels in L-NAME-treated rats (Bunaim et al. 2021). Furthermore, daily treatment of 30 mg/kg of asiatic acid for 4 weeks also partially restored blood pressure levels of hypertensive rats by interfering with the activation of renin-angiotension-aldosterone system (Maneesai et al. 2017).

Collectively, these animal studies point toward a crucial role of NO, a potent endothelium-derived relaxing factor, in mediating anti-hypertensive effect of *C. asiatica* triterpenoids. Therefore, NO could appear as one promising therapeutic target of *C. asiatica*. *C. asiatica* and its triterpenoid compounds also modulate the renin-angiotension-aldosterone system. Further investigation of the mechanisms underlying the anti-hypertensive effect of *C. asiatica* should focus on exploring other possible approaches such as vascular smooth muscle contractile mechanism.

6.10 IMPROVEMENT OF VENOUS INSUFFICIENCY

Venous insufficiency is due to improper back-flow of blood to the heart, which is usually caused by varicose veins and blood clots. Previous studies demonstrated that *C. asiatica* is effective in treatment of venous insufficiency, and this is associated with anti-inflammatory and wound-healing properties of the plant. A highly refined ethanol extract of *C. asiatica,* which contains a large amount of triterpenoids, is the most well-studied extract, and this refined extract is generally known as titrated extract or total triterpenic fraction of *C. asiatica.* It has been reported that titrated extract of *C. asiatica* contains approximately 60% triterpenic genins (29–30% asiatic acid, 29–30% madecassic acid, 1% madasiatic acid) and 40% asiaticoside. These extracts or fractions were either examined alone or in combination with other plant extracts for treatment of venous sufficiency. A recent study has confirmed the synergistic effect of *C. asiatica* and grapevine (*Vitis vinifera*) in prevention of venous insufficiency *in vitro* and *in vivo* (Seo et al. 2021).

Clinical studies also showed that titrated extract of *C. asiatica* caused significant improvements of both subjective symptoms and plethysmographic parameters in chronic venous insufficiency patients. Symptoms include oedema, swelling, pains, cramps, leg and lower limb heaviness and ankle circumference were relieved following *C. asiatica* treatment (Pointel et al. 1987), whereas parameters such as venous reflux, venous distensibility, venous flow and volume in leg, vascular tone, reduction in venous pressure, reabsorption of the leaked fluid, capillary filtration and permeability were significantly improved in the patients (De Sanctis et al. 2001; Belcaro et al. 1990). Besides, several studies have demonstrated the protective effect of *C. asiatica* titrated extract in blood vessels by improving microcirculatory parameters in terms of resting flux, standing flux, transcutaneous pO_2 and pCO_2 and leg volumetry (Cesarone et al. 2001; Lichota et al. 2019). Using the Laser Doppler flowmetry method, total triterpenic fraction of *C. asiatica* was also reported to alleviate venous hypertensive microangiopathy, which is a hypertensive condition caused by chronic venous insufficiency (Incandela et al. 2001).

6.11 ENHANCEMENT OF ENDOTHELIAL BARRIER FUNCTION

Endothelial barrier dysfunction, which is characterised by an increase in endothelial permeability, is an early key event in the development of atherosclerosis. Therefore, the endothelium is now known as a potential target for early prevention of atherosclerosis. In the past, a few *in vitro* studies have reported the protective effect of *C. asiatica* triterpenoids in endothelial barrier dysfunction. Asiaticoside, at doses of 6.25–50 µM, prevented TNF-α-induced increased endothelial permeability and this was found in parallel with inhibition of stress fibre formation (Fong et al. 2015). Other researchers also demonstrated anti-hyperpermeability effect of asiaticoside in oxidized low-density lipoprotein-induced human umbilical vein endothelial cells (Jing et al. 2018). In human aortic endothelial cells, pretreatment of asiatic acid at 40 µM has been shown to suppress an increase in permeability and an upregulated vascular cell adhesion molecule 1 (VCAM-1) expression. In addition, asiatic acid also diminishes NF-κB activation stimulated by TNF-α (Fong et al. 2016). Asiatic acid is also found to stabilise F-actin and diphosphorylated myosin light chain (pp-MLC) in endothelial cells, although this does not contribute to the barrier protective effect of asiatic acid (Fong et al. 2019). Instead, asiatic acid improves endothelial barrier integrity via prevention of adherens junction reorganization and tight junction disassembly. More *in vivo* evidence is needed to support the beneficial role of *C. asiatica* triterpenes in preserving the endothelial barrier function.

The signalling pathways and mechanisms involved in vascular protective effect of *C. asiatica* are summarized in Table 6.2.

6.12 OTHER FOODS, HERBS, SPICES AND BOTANICALS USED IN CARDIOVASCULAR HEALTH AND DISEASE

Herbal or medicinal plants serve as natural resources of medicine. Some native plants in Asian countries have long been recognised as medicinal plants which possess cardiovascular-protective effects (Table 6.3). It is also worth highlighting that a number of clinical trials have been conducted

TABLE 6.2
Protective Effect of *C. asiatica* and Its Active Constituents on Vascular Diseases

Protective Effect	Extract/Compound	Model	Signalling Pathway/Major Finding	Reference
Anti-atherosclerotic	Combined standardized Pycnogenol® and *C. asiatica* extracts	Registry study	Inhibition of oxidative stress-related marker	(Belcaro and Cornelli 2017; Belcaro et al. 2020; Hu, Belcaro, et al. 2020)
		Clinical study		(Belcaro et al. 2017)
		Observational study		(Belcaro et al. 2015)
Anti-hypertensive	*C. asiatica* tea	Randomised controlled study	Decreases systolic and diastolic blood pressure	(Astutik et al. 2021)
	Asiatic acid	*In vivo*	• eNOS • p47phox	(Bunbupha et al. 2014)
	Asiaticoside	*In vivo*	PI3K/Akt/eNOS	(Wang et al. 2018)
	C. asiatica ethanol extract	*In vivo*	NO	(Bunaim et al. 2021)
	Asiatic acid	*In vivo*	AngII/AT$_1$R/gp91phox/NF-κB	(Maneesai et al. 2017)
Improvement of venous insufficiency	Combined *C. asiatica* and *V. vinifera* leaf extracts	*In vitro*	NF-κB	(Seo et al. 2021)
	Titrated extract of *C. asiatica*	Randomised controlled study	Relieves leg heaviness and oedema	(Pointel et al. 1987)
	Total triterpenic fraction of *C. asiatica*	Randomised, placebo-controlled study	Suppression of capillary filtration and ankle oedema	(De Sanctis et al. 2001)
		Clinical study	Decreased capillary permeability and improved microcirculation	(Belcaro et al. 1990)
		Randomised study	Alleviates venous hypertension microangiopathy	(Cesarone et al. 2001; Incandela et al. 2001)
Enhancement of endothelial barrier function	Asiaticoside	*In vitro*	Inhibition of stress fibre formation	(Fong et al. 2015)
	Asiaticoside	*In vitro*	Reduction of adhesion molecule expressions	(Jing et al. 2018)
	Asiatic acid	*In vitro*	• NF-κB • pp-MLC	(Fong et al. 2016; Fong et al. 2019)

to investigate the beneficial effects of these herbal plants in the treatment and secondary prevention of cardiovascular diseases.

6.13 TOXICITY AND CAUTIONARY NOTES

In clinical trials, combined supplements of *C. asiatica* (450 mg/day) and Pycnogenol® (150 mg/day) in asymptomatic patients with atherosclerotic plaques were shown to produce no toxicity and tolerability issues (Belcaro et al. 2020). Administration of 250 mg and 500 mg of a

TABLE 6.3

Other Foods, Herbs and Botanicals Used in Cardiovascular Health and Disease

Name of Foods/Herbs/Botanicals	Beneficial Effect	Reference
Danshen (*Salvia miltiorrhiza*)	• Protects against myocardial ischemia and cardiac injury • Inhibits cardiac remodelling • Anti-atherosclerosis	(Li et al. 2018)
Hawthorn (*Crataegus sp.*)	• Anti-atherosclerosis • Anti-hyperlipidaemia • Improvement of vascular function	(Wu et al. 2020)
Jiaogulan (*Gynostemma pentaphyllum*)	• Anti-atherosclerosis • Improvement of ischaemia/reperfusion injury • Anti-hyperlipidaemia • Anti-obesity • Inhibition of platelet aggregation	(Shaito et al. 2020)

standardised extract of *C. asiatica* (ECa 233) were shown to be well-tolerated with no severe side effects (Songvut et al. 2021; Songvut et al. 2019). However, this standardised extract has been reported to cause gastrointestinal problems such as mild abdominal discomfort, flatulence, constipation, where symptoms may vary depending on the dosage regimen. In addition, mild to severe drowsiness were reported but the symptoms were unlikely to be caused by the extract (Songvut et al. 2021). Using transporter-certified cryopreserved human hepatocytes in sandwich culture and human liver microsomes, *C. asiatica* water extract has been demonstrated to have low potential for cytochrome P450 (CYP450)-mediated drug interactions (Wright et al. 2020). CYP450 enzyme inhibition and heavy metal content studies have also revealed the safe use of *C. asiatica* as herbal medicine (Kar et al. 2017).

Furthermore, a clinical case study reported that three women suffered from jaundice after ingestion of *C. asiatica* for 20, 30 and 60 days. The patients were also diagnosed with hepatitis but the symptom was improved after cessation of the treatment (Jorge and Jorge 2005). Consumption of *C. asiatica* with other plants as *SuperUlam* was found to have no adverse effects (Udani 2013). Furthermore, toxicity studies using rodents also demonstrated that the lethal dose of *C. asiatica* standardized extract was 2000 mg/kg and the no observable adverse effect level of the extract was 1000 mg/kg per day. The extract also did not possess mutagenicity potential in rats (Deshpande et al. 2015).

6.14 SUMMARY POINTS

- *C. asiatica* is used by local communities in culinary as green salad, curry vegetables, thin porridge or consumed as herbal tea and fresh juices.
- The earliest use of *C. asiatica* was found at least 3,500 years ago in traditional Ayurvedic medicine.
- *C. asiatica* protects against myocardial ischaemic/reperfusion injury and cardiac hypertrophy.
- *C. asiatica* inhibits cardiovascular disease-related risk factors including hyperlipidaemia, obesity and hyperglycaemia.
- Clinical trials show that supplementation of *C. asiatica* and Pycnogenol® delays the development of atherogenesis.
- Anti-hypertensive effect of *C. asiatica* is associated with increased NO bioavailability.
- *C. asiatica* alleviates chronic venous insufficiency and the associated venous hypertension in human subjects.

- Asiatic acid enhances endothelial barrier function through prevention of interendothelial junction disorganization.
- Pharmacokinetic and toxicity studies indicate that *C. asiatica* extracts are well-tolerated with no severe side effects.

6.15 ACKNOWLEDGEMENTS

This work was supported by the Ministry of Higher Education, Malaysia under the Fundamental Research Grant Scheme (Project number: FRGS/1/2018/SKK06/UTAR/02/7).

REFERENCES

Astutik, F. E. F., D. F. Zuhroh, and M. R. L. Ramadhan. 2021. The effect of gotu kola (*Centella asiatica* L.) tea on blood pressure of hypertension. *Enferm. Clin.* 31 (S2):s195–s198.

Belcaro, G. V., M. R. Cesarone, C. Scipione, V. Scipione, M. Dugall, S. Hu, B. Feragalli, R. Luzzi, M. Hosoi, C. Maione, and R. Cotellese. 2019. Pycnogenol(R)+Centellicum(R), post-stent evaluation: Prevention of neointima and plaque re-growth. *Minerva Cardioangiol* 67 (6):450–455.

Belcaro, G. V., M. R. Cesarone, C. Scipione, V. Scipione, M. Dugall, H. Shu, P. Peterzan, M. Corsi, R. Luzzi, M. Hosoi, B. Feragalli, and R. Cotellese. 2020. Delayed progression of atherosclerosis and cardiovascular events in asymptomatic patients with atherosclerotic plaques: 3-year prevention with the supplementation with Pycnogenol(R)+Centellicum(R). *Minerva Cardioangiol* 68 (1):15–21.

Belcaro, G. V., and U. Cornelli. 2017. Variations in echogenicity in carotid and femoral atherosclerotic plaques with Pycnogenol + Centella asiatica supplementation. *Int J Angiol* 26 (2):95–101.

Belcaro, G. V., M. Dugall, E. Ippolito, M. Hosoi, U. Cornelli, A. Ledda, M. Scoccianti, M. R. Cesarone, L. Pellegrini, R. Luzzi, M. Corsi, and B. Feragalli. 2017. Pycnogenol(R) and Centella asiatica to prevent asymptomatic atherosclerosis progression in clinical events. *Minerva Cardioangiol* 65 (1):24–31.

Belcaro, G. V., R. Grimaldi, and G. Guidi. 1990. Improvement of capillary permeability in patients with venous hypertension after treatment with TTFCA. *Angiology* 41 (7):533–540.

Belcaro, G. V., E. Ippolito, M. Dugall, M. Hosoi, U. Cornelli, A. Ledda, M. Scoccianti, R. D. Steigerwalt, M. R. Cesarone, L. Pellegrini, R. Luzzi, and M. Corsi. 2015. Pycnogenol(R) and Centella asiatica in the management of asymptomatic atherosclerosis progression. *Int Angiol* 34 (2):150–157.

Bian, G. X., G. G. Li, Y. Yang, R. T. Liu, J. P. Ren, L. Q. Wen, S. M. Guo, and Q. J. Lu. 2008. Madecassoside reduces ischemia-reperfusion injury on regional ischemia induced heart infarction in rat. *Biol Pharm Bull* 31 (3):458–463.

Biswas, D., S. Mandal, S. Chatterjee Saha, C. K. Tudu, S. Nandy, G. E. Batiha, M. S. Shekhawat, D. K. Pandey, and A. Dey. 2021. Ethnobotany, phytochemistry, pharmacology, and toxicity of Centella asiatica (L.) Urban: A comprehensive review. *Phytother Res* 35 (12):6624–6654.

Brinkhaus, B., M. Lindner, D. Schuppan, and E. G. Hahn. 2000. Chemical, pharmacological and clinical profile of the East Asian medical plant Centella asiatica. *Phytomedicine* 7 (5):427–448.

Bunaim, M. K., Y. Kamisah, M. N. Mohd Mustazil, J. S. Fadhlullah Zuhair, A. H. Juliana, and N. Muhammad. 2021. Centella asiatica (L.) Urb. prevents hypertension and protects the heart in chronic nitric oxide deficiency rat model. *Front Pharmacol* 12:742562.

Bunbupha, S., P. Pakdeechote, U. Kukongviriyapan, P. Prachaney, and V. Kukongviriyapan. 2014. Asiatic acid reduces blood pressure by enhancing nitric oxide bioavailability with modulation of eNOS and p47phox expression in L-NAME-induced hypertensive rats. *Phytother Res* 28 (10):1506–1512.

Calapai, G. 2012. Assessment report on Centella asiatica (L.) Urban, herba. European Medicines Agency. www.ema.europa.eu/en/documents/herbal-report/final-assessment-report-centella-asiatica-l-urban-herba-first-version_en.pdf (accessed 2 January 2022).

Cesarone, M. R., G. Belcaro, A. Rulo, M. Griffin, A. Ricci, E. Ippolito, M. T. De Sanctis, L. Incandela, P. Bavera, M. Cacchio, and M. Bucci. 2001. Microcirculatory effects of total triterpenic fraction of Centella asiatica in chronic venous hypertension: Measurement by laser Doppler, TcPO2-CO2, and leg volumetry. *Angiology* 52 Suppl 2:S45–S48.

Chen, Y. N., C. G. Wu, B. M. Shi, K. Qian, and Y. Ding. 2018. The protective effect of asiatic acid on podocytes in the kidney of diabetic rats. *Am J Transl Res* 10 (11):3733–3741.

Cox, D. N., S. V. Rajasuriya, P. E. Soysa, J. Gladwin, and A. Ashworth. 1993. Problems encounterd in the community based production of leaf concentrate as supplement for pre-school children in Sri Lanka. *Int J Food Sci Nutr* 44:123–132.

Dai, Y., Z. Wang, M. Quan, Y. Lv, Y. Li, H. B. Xin, and Y. Qian. 2018. Asiatic acid protests against myocardial ischemia/reperfusion injury via modulation of glycometabolism in rat cardiomyocyte. *Drug Des Devel Ther* 12:3573–3582.

De Sanctis, M. T., G. Belcaro, L. Incandela, M. R. Cesarone, M. Griffin, E. Ippolito, and M. Cacchio. 2001. Treatment of edema and increased capillary filtration in venous hypertension with total triterpenic fraction of Centella asiatica: A clinical, prospective, placebo-controlled, randomized, dose-ranging trial. *Angiology* 52 Suppl 2:S55–S59.

Deshpande, P. O., V. Mohan, and P. Thakurdesai. 2015. Preclinical safety assessment of standardized extract of centella asiatica (L.) Urban leaves. *Toxicol Int* 22 (1):10–20.

Fong, L. Y., C. T. Ng, Z. L. Cheok, M. A. Mohd Moklas, M. N. Hakim, and Z. Ahmad. 2016. Barrier protective effect of asiatic acid in TNF-alpha-induced activation of human aortic endothelial cells. *Phytomedicine* 23 (2):191–199.

Fong, L. Y., C. T. Ng, Y. K. Yong, M. N. Hakim, and Z. Ahmad. 2019. Asiatic acid stabilizes cytoskeletal proteins and prevents TNF-alpha-induced disorganization of cell-cell junctions in human aortic endothelial cells. *Vascul Pharmacol* 117:15–26.

Fong, L. Y., C. T. Ng, Z. A. Zakaria, M. T. Baharuldin, A. K. Arifah, M. N. Hakim, and A. Zuraini. 2015. Asiaticoside inhibits TNF-alpha-induced endothelial hyperpermeability of human aortic endothelial cells. *Phytother Res* 29 (10):1501–1508.

Giribabu, N., K. Karim, E. K. Kilari, S. R. Nelli, and N. Salleh. 2020. Oral administration of Centella asiatica (L.) Urb leave aqueous extract ameliorates cerebral oxidative stress, inflammation, and apoptosis in male rats with type-2 diabetes. *Inflammopharmacology* 28 (6):1599–1622.

Hu, S., G. Belcaro, M. R. Cesarone, B. Feragalli, R. Cotellese, M. Dugall, C. Scipione, V. Scipione, and C. Maione. 2020. Central cardiovascular calcifications: Supplementation with Pycnogenol(R) and Centellicum(R): Variations over 12 months. *Minerva Cardioangiol* 68 (1):22–26.

Hu, X., B. Li, L. Li, B. Li, J. Luo, and B. Shen. 2020. Asiatic acid protects against doxorubicin-induced cardiotoxicity in mice. *Oxid Med Cell Longev* 2020:5347204.

Incandela, L., G. Belcaro, M. T. De Sanctis, M. R. Cesarone, M. Griffin, E. Ippolito, M. Bucci, and M. Cacchio. 2001. Total triterpenic fraction of Centella asiatica in the treatment of venous hypertension: A clinical, prospective, randomized trial using a combined microcirculatory model. *Angiology* 52 Suppl 2:S61–S67.

Jamil, S., Q. Nizami, and M. Salam. 2007. Centella asiatica (Linn.) Urban: A review. *Indian J Nat Prod Resour* 6:158–170.

Jing, L., W. Haitao, W. Qiong, Z. Fu, Z. Nan, and Z. Xuezheng. 2018. Anti inflammatory effect of asiaticoside on human umbilical vein endothelial cells induced by ox-LDL. *Cytotechnology* 70 (2):855–864.

Jorge, O. A., and A. D. Jorge. 2005. Hepatotoxicity associated with the ingestion of Centella asiatica. *Rev Esp Enferm Dig* 97 (2):115–124.

Kar, A., S. Pandit, K. Mukherjee, S. Bahadur, and P. K. Mukherjee. 2017. Safety assessment of selected medicinal food plants used in Ayurveda through CYP450 enzyme inhibition study. *J Sci Food Agric* 97 (1):333–340.

Kumari, S., M. Deori, R. Elancheran, J. Kotoky, and R. Devi. 2016. In vitro and In vivo antioxidant, antihyperlipidemic properties and chemical characterization of centella asiatica (L.) extract. *Front Pharmacol* 7:400.

Kusumastuti, S. A., D. A. A. Nugrahaningsih, and M. S. H. Wahyuningsih. 2019. Centella asiatica (L.) extract attenuates inflammation and improve insulin sensitivity in a coculture of lipopolysaccharide (LPS)-induced 3T3-L1 adipocytes and RAW 264.7 macrophages. *Drug Discov Ther* 13 (5):261–267.

Li, H., X. Tian, Y. Ruan, J. Xing, and Z. Meng. 2021. Asiatic acid alleviates Ang-II induced cardiac hypertrophy and fibrosis via miR-126/PIK3R2 signaling. *Nutr Metab (Lond)* 18 (1):71.

Li, Z. M., S. W. Xu, and P. Q. Liu. 2018. Salvia miltiorrhiza Burge (Danshen): A golden herbal medicine in cardiovascular therapeutics. *Acta Pharmacol Sin* 39 (5):802–824.

Lichota, A., L. Gwozdzinski, and K. Gwozdzinski. 2019. Therapeutic potential of natural compounds in inflammation and chronic venous insufficiency. *Eur J Med Chem* 176:68–91.

Lou, J. S., D. M. Dimitrova, C. Murchison, G. C. Arnold, H. Belding, N. Seifer, N. Le, S. B. Andrea, N. E. Gray, K. M. Wright, M. Caruso, and A. Soumyanath. 2018. Centella asiatica triterpenes for diabetic neuropathy: A randomized, double-blind, placebo-controlled, pilot clinical study. *Esper Dermatol* 20 (2 Suppl 1):12–22.

Ma, Z. G., J. Dai, W. Y. Wei, W. B. Zhang, S. C. Xu, H. H. Liao, Z. Yang, and Q. Z. Tang. 2016. Asiatic acid protects against cardiac hypertrophy through activating AMPKalpha signalling pathway. *Int J Biol Sci* 12 (7):861–871.

Maneesai, P., S. Bunbupha, U. Kukongviriyapan, L. Senggunprai, V. Kukongviriyapan, P. Prachaney, and P. Pakdeechote. 2017. Effect of asiatic acid on the Ang II-AT1R-NADPH oxidase-NF-kappaB pathway in renovascular hypertensive rats. *Naunyn Schmiedebergs Arch Pharmacol* 390 (10):1073–1083.

Mohd Razali, N. N., C. T. Ng, and L. Y. Fong. 2019. Cardiovascular protective effects of centella asiatica and its triterpenes: A review. *Planta Med* 85 (16):1203–1215.

Pakdeechote, P., S. Bunbupha, U. Kukongviriyapan, P. Prachaney, W. Khrisanapant, and V. Kukongviriyapan. 2014. Asiatic acid alleviates hemodynamic and metabolic alterations via restoring eNOS/iNOS expression, oxidative stress, and inflammation in diet-induced metabolic syndrome rats. *Nutrients* 6 (1):355–370.

Pointel, J. P., H. Boccalon, M. Cloarec, C. Ledevehat, and M. Joubert. 1987. Titrated extract of Centella asiatica (TECA) in the treatment of venous insufficiency of the lower limbs. *Angiology* 38 (1 Pt 1):46–50.

Qiu, F., Y. Yuan, W. Luo, Y. S. Gong, Z. M. Zhang, Z. M. Liu, and L. Gao. 2022. Asiatic acid alleviates ischemic myocardial injury in mice by modulating mitophagy- and glycophagy-based energy metabolism. *Acta Pharmacol Sin* 43 (6):1395–1407.

Rameshreddy, P., V. V. S. Uddandrao, P. Brahmanaidu, S. Vadivukkarasi, R. Ravindarnaik, P. Suresh, K. Swapna, A. Kalaivani, P. Parvathi, P. Tamilmani, and G. Saravanan. 2018. Obesity-alleviating potential of asiatic acid and its effects on ACC1, UCP2, and CPT1 mRNA expression in high fat diet-induced obese Sprague-Dawley rats. *Mol Cell Biochem* 442 (1–2):143–154.

Ramli, S., W. J. Xian, and N. A. Abd Mutalib. 2020. A review: Antibacterial activities, antioxidant properties and toxicity profile of *Centella asiatica*. *EDUCATUM Journal of Science, Mathematics and Technology* 7 (1):9–47.

Seo, M. G., M. J. Jo, N. I. Hong, M. J. Kim, K. S. Shim, E. Shin, J. J. Lee, and S. J. Park. 2021. Anti-inflammatory and anti-vascular leakage effects by combination of centella asiatica and vitis vinifera L. Leaf extracts. *Evid Based Complement Alternat Med* 2021:7381620.

Setyaningsih, W. A. W., N. Arfian, A. S. Fitriawan, R. Yuniartha, and D. C. R. Sari. 2021. Ethanolic extract of centella asiatica treatment in the early stage of hyperglycemia condition inhibits glomerular injury and vascular remodeling in diabetic rat model. *Evid Based Complement Alternat Med* 2021: 6671130.

Shaito, A., D. T. B. Thuan, H. T. Phu, T. H. D. Nguyen, H. Hasan, S. Halabi, S. Abdelhady, G. K. Nasrallah, A. H. Eid, and G. Pintus. 2020. Herbal medicine for cardiovascular diseases: Efficacy, mechanisms, and safety. *Front Pharmacol* 11:422.

Si, L., J. Xu, C. Yi, X. Xu, C. Ma, J. Yang, F. Wang, Y. Zhang, and X. Wang. 2015. Asiatic acid attenuates the progression of left ventricular hypertrophy and heart failure induced by pressure overload by inhibiting myocardial remodeling in mice. *J Cardiovasc Pharmacol* 66 (6):558–568.

Songvut, P., P. Chariyavilaskul, P. Khemawoot, and R. Tansawat. 2021. Pharmacokinetics and metabolomics investigation of an orally modified formula of standardized Centella asiatica extract in healthy volunteers. *Sci Rep* 11 (1):6850.

Songvut, P., P. Chariyavilaskul, M. H. Tantisira, and P. Khemawoot. 2019. Safety and pharmacokinetics of standardized extract of centella asiatica (ECa 233) capsules in healthy thai volunteers: A phase 1 clinical study. *Planta Med* 85 (6):483–490.

Sun, B., L. Wu, Y. Wu, C. Zhang, L. Qin, M. Hayashi, M. Kudo, M. Gao, and T. Liu. 2020. Therapeutic potential of centella asiatica and its triterpenes: A review. *Front Pharmacol* 11:568032.

Udani, J. K. 2013. Effects of SuperUlam on supporting concentration and mood: A randomized, double-blind, placebo-controlled crossover study. *Evid Based Complement Alternat Med* 2013:238454.

Uddandrao, V. V. S., P. Rameshreddy, P. Brahmanaidu, P. Ponnusamy, S. Balakrishnan, R. N. Ramavat, K. Swapna, S. Pothani, H. Nemani, B. Meriga, S. Vadivukkarasi, R. N. P., and S. Ganapathy. 2020. Antiobesity efficacy of asiatic acid: Down-regulation of adipogenic and inflammatory processes in high fat diet induced obese rats. *Arch Physiol Biochem* 126 (5):453–462.

Wang, X., X. Cai, W. Wang, Y. Jin, M. Chen, X. Huang, X. Zhu, and L. Wang. 2018. Effect of asiaticoside on endothelial cells in hypoxiainduced pulmonary hypertension. *Mol Med Rep* 17 (2):2893–2900.

Wright, K. M., A. A. Magana, R. M. Laethem, C. L. Moseley, T. T. Banks, C. S. Maier, J. F. Stevens, J. F. Quinn, and A. Soumyanath. 2020. Centella asiatica water extract shows low potential for cytochrome P450-mediated drug interactions. *Drug Metab Dispos* 48 (10):1053–1063.

Wu, K., M. Hu, Z. Chen, F. Xiang, G. Chen, W. Yan, Q. Peng, and X. Chen. 2017. Asiatic acid enhances survival of human AC16 cardiomyocytes under hypoxia by upregulating miR-1290. *IUBMB Life* 69 (9):660–667.

Wu, M., L. Liu, Y. Xing, S. Yang, H. Li, and Y. Cao. 2020. Roles and mechanisms of hawthorn and its extracts on atherosclerosis: A review. *Front Pharmacol* 11:118.

Xu, X., L. Si, J. Xu, C. Yi, F. Wang, W. Gu, Y. Zhang, and X. Wang. 2015. Asiatic acid inhibits cardiac hypertrophy by blocking interleukin-1beta-activated nuclear factor-kappaB signaling in vitro and in vivo. *J Thorac Dis* 7 (10):1787–1797.

Yan, S. L., H. T. Yang, Y. J. Lee, C. C. Lin, M. H. Chang, and M. C. Yin. 2014. Asiatic acid ameliorates hepatic lipid accumulation and insulin resistance in mice consuming a high-fat diet. *J Agric Food Chem* 62 (20):4625–4631.

Yi, C., L. Si, J. Xu, J. Yang, Q. Wang, and X. Wang. 2020. Effect and mechanism of asiatic acid on autophagy in myocardial ischemia-reperfusion injury in vivo and in vitro. *Exp Ther Med* 20 (5):54.

Zhang, J., M. Yao, X. Jia, J. Xie, and Y. Wang. 2020. Hexokinase II upregulation contributes to asiaticoside-induced protection of H9c2 cardioblasts during oxygen-glucose deprivation/reoxygenation. *J Cardiovasc Pharmacol* 75 (1):84–90.

7 *Terminalia arjuna* and Cardiovascular Protection
A Comprehensive Overview

Aashis Dutta and Manas Das

CONTENTS

7.1 Introduction 94
7.2 Background...95
7.3 Physiological Aspects 96
7.4 Reactive Oxygen Species (ROS) and *T. arjuna*..96
7.5 Isoproterenol Induced Cardiac Hypertrophy and *T. arjuna* 98
7.6 Lipid Metabolism and *T. arjuna*...100
7.7 Clinical Trials 101
7.8 Immunomodulatory Aspects 101
7.9 Clinical Study 103
7.10 Cellular Aspects...104
7.11 Other Foods, Herbs, Spices and Botanicals Used 104
7.12 Toxicity and Cautionary Notes 105
7.13 Summary Points 105
References...106

LIST OF ABBREVIATIONS

DPPH	2,2-Diphenyl-1-Picrylhydrazyl
AP-1	Activator Protein-1
ALT	Alanine Transaminase
ARE	Antioxidant Response Element
AST	Aspartate Transaminase
BNP	Brain Natriuretic Peptide
Cd	Cadmium
CVD	Cardiovascular Disease
CAT	Catalase
CAM	Cell Adhesion Molecule
Col1α	Collagen 1α
Col3α	Collagen 3α
CHF	Congestive Heart Failure
CTGF	Connective Tissue Growth Factor
CAD	Coronary Artery Disease
CK-MB	Creatine Kinase-Myocardial Band
COX-2	Cyclooxygenase 2
DPP-IV	Dipeptidyl peptidase-IV
DOX	Doxorubicin
ET	Endothelin
GSH	Glutathione

DOI: 10.1201/9781003220329-9

GPx	Glutathione Peroxidase
GAPDH	Glyceraldehyde 3-Phosphate Dehydrogenase
HDL-C	High-Density Lipoprotein-Cholesterol
HFD	High Fat Diet
HAEC	Human Aortic Endothelial Cells
ICAM-1	Intercellular Adhesion Molecule-1
ISO	Isoproterenol
LDH	Lactate Dehydrogenase
LVEF	Left Ventricular Ejection Fraction
LVEDP	Left Ventricular End Diastolic Pressure
LVP	Left Ventricular Pressure
LPS	Lipopolysaccharide
LXR-α	Liver X Receptor-α
LDL-C	Low-Density Lipoprotein Cholesterol
MDH	Malate Dehydrogenase
MDA	Malonialdehyde
MMP	Matrix Metalloproteinase
NPP	Natriuretic Peptide
Nrf2	Nuclear Factor erythroid 2 – related factor 2
NF-Kb	Nuclear Factor kappa B
PPAR-γ	Peroxisome Proliferator Activated Receptor-γ
ROS	Reactive Oxygen Species
SR	Sarcoplasmic Reticulum
SGOT	Serum Glutamic Oxaloacetic Transaminase
STAT-3	Signal Transducer and Activator of Transcription 3
STZ	Streptozotocin
SOD	Superoxide Dismutase
TUNEL	Terminal deoxynucleotidyl transferase dUTP nick end labeling assay
TAAE	*Terminalia arjuna* aqueous extract
TACMCE	*Terminalia arjuna* carboxy methyl cellulose extract
TAEE	*Terminalia arjuna* ethanolic extract
TAME	*Terminalia arjuna* methanolic extract
TC	Total Cholesterol
TGF-β1	Transforming Growth Factor β1
TG	Triglyceride
TGF-β	Tumor Growth Factor-β
TNF-α	Tumor Necrosis Factor-α
VCAM-1	Vascular Cell Adhesion Molecule-1
VLDL-C	Very Low-Density Lipoprotein Cholesterol

7.1 INTRODUCTION

Terminalia arjuna (Roxb.) Wight and Arn is a unique, popular and valuable medicinal plant in traditional systems of medicine and is used as a remedy for various cardiovascular diseases (CVDs). It is a deciduous tree found throughout India, Sri Lanka, Mauritius and Burma, attaining a height of 60–80 feet with strengthened trunk and hanging branches. The sub-Indo-Himalayan tracts of Uttar Pradesh, West Bengal, Orissa, Punjab, Deccan, South Bihar and Madhya Pradesh harbors this medicinal plant which is widely known as Arjuna, Indraru, Partha and Veeravriksha. The bark of the stem is simple, flattened and pinkish grey in outward view while internally it is soft and reddish in color. The leaves are simple, acute or obtuse at the apex with the upper face being pale or dark green while the lower face is pale brown. The tree bears white, immobile bisexual flowers in short

TABLE 7.1
The Phytoconstituents Present in Different Plant Parts with Their Therapeutic Potential

Types of Phytoconstituents	Plant Part Present	Therapeutic Potential	References
Flavonoids (Gallic acid, ellagic acid, ethyl gallate, (+)-catechin, (+)-gallocatechin, (-)-epigallocatechin)	Stem bark, Fruits, Leaves and Seeds	• Inhibition of LDL oxidation, Endothelial activation and platelet aggregation. • Antioxidant activity (free radical scavenging property)	(Carluccio et al. 2003; Pettit et al. 1996; Bajpai et al. 2005)
Tannins (Castalagin, casuariin, casuarinin, punicallin, pyrocatechol)	Stem bark	• Hypotensive • Antioxidant activity	(Kolodziej and Kiderlen 2005; Chaudhari and Mengi 2006)
Terpenoids and glycosides (Arjunin, arjunic acid, arjungenin, arjunolic acid, oleanolic acid, arjunetin, arjunolone, arjunaphthanoloside, termiarjunoside I, termiarjunoside II)	Stem bark, roots, fruits, leaves and seeds	• Antioxidant activity • Inhibits NO production in LPS induced rat peritoneal macrophages • Inhibits superoxide release from macrophages • Inhibits platelet aggregation	(Ali et al. 2003; Alam et al. 2008; Patnaik et al. 2007)

auxiliary spikes or in a terminal panicle positioning. The fruits are elliptical, fibrous-woody and smooth having five hard wings or angles curved upwards. The major phytochemicals in bark, root, stem, fruits, seeds and leaves have been differentially characterized and these plant parts are found to contain triterpenoids (arjunin, arjunic acid, arjunolic acid), glycosides (arjunetin, arjunolone, arjunolitin), flavonoids and phenolics (arjunone, luteolin, gallic acid, kaempferol), tannins (pyrocatechols, punicallin), minerals (calcium, magnesium, aluminum) that are attributing the antioxidant, anti-inflammatory, immunomodulatory, anti-carcinogenic, anti-microbial, anti-hypertensive and anti-hypertrophic property of the plant (Amalraj and Gopi 2016).

Cardiovascular diseases (CVDs) are the most prevalent cause of death worldwide with significant prominence due to the recent alterations in lifestyle, food habits and environmental pollution. The imperfectly maintained CVDs can result in prolonged disability from their complications (Khaliq and Fahim, 2018). The different CVDs like myocardial infarction, congestive heart failure (CHF), ischemic mitral regurgitation (IMR), rheumatic heart disease, platelet aggregation, cardiomyopathy, dyslipidemia and thrombotic condition has taken a widespread toll on human lives. Although there are several factors like obesity, hyperlipidemia, hypertension, tobacco, diabetes that increase the incidence towards the occurrence of these disorders, proper scientific management in the dietary intake of food, food habits and also of our lifestyle can aid in the prevention and early detection of such CVDs. Speaking of the medicinal plants that have been in use since ancient times, *T. arjuna* stands out in itself as being one of the most sought-after herbal plants in the treatment of these disorders. Detailed scientific investigations of *T. arjuna* have been thoroughly reported and discussed through exploration of physiological, molecular and cellular effects with the help of various available clinical and pre-clinical literature.

7.2 BACKGROUND

The ancient Indian physician Charaka in his work *Charak Samhita* mentioned the therapeutic usage of *T. arjuna*, particularly the bark for cardiac ailments. His successive Ayurvedic practitioners including Chakradatta, Bhava Mishra were also pivotal in utilizing the bark to its therapeutic potential. Even the present-day Ayurvedic physicians do not make an exception to it in following the age-old traditions. The Ayurveda proposes two main bark powder formulations for patients –one known as Ghrita (bark powder in fat) and the other known as Kshirpaak (bark powder boiled in milk). These physicians endorsed the usage of the plant for a variety of cardiopathological conditions ranging from angina pectoris to heart failure although evidence based on clinical and pre-clinical reports have only been made recently (Maulik and Talwar 2012). The pre-clinical studies were performed using different solvent extracts (water, hydroalcohol, ethanol, hexane, acetone, dichloromethane, ethyl acetate, methanol). In one such study, it was demonstrated that the aqueous extract was capable of inducing adult rat ventricular myocytes by elevating sarcoplasmic reticulum (SR) function and reducing the occurrence of arrhythmias than the organic extract that caused excitability loss and arrhythmias indicative of the aqueous extract being a better cardiotonic substance (Oberoi et al. 2011). On the other hand, clinical studies were conducted on patients with different CVDs like angina pectoris, endothelial dysfunction, hypertension and heart failure. Most of these studies are arbitrary, double blind and placebo controlled but some of these studies have limitations, like the scarcity of information of the source, method for extract identification, botanical identification and its standardization (Maulik and Talwar 2012).

7.3 PHYSIOLOGICAL ASPECTS

The *T. arjuna* tree, particularly the stem bark, exerts profound beneficial physiological effects on the cardiovascular system of the body. These scientific validations have involved the usage of the different solvent extracts of the bark (primarily the ethanolic and methanolic extract) in demonstrating its cardioprotective and cardiotonic behavior.

7.4 REACTIVE OXYGEN SPECIES (ROS) AND *T. ARJUNA*

Oxidative stress is mostly defined as an instability causing the generation of ROS against the antioxidant system in the body. The mechanism of ROS generation is still elusive. Mitochondria is the prime organelle for the production of superoxide radicals and other ROS, particularly the complex I and complex II. The ROS are degraded or the peroxidation products are counterbalanced by the natural antioxidant defense systems constituted by mitochondrial (manganese-containing) and cytosolic (containing Cu and Zn) superoxide dismutases (Mn- and Cu-Zn-SOD respectively), glutathione peroxidase (GPx) and phospholipid hydroperoxide glutathione peroxides. The lethal effect of ROS involves the lipid peroxidation, particularly phospholipids of biomembranes and oxidative damage to proteins and DNA. *Terminalia arjuna* aqueous extract (TAAE) was capable of scavenging the 2,2-diphenyl-1-picrylhydrazyl (DPPH) radical and as such demonstrated its cardioprotective nature. In an experiment, the copper ascorbate (Cu-ascorbate) was found to cause oxidative damage by elevating tissue lipid peroxidation, protein carbonyl content and decreasing tissue reduced glutathione (GSH) levels. Even oxidized proteins can aggregate and lead to cellular damage. The TAAE was capable of removing the reactive intermediate and toxic free radicals or by chelation with the redox-active transition/non-transition heavy metal divalent cations, thereby preventing the proteins from getting oxidized. The action of Mn-SOD, catalase (CAT), GPx, glutathione reductase was markedly depleted following Cu-ascorbate treatment while TAAE restored the activity of all the aforementioned enzymes. Even the altered activity of the enzymes of the Krebs cycle, like α-ketoglutarate dehydrogenase, isocitrate dehydrogenase and succinate dehydrogenase, along with the enzymes of ETC like NADH cytochrome c oxidoreductase and cytochrome c oxidase, was reinstated by TAAE which is indicative of the fact that the extract has some chelating properties or is capable of preserving the activity of mitochondria by itself being an absorber of ROS (Figure 7.1) (Dutta et al. 2013).

A highly effective chemotherapeutic agent, Doxorubicin (DOX) induces oxidative stress by stimulating the generation of ROS and causes elevation in mitochondrial oxidation primarily by superoxide anions. The aqueous extract (i.e. TAAE) alone could inhibit the DOX-stimulated superoxide-associated oxidative stress and cell damage in a concentration-dependent manner

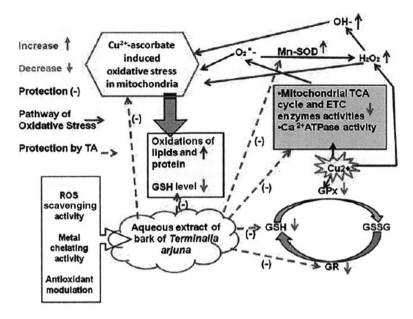

FIGURE 7.1 Scheme showing the probable mechanism of protection offered by aqueous bark extract of *Terminalia arjuna* against copper-ascorbate induced oxidative stress in vitro in goat heart mitochondria.

Source: Dutta et al. (2013).

(Bishop and Liu 2017). The chemotherapeutic agent also decreased the mitochondrial membrane potential indicative of defective cell bioenergetics homeostasis (Berthaiume and Wallace 2007). This lowering of mitochondrial membrane potential was restored by the TAAE which might be due to the flavonoids present in it counterbalancing the elevated superoxide free radicals or chelating/reducing iron in mitochondria (Ichikawa et al. 2014). Furthermore, the impairment in SR functioning that disturbs the Ca^{2+} cell homeostasis is correlated with DOX-stimulated cardiotoxicity (Arai et al. 2000). The TAAE is capable of ameliorating the SR function in isolated ventricular myocytes and likewise the protective effect of the extract against DOX induced cardiotoxicity occurs as a result of its action on prohibiting SR dysfunction or ameliorating the SR function. The extract administration prevented DOX-stimulated left ventricle (LV) systolic dysfunction thereby augmenting the LV myocyte contraction (Oberoi et al. 2011). The *Terminalia arjuna* ethanolic extract (TAEE) was found to possess higher antioxidant potential as compared to TAAE (Shastry Viswanatha et al. 2010). Cadmium (Cd) is considered to be yet another ubiquitous toxic heavy metal that might cause an elevation in the generation of ROS such as hydroxyl radical (·OH), superoxide anion free radical (O_2·−), nitric oxide radical and hydrogen peroxide (H_2O_2), thereby stimulating oxidative stress. The increased concentration of Xanthine Dehydrogenase (XDH) and Xanthine Oxidase (XO) on Cd treatment implicates enhanced generation of O_2·− in cardiac tissues which was later reinstated by the action of TAAE. Similar is the case with cardiac marker enzymes like Serum Glutamic Pyruvic Transaminase (SGPT), Alkaline Phosphatase (ALP), Creatine Kinase-Myocardial Band (CK-MB), GPx, Serum Glutamic Oxaloacetic Transaminase (SGOT), Lactate Dehydrogenase-1 (LDH1) and LDH5 whose levels were elevated by Cd treatment while TAAE restored them. The activities of Cu-Zn SOD and Mn-SOD were found to decline in the cardiac tissue which might be due to the deactivation of SOD either by Cd induced lipid peroxidation or directly by the interplay of Cd with enzyme, thereby disrupting the enzyme structure while the activity of CAT is reported to be increased, perhaps due to overproduction of O_2·−, leading to the formation of H_2O_2 which might have deactivated the enzyme activity. All these enzyme activities were reinstated by the action of TAAE. Even the enzymes of ETC like isocitrate dehydrogenase, α-ketoglutarate dehydrogenase, succinate dehydrogenase portray the same story. The alteration in the ETC enzymes influences the inner mitochondrial permeability of protons that leads to the destruction of electrochemical gradient. This alteration was prevented to a considerable extent by the application of TAAE. The levels of the oxidative stress biomarkers such as peroxidation of lipids and protein carbonyl content are enhanced by Cd treatment but again lowered by TAAE (Bhattacharjee et al. 2019). Furthermore, the administration of 500 mg/kg dose of *T. arjuna* carboxy methyl cellulose bark extract (TACMCE) delivered better results in ischemic reperfused rat hearts when it came to amelioration of the antioxidant system (increase in SOD, GSH and CAT levels) as compared to the 750 mg/kg dosage (which caused increase in only CAT level). The former dose gave better oxidative stress protection while the latter dose failed to do so thereby leaving us in the dark for the occurrence of such a phenomenon (Gauthaman et al. 2001). Besides the dose of 40 mg/kg TAAE caused a remarkable decline in the blood pressure, the duration of which lasted for 90 minutes in anesthetized dogs. The decline in the blood pressure was brought about by improving the autonomic behavior of the body (Bhatia et al. 2000). A colorless, volatile and very stable chlorinated hydrocarbon, carbon tetrachloride (CCl_4), when administered to mice caused depletion in the activities of antioxidant enzymes like SOD, CAT and GST and also in the level of GSH in cardiac tissue while simultaneously elevating the magnitude of lipid peroxidation and the concentration of oxidized glutathione (GSSG). The pretreatment with the active constituents of TAEE prior to CCl_4 administration reinstated the action of all the antioxidant enzymes along with the concentration of GSH and reduced the lipid peroxidation end products. It was found that half the concentration of TAEE (i.e. 50 mg/kg) was capable of bringing about the equivalent effect compared to vitamin C dose (100 mg/kg). It has been argued that CCl_4, being a free radical inducer, stimulates cardiac damage via formation of abundant free radicals like $^{\bullet}CCl_3$ and $^{\bullet}OOCCl_3$ through major pathways, and as such the phytochemical constituents of TAEE were capable of reverting oxidative stress through free radical scavenging activity (Manna et al. 2007). The TAEE exhibited cardioprotection via stimulation of cardiac intracellular antioxidant activity and prevented murine hearts from undergoing the damage caused by sodium fluoride stimulated oxidative stress (Sinha et al. 2008). Prophylactic and therapeutic administration of *Terminalia arjuna* ameliorated cardiac functions and baroreflex responsiveness along with impoverishment of left ventricular hypertrophy and fibrosis (Parveen et al. 2012). The cardiotonic property of *T. arjuna* may also be attributed to its Dipeptidyl peptidase-IV (DPP-IV) inhibitory action which is due to the presence of its phytoconstituents like arjunetin, arjungenin, arjunic acid, arjunone, ellagic acid, gallic acid demonstrated through in silico docking studies. Arjunetin and arjunone bind to the DPP-IV enzyme active site while arjunetin prefers to attach itself to the interface of DPP-IV as its biological active form is a homodimer and attaches to the same amino acid ASP 379 (Mohanty et al. 2019).

7.5 ISOPROTERENOL INDUCED CARDIAC HYPERTROPHY AND *T. ARJUNA*

Isoproterenol (ISO) is an β-adrenergic agonist and an excellent synthetic catecholamine causing extreme myocardial stress resulting in necrosis-like conditions. It has a strong stimulatory influence on the heart thereby elevating the cardiac output (Das and Dutta 2020). The chemical was utilized to induce ischemic reperfusion in rats followed by the treatment with different doses of 90 % TAEE (3.4 mg/kg; 6.75 mg/kg; 9.75 mg/kg). The 6.75 mg/kg dose turned out to be the most optimum one for effective enhancement of GSH, SOD and CAT levels as compared to the other two doses (3.4 mg/kg and 9.75 mg/kg) correlated with in vivo reperfusion injury. The optimum dose is perfectly capable of surviving the oxidative stress while the 3.4 mg/kg dosage administered rats declined to survive the stress. Elevation in cellular SOD without rise in CAT is injurious as it favors H_2O_2 production. The 9.75 mg/kg dosage increased both the GSH and CAT levels but not SOD and the mechanism behind the occurrence of this phenomenon is not fully understood (Karthikeyan et al. 2003). Although it has been reported by various scientists that the bark extract elevates CAT activity in in vivo studies with animal models, but TAEE, amongst all other solvent extracts like acetone, water, ethyl acetate, chloroform and hexane, was found to exhibit a specific and rare competitive–non-competitive type of inhibition of CAT activity and as such the bark extract does not enhance CAT activity in vitro (Padma Sree et al. 2007). In another experiment conducted on wistar albino rats, TAEE demonstrated a prominent elevation in endogenous antioxidants like SOD and GSH in RBCs and this effect was more marked when α-tocopherol was used in combination. The pre-administered dose of the extract along with α-tocopherol lowered the ISO elevated malondialdehyde (MDA) level significantly (Shukla, Sharma and Singh et al. 2015; Shukla, Sharma, Singh, Ahmad et al. 2015). Substantiating the results of the aforementioned experiment, the elevated concentration of major lipid peroxidant end product, MDA, and the depleted activity of the antioxidant system by ISO administration was reinstated by the administration of the dosage of 50% TAEE. The enhanced level of pro-inflammatory cytokine, Tumor Necrosis Factor-α (TNF-α), is found to be decreased by the aforementioned extract treatment (Parveen et al. 2011; Parveen et al. 2012). The serum markers of cardiac damage, SGOT, CK-MB, Troponin I and LDH were enhanced in ISO-treated rats which is reflective of the extent of necrotic damage to the myocardial membrane. The TAEE alone and in combination with α-tocopherol was capable of reverting the damage induced by the dose of ISO (Shukla, Sharma, and Singh et al. 2015; Shukla, Sharma, Singh, Ahmad et al. 2015). However, both the ethanolic and the aqueous extracts were capable of reverting the lipid profile and serum LDH, ALT and AST back to normal after being elevated by ISO treatment (Sivakumar and Rajeshkumar 2014). The ISO induced alterations in the action of cardiac marker enzymes (CK-MB, ALT, AST and LDH) and antioxidant enzymes (SOD, CAT) were reinstated by the gemmomodified bark extract (mixture of glycerin and methanol in the ratio of 1:2) of *T. arjuna* (Jahan et al. 2012). In case of creatine kinase isoenzyme-MB (CK-MB), the ISO caused the leakage of the enzyme from the plasma membrane, thereby destroying its integrity and permeability and led to the increase in the elevation of serum enzyme level. The TAEE administration reverted the entire phenomenon by stabilizing the membrane integrity thus inhibiting the escape of the CK-MB (Parveen et al. 2011; Parveen et al. 2012). Besides, the action of 50% TAEE dosage was comparable to that of fluvastatin in preserving the left ventricular function as demonstrated in its remarkable restoration of left ventricular pressure (LVP) and left ventricular end diastolic pressure (LVEDP). The restoration (elevation in case of LVEDP and decline in case of LVP to normal physiological level) manifests an increase in myocardial contractility and relaxation with amelioration of left ventricular dysfunction caused by ISO. The extract caused the blood to flow at normal rate in the myocardium and even lowered the left ventricle weight to body weight index (Parveen et al. 2012). Moreover, both the ethanolic and aqueous extracts (i.e. TAEE and TAAE) blocked the lipid peroxidation and the action of HMG coA reductase along with reduction in the ROS generation in human monocyte cells by stimulating the action of CAT, GPx activities, thereby maintaining reducing property of the cell (Kokkiripati et al. 2013). The ISO induced cardiac fibrosis demonstrated enhanced RNA levels of pro-fibrotic genes like Collagen 1α (Col1α), Collagen 3α (Col3α), Transforming Growth Factor-β1(TGF-β1) and Connective Tissue Growth Factor (CTGF) while TAAE prevents cardiac remodeling through downregulation of pro-fibrotic cytokines and collagen content. The elevated DNA binding action of the redox sensitive transcription factors, nuclear factor kappa-light-chain-enhancer of activated B cells (NF-κB) and activator protein 1 (AP-1) in ISO treated heart was partly reverted by TAAE. Nuclear factor erythroid 2 – related factor 2 (Nrf2) is a well-known transcription factor which is present in cytosol along with Keap1. In presence of ROS, certain cysteine residues in Keap1 are oxidized causing its dissociation from Nrf2 accompanied by its trafficking into the nucleus where it attaches itself with antioxidant response element (AREs) and modulates the antioxidant response. The activity of Nrf2 was enhanced by TAAE in ISO induced fibrotic heart (Santosh et al. 2017). The ISO is capable of interfering with the c-Jun N-terminal kinase (JNK) signaling pathway as its administration stimulates the phosphorylation of JNK causing cardiac hypertrophy while the treatment with ethanolic extract regulates the pathway by inducing JNK by prohibiting JNK1/2 and c-Jun phosphorylation followed by stimulation of caspase-3. Simultaneously, TAEE stimulates the anti-apoptotic genes such as Bcl-2 and prohibits the inducible nitric oxide synthase (iNOS) causing a decline in the liberation of ROS and oxidative stress stimulated cytochrome c and caspase-3. An alteration in cardiac apoptotic protein expression (i.e. downregulation of Bcl-2 and upregulation of Bax, p-JNK and p-Jun) was noticeable by treatment with ISO while TAEE restored the normal expression levels of these apoptotic proteins (Thangaraju et al. 2020). Transcriptomic analysis revealed the capability of ISO in elevating the expression of key genes associated with angiogenesis, inflammation and drug metabolism like Vascular Endothelial Growth factor D (VEGF-D), Interleukin-18 (IL-18), Cyt P450 while lowering ATP synthase, Succinate dehydrogenase flavoprotein subunit (Sdha1), Acetyl-CoA metabolism like Acetyl-CoA acyltransferase (i.e. the genes involved in oxidative phosphorylation and Acetyl CoA metabolism). However, TAAE was capable of restoring the gene regulatory network disturbed by ISO administration in cardiac hypertrophied rats (Kumar et al. 2019). The TAAE significantly ameliorated oxidative stress and depletion in antioxidant level but the enhancement in heart weight to body weight ratio was not improved by the extract which only proves that it only inhibited ISO induced myocardial alterations (Kumar et al. 2009). When the three different *Terminalia arjuna* bark extracts (i.e. ethyl acetate, ethanol and diethyl ether) were used to figure out the cardioprotective effect in poloxamer (PX)-407 stimulated hyperlipidemic male wistar rats in two different doses (175 mg/kg and 350 mg/kg), the anti-hyperlipidemic and antioxidant effect exhibition followed the order, ethanolic, diethyl ether and ethyl acetate (Subramaniam et al. 2011). The aqueous bark extract was demonstrated to possess enhanced capacity to induce ventricular myocytes of adult rats, increased functionality of SR and lowered the chances of occurrence of arrhythmias as compared to the different organic extracts (Oberoi et al. 2011). Along with ISO, anti-neoplastic chemicals like streptozotocin (STZ) when administered produced myocardial alterations in wistar albino rats which involved fall in LVP, maximal rate of increase and decrease in LVP, cardiac contractile index and elevation in LVEDP, all of which were prominently ameliorated by TAEE cementing the position of *Terminalia arjuna* as a cardioprotective agent (Khaliq, Parveen, Singh, Gondal et al. 2013). Substantiating the outcome of the aforementioned experiment, it was noticed that the TAEE even ameliorated baroreflex responsiveness in STZ induced diabetic rats, probably by sustaining endogenous antioxidant enzyme system and lowering cytokine levels (Khaliq, Parveen et al. 2013).

7.6 LIPID METABOLISM AND *T. ARJUNA*

Lipids are known to play a pivotal role in cardiovascular diseases such as hyperlipidemia and hypercholesterolemia that ultimately culminate in the occurrence of heart failure. Malfunctioning in lipid metabolism will result in cardiac dysfunction by altering the composition, structure and stability of cellular membranes that result in cell death. Amongst the different solvent extracts (solvent ether, petroleum ether, ethanol and water) used, the ethanolic extract stood out in exerting anti-hyperlipidemic activity followed by solvent ether and petroleum ether as it displayed distinctive lipid lowering effect in its capacity to revert the plasma levels of total cholesterol (TC), triglycerides (TG) and plasma lipids which were elevated by triton WR-1339 in rats and fructose rich high fat diet (HFD) in hamsters (Chander et al. 2004). The elevation in serum low-density lipoprotein cholesterol (LDL-C) and very low-density lipoprotein cholesterol (VLDL-C) noticeable in ISO treated rats was successfully reversed by TAEE dosage (Parveen et al. 2011; Parveen et al. 2012). The extract even inhibited the development of atherosclerosis in white New Zealand rabbits fed with HFD by lowering TC, LDL-C and TG levels while simultaneously elevating the HDL-C level. The atherosclerotic lesions in the aorta were also reduced by the extract (Subramaniam et al. 2011). Similar lipid lowering action of the ethanolic extract of *T. arjuna* was also visualized in case of the caffeine induced coronary heart diseased rats, hyperlipidemic male Charles Foster rats, triton induced hyperlipidemic male rats and hypercholesterolemic albino wistar rats (Asha and Taju 2011; Chander et al. 2004). This hypolipidemic property is modulated via the suppression of hepatic cholesterol biosynthesis, enhanced fecal bile acid like cholic acid and deoxycholic acid removal and elevated plasma lecithin:cholesterol acyltransferase action and induction of receptor mediated catabolism of

LDL-C (Khanna et al. 1996). Though the ethanolic extract was superior in manifesting hypolipidemic property, the aqueous extract (i.e. TAAE) was also capable of causing a statistically remarkable lowering of atherogenic lipids but simultaneously an elevation in HDL-C concentration in IL-18 treated mice (Bhat et al. 2017).

7.7 CLINICAL TRIALS

After understanding the demonstration of cardiotonic behavior of *T. arjuna* in pre-clinical studies, diving into the clinical trials would definitely give us a better insight of its proposed behavior. The clinical experimental design involving treatment of patients with refractory chronic congestive heart failure with the aqueous extract (i.e. TAAE) demonstrated amelioration in cardiac functions including decline in left ventricular end diastolic and end systolic volume indices, elevation in left ventricular stroke volume index and left ventricular ejection fractions (LVEF) (Bharani et al. 1995). Similar results were also reported in a case study involving 30 rheumatic valvular heart diseased patients using the aqueous extract (Antani et al. 1991). In another study involving 10 patients with chronic heart disease and hypertension, a herbo-mineral preparation containing *T. arjuna* called Abana significantly prohibits platelet adhesion and adrenaline-stimulated platelet aggregation (Wahal 1991). The administration of bark powder along with other anti-anginal drugs causes amelioration in exercise tolerance and decrease in frequency of angina attacks in coronary artery disease (CAD) patients. Decline in angina frequency and left ventricular mass along with improvement in LVEF was noticeable in patients with post-myocardial infarction and ischemic cardiomyopathy. Even promising results have been obtained in case of hypertensive patients where a decline in echocardiographic left ventricular internal diameter, systolic blood pressure, left posterior wall thickness and interventricular septum was observed by administration of bark extract of *T. arjuna* in a polyherbal formulation (Ygnanarayan et al. 1997). The lipid profile (TC, LDL-C) has been lowered along with lipid peroxides in patients with Coronary Heart Disease (CHD) and also in CAD patients by the administration of *T. arjuna* bark powder (Gupta et al. 2001). The administration of capsules of *T. arjuna* as an adjuvant therapy decreased the expression of different immuno-inflammatory markers like IL-8, IL-1β, NF-kappa-B inhibitor zeta (NF-κBIZ), FOS (Fos Proto-Oncogene, AP-1 Transcription Factor Subunit), JUN (Jun Proto-Oncogene, AP-1 Transcription Factor Subunit), cAMP Response Element Binding Protein (CREB-1) and IL-6R in CAD patients (Kapoor et al. 2015).

7.8 IMMUNOMODULATORY ASPECTS

T. arjuna is also capable of exerting its influence on the expression of various genes like Heat Shock Protein (HSP), Aquaporins (AQPs), Matrix Metalloproteinases (MMPs) both at transcriptional and translational level by upregulating and downregulating the necessary genes which in turn facilitates its cardiotonic behavior. For instance, the stimulation of myocardial HSP72 was brought about by the dose of 500–750 mg/kg/day TACMCE in ischemic reperfused rats (Gauthaman et al. 2005). Moreover both the aqueous and the ethanolic extracts (i.e. TAAE and TAEE) were capable of lowering the amounts of typical inflammatory marker proteins – viz LPS induced TNF-α released by human monocytic (THP-1) cells and TNF-α stimulated cell surface adhesion protein molecules on human aortic endothelial cells (HAECs), namely vascular cell adhesion molecule-1 (VCAM-1) and E-selectin (Kokkiripati et al. 2013). IL-18 is a powerful pro-inflammatory cytokine with pleiotropic characteristics generated constitutively by various cell types. Enhanced amounts of IL-18 are correlated with the presence of atherosclerosis. IL-18 acts by attaching itself to the interleukin-18 receptor α (IL-18Rα) expressed on numerous cells and modulates its signaling through stimulation of nuclear factor kappa-light-chain-enhancer of activated B cells (NF-κB) and also through p38 mitogen-activated protein kinase (p38 MAPK) pathway. The administration of TAAE caused prominent downregulation of NF-κB in IL-18 treated mice. The extract also causes

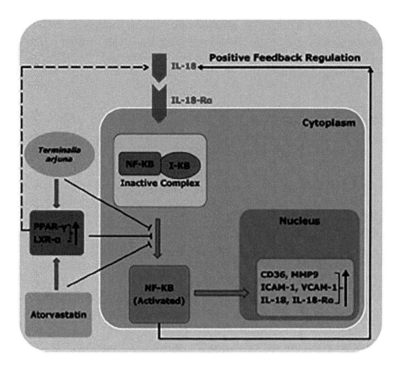

FIGURE 7.2 Scheme demonstrating the protection exhibited by TAAE against IL-18 induced atherosclerosis via NF-κB/PPAR-γ mediated pathway.

Source: Bhat et al. (2017).

improvement of cholesterol trafficking regulator genes including peroxisome proliferator-activated receptor-γ (PPAR-γ) and liver X receptor-α (LXR-α). The downregulation of NF-κB decreases IL-18 action and its further stimulation along with the inhibition of expression of cytokines, chemokines and adhesion molecules thereby blocking the occurrence of atherosclerotic lesions. Thus, the herb *T. arjuna* has an innate capacity to reduce the inflammatory cascade through pleiotropic stimulation of PPAR-γ and LXR-α that might be responsible for cardiotonic property. The TAAE also caused a prominent reduction of MMP-9 expression in IL-18 treated mice which might be due to the decreased oxidized LDL-C levels (Ox-LDL) leading to decreased atherosclerotic lesion progression. A prominent downregulation of the cell adhesion molecules (CAMs) including VCAM-1 and intercellular adhesion molecule 1 (ICAM-1) at RNA and protein levels was demonstrated by TAAE dose in IL-18 treated mice. As activated PPAR-γ is found to prohibit the TNF-α stimulated CAMs through blockage of NF-κB action, thus it is highly likely that downregulation of IL-18 stimulated CAMs by TAAE might be modulated through PPAR-γ/NF-κB pathway (Figure 7.2) (Bhat et al. 2017).

These findings can be well correlated with the outcome of an experiment in which the aqueous extract (i.e. TAAE) alone was capable of significantly prohibiting the expression of interleukin-18 (IL-18), along with Matrix Metalloproteinase-2 (MMP-2) and Cyclooxygenase 2 (COX-2) at both the RNA and protein level. The marker mRNAs for cardiac hypertrophy including β-Myosin Heavy Chain (MHC), skeletal α-actin, brain natriuretic peptide (BNP) and TGF-β were analyzed and were found to be elevated in ISO induced hypertrophied rats. The TAAE extract was capable of reinstating their levels to a great extent. Even the level of nodal signaling kinase, extracellular signal-regulated kinase (ERK) enhanced by ISO was restored to one-third the baseline level by aqueous dose. Similar results were witnessed in case of survival kinase Akt, ER stress marker glucose regulated protein 78 (GRP-78) and epigenetic regulator histone deacetylase 5 (HDAC 5) where the extract restored their levels to various extent (Kumar et al. 2017). Although NF-κB was regarded as a pro-hypertrophic transcription factor, it has been found to exert an anti-hypertrophic effect. ISO treatment enhanced their levels but TAAE further caused its level to shoot up which is indicative of successful gene expression reprogramming by the extract. Furthermore, proteomic study reflected the capability of TAAE in restoring the levels of purinergic receptor, phosphoinositide 3-kinase (PI3K), myosin light chain 3 (MLC3) and tropomyosin α-1. Even the levels of proteins like GAPDH, mitochondrial malate dehydrogenase (MDH), carnosine dipeptidase modulated by ISO were reinstated by TAAE. However there are certain proteins which were overexpressed by ISO but not reinstated by the aqueous extract. Amongst these proteins are ADP ribosyltransferase, ornithine transferase, C type lectin domain family 12, C type natriuretic peptide (NPP), Serpine 1-mRNA binding protein and COMM domain containing 7. Thus, the ameliorative influence of TAEE seems to be wide yet selective as it is incapable of restoring the amounts of aforementioned proteins (Kumar et al. 2017). The extract is demonstrated to prohibit the expression of activator protein 1 (AP-1), GATA-binding factor 1 (GATA-1), signal transducer and activator of transcription 3 (STAT-3) and cAMP Response Element-Binding Protein (CREB) and target DNA elements like NF-κB (Lampronti et al. 2008). AQPs are a group of integral membrane proteins that are selectively expressed in the myocardium and facilitates the transportation of water and solutes like urea and glycerol. Transcriptional analysis revealed the overexpression of distinctive aquaporin sub-types like *aqp1*, *aqp4*, *aqp5* and *aqp7* in ISO induced myocardial infarcted group of rats. The dose of *Terminalia arjuna* methanolic extract (TAME) was capable of downregulating these genes suggesting a possible role of the extract in cardioprotection as their upregulation was associated with the process of edema formation and cardiac dysfunction (Das and Dutta 2020). Proteomic analysis using TAAE in hypercholesterolemic rabbits involved the downregulation of various proteins like TNF-α, COX-2, MMP-9, HSP60, ICAM-5, Endothelin-3 (ET-3), Vimentin, Protein S100-A9, which are known for being correlated with endothelial dysfunction, plaque rupture, inflammation and immune imbalance (Rather et al. 2016). Malfunctioning of the vascular endothelium is a common observation leading to the occurrence of cardiovascular diseases. Endothelin-1 (ET-1) is correlated with elevated oxidative stress and endothelial dysfunction in humans. The concentration of ET-1 is found to be elevated in various cells like endothelial cells, cardiac myocytes and inflammatory cells like macrophages under different pathophysiological conditions. The enhanced concentration of ET-1 causes activation of macrophages leading to secretion of pro-inflammatory and chemotactic mediators including IL-1, IL-6, IL-8 and TNF-α that play a role in atherosclerotic process. TAEE was able to reduce the levels of both ET-1 and inflammatory cytokine levels (Khaliq, Parveen, Singh, Gondal et al. 2013). The ethanolic extract when compared with atorvastatin (a statin medication) was found to be more effective in lowering TNF-α level while atorvastatin was more capable in declining IL-18 levels in hypercholesterolemic rabbits. The expression level of High-sensitivity C-reactive protein (hsCRP), a biomarker of inflammation that is capable of predicting the incident myocardial infarction, peripheral arterial disease, stroke and sudden cardiac death, was reduced significantly by TAEE in these rabbits (Rather et al. 2015).

7.9 CLINICAL STUDY

The successful pre-clinical trials called for the clinical trials in patients to look further into the immunomodulatory aspects associated with the administration of the *T. arjuna* extracts. A striking clinical case cites the capability of the ethanolic extract (i.e. TAEE) in suppressing 50% of platelet aggregation in CAD patients which might be due to its antioxidant activity either by prohibiting the generation of endogenous mediators derived from phospholipid peroxidation or by decreasing platelet responsiveness to agonists by blocking the occurrence of lipid peroxidation (Malik et al. 2009). The bark extract prominently reduces the LPS stimulated expression of inflammatory genes such as IL-18, COX-2, Receptor for advanced glycation end products (RAGE) and MMP-2 in peripheral blood mononuclear cells (PBMCs) of CADs (Bhat et al. 2017). It was also found that action of aortic prostaglandin E_2 (PGE2), known to generate coronary vasodilation and enhanced coronary flow in CAD patients, was elevated after the dose of *T. arjuna* (Bhatia et al. 1998). The enhanced systolic and diastolic blood pressure was decreased to the basal levels in CAD patients after month-long *T. arjuna* therapy while the lipid profile also showed positive results. The pulse rate and the total platelet count also showed a sharp decline in these patients. Molecular docking analysis unfolds the triterpenoid arjunolic acid as a potential phytocompound for developing therapeutic targeting Apo lipoprotein-E (APOE) in CAD patients (Hazarika et al. 2021).

7.10 CELLULAR ASPECTS

The studies concerned with the demonstration of the cardioprotective behavior in terms of reinstatement of the histopathological alterations through various experiments further cements its position as a miraculous medicinal plant affecting the different levels of organization inside living organisms. If the case of the histopathological changes due to the ISO induced ischemic reperfusion in rats is taken into consideration, it was found that TAAE reversed the condition and caused the restoration of the normal architecture of myofibrillar striated structure with complete preservation of cardiac muscle fibers (Karthikeyan et al. 2003). Similar results were also reported in case of myocardial infarcted rats induced by ISO where TAEE and TAAE helped to reverse the histopathological alterations in the rat myocardium (Sivakumar and Rajeshkumar 2014). The unnatural fine structural changes, alterations in myocardial structure, cardiac myocyte hypertrophy, interstitial edema, fibrosis brought about by CCl_4 treatment and ISO treatment respectively, were restored back to their normal conditions by the administration of TAEE (Manna et al. 2007). Consistent with the aforementioned findings was the outcome of the experiment demonstrating the capability of the TAME in reverting the ISO induced muscle separation and lymphocyte infiltration in myocardial infarcted group of rats (Das and Dutta 2020). The highly effective chemotherapeutic agent, DOX, induced shrinkage of epicardium and reduced the density of myocardium along with hyalinization. Vacuolated enlarged endocardium are prominent along with the loss of myofibrils or functional cardiomyocytes and are responsible for LV dysfunction. These visualizable structural alterations are also blocked by co-treatment with TAAE (Bishop and Liu 2017). The extract was also capable of limiting the appearance of atherosclerotic lesions in IL-18 treated mice thereby concentrating the lesions only to the base of the aorta while making the descending aorta completely devoid of such lesions (Bhat et al. 2017). Collagen deposition is considered to be a trademark of pathological hypertrophy. Enhancement in collagen content and its progressive maturation is responsible for myocardial dysfunction. The antioxidant feature of TAAE is correlated with the inhibition of elevation in myocardial collagen content as evident from light microscopy studies. Similarly, the TAAE also exhibited comparable results with histopathological alteration brought about by Cd administration (Bhattacharjee et al. 2019). The anti-apoptotic evaluation performed by using Terminal deoxynucleotidyl transferase dUTP nick end labeling (TUNEL) assay and the localization of Bax and Bcl-2 proteins to characterize the association of apoptosis in ISO-administered rats demonstrated the occurrence of apoptosis while pre-treatment with TAEE and α-tocopherol decreased apoptotic cell number and ameliorated Bax expression simultaneously (Shukla, Sharma and Singh, 2015).

7.11 OTHER FOODS, HERBS, SPICES AND BOTANICALS USED

The incorporation of *T. arjuna* in different products has been found in the present-day world. The first of its use comes in the form of herbal ghee which is marketed globally today as medicinal ghee. This possesses a typical flavor, a bitter or pungent taste and a dark color, and is not suitable for daily consumption. Arjuna ghee has been developed for having cardioprotective property against CVDs and the product was more resistant to oxidative degradation compared to conventional ghee. The consumer acceptability of the product is incredibly high (Upadhyay et al. 2001). The incorporation

Terminalia arjuna and Cardiovascular Protection

of 2% of *T. arjuna* bark extract to buffalo meat rolls increased hardness, springiness and cohesiveness of the developed product and consequently, buffalo male calf meat rolls with excellent textural properties can be developed (Verma et al. 2012). The development of herbal green tea with *T. arjuna* bark in conjugation with *Withania somnifera* stem, Cinnamon bark, *Tinospora cordifolia* stem is yet another excellent source of nutraceuticals and flavoring agents with numerous health benefits, making it a perfect physical and psychological health rejuvenator (Wang et al. 2010). The blending of encapsulated *T. arjuna* in vanilla chocolate dairy drink added therapeutic benefits as it exhibited hypolipidemic and antioxidant activities for treating CVDs (Sawale et al. 2016).

7.12 TOXICITY AND CAUTIONARY NOTES

In majority of the studies, *T. arjuna* is being reported as a safe medicinal plant with tremendous medicinal benefits and few side effects on health. However, moderate complications like nausea, gastritis, headache, bodyaches, constipation have been reported. There have been no cases of hematological, renal or metabolic toxicity reported so far, even after 24 long months of its administration (Dwivedi et al. 1989; Bharani et al. 1995). In a study, administration of TAEE caused decrease in thyroid function and cardiac lipid peroxidation, which suggests that its cardioprotective nature might be exhibited via prohibition of thyroid function. This view is also being backed by the fact that hyperthyroidism causes tachycardia, hypertension and cardiac hypertrophy. As both the thyroid hormones, triiodothyronine (T_3) and tetraiodothyronine (T_4) were lowered, it seems that the extract is able to block thyroid function both at glandular (major source of T_4 synthesis) and at peripheral level of T_4 to T_3 conversion. This extract enhanced hepatic lipid peroxidation in euthyroid animals, indicating its toxic nature. Lower dose has no effect on thyroid functions or cardiac lipid peroxidation while higher concentration may be hepatotoxic and as such consumption of higher doses should be avoided. Furthermore, this plant extract must not be ingested by healthy individuals as it might cause hepatotoxicity and hypothyroidism (Parmar et al. 2006). To date this is an isolated report in the literature citing its toxic effects. Acute and oral toxicological study demonstrated that limited oral dosage of 2000 mg/kg did not cause toxicity and death in animals. Thus, the long-term usage of *T. arjuna* needs to be elucidated and there is an urgency for well-maintained multi-centric clinical trials in huge subject set-up with a standardized product for figuring out the real therapeutic potential of *T. arjuna*.

7.13 SUMMARY POINTS

- *Terminalia arjuna* (Roxb.) Wight and Arn is a valuable medicinal plant in use in different systems of medicine like Ayurveda, Unani and Homeopathy since ancient times for the remedy of a number of cardiovascular diseases like congestive heart failure, heart attack, cardiomyopathy, rheumatic heart disease and ischemic mitral regurgitation.
- Arjuna, a deciduous tree which attains a height of 60–80 feet with strengthened trunk, hanging branches, simple leaves, immobile bisexual flowers and elliptical fibrous woody fruits, is found throughout India, Burma, Mauritius and Sri Lanka.
- The different solvent extracts primarily of the bark, like ethanolic and aqueous extract, were capable of inhibiting ROS generation by enhancing the activity of antioxidant enzymes like Mn-Zn-SOD, CAT, GPx, GST thereby strengthening the antioxidant defense system of the body.
- The alterations in the mitochondrial membrane potential (indicative of defective cell bioenergetics homoeostasis) and also in the amount of cardiac marker enzymes like CK-MB, SGPT, ALP, SGOT, LDH5 brought about by the action of DOX and Cd administration respectively was reinstated by the action of the aqueous extract.
- Most studies on the occurrence of CVDs in in vivo models have been concerned with the β-adrenergic agonist called Isoproterenol (ISO), the administering of which not only

causes changes in cardiac marker enzymes and antioxidant enzymes but also in the LVP and LVEDP. The restoration is being carried out by the dosage of ethanolic extract of the bark with clinical trials involving CHF patients substantiating pre-clinical trials.

- The ISO also causes interference in the JNK signaling pathway by stimulating the phosphorylation of JNK while the ethanolic extract reverted all these physiological imbalances done to the body.
- The anti-hyperlipidemic property of the plant has been well manifested both in clinical and pre-clinical trials as the extracts are well capable of depleting the levels of TG, TC, LDL-C while elevating the levels of HDL-C. Even the extracts were efficient enough in reviving the normal architecture of the heart in hypertensive patients involving decrease in echocardiographic left ventricular internal diameter and left posterior wall thickness and interventricular septum.
- The bark extracts demonstrated their cardiotonic behavior even at the molecular level by enhancing and suppressing the expression of genes like MMP-2, COX-2, GATA-1, IL-18, STAT-3, MHC, BNP, CREB, TGF-β, AP-1, AQPs both at transcriptional and translational levels.
- The marked histopathological modifications brought about by the administration of chemicals like CCl_4, ISO or DOX, like damage to the architecture of the heart including cardiac myocyte hypertrophy, interstitial edema and fibrosis, was also brought back to normal condition by the application of the extracts.
- *T. arjuna* has found application in the form of different products in the market like Arjuna ghee or herbal green tea developed in conjugation with *Withania somnifera* stem, Cinnamon bark, *Tinospora cordifolia* stem or blended vanilla chocolate dairy drink.
- *T. arjuna* is regarded as a safe medicinal plant with magnanimous health benefits and minimum side effects involving blockage of thyroid function and lowering of T_3 and T_4 hormones. However, the therapeutic potential of the plant overpowers these effects and makes it a consumable plant, especially for patients with CVDs.

REFERENCES

Alam, M. S., Kaur, G., Ali, A., Hamid, H., Ali, M., and M. Athar. 2008. Two new bioactive oleanane triterpene glycosides from Terminalia arjuna. Natural Product Research 22, no. 14: 1279–1288. doi: 10.1080/14786410701766380.

Ali, A., Kaur, G., Hamid, H., Abdullah, T., Ali, M., Niwa, M., and M. S. Alam. 2003. Terminoside A, a new triterpene glycoside from the bark of Terminalia arjuna inhibits nitric oxide production in murine macrophages. Journal of Asian Natural Products Research 5, no. 2 (June): 137–142. doi: 10.1080/1028602031000066834.

Amalraj, A., and S. Gopi. 2016. Medicinal properties of *Terminalia arjuna (Roxb.) Wight & Arn.*: A review. Journal of Traditional and Complementary Medicine 7, no. 1 (March): 65–78. doi: 10.1016/j.jtcme.2016.02.003.

Antani, J. A., Gandhi, S., and N. J. Antani. 1991. Terminalia arjuna in congestive heart failure (Abstract). Journal of Association of Physicians of India 39, no. 801.

Arai, M., Yoguchi, A., Takizawa, T., Yokoyama, T., Kanda, T., Kurabayashi, M., and R. Nagai. 2000. Mechanism of doxorubicin-induced inhibition of sarcoplasmic reticulum Ca(2+)-ATPase gene transcription. Circulation Research 86, no. 1 (January): 8–14. doi: 10.1161/01.res.86.1.8.

Asha, S and G. Taju. 2011. Cardioprotective effect of Terminalia arjuna on caffeine induced coronary heart disease. International Journal of Pharmaceutical Sciences and Research 3, no. 1 (November): 150–153. https://ijpsr.com/bft-article/cardioprotective-effect-of-terminalia-arjuna-on-caffeine-induced-coronary-heart-disease/.

Bajpai, M., Pande, A., Tewari, S. K., and D. Prakash. 2005. Phenolic contents and antioxidant activity of some food and medicinal plants. International Journal of Food Sciences and Nutrition 56, no. 4 (June): 287–291. doi: 10.1080/09637480500146606.

Berthiaume, J. M., and K. B. Wallace. 2007. Adriamycin-induced oxidative mitochondrial cardiotoxicity. Cell Biology and Toxicology 23, no. 1 (January): 15-25. doi: 10.1007/s10565-006-0140-y.

Bharani, A., Ganguly, A., and K. D. Bhargava. 1995. Salutary effect of Terminalia Arjuna in patients with severe refractory heart failure. International Journal of Cardiology 49, no. 3 (May): 191–199. doi: 10.1016/0167-5273(95)02320-v.

Bhat, O. M., Kumar, P. U., Rao, K. R., Ahmad, A., and V. Dhawan. 2017. Terminalia arjuna prevents Interleukin-18-induced atherosclerosis via modulation of NF-κB/PPAR-γ-mediated pathway in Apo E-/- mice. Inflammopharmacology 26, no. 2 (April): 583–598. doi: 10.1007/s10787-017-0357-9.

Bhatia, J., Bhattacharya, S. K., Mahajan, P., and S. Dwivedi. 1998. Effect of Terminalia arjuna on coronary flow: An experimental study (Abstract). Indian Journal of Pharmacology 30, no. 118.

Bhatia, J., Bhattacharya, S. K., Mahajan, P., and S. Dwivedi. 2000. Effect of Terminalia arjuna on blood pressure of anaesthetised dogs (Abstract). Indian Journal of Pharmacology 32 (January): 159–160. www.researchgate.net/publication/284669329_Effect_of_Terminalia_arjuna_on_blood_pressure_of_anaesthetised_dogs.

Bhattacharjee, B., Pal, P. K., Ghosh, A. K., Mishra, S., Chattopadhyay, A., and D. Bandyopadhyay. 2019. Aqueous bark extract of Terminalia arjuna protects against cadmium-induced hepatic and cardiac injuries in male Wistar rats through antioxidative mechanisms. Food and Chemical Toxicology 124:249–264. doi: 10.1016/j.fct.2018.12.008.

Bishop, S., and S. J. Liu. 2017. Cardioprotective action of the aqueous extract of Terminalia arjuna bark against toxicity induced by doxorubicin. Phytomedicine 36 (December): 210–216. doi: 10.1016/j.phymed.2017.10.007.

Carluccio, M. A., Siculella, L., Ancora, M. A., Massaro, M., Scoditti, E., Storelli, C., Visioli, F., Distante, A., and R. De Caterina. 2003. Olive oil and red wine antioxidant polyphenols inhibit endothelial activation: Antiatherogenic properties of Mediterranean diet phytochemicals. Arteriosclerosis, Thrombosis, and Vascular Biology 23, no. 4 (February): 622–629. doi: 10.1161/01.ATV.0000062884.69432.A0.

Chander, R., Singh, K., Khanna, A. K., Kaul, S. M., Puri, A., Saxena, R., Bhatia, G., Rizvi, F., and A. K. Rastogi. 2004. Antidyslipidemic and antioxidant activities of different fractions of Terminalia arjuna stem bark. Indian Journal of Clinical Biochemistry 19, no. 2 (July): 141–148. doi: 10.1007/BF02894274.

Chaudhari, M., and S. Mengi. 2006. Evaluation of phytoconstituents of Terminalia arjuna for wound healing activity in rats. Phytotherapy Research 20, no. 9 (September): 799–805. doi: 10.1002/ptr.1857.

Das, M., and A. Dutta. 2020. Expression patterns of different isoforms of aquaporins in isoproterenol induced myocardial infarction model in rat treated with Terminalia arjuna Bark extract. Medicinal Plants: International Journal of Phytomedicines and Related Industries 12, no. 2: 265. 10.5958/0975-6892.2020.00035.0.

Dutta, M., Ghosh, A., Basu, A. K., Bandyopadhyay, D., and A. Chattopadhyay. 2013. Protective effect of aqueous bark extract of Terminalia arjuna against copper-ascorbate induced oxidative stress in vitro in goat heart mitochondria. International Journal of Pharmacy and Pharmaceutical Sciences 5, no. 2 (January): 439–447. www.scinapse.io/papers/2575539990.

Dwivedi, S., Chansouria, J. P. N., Somani, P. N., and K. N. Udupa. 1989. Effect of Terminalia arjuna on ischaemic heart disease. Alternative Medicine 3, no. 2: 115–122.

Gauthaman, K., Banerjee, S., Dinda, A. K., Ghosh, C. C, and S. K. Maulik. 2005. Terminalia arjuna (Roxb.) protects rabbit heart against ischemic-reperfusion injury: Role of antioxidant enzymes and heat shock protein. Journal of Ethnopharmacology 96, (October): 403–409. doi: 10.1016/j.jep.2004.08.040.

Gauthaman, K., Maulik, M., Kumari, R., Manchanda, S. C., Dinda, A. K., and S. K. Maulik. 2001. Effect of chronic treatment with bark of Terminalia arjuna: A study on the isolated ischemic-reperfused rat heart. Journal of Ethnopharmacology 75, no. 2–3 (May): 197–201. doi: 10.1016/s0378-8741(01)00183-0.

Gupta, R., Singhal, S., Goyle, A., and V. N. Sharma. 2001. Antioxidant and hypocholesterolaemic effects of Terminalia arjuna tree-bark powder: A randomised placebo-controlled trial. Journal of the Association of Physicians of India 49, February:231–235. www.researchgate.net/publication/12106586_Antioxidant_and_hypocholesterolaemic_effects_of_Terminalia_arjuna_tree-bark_powder_a_randomised_placebo-controlled_trial.

Hazarika, L., Sen, S., and J. Doshi. 2021. Molecular docking analysis of arjunolic acid from Terminalia arjuna with a coronary artery disease target APOE4. Bioinformation 17, no. 11 (October): 949–958. www.bioinformation.net/017/97320630017949.pdf.

Ichikawa, Y., Ghanefar, M., Bayeva, M., Wu, R., Khechaduri, A., Naga Prasad, S. V., Mutharasan, R. K., Naik, T. J., and H. Ardehali. 2014. Cardiotoxicity of doxorubicin is mediated through mitochondrial iron accumulation. Journal of Clinical Investigation 124, no. 2: 617–630. doi: 10.1172/JCI72931.

Jahan, N., Rahman, K., Ali, S., Asi, M. R., and A. Akhtar. 2012. Cardioprotective potential of gemmomodified extract of terminalia arjuna against chemically induced myocardial injury in rabbits. Pakistan Veterinary Journal 32, no. 2 (January): 255–259. https://doaj.org/article/957c09e66c754293abac4eb44d8ef6c4.

Kapoor, D., Trikha, D., Vijayvergiya, R., Parashar, K. K., Kaul, D., and V. Dhwan. 2015. Short-term adjuvant therapy with terminalia arjuna attenuates ongoing inflammation and immune imbalance in patients with stable coronary artery disease: In Vitro and In Vivo evidence. Journal of Cardiovascular Translational Research 8, 3 (April): 173–186. doi: 10.1007/s12265-015-9620-x.

Karthikeyan, K., Bai, B. R., Gauthaman, K., Sathish, K. S., and S. N. Devaraj. 2003. Cardioprotective effect of the alcoholic extract of Terminalia arjuna bark in an in vivo model of myocardial ischemic reperfusion injury. Life Science 73, no. 21 (October): 2727–2739. doi: 10.1016/s0024-3205(03)00671-4.

Khaliq, F., and M. Halim. 2018. Role of Terminalia Arjuna in improving cardiovascular functions: A review. Indian Journal of Physiology and Pharmacology 62, no. 1 (January): 8–19. https://ijpp.com/IJPP%20archives/2018_62_1/8-19.pdf.

Khaliq, F., Parveen, A., Singh, S., Gondal, R., Hussain, M. E., and M. Fahim. 2013. Improvement in myocardial function by Terminalia arjuna in streptozotocin-induced diabetic rats: Possible mechanisms. Journal of Cardiovascular Pharmacology and Therapeutics 18, no. 5 (September): 481–489. doi: 10.1177/1074248413488831.

Khaliq, F., Parveen, A., Singh, S., Hussain, M. E., and M. Fahim. 2013. Terminalia arjuna improves cardiovascular autonomic neuropathy in streptozotocin-induced diabetic rats. Cardiovascular Toxicology 13, no. 1 (March): 68–76. doi: 10.1007/s12012-012-9187-6.

Khanna, A. K., Chander, R., and N. K. Kapoor. 1996. Terminalia arjuna: An ayurvedic cardiotonic, regulates lipid metabolism in hyperlipaemic rats. Phytotherapy Research 10, no. 8 (December): 663–665. https://doi.org/10.1002/(SICI)1099-1573(199612)10:8<663::AID-PTR935>3.0.CO;2-W.

Kokkiripati, P. K., Kamsala, R. V., Bashyam, L., Manthapuram, N., Bitla, P., Peddada, V., Raghavendra, A. S., and S. D. Telai. 2013. Stem-bark of Terminalia arjuna attenuates human monocytic (THP-1) and aortic endothelial cell activation. Journal of Ethnopharmacology 146, no. 2 (March): 456–464. doi: 10.1016/j.jep.2012.12.050.

Kolodziej, H., and A. F. Kiderlen. 2005. Antileishmanial activity and immune modulatory effects of tannins and related compounds on Leishmania parasitised RAW 264.7 cells. Phytochemistry 66, no. 17 (September): 2056–2071. doi: 10.1016/j.phytochem.2005.01.011. PMID: 16153409.

Kumar, G., Saleem, N., Kumar, S., Maulik, S. K., Ahmad, S., Sharma, M., and S. K Goswami. 2019. Transcriptomic validation of the protective effects of aqueous bark extract of Terminalia arjuna (Roxb.) on isoproterenol-induced cardiac hypertrophy in rats. Frontiers in Pharmacology 10, no. 10 (December): 1443. doi: 10.3389/fphar.2019.01443.

Kumar, N. 2014. Phytopharmacological overview on Terminalia arjuna Wight and Arn. World Journal of Pharmaceutical Sciences 2, no. 11 (October): 1557–1566. www.semanticscholar.org/paper/Phytopharmacological-overview-on-Terminalia-arjuna-Kumar/739058671200fd4d9c6ed866f7d2764a3e419853.

Kumar, S., Enjamoori, R., Jaiswal, A., Ray, R., Seth, S., and S. K. Maulik. 2009. Catecholamine-induced myocardial fibrosis and oxidative stress is attenuated by Terminalia arjuna (Roxb.). J Journal of Pharmacy and Pharmacology 61, no. 11 (November):1529–36. doi: 10.1211/jpp/61.11.0013.

Kumar, S., Jahangir Alam, Md., Prabhakar, P., Ahmad, S., Maulik, S. K., Sharma, M., and S. K. Goswami. 2017. Proteomic analysis of the protective effects of aqueous bark extract of Terminalia arjuna (Roxb.) on isoproterenol-induced cardiac hypertrophy in rats. Journal of Ethnopharmacology 23, no. 198 (February): 98–108. doi: 10.1016/j.jep.2016.12.050.

Lampronti, I., Khan, M. T., Borgatti, M., Bianchi, N., and R. Gambari. 2008. Inhibitory effects of Bangladeshi medicinal plant extracts on interactions between transcription factors and target DNA sequences. Evidence-Based Complementary and Alternative Medicine 5, no. 3 (September): 303–312. doi: 10.1093/ecam/nem042.

Malik, N., Dhawan, V., Bahl, A., and D. Kaul. 2009. Inhibitory effects of Terminalia arjuna on platelet activation in vitro in healthy subjects and patients with coronary artery disease. Platelets. 20, no. 3 (May): 183–190. doi: 10.1080/09537100902809004.

Manna, P., Sinha, M., and P. C. Sil. 2007. Phytomedicinal activity of Terminalia arjuna against carbon tetrachloride induced cardiac oxidative stress. Pathophysiology 14, no. 2 (May): 71–78. doi: 10.1016/j.pathophys.2007.05.002.

Maulik, S. K., and K. K. Talwar. 2012. Therapeutic potential of Terminalia arjuna in cardiovascular disorders. American Journal of Cardiovascular Drugs 12, no. 3 (June): 157–163. https://link.springer.com/article/10.2165/11598990-000000000-00000.

Mohanty, I. R., Borde, M., Kumar, C. S., and U. Maheshwari. 2019. Dipeptidyl peptidase IV inhibitory activity of Terminalia arjuna attributes to its cardioprotective effects in experimental diabetes: In silico, in vitro and in vivo analyses. Phytomedicine 57: 158–165. doi: 10.1016/j.phymed.2018.09.195.

Oberoi, L., Akiyama, T., Lee, K. H., and S. J. Liu. 2011. The aqueous extract, not organic extracts, of Terminalia arjuna bark exerts cardiotonic effect on adult ventricular myocytes. Phytomedicine 18, no. 4: 259–265. doi: 10.1016/j.phymed.2010.07.006.

Padma Sree, T. N., Krishna Kumar, S., Senthilkumar, A., Aradhyam, G. K., and S. Gummadi. 2007. In vitro effect of Terminalia arjuna bark extract on antioxidant enzyme catalase. Journal of Pharmacology and Toxicology 2: no. 8 (August): 698–708. doi: 10.3923/jpt.2007.698.708.

Parmar, H. S., Panda, S., Jatwa, R., and A. Kar. 2006. Cardio-protective role of Terminalia arjuna bark extract is possibly mediated through alterations in thyroid hormones. Pharmazie 61, no. 9 (September): 793–795. www.ingentaconnect.com/contentone/govi/pharmaz/2006/00000061/00000009/art00013?crawler=true.

Parveen, A., Babbar, R., Agarwal, S., Kotwani, A., and M. Fahim. 2011. Mechanistic clues in the cardioprotective effect of Terminalia arjuna bark extract in isoproterenol-induced chronic heart failure in rats. Cardiovascular Toxicology 11, no. 1 (March): 48–57. doi: 10.1007/s12012-010-9099-2.

Parveen, A., Babbar, R., Agarwal, S., Kotwani, A., M. Fahim. 2012. Terminalia arjuna enhances baroreflex sensitivity and myocardial function in isoproterenol-induced chronic heart failure rats. Journal of Cardiovascular Pharmacology and Therapeutics 17, no. 2 (June): 199–207. doi: 10.1177/1074248411416816.

Patnaik, T., Dey, R. K., and P. Gouda. 2007. Isolation of triterpenoidglycoside from bark of Terminalia arjuna using chromatographic technique and investigation of pharmacological behavior upon muscle tissues. European Journal of Advanced Chemistry Research 4: 474–479.

Pettit, G. R., Hoard, M. S., Doubek, D. L., Schmidt, J. M., Pettit, R. K., Tackett, L. P., and J. C Chapuis. 1996. Antineoplastic agents 338. The cancer cell growth inhibitory. Constituents of Terminalia arjuna (Combretaceae). Journal of Ethnopharmacology 53, no. 2 (August): 57–63. doi: 10.1016/S0378-8741(96)01421-3.

Rather, R. A., Dhawan, V., and D. Trikha. 2015. Effect of ethanolic fraction of Terminalia arjuna on inflammatory markers in hypercholesterolemic rabbits. Atherosclerosis 241, no. 1 (July): e55–56. https://doi.org/10.1016/j.atherosclerosis.2015.04.197.

Rather, R. A., Malik, V. S., Trikha, D., Bhat, O., and V. Dhawan. 2016. Aqueous Terminalia arjuna extract modulates expression of key atherosclerosis-related proteins in a hypercholesterolemic rabbit: A proteomic-based study. Proteomics: Clinical Applications 10, no. 7 (July): 750–759. doi: 10.1002/prca.201500114.

Santosh, K. C., Jahangir, M. A., Pankaj, P., Subir, K. M., and K. G. Shyama. 2017. Terminalia arjuna (Roxb.) reverses themolecular signature of fibrosis induced byisoproterenol in rat heart. American Journal of Phytomedicine and Clinical Therapeutics 5, no. 3 (November): 22. www.imedpub.com/articles/terminalia-arjuna-roxb-reverses-themolecular-signature-of-fibrosis-induced-byisoproterenol-in-rat-heart.php?aid=21258.

Sawale, P. D., Pothuraju, R., Abdul Hussain, S., Kumar, A., Kapila, S., and G. R. Patil. 2016. Hypolipidaemic and anti-oxidative potential of encapsulated herb (Terminalia arjuna) added vanilla chocolate milk in high cholesterol fed rats. Journal of the Science of Food and Agriculture 96, 4 (March): 1380–1385. doi: 10.1002/jsfa.7234.

Shastry Vishwanatha, G. L., Vaidya, S. K., C. R., Krishnadas, N., and S. Rangappa. 2010. Antioxidant and antimutagenic activities of bark extract of Terminalia arjuna. Asian Pacific Journal of Tropical Medicine 3, no. 12 (December): 965–970. www.researchgate.net/publication/236616376_Antioxidant_and_anti-mutagenic_activities_of_bark_extract_of_Terminalia_arjuna.

Shukla, S. K., Sharma, S. B., and U. R. Singh. 2015. Pre-treatment with α-tocopherol and Terminalia arjuna ameliorates, pro-inflammatory cytokines, cardiac and apoptotic markers in myocardial infracted rats. Redox Report 20. no. 2 (March): 49–59. doi: 10.1179/1351000214Y.0000000104.

Shukla, S. K., Sharma, S. B., Singh, U. R., Ahmad, S., and S. Dwivedi. 2015. Terminalia arjuna (Roxb.) Wight & Arn. augments cardioprotection via antioxidant and antiapoptotic cascade in isoproterenol induced cardiotoxicity in rats. Indian Journal of Experimental Biology 53, no. 12 (December): 810–818.

Sinha, M., Manna, P., and P. C. Sil. 2008. Terminalia arjuna protects mouse hearts against sodium fluoride-induced oxidative stress. Journal of Medicinal Food 11, no. 4 (December): 733–740. doi: 10.1089/jmf.2007.0130.

Sivakumar, V., and S. Rajeshkumar. 2014. Screening of cardioprotective effect of Terminalia arjuna Linn bark in isoproterenol: Induced myocardial infarction in experimental animals. International Journal of Pharma Sciences and Research 5, no. 6 (June): 262–268. www.ijpsr.info/docs/IJPSR14-05-06-004.pdf.

Subramaniam, S., Ramachandran, S., Uthrapathi, S., Gnamanickam, V. R., and G. P. Dubey. 2011. Anti-hyperlipidemic and antioxidant potential of different fractions of Terminalia arjuna Roxb. bark against PX-407 induced hyperlipidemia. Indian Journal of Experimental Biology. 49, no. 4 (April): 282–288. http://nopr.niscair.res.in/bitstream/123456789/11387/1/IJEB%2049(4)%20282-288.pdf.

Thangaraju, M. M., Tamatam, A., Bhat, P. V., Deshetty, U. M., Babusha, S. T., and F. Khanum, 2020. Terminalia arjuna extract attenuates isoproterenol-induced cardiac stress in wistar rats via an anti-apoptotic pathway. Proceedings of the National Academy of Sciences, India Section B: Biological Sciences 90, no. 3 (June). https://pubag.nal.usda.gov/catalog/7184051.

Upadhyay, R. K., Pandey, M. B., Jha, R. N., Singh, V. P., and V. B. Pandey. 2001. Triterpene glycoside from Terminalia arjuna. Journal of Asian Natural Products Research 3, no. 3 (October): 207–212. doi: 10.1080/10286020108041392.

Verma, S. C., Jain, C. L., Padhi, M. M., and R. B. Devalla. 2012. Microwave extraction and rapid isolation of arjunic acid from Terminalia arjuna (Roxb. ex DC.) stem bark and quantification of arjunic acid and arjunolic acid using HPLC-PDA technique. Journal of Separation Science 35, no. 13 (July): 1627–1633. doi: 10.1002/jssc.201200083.

Wahal, P. K. 1991. A preliminary report on the inhibitory effect of abana on platelet aggregation and adhesiveness in cases of coronary heart disease and hypertension. Probe 30: 312–315.

Wang, W., Ali, Z., Shen, Y., Li, X. C., and I. A. Khan. 2010. Ursane triterpenoids from the bark of Terminalia arjuna. Fitoterapia 81, no. 6 (September): 480–484. doi: 10.1016/j.fitote.2010.01.006.

Ygnanarayan, R., Sangle, S. A., Sirsikar, S. S., and D. K. Mitra. 1997. Regression of cardiac hypertrophy in hypertensive patients: Comparison of abana with propanolol. Phytotherapy Research 11: 257–259.

8 Baicalein Extract from Chinese Herbal Medicine to Use in Cardiovascular Diseases
Focus on Myocardial Ischemia/ Reperfusion Injury

Ramona D'Amico, Salvatore Cuzzocrea and Rosanna Di Paola

CONTENTS

8.1 Introduction 112
8.2 Source of Baicalein 113
    8.2.1 Extraction and Purification 113
    8.2.2 Absorption, Metabolism and Excretion of Baicalein 113
8.3 Use of Baicalein in Cardiovascular Disease 114
    8.3.1 Atherosclerosis 115
    8.3.2 Hypertension 115
    8.3.3 Heart Failure 116
8.4 Myocardial Ischemia/Reperfusion Injury: Molecular Mechanisms and Therapeutic Potential of Baicalein 117
    8.4.1 Inhibition of Oxidative Stress 117
    8.4.2 Mitigation of Inflammatory Response 118
    8.4.3 Modulation of Apoptosis Process 118
    8.4.4 Vascular Action 119
8.5 Conclusion 120
8.6 Toxicity and Cautionary Notes 120
8.7 Summary Points 120
References 121

LIST OF ABBREVIATIONS

Ang II   Angiotensin II
ARE   Antioxidant response element
AS   Atherosclerosis
CHM   Chinese herbal medicine
CRP   C-reactive protein
CVDs   Cardiovascular diseases
ECM   Extracellular matrix
ERK   Extracellular signal-regulated kinase
IL   Interleukin
I/R   Ischemia/Reperfusion
MAPK   Mitogen-activated protein kinase
MnSOD   Manganese superoxide dismutase

DOI: 10.1201/9781003220329-10

NF-kB   Nuclear factor-kB
Nrf2   Nuclear factor-erythroid 2-related factor 2
NO   Nitric oxide
ROS   Reactive oxygen species
TCM   Traditional Chinese medicine
TNF-α   Tumor necrosis factor-α

8.1 INTRODUCTION

Traditional Chinese medicine (TCM), which originated from more than 2500 years of Chinese medical practice, differs from Western medicine. Compared with modern medicine, experts believe that TCM has fewer side effects, is safe and has ideal effects in treating refractory chronic diseases (Xiao and Tao 2017). In addition, TCM can be co-administered with modern medicine or other traditional medicine to reduce toxicity. To date, TCM is a fully institutionalized part of Chinese health care and widely used with Western medicine. TCM encompasses many different practices (see Figure 8.1), but Chinese herbal medicine (CHM) is the principal form of TCM practice (Zhou et al. 2019). CHM consists in the use of plants (including berries, roots, seeds, bark, leaves or flowers) and other natural substances to treat and prevent disease. The use of herbal medicinal products and supplements has increased dramatically over the past 40 years as scientists have extracted and modified active ingredients from plants. In this regard, in recent years, flavonoids have attracted increasing interest because of their various beneficial biological activities to human health. Flavonoids are a group of various phytonutrients found in almost all plants and possess strong antioxidant properties. Baicalein is one of the flavonoids isolated from the root of *Scutellaria baicalensis* Georgi (Huang Qin in Chinese), which has a long history of practice in TCM. In addition to its antioxidant effects, baicalein exhibits multiple biological effects to alleviate or prevent some human diseases including cancers, autoimmune disorders, neurological disorders and inflammatory diseases (Xu et al. 2018; Mutha, Tatiya, and Surana 2021). Recently, many researchers have paid special attention to the cardioprotective properties of baicalein.

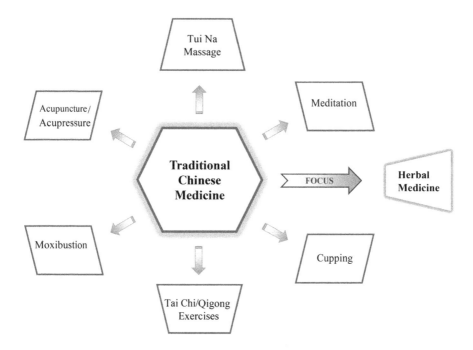

FIGURE 8.1 Representative practices of traditional Chinese medicine: focus on herbal medicine.

Baicalein Extract from Chinese Herbal Medicine 113

In this chapter, we introduce the biological effects of baicalein and discuss its cardioprotective features in cardiovascular diseases (CVDs) and in myocardial ischemia/reperfusion (I/R) injury, examining the underlying mechanisms involved in this property.

8.2 SOURCE OF BAICALEIN

Baicalein (5,6,7-trihydroxyflavone) is an aglycone derivative from baicalin (Dinda et al. 2017). The most important structural characteristic of baicalein is the presence of a di-*ortho*-hydroxyl functional group on ring-A (see Figure 8.2). The most researched source of baicalein is the root of *Scutellaria baicalensis* Georgi (*S. baicalensis*). This plant is native to East Asian countries, and it has been employed in traditional medical systems since ancient times (Zhao, Chen, and Martin 2016). The root of *S. baicalensis* is extensively used in TCM to treat a variety of conditions such as hyperlipidemia, dysentery, atherosclerosis, hypertension and respiratory disorders. Baicalein is also found in other Scutellaria species, *S. lateriflora*, *S. galericulata*, and *S. rivularia*. In addition, baicalein has also been found in the seed, fruit, root bark and leaf parts of *Oroxylum indicum* (Nik Salleh et al. 2020).

8.2.1 EXTRACTION AND PURIFICATION

Several methods have been used to extract baicalein from the dried root of *S. baicalensis*, including dynamic ultrasonic extraction, infrared-assisted self-enzymolysis extraction, ionic liquid-based microwave-assisted extraction, traditional extraction method and supercritical fluid extraction (Wang et al. 2017; Zhang et al. 2015). The latter two methods are the most applied to extract baicalein (Li, Jiang, and Chen 2004). The traditional extraction procedure is used to ground the raw material (dried root) into fine powder (Figure 8.3), after which 70% ethanol is used to collect the filtrate; this process is repeated numerous times. On the other hand, supercritical fluid extraction uses both methanol and ethanol to collect the extracts, as the highest flavonoid solubility is obtained in those solvents. The purity of the filtrate or extracts gained by these two methods are finally evaluated via high-performance liquid chromatography (Gao et al. 2016). Over 295 compounds, classified into flavonoids, phenylethanoid glycosides, iridoid glycosides, diterpenes, triterpenoids, alkaloids, phytosterols, polysaccharides, and other biocomponents, are isolated from *S. baicalensis* (Liang, Huang, and Chen 2017). Baicalein and its metabolite baicalin are the major bioactive components in *S. baicalensis*.

8.2.2 ABSORPTION, METABOLISM AND EXCRETION OF BAICALEIN

Baicalein is well absorbed from the stomach and small intestine as compared to the colon (Tuli et al. 2020). Importantly, the major route of metabolism for baicalein in plasma and urine is conjugated metabolism. Several studies showed that the intact levels of baicalein in plasma were negligible

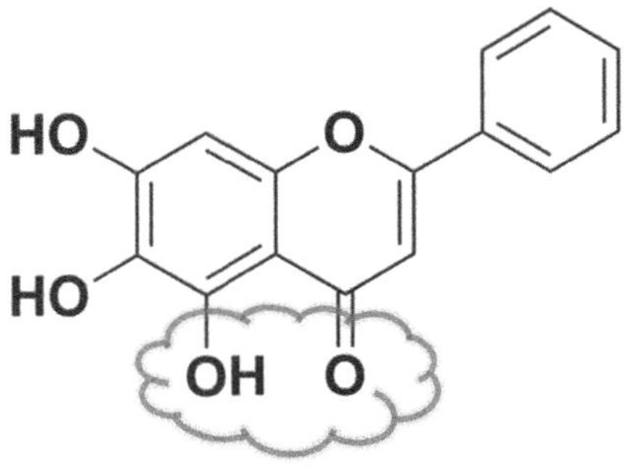

FIGURE 8.2 Chemical structure of baicalein with the di-ortho-hydroxyl functional group on ring-A in evidence.

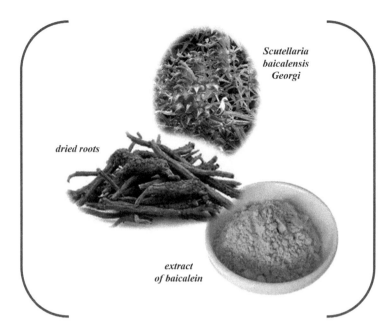

FIGURE 8.3 The dried root, principal medicinal part of *Scutellaria baicalensis* Georgi, and extract of baicalein.

following oral dosing of baicalein; on contrary, the conjugates of baicalein with glucuronides and sulfate examined in the plasma (Tuli et al. 2020; Fong et al. 2012). Following intravenous dosing of baicalein, about 76% of the baicalein was converted into the conjugated forms. Glucuronidation, glucosidation metabolites were abundant in the small intestine sample, dehydroxylation metabolites were abundant in the large intestine sample and methylation, sulfation metabolites were abundant throughout the intestine (Li et al. 2011; Zhang et al. 2013). It can be inferred that gut microbiota is responsible for various metabolites present in different intestinal tissue. Apart from the intestines, even the liver is able to metabolize baicalein, contributing to the first pass effect (Zhang et al. 2011). Therefore, the absolute systemic bioavailability of baicalein in its parent form is almost zero. Thus, the conjugate metabolites of baicalein are responsible for its *in vivo* effects.

8.3 USE OF BAICALEIN IN CARDIOVASCULAR DISEASE

Life-threatening conditions like congenital heart diseases, coronary heart disease, cerebrovascular, peripheral arterial, and pulmonary embolism are caused by impairment of the heart and blood vessels, and they are collectively known as cardiovascular diseases (CVDs). The World Health Organization has reported that CVDs are the primary cause of mortality worldwide, with an estimated 17.9 million deaths in 2019 (Sahin and Ilgun 2022), representing 32% of all global deaths. Of these deaths, 85% were due to heart attack and stroke. Patients with CVDs are treated by various medications to reduce hypertension, palpitation, cholesterol and blood vessel narrowing. While these treatments assist to reduce the severity of the diseases, they can cause serious side effects such as fatigue, headaches, shortness of breath and dizziness (Crea 2021; Aguilar-Ballester et al. 2021). For example, statins are the most effective drugs in the treatment of lowering low-density lipoproteins and coronary heart disease. However, they do cause cardiomyopathy or rhabdomyolysis and polyneuropathy with adverse side effects (Kukes et al. 2020). Hence, there is an urgent need for research and development to design new therapeutic agents with low side effects for the treatment of cardiovascular diseases. Recently, many researchers have paid special attention to the cardioprotective properties of baicalein. The natural polyphenols exert a vasodilator effect and are able to manage lipid profiles in the human system (Behl et al. 2020). So, it is rational to propose that baicalein might play an essential role in the pathogenesis of CVDs.

8.3.1 ATHEROSCLEROSIS

Atherosclerosis (AS) is the principal pathological basis of CVDs, which can lead to serious clinical events including unstable angina or myocardial infarction. The pathophysiological factors involving AS are lipid deposition, immune inflammatory response, oxidative stress damage, endothelial dysfunction and platelet aggregation (Wolf and Ley 2019). Sustained inflammation contributes to the overproduction of reactive oxygen species (ROS), which in turn exacerbates the inflammatory process and perturbs the function of the vasculature, triggering the atherosclerotic cascade (Marchio et al. 2019). Several biological processes associated with baicalein are involved in lipid regulation activities, including inhibition of accumulation of cholesterol and delayed transformation of macrophages into foam cells, which occurs in the early phases of AS (Tsai et al. 2016). Additionally, experimental data confirmed that baicalcin improves the state of blood lipid disorders, associated with decreasing the levels of serum markers of AS (total cholesterol, triacylglycerol, low-density lipoprotein cholesterol and apolipoproteins) (Seo et al. 2014; Chan et al. 2016). Thus, baicalein seems to exert protective effects against AS by targeting these proatherogenic processes (Figure 8.4).

8.3.2 HYPERTENSION

Hypertension is a complex condition in which the long-term force of the blood against your artery walls is high enough that it may eventually cause cardiovascular disease, including stroke, heart attack, heart failure and aneurysm (McManus et al. 2020). Recently, the oxidative stress and inflammatory response have been shown to play an essential role in the pathogenesis of hypertension. Many inflammatory markers such as C-reactive protein (CRP), cytokines and adhesion molecules have been found to be elevated in hypertensive patients supporting the role of inflammation in the hypertension (Angeli, Reboldi, and Verdecchia 2021). Another potential mechanism involved

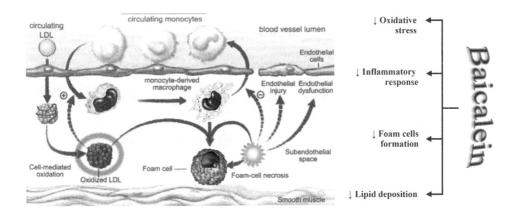

FIGURE 8.4 Schematic representation of sequential events involved in atherosclerosis.

Note: Monocytes are critical mediators in all stages of atherosclerosis. When they gain entry into the subendothelial spaces, the infiltrating monocytes transform into macrophages. Simultaneously, circulating LDL cholesterol also moves into the subendothelial space. Here, LDL are subjected to oxidative modification and are taken up by macrophages. These macrophages transform themselves into foam cells which become necrotic due to the accumulation of oxidized LDL. This leads to endothelial dysfunction, lipid deposition and injury. Baicalein, targeting these proatherogenic processes, is able to reduce atherosclerosis.

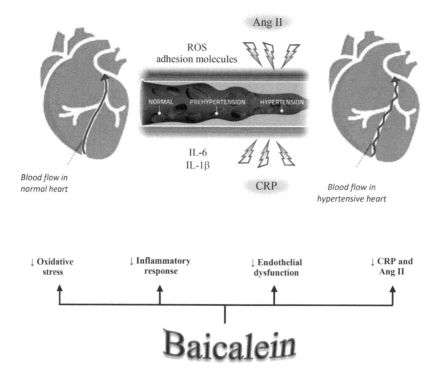

FIGURE 8.5 Schematic illustration of factors involved in hypertension.

Note: ROS, inflammatory cytokines and increased adhesion molecules are the principal features of hypertension. In particular, C-reactive protein (CRP) and angiotensin II (Ang II) induce endothelial dysfunction, activate platelets and aggravate stress-induced alterations in cardiac function. High levels of CRP are directly involved in vascular pathology via its effects on macrophages, endothelial cells and vascular smooth muscle cells. Angiotensin II, locally produced, raises blood pressure by promoting vasoconstriction and causing hypertension. Baicalein, due to its antioxidant and anti-inflammatory capability, ameliorates hypertension.

in the hypertension is enhancing angiotensin II (Ang II), as the main active peptide of the renin-angiotensin system that induces oxidative stress and apoptosis leading to endothelial dysfunction (Jackson 1989; Wu et al. 2021). Cumulative studies demonstrate that baicalein was able to reduce the endothelial dysfunction and oxidative stress induced by Ang II, as well as decrease the serum levels of high-sensitivity CRP, interleukin (IL)-6 and IL-1β in spontaneously hypertensive rats (Wang et al. 2015; Huang et al. 2005). Targeting these pathogenesis processes would explain the cardioprotective effects of baicalein on the improvement of hypertension (Figure 8.5).

8.3.3 Heart Failure

Heart failure is a serious disease resulting from inadequate cardiac output and subsequent dysregulation in compensatory mechanisms. The key histopathological features of heart failure are myocardial remodeling, hypertrophy and fibrosis (Bauersachs and Soltani 2021). Cardiac fibrosis is characterized by interstitial fibroblast proliferation and excessive production and deposition of myocardial extracellular matrix (ECM) proteins, due to over-expression of MMP-9 via induction of ERK phosphorylation (Prabhu and Frangogiannis 2016). Possibly, 12-LOX plays a key role in collagen deposition by elevating the expression of 12-HETE from arachidonic acid, which, in turn, enhances the extracellular signal-regulated kinase (ERK) phosphorylation and initiates both MMP-9 and TIMP-2 synthesis for collagen production and inhibition of its degradation (Dinda et al. 2017). The antifibrotic effects

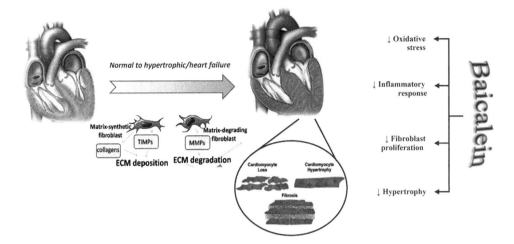

FIGURE 8.6 Mechanisms involved in heart failure.

Note: Extracellular matrix (ECM) remodeling and crosslinking play a crucial role in heart failure. After injury, activated cardiac fibroblasts induce collagen synthesis and production of antiproteases (such as TIMPs [tissue inhibitor of metalloproteinase]). Prolonged pressure overload may be associated with transition of infiltrating fibroblasts to a matrix-degrading phenotype that produces MMPs (matrix metalloproteinases), thus causing ECM degradation and generating matrix fragments. Baicalein is able to reduce cardiac fibroblasts activation, collagens deposition and contractile dysfunction, demonstrating antifibrotic effects.

of baicalein are demonstrated by reduction of fibroblast proliferation and ECM accumulation, and downregulation of fibrosis genes expression (Zhao et al. 2016; Kong et al. 2011), suggesting this flavonoid as potential treatment for the cardiac fibrosis in HF (Figure 8.6).

8.4 MYOCARDIAL ISCHEMIA/REPERFUSION INJURY: MOLECULAR MECHANISMS AND THERAPEUTIC POTENTIAL OF BAICALEIN

Ischemia/reperfusion (I/R) injury is characterized by myocardial damage caused by the ischemic insult followed by reperfusion injury. While the primary damage depends principally on the time frame and the gravity of blood flow restriction, reperfusion injury is the consequence of a series of complex mechanisms, some of which are not yet completely understood (D'Amico et al. 2019). Reperfusion injury has been linked to inflammatory processes, the overproduction of ROS, apoptotic cell death, leading to irreversible myocyte damage (Di Paola et al. 2018). Thus, timely reperfusion is mandatory to salvage the ischemic myocardium from infarction, but cardioprotection is needed to reduce infarct size and to improve the prognosis of patients with acute myocardial infarction. Numerous studies have confirmed that baicalein has a protective effect in myocardial infarction and myocardial ischemia/reperfusion, and its main mechanism of action includes inflammation regulation, inhibition of oxidative stress and reduction of apoptosis (D'Amico et al. 2019).

8.4.1 INHIBITION OF OXIDATIVE STRESS

At least half of myocardial damage resulting from myocardial infarction is associated with reperfusion injury. Once the blood supply to an organ is interrupted (ischemia) and re-established (reperfusion), this kind of situation leads to a "burst" of ROS generation from mitochondria (Xin et al. 2020). Oxygen free radicals are highly toxic compounds that cause peroxidation of lipids and proteins;

therefore, intracellular generation of ROS worsens cellular injury during ischemia and reperfusion in cardiac tissues (Huang et al. 2005; Kemp-Harper et al. 2021). Increased endogenous ROS may act as intracellular mediators or second messengers to activate redox-sensitive kinases (such as mitogen-activated protein kinase family and ERK cascade) and phosphorylate transcription factors (such as NF-kB) (Krylatov et al. 2018), which play an important role in the inflammatory process, as described in the next paragraph. It is well known that baicalein, and flavonoids in general, exerts an antioxidant effect mainly mediated by scavenging primary and secondary free radicals, including superoxide and H_2O_2, during oxidative stress (Wang et al. 2020). This is mainly due to the fact that flavonoids contain multiple hydroxyl substitutions that exhibit radical scavenging activity. In particular, baicalein has the 5,6,7-trihydroxy structure on ring-A, which attributes it these strong antioxidant properties (Li, Zhao, and Holscher 2017). In addition to scavenging free radicals, baicalein has the ability to boost antioxidant capabilities by recovering activities of endogenous antioxidant enzymes and upregulating their gene expression.

One of the mechanisms that cardiac cells have adapted to protect themselves against oxidative stress is the nuclear factor-erythroid 2-related factor 2 (Nrf2) pathway and its binding with the antioxidant response element (ARE) in the regulatory region of many genes, which leads to the expression of several enzymes with antioxidant and detoxification capacities (Li, Zhao, and Holscher 2017). Notably, manganese superoxide dismutase (MnSOD) is an important antioxidant enzyme in mitochondria against oxidative stress. It was found that baicalein restored both MnSOD and nuclear Nrf2 protein expression (Lee et al. 2011). Therefore, baicalein could be considered a potential therapeutic approach to prevent reperfusion-associated oxidative stress.

8.4.2 Mitigation of Inflammatory Response

Inflammation is an important process in the pathophysiology of myocardial I/R injury. Under inflammatory conditions, signaling pathways like mitogen-activated protein kinases (MAPKs) and nuclear factor-kB (NF-kB) are activated, inducing the transcription of various cytokines and chemokines such as tumor necrosis factor (TNF)-α, IL-1β, IL-6, and IL-18, and anti-inflammatory cytokines such as IL-10 which protect cardiac function (Li, Fang, et al. 2021). Data suggest that the likely mechanism by which baicalein inhibits inflammation is related to the inhibition of NF-kB signaling pathways and consequently cytokines release (Li et al. 2016; Yuan et al. 2020). Similarly, MAPKs cascades, especially ERK, c-Jun N-terminal kinase/stress-activated protein kinase (JNK/SAPK) and p38, play a pivotal role in the amelioration of ischemic insults. Thus, the cardioprotective effect of baicalein could also be due to the activation of ERK and suppression of JNK and p38 activity (Chen et al. 2014). Therefore, targeting the inflammatory cascade and related inflammatory cytokines, baicalein plays a protective role in myocardial I/R damage.

8.4.3 Modulation of Apoptosis Process

Baicalein also exerts cardioprotective effects via regulating several signaling pathways and apoptosis regulators. Apoptosis and mitochondrial dysfunction-mediated apoptosis are considered the most important forms of cardiac cell death following myocardial I/R. Bax and Bcl-2 belong to the same apoptosis gene family, but they have opposite effects; Bcl-2 inhibits cell apoptosis, while Bax promotes it. Caspase-3 is an important apoptosis executor in the caspase family, and upregulating the expression of caspase-3 gene promotes myocardial apoptosis (Korshunova et al. 2021). It was demonstrated that baicalein can improve I/R damage by upregulating the expression of Bcl-2 and downregulating Bax. Additionally, baicalein seems to inhibit caspase-3 activity and protein expression, protecting the heart from I/R damage (Li et al. 2020; Jie, Xiujian, and Jin 2019). The specific mechanism involved might be related to the activation of survival kinases including ERK and the inhibition of apoptotic kinases such as JNK and p38 (Xin et al. 2020). However, whether it is directly related to ischemia and reperfusion remains to be verified. Understanding the effects of baicalein in mediating functions of anti-apoptotic activity would supply newly insights for the management of myocardial I/R injury.

8.4.4 VASCULAR ACTION

It is worth pointing out that baicalein exerts direct vasorelaxant effects, thus indicating the involvement of endothelium-derived vasoactive factors (Wang et al. 2015). However, the mechanisms involved are unknown. To date, studies indicate that baicalein increases the evoked contractile responses likely through inhibition of NO formation and/or release in the endothelium, without affecting gene expression of endothelial NOS. This flavonoid markedly inhibits acetylcholine-induced endothelial NO-mediated vasorelaxation and decreases the tissue content of cyclic GMP (indicative of NO production) (Tsang et al. 2000; Huang et al. 2004).

Additionally, arachidonic acid released from tissue lipids around blood vessels is metabolized via COX, lipoxygenase and cytochrome P-450 pathways to form various vasoactive products. Interestingly, inhibition of the lipoxygenase pathway in arachidonic acid metabolism can prevent the development of elevated blood pressure, suggesting to play a key role in I/R injury and cardiovascular diseases (Figure 8.7). Baicalein is a potent inhibitor of 5-, 12- and 15-lipooxygenase (Lapchak et al. 2007; Hsieh et al. 2007). This property gives baicalein a role as a valuable agent in determining the physiological role of lipoxygenase-dependent pathways that regulate vessel tone and blood flow. This mechanism in part explains the cardioprotective effect of baicalein.

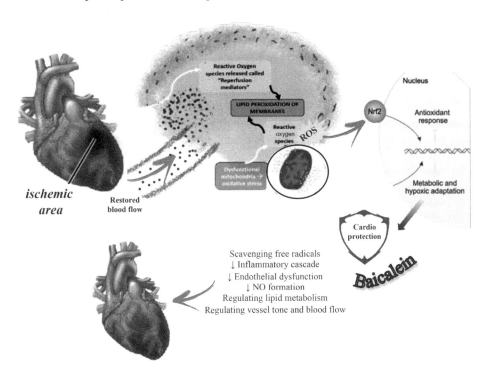

FIGURE 8.7 Cellular and molecular mechanisms underlying the beneficial effects of baicalein in myocardial I/R injury.

Note: Ischemia following by reperfusion causes a "burst" of ROS generation from mitochondria. In response to oxidative stress, Nrf2 translocates to the nucleus to bind to antioxidant response element (ARE), causing activation of antioxidant mechanisms involved in antioxidant/oxidant homeostasis. Baicalein acts as a potent antioxidant, attenuating oxidative stress and scavenging ROS, thus helps to preserve endothelial function. Additionally, baicalein inhibits inflammatory cascades, inducible NO biosynthesis, as well as regulates lipid metabolism and blood flow.

8.5 CONCLUSION

In conclusion, *in vitro/vivo* studies have provided evidence that baicalein, a naturally occurring bioactive compound in *S. baicalensis* Georgi, is a promising therapeutic agent for cardiovascular protection. To summarize, baicalein exerts therapeutic effects in cardiovascular disorders via mechanisms involving in regulating lipid metabolism, reducing inflammation-induced damage, inhibiting oxidative stress, reducing apoptosis and helping immune regulation.

Although a great deal of knowledge has been acquired regarding the benefits of baicalein on CVDs from experimental data, it is worth noting that the specific underlying mechanisms are still relatively unexplained. As the next step, clinical trials evaluating the effects in patients with cardiovascular disorders need to be initiated to test its safety and efficacy in clinical applications. The pleiotropic activities of baicalein suggest it has great potential for clinical application in the prevention and treatment of CVDs, in particular in myocardial I/R.

8.6 TOXICITY AND CAUTIONARY NOTES

To date, numerous studies have been conducted to evaluate the pharmacokinetic profile and bioavailability of baicalein for its safety and efficacy in clinical applications (Li, Zhao, and Holscher 2017; Pan et al. 2021). Notably, two phase I clinical trials of baicalein chewable tablets in healthy volunteers have been completed in China (Pang et al. 2016; Li, Gao, et al. 2021). Samples of blood, urine and feces were collected at regular intervals up to 48 h after administration of the drug. The drug concentration was then analyzed using liquid chromatography – tandem mass spectrometry. Physical examinations, vital signs, electrocardiogram findings, hematology and urinalysis were monitored before and at regular intervals after administration of the drug. There were no clinically relevant changes in blood pressure or electrocardiogram findings in individuals during the study. Additionally, no serious adverse events occurred, and clinical laboratory assessments showed no signs of toxicity in the liver or kidney (Li et al. 2014). In conclusion, in a dose range of 200–800 mg, multiple-dose oral baicalein administration was safe and no serious accumulation of baicalein was observed (Li, Gao, et al. 2021). Although these phase I clinical trials have indicated that oral baicalein is safe and well tolerated, clinical trials for other dosages for baicalein are not reported, and further phase II and III clinical trials of baicalein in patients will have to be conducted to prove its efficacy. Furthermore, clinical trials to evaluate the therapeutic potential of baicalein in patients with cardiovascular disease are necessary.

8.7 SUMMARY POINTS

- Cardiovascular diseases are the primary cause of mortality worldwide.
- This chapter focuses on cardioprotective effects of baicalein.
- Baicalein is a flavonoid isolated from the root of *Scutellaria baicalensis* Georgi.
- The major route of metabolism for baicalein is conjugated metabolism, responsible for its *in vivo* effects.
- Baicalein exerts protective effects in atherosclerosis by targeting proatherogenic processes. Baicalein reduces the endothelial dysfunction and oxidative stress, improving hypertension.
- Baicalein possesses antifibrotic effects, suggesting it as potential approach in heart failure.
- Baicalein has a protective effect in myocardial ischemia/reperfusion, through inflammation regulation, inhibition of oxidative stress and reduction of apoptosis.
- Clinical trials are needed to evaluate the therapeutic potential of baicalein in cardiovascular disease.

REFERENCES

Aguilar-Ballester, M., G. Hurtado-Genoves, A. Taberner-Cortes, A. Herrero-Cervera, S. Martinez-Hervas, and H. Gonzalez-Navarro. 2021. "Therapies for the treatment of cardiovascular disease associated with type 2 diabetes and dyslipidemia." *Int J Mol Sci* 22 (2). doi: 10.3390/ijms22020660.

Angeli, F., G. Reboldi, and P. Verdecchia. 2021. "The link between inflammation and hypertension: Unmasking mediators." *Am J Hypertens* 34 (7):683–685. doi: 10.1093/ajh/hpab034.

Bauersachs, J., and S. Soltani. 2021. "Guidelines of the ESC 2021 on heart failure." *Herz*. doi: 10.1007/s00059-021-05084-5.

Behl, T., S. Bungau, K. Kumar, G. Zengin, F. Khan, A. Kumar, R. Kaur, T. Venkatachalam, D. M. Tit, C. M. Vesa, G. Barsan, and D. E. Mosteanu. 2020. "Pleotropic effects of polyphenols in cardiovascular system." *Biomed Pharmacother* 130:110714. doi: 10.1016/j.biopha.2020.110714.

Chan, S. H., C. H. Hung, J. Y. Shih, P. M. Chu, Y. H. Cheng, Y. J. Tsai, H. C. Lin, and K. L. Tsai. 2016. "Baicalein is an available anti-atherosclerotic compound through modulation of nitric oxide-related mechanism under oxLDL exposure." *Oncotarget* 7 (28):42881–42891. doi: 10.18632/oncotarget.10263.

Chen, H. M., J. H. Hsu, S. F. Liou, T. J. Chen, L. Y. Chen, C. C. Chiu, and J. L. Yeh. 2014. "Baicalein, an active component of Scutellaria baicalensis Georgi, prevents lysophosphatidylcholine-induced cardiac injury by reducing reactive oxygen species production, calcium overload and apoptosis via MAPK pathways." *BMC Complement Altern Med* 14:233. doi: 10.1186/1472-6882-14-233.

Crea, F. 2021. "How epidemiology can improve the understanding of cardiovascular disease: From mechanisms to treatment." *Eur Heart J* 42 (44):4503–4507. doi: 10.1093/eurheartj/ehab797.

D'Amico, R., R. Fusco, E. Gugliandolo, M. Cordaro, S. Siracusa, D. Impellizzeri, A. F. Peritore, R. Crupi, S. Cuzzocrea, and R. Di Paola. 2019. "Effects of a new compound containing Palmitoylethanolamide and Baicalein in myocardial ischaemia/reperfusion injury in vivo." *Phytomedicine* 54:27–42. doi: 10.1016/j.phymed.2018.09.191.

Dinda, B., S. Dinda, S. DasSharma, R. Banik, A. Chakraborty, and M. Dinda. 2017. "Therapeutic potentials of baicalin and its aglycone, baicalein against inflammatory disorders." *Eur J Med Chem* 131:68–80. doi: 10.1016/j.ejmech.2017.03.004.

Di Paola, R., R. Fusco, E. Gugliandolo, R. D'Amico, M. Campolo, S. Latteri, A. Carughi, G. Mandalari, and S. Cuzzocrea. 2018. "The antioxidant activity of pistachios reduces cardiac tissue injury of acute Ischemia/Reperfusion (I/R) in diabetic streptozotocin (STZ)-induced hyperglycaemic rats." *Front Pharmacol* 9:51. doi: 10.3389/fphar.2018.00051.

Fong, Y. K., C. R. Li, S. K. Wo, S. Wang, L. Zhou, L. Zhang, G. Lin, and Z. Zuo. 2012. "In vitro and in situ evaluation of herb-drug interactions during intestinal metabolism and absorption of baicalein." *J Ethnopharmacol* 141 (2):742–753. doi: 10.1016/j.jep.2011.08.042.

Gao, Y., S. A. Snyder, J. N. Smith, and Y. C. Chen. 2016. "Anticancer properties of baicalein: A review." *Med Chem Res* 25 (8):1515–1523. doi: 10.1007/s00044-016-1607-x.

Hsieh, Y. C., S. J. Hsieh, Y. S. Chang, C. M. Hsueh, and S. L. Hsu. 2007. "The lipoxygenase inhibitor, baicalein, modulates cell adhesion and migration by up-regulation of integrins and vinculin in rat heart endothelial cells." *Br J Pharmacol* 151 (8):1235–1245. doi: 10.1038/sj.bjp.0707345.

Huang, Y., S. Y. Tsang, X. Yao, and Z. Y. Chen. 2005. "Biological properties of baicalein in cardiovascular system." *Curr Drug Targets Cardiovasc Haematol Disord* 5 (2):177–184. doi: 10.2174/1568006043586206.

Huang, Y., C. M. Wong, C. W. Lau, X. Yao, S. Y. Tsang, Y. L. Su, and Z. Y. Chen. 2004. "Inhibition of nitric oxide/cyclic GMP-mediated relaxation by purified flavonoids, baicalin and baicalein, in rat aortic rings." *Biochem Pharmacol* 67 (4):787–794. doi: 10.1016/j.bcp.2003.10.002.

Jackson, E. K. 1989. "Relation between renin release and blood pressure response to nonsteroidal anti-inflammatory drugs in hypertension." *Hypertension* 14 (5):469–471. doi: 10.1161/01.hyp.14.5.469.

Jie, Z., W. Xiujian, and L. Jin. 2019. "Pharmacological mechanism and apoptosis effect of baicalein in protecting myocardial ischemia reperfusion injury in rats." *Pak J Pharm Sci* 32 (1(Special)):407–412.

Kemp-Harper, B. K., A. Velagic, N. Paolocci, J. D. Horowitz, and R. H. Ritchie. 2021. "Cardiovascular therapeutic potential of the redox siblings, Nitric Oxide (NO*) and Nitroxyl (HNO), in the setting of reactive oxygen species dysregulation." *Handb Exp Pharmacol* 264:311–337. doi: 10.1007/164_2020_389.

Kong, E. K., S. Yu, J. E. Sanderson, K. B. Chen, Y. Huang, and C. M. Yu. 2011. "A novel anti-fibrotic agent, baicalein, for the treatment of myocardial fibrosis in spontaneously hypertensive rats." *Eur J Pharmacol* 658 (2–3):175–181. doi: 10.1016/j.ejphar.2011.02.033.

Korshunova, A. Y., M. L. Blagonravov, E. V. Neborak, S. P. Syatkin, A. P. Sklifasovskaya, S. M. Semyatov, and E. Agostinelli. 2021. "BCL2 regulated apoptotic process in myocardial ischemiareperfusion injury (Review)." *Int J Mol Med* 47 (1):23–36. doi: 10.3892/ijmm.2020.4781.

Krylatov, A. V., L. N. Maslov, N. S. Voronkov, A. A. Boshchenko, S. V. Popov, L. Gomez, H. Wang, A. S. Jaggi, and J. M. Downey. 2018. "Reactive oxygen species as intracellular signaling molecules in the cardiovascular system." *Curr Cardiol Rev* 14 (4):290–300. doi: 10.2174/1573403X14666180702152436.

Kukes, V., N. Chebyshev, L. Pavlova, I. Berechikidze, T. Degtyarevskaya, and L. Badriddinova. 2020. "Clinical case: The side effects of statins." *Georgian Med News* (299):75–78.

Lapchak, P. A., P. Maher, D. Schubert, and J. A. Zivin. 2007. "Baicalein, an antioxidant 12/15-lipoxygenase inhibitor improves clinical rating scores following multiple infarct embolic strokes." *Neuroscience* 150 (3):585–591. doi: 10.1016/j.neuroscience.2007.09.033.

Lee, I. K., K. A. Kang, R. Zhang, B. J. Kim, S. S. Kang, and J. W. Hyun. 2011. "Mitochondria protection of baicalein against oxidative damage via induction of manganese superoxide dismutase." *Environ Toxicol Pharmacol* 31 (1):233–241. doi: 10.1016/j.etap.2010.11.002.

Li, C., M. Fang, Z. Lin, W. Wang, and X. Li. 2021. "MicroRNA-24 protects against myocardial ischemia-reperfusion injury via the NF-kappaB/TNF-alpha pathway." *Exp Ther Med* 22 (5):1288. doi: 10.3892/etm.2021.10723.

Li, C., L. Zhang, G. Lin, and Z. Zuo. 2011. "Identification and quantification of baicalein, wogonin, oroxylin A and their major glucuronide conjugated metabolites in rat plasma after oral administration of Radix scutellariae product." *J Pharm Biomed Anal* 54 (4):750–758. doi: 10.1016/j.jpba.2010.10.005.

Li, H. B., Y. Jiang, and F. Chen. 2004. "Separation methods used for Scutellaria baicalensis active components." *J Chromatogr B Analyt Technol Biomed Life Sci* 812 (1–2):277–290. doi: 10.1016/j.jchromb.2004.06.045.

Li, J., J. Ma, K. S. Wang, C. Mi, Z. Wang, L. X. Piao, G. H. Xu, X. Li, J. J. Lee, and X. Jin. 2016. "Baicalein inhibits TNF-alpha-induced NF-kappaB activation and expression of NF-kappaB-regulated target gene products." *Oncol Rep* 36 (5):2771–2776. doi: 10.3892/or.2016.5108.

Li, L., H. Gao, K. Lou, H. Luo, S. Hao, J. Yuan, Z. Liu, and R. Dong. 2021. "Safety, tolerability, and pharmacokinetics of oral baicalein tablets in healthy Chinese subjects: A single-center, randomized, double-blind, placebo-controlled multiple-ascending-dose study." *Clin Transl Sci* 14 (5):2017–2024. doi: 10.1111/cts.13063.

Li, M., A. Shi, H. Pang, W. Xue, Y. Li, G. Cao, B. Yan, F. Dong, K. Li, W. Xiao, G. He, G. Du, and X. Hu. 2014. "Safety, tolerability, and pharmacokinetics of a single ascending dose of baicalein chewable tablets in healthy subjects." *J Ethnopharmacol* 156:210–215. doi: 10.1016/j.jep.2014.08.031.

Li, Q., Z. Yu, D. Xiao, Y. Wang, L. Zhao, Y. An, and Y. Gao. 2020. "Baicalein inhibits mitochondrial apoptosis induced by oxidative stress in cardiomyocytes by stabilizing MARCH5 expression." *J Cell Mol Med* 24 (2):2040–2051. doi: 10.1111/jcmm.14903.

Li, Y., J. Zhao, and C. Holscher. 2017. "Therapeutic potential of baicalein in Alzheimer's disease and parkinson's disease." *CNS Drugs* 31 (8):639–652. doi: 10.1007/s40263-017-0451-y.

Liang, W., X. Huang, and W. Chen. 2017. "The effects of baicalin and baicalein on cerebral ischemia: A review." *Aging Dis* 8 (6):850–867. doi: 10.14336/AD.2017.0829.

Marchio, P., S. Guerra-Ojeda, J. M. Vila, M. Aldasoro, V. M. Victor, and M. D. Mauricio. 2019. "Targeting early atherosclerosis: A focus on oxidative stress and inflammation." *Oxid Med Cell Longev* 2019:8563845. doi: 10.1155/2019/8563845.

McManus, R., M. Constanti, C. N. Floyd, M. Glover, A. S. Wierzbicki, and Health National Institute for, and Group Care Excellence Hypertension Guideline Development. 2020. "Managing cardiovascular disease risk in hypertension." *Lancet* 395 (10227):869–870. doi: 10.1016/S0140-6736(20)30048-9.

Mutha, R. E., A. U. Tatiya, and S. J. Surana. 2021. "Flavonoids as natural phenolic compounds and their role in therapeutics: An overview." *Futur J Pharm Sci* 7 (1):25. doi: 10.1186/s43094-020-00161-8.

Nik Salleh, N. N. H., F. A. Othman, N. A. Kamarudin, and S. C. Tan. 2020. "The biological activities and therapeutic potentials of baicalein extracted from oroxylum indicum: A systematic review." *Molecules* 25 (23). doi: 10.3390/molecules25235677.

Pan, L., K. S. Cho, I. Yi, C. H. To, D. F. Chen, and C. W. Do. 2021. "Baicalein, baicalin, and wogonin: Protective effects against ischemia-induced neurodegeneration in the brain and retina." *Oxid Med Cell Longev* 2021:8377362. doi: 10.1155/2021/8377362.

Pang, H., W. Xue, A. Shi, M. Li, Y. Li, G. Cao, B. Yan, F. Dong, W. Xiao, G. He, G. Du, X. Hu, and G. Cheng. 2016. "Multiple-ascending-dose pharmacokinetics and safety evaluation of baicalein chewable tablets in healthy Chinese volunteers." *Clin Drug Investig* 36 (9):713–724. doi: 10.1007/s40261-016-0418-7.

Prabhu, S. D., and N. G. Frangogiannis. 2016. "The biological basis for cardiac repair after myocardial infarction: From inflammation to fibrosis." *Circ Res* 119 (1):91–112. doi: 10.1161/CIRCRESAHA.116.303577.

Sahin, B., and G. Ilgun. 2022. "Risk factors of deaths related to cardiovascular diseases in World Health Organization (WHO) member countries." *Health Soc Care Community* 30 (1):73–80. doi: 10.1111/hsc.13156.

Seo, M. J., H. S. Choi, H. J. Jeon, M. S. Woo, and B. Y. Lee. 2014. "Baicalein inhibits lipid accumulation by regulating early adipogenesis and m-TOR signaling." *Food Chem Toxicol* 67:57–64. doi: 10.1016/j.fct.2014.02.009.

Tsai, K. L., C. H. Hung, S. H. Chan, J. Y. Shih, Y. H. Cheng, Y. J. Tsai, H. C. Lin, and P. M. Chu. 2016. "Baicalein protects against oxLDL-caused oxidative stress and inflammation by modulation of AMPK-alpha." *Oncotarget* 7 (45):72458–72468. doi: 10.18632/oncotarget.12788.

Tsang, S. Y., Z. Y. Chen, X. Q. Yao, and Y. Huang. 2000. "Potentiating effects on contractions by purified baicalin and baicalein in the rat mesenteric artery." *J Cardiovasc Pharmacol* 36 (2):263–269. doi: 10.1097/00005344-200008000-00018.

Tuli, H. S., V. Aggarwal, J. Kaur, D. Aggarwal, G. Parashar, N. C. Parashar, M. Tuorkey, G. Kaur, R. Savla, K. Sak, and M. Kumar. 2020. "Baicalein: A metabolite with promising antineoplastic activity." *Life Sci* 259:118183. doi: 10.1016/j.lfs.2020.118183.

Wang, A. W., L. Song, J. Miao, H. X. Wang, C. Tian, X. Jiang, Q. Y. Han, L. Yu, Y. Liu, J. Du, Y. L. Xia, and H. H. Li. 2015. "Baicalein attenuates angiotensin II-induced cardiac remodeling via inhibition of AKT/mTOR, ERK1/2, NF-kappaB, and calcineurin signaling pathways in mice." *Am J Hypertens* 28 (4):518–526. doi: 10.1093/ajh/hpu194.

Wang, L., H. Duan, J. Jiang, J. Long, Y. Yu, G. Chen, and G. Duan. 2017. "A simple and rapid infrared-assisted self enzymolysis extraction method for total flavonoid aglycones extraction from Scutellariae Radix and mechanism exploration." *Anal Bioanal Chem* 409 (23):5593–5602. doi: 10.1007/s00216-017-0497-1.

Wang, Y., L. Li, G. Liu, T. Xu, D. Xiao, L. Zhang, Q. Wan, W. Chang, Y. An, and J. Wang. 2020. "Baicalein protects cardiomyocytes from oxidative stress induced programmed necrosis by stabilizing carboxyl terminus of Hsc70-interacting protein." *Int J Cardiol* 311:83–90. doi: 10.1016/j.ijcard.2020.03.035.

Wolf, D., and K. Ley. 2019. "Immunity and inflammation in atherosclerosis." *Circ Res* 124 (2):315–327. doi: 10.1161/CIRCRESAHA.118.313591.

Wu, Y., Y. Ding, T. Ramprasath, and M. H. Zou. 2021. "Oxidative stress, GTPCH1, and endothelial nitric oxide synthase uncoupling in hypertension." *Antioxid Redox Signal* 34 (9):750–764. doi: 10.1089/ars.2020.8112.

Xiao, L. J., and R. Tao. 2017. "Traditional Chinese Medicine (TCM) therapy." *Adv Exp Med Biol* 1010:261–280. doi: 10.1007/978-981-10-5562-1_13.

Xin, L., J. Gao, H. Lin, Y. Qu, C. Shang, Y. Wang, Y. Lu, and X. Cui. 2020. "Regulatory mechanisms of baicalin in cardiovascular diseases: A review." *Front Pharmacol* 11:583200. doi: 10.3389/fphar.2020.583200.

Xu, J., J. Liu, G. Yue, M. Sun, J. Li, X. Xiu, and Z. Gao. 2018. "Therapeutic effect of the natural compounds baicalein and baicalin on autoimmune diseases." *Mol Med Rep* 18 (1):1149–1154. doi: 10.3892/mmr.2018.9054.

Yuan, Y., W. Men, X. Shan, H. Zhai, X. Qiao, L. Geng, and C. Li. 2020. "Baicalein exerts neuroprotective effect against ischaemic/reperfusion injury via alteration of NF-kB and LOX and AMPK/Nrf2 pathway." *Inflammopharmacology* 28 (5):1327–1341. doi: 10.1007/s10787-020-00714-6.

Zhang, L., C. Li, G. Lin, P. Krajcsi, and Z. Zuo. 2011. "Hepatic metabolism and disposition of baicalein via the coupling of conjugation enzymes and transporters-in vitro and in vivo evidences." *AAPS J* 13 (3):378–389. doi: 10.1208/s12248-011-9277-6.

Zhang, Q., S. H. Zhao, J. Chen, and L. W. Zhang. 2015. "Application of ionic liquid-based microwave-assisted extraction of flavonoids from Scutellaria baicalensis Georgi." *J Chromatogr B Analyt Technol Biomed Life Sci* 1002:411–417. doi: 10.1016/j.jchromb.2015.08.021.

Zhang, Z. Q., W. Liua, L. Zhuang, J. Wang, and S. Zhang. 2013. "Comparative pharmacokinetics of baicalin, wogonoside, baicalein and wogonin in plasma after oral administration of pure baicalin, radix scutellariae and scutellariae-paeoniae couple extracts in normal and ulcerative colitis rats." *Iran J Pharm Res* 12 (3):399–409.

Zhao, F., L. Fu, W. Yang, Y. Dong, J. Yang, S. Sun, and Y. Hou. 2016. "Cardioprotective effects of baicalein on heart failure via modulation of Ca(2+) handling proteins in vivo and in vitro." *Life Sci* 145:213–223. doi: 10.1016/j.lfs.2015.12.036.

Zhao, Q., X. Y. Chen, and C. Martin. 2016. "Scutellaria baicalensis, the golden herb from the garden of Chinese medicinal plants." *Sci Bull (Beijing)* 61 (18):1391–1398. doi: 10.1007/s11434-016-1136-5.

Zhou, X., C. G. Li, D. Chang, and A. Bensoussan. 2019. "Current status and major challenges to the safety and efficacy presented by Chinese herbal medicine." *Medicines (Basel)* 6 (1). doi: 10.3390/medicines6010014.

9 Balloon Vine (*Cardiospermum halicacabum* L.) and Cardiovascular Protection
Cellular, Molecular and Metabolic Aspects

A. Rajasekaran, R. Arivukkarasu and G. Venkatesh

CONTENTS

9.1 Introduction 127
9.2 Background 129
9.3 Traditional Uses of CH 129
    9.3.1 Aerial Parts 129
    9.3.2 Leaves 130
    9.3.3 Seed 130
    9.3.4 Roots 130
9.4 Phytoconstituents of CH 131
    9.4.1 Leaves 131
    9.4.2 Seeds 131
    9.4.3 Roots 131
9.5 Risks Associated with CH 131
9.6 Cardioprotective Role of CH – A Possible Approach 132
9.7 Vali Thamaraga Noi 133
9.8 Azhal Thamaraga Noi 133
9.9 Iyya Thamaraga Noi 133
9.10 Mukkutra Thamaraga Noi 133
9.11 Cardio-Cerebral Approach 133
9.12 Cellular and Molecular Aspects of Cardioprotective Action of Flavonoids in CH 135
9.13 Influence of Nitric Oxide Synthase in Cardioprotection by CH Flavonoids 137
9.14 Modification of Cell Membrane Properties 137
9.15 Modulation of Ion Channels 137
9.16 Receptor Perspective 138
9.17 Transporter Mechanism 138
9.18 Antioxidant Approach 138
9.19 Inhibition of Enzymatic Activity 138
9.20 Metabolic Aspects 140
9.21 Toxicity and Cautionary Notes 140
9.22 Summary Points 141
References 141

DOI: 10.1201/9781003220329-11

LIST OF ABBREVIATIONS

ABCA1	ATP-binding cassette transporter
ACE	Angiotensin-converting enzyme
AKT	Apoptotic key protein or protein kinase B
AMPK	AMP-activated protein kinase
ASK	Apoptosis signal-Regulating kinase
BAX	BCL2 Associated X, Apoptosis Regulator
Bcl-2	B-cell lymphoma 2
CaMKII	Calmodulin-dependent protein kinase II
CH	*Cardiospermum halicacabum*
CK-MB	Creatine kinase-MB
COMT	Catechol-O-methyl transferase
CPK	Creatinine phosphokinase
CRP	C-reactive protein
CVD	Cardiovascular disease
DMARDs	Disease modifying anti-rheumatic drugs
ECs	Endothelial cells
eNOS	Endothelial nitric oxide synthase
ERK	Extracellular-signal-regulated kinase
H9C2	Cardiomyoblast cell
HASMC	Human Aortic Smooth Muscle Cells
HMG-CoA	3-hydroxy-3-methylglutaryl-coenzyme A reductase
iNOS	Inducible nitric oxide synthase
JNK	c-Jun N-terminal kinase
LDH	Lactate dehydrogenase
LDL	Low-density lipoprotein
LOX	Lipoxygenase
MAPK	Mitogen-activated protein kinase
NADPH	Nicotinamide adenine dinucleotide phosphate
NF-kB	Nuclear factor kappa-B
NO	Nitric oxide
Nrf2	Nuclear factor erythroid 2
PCSK9	Proprotein convertase subtilisin/kexin type 9
PDGF	Platelet-derived growth factor
PHLPP1	PH Domain And Leucine Rich Repeat Protein Phosphatase 1
POPC	1-palmitoyl-2-oleoyl-sn-glycero-3-phosphocholine
POPE	1-palmitoyl-2-oleoyl-*sn*-glycero-3-phosphoethanolamine
POPS	1-palmitoyl-2-oleoyl-*sn*-glycero-3-[phospho-L-serine]
PPAR	Peroxisome proliferator-activated receptor
RA	Rheumatoid arthritis
ROS	Reactive oxygen species
SERCA2a	Cardiac sarcoplasmic reticulum
Sp1	Specificity protein 1
SULTs	Sulfotransferases
TNF-α	Tumor necrosis factor-α
UGTS	Uridine diphospho-glucuronosyl transferases
VSMCs	Vascular smooth muscle cells

9.1 INTRODUCTION

Cardiospermum halicacabum L. is named balloon vine due to its lightweight, inflated or balloon-like fruits (Figure 9.1).

"Cardio" means "heart" and "spermum" means "seed" and hence it is commonly called heart seed. Halicacabum is derived from the Latin word halicacabus, a plant with inflated fruits. *Cardiospermum halicacabum* is also called balloon plant, blister creeper, frolitos, love in a puff, heart seed vine, heart pea, mudakathaan, natural cortisone, orfutki, winter cherry. "Modaku" means crippling joint pain; "thon" means remedy. In the Ayurvedic system of medicine, it is called Kaakatiktaa, Kaakaadani, Karnasphota, Shatakratulataa or Indravalli. In folklore, it is

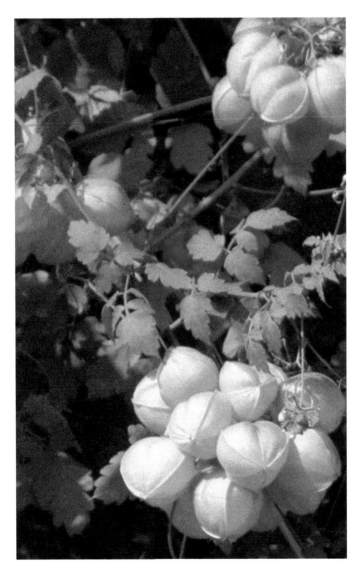

FIGURE 9.1 *Cardiospermum halicacabum* L. plant with inflated balloon fruit.

called Kanphotaa, Kanphuti or Lataaphatakari; in the Unani system, it is called Habb-e-Qilqil. The ornamental attraction of this species is mainly due to its inflated balloon-shaped fruit. It is considered to be a significant environmental weed in many countries. It was reported that inflated fruits float in sea water and stay viable for long periods of time, facilitating long distance dispersal.

The various species of *Cardiospermum* are *Cardiospermum anomalum* Cambess, *Cardiospermum bahianum* Ferruccci and Urdampill, *Cardiospermum barbicaule* Baker, *Cardiospermum corundum* Linnaeus (South African origin) (synonymically known as *Cardiospermum canescens* Wall), Cardiospermum cristobaliae Ferrucci, *Cardiospermum dissectum* (S. Watson) *Radik*, (synonymically called *Cardiospermum pechuelii*) (native of Namibia), *Cardiospermum grandiflorum* Swartz (native to Mexico), *Cardiospermum cuchujaquense* Ferrucci and Acevedo-Rodríguez, *Cardiospermum heringeri* Ferrucci, *Cardiospermum hirsutum* Willd, Cardiospermum integerrimum Radik, *Cardiospermum oliveirae* Ferrucci, *Cardiospermum ovatum* Wall, Cardiospermum procumbens Radik, *Cardiospermum pterocarpum* Radik, Cardiospermum pygmaeum, *Cardiospermum strictum* Radik, *Cardiospermum tortuosum* Benth, Cardiospermum urvilleoides (Radik) Ferrucci and Acevedo-Rodríguez *Cardiospermum vesicarium* Humb.

Among 1200 species available worldwide, the most commonly distributed species are *Cardiospermum corindum*, *Cardiospermum grandiflorum* and *Cardiospermum halicacabum*. Synonymical and vernacular names of *Cardiospermum halicacabum* L. by country are provided in Table 9.1 and Table 9.2 respectively.

TABLE 9.1
Synonyms of *Cardiospermum halicacabum* L.

S. No.	Synonyms	References
1	*Cardiospermum acuminatum* Miq	Ductu ET Consilio et al., 1941
2	*Cardiospermum corycodes* Kuntze	Ductu ET Consilio et al., 1941.
3	*Cardiospermum glabrum* Schumach. and Thonn.	Beskr. Guin. Pl. 1827, 197–198.
4	*Cardiospermum inflatum* Salisb	In Prodr. Stirp. Chap. Allerton: 279 (1796)
5	*Cardiospermum luridum* Blume	In Rumphia 3: 184 (1847)
6	*Cardiospermum moniliferum* Swartz. ex Steud.	Nomencl. Bot. ed. 2, 1840, 1: 150
7	*Cardiospermum truncatum* A. Rich.	Tent. Fl. Abyss. 1: 101
8	*Corindum halicacabum* (L.) Medik.	In Malvenfam.: 110 (1787) Pl.197 (1827)
9	*Cardiospermum microcarpum* Kunth	The European Agency 1999

TABLE 9.2
Vernacular Names of *Cardiospermum halicacabum* L. by Country

SN	Country	Regional or Vernacular Names (Kirthikar and Basu 1984)
1	Bangladesh	Futka
2	Burma	Malamai
3	China	Jiahugua, Dao di ling, Feng chuange, Jinsikulianteng, Ye kugua, Bao fu cao, Tao ti ling
4	Cuba	Farolito
5	France	Cardiosperme, Corinde or Pois de merveille
6	Germany	Herzsamen, Ballonrebe or Blasenerbse
7	India Tamil Nadu	Modakathon
8	Indonesia	Ketipes, Pari gunung, Cenet

TABLE 9.2 *(Continued)*
Vernacular Names of *Cardiospermum halicacabum* L. by Country

SN	Country	Regional or Vernacular Names (Kirthikar and Basu 1984)
9	Italy	Vesicaria del cuore
10	Madagascar	Masontsokina
11	Malaysia	Peria buian, Uban kayu, Bintang berahi
12	Netherlands	Blaaserwt
13	North America	Climbing balloon or balloon vine
15	Philippines	Parol-paralon or Barcolon
16	Portuguese	Balaozinho
17	Sri Lanka	Mudakottam
18	South Africa	Balloon vine
19	Spain	Revienta caballo
20	Thailand	Kokkraorm
21	Vietnam	T[aaf]m phong, Ch[uf]m phong

9.2 BACKGROUND

Cardiospermum halicacabum L. belongs to the family **Sapindaceae**, is a perennial plant, and different parts of it are used as food and in the treatment of many diseases. It is a deciduous, branched, herbaceous larger creeper with wiry stems and is distributed throughout the plains of India, South America and Africa (Joshi et al. 1992). Sturdy stems and tendrils enable it to climb upon other plants where it grows about 4 m in height and may climb over 10 m from the ground. In Tamil Nadu, (India) leaves of *Cardiospermum halicacabum* are consumed as a vegetable and also in the form of soup, kanji, kashayam, thokku, thuvaial, dosa, adai and rasam (used to ease constipation and gas) (Pieroni et al. 2012). In the southern state of India, Tamil Nadu, it is called Mudakathaan in the Tamil language as Mudakathaan. "Mudakku" means arthritis, "athan" means "relief". The leaves and the oil from the seed are used as hair oil and hair wash.

CH is one of the plants used for worship in religious rituals in India such as "Ashtamangalya", "Sahasra kalasam", "Prathishta mahotsava" and is worn on the head by women on "thiruvathira" day of "Dhanu" for prosperity. CH is a member of ten sacred plants of Dasapushpa (dasa means ten). In addition to these, the members are used for the worship of Lord Ganesha. "Mukkutticharthu", Karuka archana, last rites, etc. The members of Dasapushpa are *Aerva lanata* L. (Amaranthaceae), *Biophytum sensitivum* L. (Oxalidaceac), *Cardiospermum halicacabum* L. (**Sapindaceae**), *Curculigo orchioides* Gaertn. (Hypoxidaceae), *Cynodon dactylon* L. (Poaceae), *Eclipta prostrate* L. (Asteraceae), *Emiliasonchifolia* L. (Asteraceae), *Evolvulusalsinoides* L. (Convolvulaceae), *Ipomoea obscura* L. (Convolvulaceae) and *Vernonia cinarea* L (Asteraceae).

Low cost, high abundance and ready availability of CH developed interest among scientists to pursue research of this plant and hence various formulations of CH as gel, cream, shampoo and spray were developed and used for the treatment of dry itchy skin, inflammatory dermatitis, hives and insect bites (Fai et al. 2020).

9.3 TRADITIONAL USES OF CH

9.3.1 AERIAL PARTS

Balloon vine is used in the treatment of rheumatism, nervous diseases, stiffness of the limbs and snakebite (Chopra et al. 1986). Esakkimuthu et al. (2021) reported that CH is used internally by Siddha practitioners to treat various musculoskeletal ailments. Homeopathic remedy

Cardiospermum halica mother tincture is recommended for the treatment of kidney disorders, and to improve memory, headache, flatulence and congestion in the chest (Riley 2018). CH in traditional medicine is used both orally and dermally for itchy skin in African and Asian countries. In traditional practice, CH was used for the treatment of fever and inflammation (Sheeba and Asha 2009) and various diseases due to the presence of diverse phytochemical constituents (Naik et al. 2014).

9.3.2 Leaves

Decoction of the leaves and stems are used in the treatment of diarrhea, dysentery and headache. Juice of the leaves is used for ear ache. Leaves are crushed and made into tea for itchy skin. Salted leaves are used as a poultice on swellings (Ragupathy et al. 2007). Ethnomedical information revealed that leaves of CH were mainly used in the treatment of rheumatoid arthritis. Mudakathan oil, prepared by mixing equal parts of CH leaves, chitramoolaver patai, omamam, sesame oil and karpuram (camphor), is used for the ailment of arthritis. Arthritis is one of the major health-related issues for aged population around the world. In Greek "artho" means joint and "itis" means inflammation and so arthritis is a form of joint disorder that involves inflammation of joints. Among 100 different forms of arthritis, osteoarthritis, rheumatoid arthritis, psoriatic arthritis and related autoimmune disease, septic arthritis are the most common forms that are primarily caused by joint infection. Due to lack of evidence-based medicine, no targeted specific therapy is being offered for arthritis to date and hence pharmaceutical companies are urged to develop a novel potential drug candidate for the permanent cure of RA.

Opioids, non-opioid anti-inflammatory agents, DMARDs, immunomodulators and immunosuppressant drugs are being commonly prescribed to deal with the RA condition. Though the purpose of prescribing these agents is to relieve pain and suppress joint inflammation and destruction, restore function of disabled joints, these drugs are known to produce expected and unexpected side effects based on the patient's condition. The most prominent and harmful undesired effects caused by non-steroidal anti-inflammatory agents are gastric erosions, ulceration, bleeding, perforation, acute renal failure and fatal liver toxicity. The Siddha and Ayurvedic systems of medicine are progressively documented as an alternative therapy for RA treatment. The Irula community from Thanjavur district, Tamil Nadu, India, has exploited CH for treating RA for many years, which is being followed by the present traditional practitioners (Kirtikar and Basu 1984; Nadkarni 1976).

Leaves of CH are consumed in the form of rasam to cure Vatha disease (Ramanathan 2002). Soup prepared with leaves of CH, pepper, cumin seeds, salt cooked in 100 ml of water for 5–10 min was given to children for the relief of cold and cough. Fried leaves are applied on the stomach for menstrual disorders and related stomach pain. A paste of leaves are applied and tied over the lower abdomen of a woman who has recently given birth for one week after delivery to expel undesired contents out of the uterus. For andavaatham or (hydrocele) the leaves can be applied as an external paste over the scrotum.

9.3.3 Seed

The oil, rich in unsaturated fatty acids, is used in the prevention of CVDs. Flour from the inner parts of the seed mixed with cereal flours is used for baking (Ferrara 2018). Alkaloidal fraction of the seeds decreased the blood pressure, pacemaker activity and cardiac inhibition in preclinical study (Khare 2007).

9.3.4 Roots

Decoction of the roots is used to control excess sweating, natriuresis, emesis, evacuation of the bowels and also is used as emmenagogue, laxative and rubefacient (Chopra et al. 1986). CH roots have been indicated in the folklore system for anxiety and epilepsy (Venkatesh Babu and Krishnakumari 2006). Roots are used in the treatment of throat infection, CNS ailments and headache (Muthu et al. 2006). The decoction of roots or the whole plant of CH (20 g of paste is boiled in 200 ml of water until it is reduced to 50 ml) is used for piles twice daily.

9.4 PHYTOCONSTITUENTS OF CH

CH is known to contain flavonoids, triterpenoids, tannins, saponins, glycosides, fatty acids, alkaloids, proanthocyanides and steroids. The following flavonoids (Figure 9.2) were reported to be present in CH (Cheng et al. 2013).

1. Apigenin
2. Apigenin-7-O-glucuronide
3. Apigenin 7-O-glucuronide methyl ester
4. Apigenin 7-O-glucuronide ethyl ester
5. Apigenin-7-glucoside
6. Chrysoeriol
7. Chrysoeriol-7-glucuronide
8. Kaempferol
9. Kaempferol-3-O-rhamnoside
10. Luteolin
11. Luteolin-7-O-glucuronide
12. Luteolin-6-C-glucoside
13. Luteolin-7-glucoside (cynaroside)
14. Luteolin-8-C-glucoside
15. Quercetin
16. Quercetin-3-O-rhamnoside
17. Rutin

CH is also reported to contain the phenolic phytoconstituents quebrachitol, methyl 3,4-dihydroxybenzoate, p-coumaric acid, 4-hydroxybenzoic acid, hydroquinone, protocatechuic acid and gallic acid (Dass 1966, Khan et al. 1990, Srinivas et al. 1998).

9.4.1 LEAVES

Leaves of CH are reported to contain β-sitosterol, D-glucose, oxalic acid, amino acids, alkaloids, pinitol, apigenin, luteolin and chrysoeriol (Khare 2007).

9.4.2 SEEDS

Seeds contain 33% fatty acids; out of these 55% are cyanolipids. The major component reported to be present in the seed oil is 11-eicosenoicacid (Chisholmm and Hopkins 1958). The other components of the oil are oleic acid, arachidic acid, linolenic acid, linoleic acid, palmitic acid, steric acid, erucic acid, octanoic acid, behenic acid and n-hexadecanoic acid (Shareef et al. 2012).

9.4.3 ROOTS

Roots contain β-sitosterol, phlobaphene, phloba-tannin and proanthocyanidine.

9.5 RISKS ASSOCIATED WITH CH

No study has been reported on human health risks associated with CH; however, it may cause vomiting in humans and animals. Children may have gagging or choking if a piece of plant is consumed.

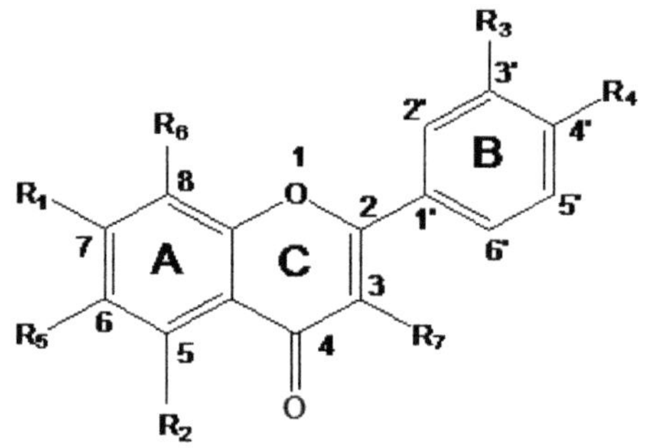

FIGURE 9.2 Chemical structures of flavonoids in *Cardiospermum halicacabum* L.

Name of the flavonoid	R_1	R_2	R_3	R_4	R_5	R_6	R_7
Apigenin	OH	OH	H	OH	H	H	H
Apigenin-7-*O*-glucuronide	O-Glucuronide	OH	H	OH	H	H	H
Apigenin-7-*O*-glucuronide methyl ester	O-Glucuronide methyl ester	OH	H	OH	H	H	H
Apigenin-7-*O*-glucuronide ethyl ester	O-Glucuronide ethyl ester	OH	H	OH	H	H	H
Apigenin-7-glucoside	O-Glucoside	OH	H	OH	H	H	H
Chrysoeriol	OH	OH	OCH$_3$	OH	H	H	H
Chrysoeriol-7-glucuronide	O-Glucuronide	OH	OCH$_3$	OH	H	H	H
Kaempferol	OH	OH	H	OH	H	H	OH
Kaempferol-3-*O*-rhamnoside	OH	OH	H	OH	H	H	O-Rhamnoside
Luteolin	OH	OH	OH	OH	H	H	H
Luteolin-7-*O*-glucuronide	O-Glucuronide	OH	OH	OH	H	H	H
Luteolin-6-*C*-glucoside	OH	OH	OH	OH	Glucoside	H	H
Luteolin-7-glucoside	Glucoside	OH	OH	OH	H	H	H
Luteolin-8-*C*-glucoside	OH	OH	OH	OH	H	Glucoside	H
Quercetin	OH	OH	OH	OH	H	H	OH
Quercetin-3-*O*-rhamnoside	OH	OH	OH	OH	H	H	O-Rhamnoside
Rutin	OH	OH	OH	OH	H	H	O-Rutinose

Invasion of *Cardiospermum* species have a wide range of financial significance on the sugarcane and soybean industry (Subramanyam et al. 2007). In a study in Brazil, CH decreased the yield of soybean crop by 26% (Brighenti et al. 2003), which clearly indicates economic threat to agricultural crop production by CH species.

9.6 CARDIOPROTECTIVE ROLE OF CH – A POSSIBLE APPROACH

The heart is the important organ in the body that supplies blood and oxygen to other parts of the body. It contains enzymes like xanthine oxido-reductase, nitric oxide synthase, NADPH oxidase, cytochrome P-450 enzymes and monoamine oxidases, which are critical in regulating homeostatic processes of the heart (Pavek and Dvorak 2008). Globally, one-third of all deaths are mainly caused by CVDs. CVDs include hypertension, angina pectoris, myocardial infarction, valvular heart disease, inflammatory/congestive cardiac failure, arrhythmic heart diseases and congenital heart

Balloon Vine and Cardiovascular Protection 133

diseases. Oxidative stress has been proposed as the major cause in the pathogenesis of cardio-vascular disease, myocardial infarction, atherosclerosis, hypertension, ischemia/reperfusion injury. Elevated levels of cardiac enzymes, troponin and CPK (known as creatine kinase) in the blood stream are the indication of damage of heart muscle and the symptoms of heart diseases. C-reactive protein, homocysteine and soluble CD40 ligand is the indication that inflammation of the heart may be due to atherosclerosis.

In Siddha system, CVDs are known as thamaraga noi (disease) and are caused by deranged vatha and kabam. Vatha is classified into four types: 1) Vali, 2) Azhal, 3) Iyyam and 4) Mukkutram.

9.7 VALI THAMARAGA NOI

In the Siddha system, vali thamaraga noi is due to increase in prominent vatha humor and produces symptoms of sore throat, fever, anemia, edema, palpitation, heaviness of the chest, breathing difficulty, coughing and vomiting, which are correlated with modern cardiac disorders of rheumatic valvular heart diseases. Vali thamaraga noi is treated with internal Siddha medicines (viz. Kudineer, Chooranam, Mathirai, Manapagu, Rasayanam, Vadagam) and externally by taking an oil bath.

9.8 AZHAL THAMARAGA NOI

Azhal thamaraga noi is due to chest pain, palpitation, breathlessness, dyspnea, sweating, giddiness and is correlated with modern cardiac ischemic heart diseases. Azhal thamaraga noi is treated with internal Siddha medicines (viz. Kudineer, Chooranam, Mathirai, Rasayanam, Manapagu, Parpam, Chendooram, Mezhugu, Thravagam, Kattu) and externally by taking an oil bath.

9.9 IYYA THAMARAGA NOI

Iyya thamaraga noi is due to heaviness of chest, difficulty breathing, sweating pain radiating to the left upper limb to the fingertips, dyspnea, restlessness that is correlated with modern cardiac diseases of myocardial infraction. Iyya thamaraga noi is treated with internal Siddha medicines (viz. Kudineer, Chooranam, Mathirai, Rasayanam, Manapagu, Parpam, Chendooram, Mezhugu, Thravagam, Kattu) and externally by taking an oil bath.

9.10 MUKKUTRA THAMARAGA NOI

Mukkutra thamaraga noi is due to rheumatism, hypertension, diabetes, renal diseases it also comes like fever (kabavathasuram) correlated with modern cardiac disease of congestive cardiac failure/arrhythmia. Mukkutra thamaraga noi is treated with internal Siddha medicines viz. Kudineer, Chooranam, Mathirai, Rasayanam, Manapagu, Parpam, Chendooram, Mezhugu, Thravagam, Kattu and externally by taking Oil bath.

As per Siddha system of practice, cardiac diseases occur due to excessive intake of vatha diet, bad habits, sexually transmitted diseases and aggravation of uthanavayu (Mel nokkunkal), Viyanavayu (Paravukal) that can be prevented and cured by lifestyle modification and rejuvenation drugs.

9.11 CARDIO-CEREBRAL APPROACH

Pakkavatham (stroke) is a neurodegenerative condition that can cause speech disability, or part of the body can become paralyzed due to blockade of cerebral blood flow, or the rupture of the cerebral artery which supplies oxygen or energy to the brain. Stroke is recognized by the symptoms of numbness of the face, arm or leg, giddiness, confusion and loss of balance.

Siddha medicines (viz. Choornam, Ilagam, Thylum (medicated oil), Parpam (calcined oxide), Chendooram (calcined red oxides/sulfide), Mezhugu, Pathangam (sublimate), Mathirai (tablet)) are taken internally. Thokkanam oil, which posses anti-Vaatham properties are applied over the affected region with the procedures of Azhthudhal (pressing), Izhuthal (pulling), Pidithal (grasping/gripping) and Varmam. Patients are advised to take the dietary supplements Kaththari Pinchu (*Solanum melongena*), Avarai Pinchu (*Dolichos lablab*), Aththipinchu (*Ficus racemosa*), Mudakkarran (*Cardiospermum halicacabum*), Ponnakaanik Keerai (*Alternanthera sessilis*), Thoothuvealaik Keerai (*Solanum trilobatum*), Mookkirattai Keerai (*Boerhaavia diffusa*), Vealaikkeerai (*Cleome viscosa*) for the management of stroke (Kuppusamy Mudaliar 1987).

Flavonoids are the most widely present secondary metabolite and nutraceutical ingredient in plants that are reported for cardioprotective effects (Figure 9.3) mainly due to the phenolic components (Van Dam et al. 2013).

CH extracts were reported as a major source of phytochemicals for treating oxidative stress which is the most important factor for CVDs. CH extract caused fall of blood pressure and bradycardia in

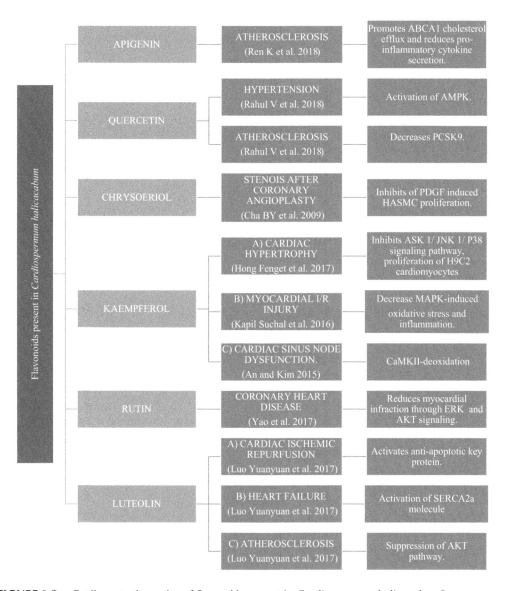

FIGURE 9.3 Cardioprotective action of flavonoids present in *Cardiospermum halicacabum* L.

Balloon Vine and Cardiovascular Protection 135

rats and anesthetized dogs. Venkatesh Babu and Krishnakumari (2006) reported that the ethanol extract of CH subdues the release of NO in T cells, B cells, NK cells and monocytic cells of human blood.

Luteolin, a major phytoconstituent of CH, containing two aromatic rings connected by a heterocyclic pyran ring, is used in traditional Chinese medicine for hypertension and provides a cardioprotective effect against ischemia and reperfusion injury (Marijan-Jankovic 1957).

Flavonoids consist of C_6-C_3-C_6 rings, namely rings A and B linked by three-carbon-ring C. Presence of catechol moiety in ring B, substitution of methoxyl group in 5'-position in ring B, double bond between C_2 and C_3 in ring C, 4-carbonyl group in ring C, and 3-hydroxyl group in ring C enhances the cardioprotective activity. All these structural features are reported to be essential for eNOS and ET-1 expression (apigenin vs. naringenin). Hydroxylation or glycosylation in position 5 may decrease eNOS/ET-1 expression by 2 times (quercetin/rutin vs. luteolin). Presence of double bond between C_2 and C_3 in ring C, 4-carbonyl oxygen and 3-hydroxyl group is important for protein binding (Atrahimovich et al. 2013).

Quercetin and rutin, due to their anti-aggregating properties and stimulatory effect activate vascular dilation, and thus help in blood pressure regulation. Pinitol present in plants is reported to be used in the treatment of hypertension and CVDs. High amounts of unsaturated fatty acid present in the oil of CH is reported to protect from CVDs (Ferrara 2018).

9.12 CELLULAR AND MOLECULAR ASPECTS OF CARDIOPROTECTIVE ACTION OF FLAVONOIDS IN CH

No scientific study is reported for cardioprotective effect of CH in molecular and cellular aspects. But, in general, medicinal plants/herbs exert beneficial pharmacological action through a sequence of processes including the inhibition, stimulation, modulation and expression of various genes, proteins and ions at the intracellular and extracellular level.

Largely, the cardioprotective effect of plant and herbal preparations have been explicated by improving the actions of myocardial cells, endothelial cells (ECs), VSMCs and macrophages and monocytes (Table 9.3). Some of them express their protective role through the regulation of K^+ATP channel, atrial natriuretic peptide, oxidative stress, and apoptosis. They also display cardioprotection by controlling inflammation, endothelial nitric oxide signaling pathway, angiogenesis and endothelial permeability.

In VSMCs, those preparations demonstrate the beneficial action on the heart by controlling structural and contractile proteins, proliferation and migrations of extracellular matrixes, regulation of calcium channel and mitochondrial functions (Huang 2016).

TABLE 9.3

Potential Herbs Used in Cardiovascular Diseases

Name of the Herb (Family)	Phytoconstituents	Mechanism of Action	References
Aegle marmelos (Rutaceae)	Fruit-Marmesin	Inhibiting the release of beta-glucuronidase	Vimal and Devaki 2004
Allium sativum (Liliaceae)	Allicin, ajoene, S-allyl-L-cysteine, diallyl disulfides, methyl thiosulfonate and diallyl trisulfides	• NF-κB pathway • ACE inhibition	Wai et al. 2020
Amaranthus viridis (Amaranthaceae)	Flavonoids, alkaloids, phenols, steroids, terpenoids, saponins, cardiac glycosides, tannins	Regulation of LDH and CPK	Saravanan et al. 2013

(Continued)

TABLE 9.3 *(Continued)*
Potential Herbs Used in Cardiovascular Diseases

Name of the Herb (Family)	Phytoconstituents	Mechanism of Action	References
Asparagus racemosus (Asparagaceae)	Saponin-shatavarins 1–1V	Inhibition of CK-MB and LDH release	Bopana and Saxena 2007
Andrographis aniculata (Acanthaceae)	Andrographolide, 14-deoxy-11,12-didehydro andrographolide	ACE inhibition	Zhang and Tan et al. 1996
Camellia sinensis (Theaceae)	Epicatechin, Epigallocatechin, and Epigallocatechin-3-gallate.	Endothelial NO Release	Huang et al. 2000
Cinnamomum zeylanicum (Lauraceae)	Cinnamaldehyde	Inhibition of endothelin-1 receptor NO stimulation Activation of Ca^{2+} activated K^+ channels	Zhang and Liu et al. 2020
Coriandum sativum (Umbelliferae)	Linalool, geranyl acetate and gamma-terpinene	Inhibition of myocardial Ca(2+) channel	Jabeen et al. 2009
Curcuma longa (Zingiberaceae)	Curcuminoids, terpinolene, p-cymene, undecanol 1, 8-cineole, α-turmerone	Inhibition of CK-MB and LDH release Activation of endothelial NO release	Eman et al. 2011
Digitalis purpurea (Scrophulariaceae)	Digitoxin, gitoxin, digitoxigenin, gitoxigenin, digipurpurin, diginin, digitalonin	Inhibition of Na+ K+ ATPase activation	Dec 2003.
Garcinia mangostana (Guttiferae)	Mangostin	Inhibition of LDH, CPK markers	Devi Sampath and Vijayaraghavan 2007
Matricaria chamomilla (Asteraceae)	Apigenin, Luteolin, Quercetinpolyacetylenes, Terpenoid α-Bisabolol, Chamazulene	ACE inhibition	Awaad et al. 2018.
Morus alba (Moraceae)	Morin	Inhibition of Beta Adrenergic	Pogula et al. 2012
Ocimum sanctum (Laminaceae)	Oleanolic acid, rosmarinic acid, ursolic acid eugenol, linalool, carvacrol, β elemene, β caryophyllene, germacrene	Inhibition of lactate dehydrogenase activity	Sharma et al. 2001
Rauwolfia serpentina (Apocyanceae)	Reserpine, ajmalinine, ajmalidine, ajmalicine, ajmaline	Activation of endothelial NO release	Soni et al. 2016.
Strophanthus gratus (Apocynaceae)	Cardiac glycosides Ouabain binds with Na+ K+-ATPase pump and inhibits its action, thereby causing a rise in intracellular sodium ions and enhancing cardiac ionotropy	Stimulation of cardiac Na+/K+ pumps	Gao et al. 2002
Terminalia arjuna (Combretaceae)	Flavonoids	• Oxidative stress pathway • Increases the NO release	Navjot et al. 2014
Vitis vinifera (Vitaceae)	Resveratrol	Upregulation of NO production	Hung et al. 2000
Zingiber officinale (Zingiberaceae)	Gingerols, shogaols, paradols, β-bisabolene, zingiberene	Activation of the Nrf2/HO-1 pathway	Liu et al. 2015

9.13 INFLUENCE OF NITRIC OXIDE SYNTHASE IN CARDIOPROTECTION BY CH FLAVONOIDS

Nitric oxide is synthesized by various isoforms of nitric oxide synthases, namely neuronal nitric oxide synthases, endothelial nitric oxide synthases and inducible nitric oxide synthases enzymes (Forstermann et al. 1995) involving maintenance of cardiovascular and renal homeostasis. Neuronal NOS decreases cardiac contractility via inhibition of L-type Ca^{2+} channel activated impulse generation and the intracellular Ca^{2+} ion movement, where both mitochondrial cells and xanthine oxidoreductase enzyme have been recognized as effective targets for neuronal NOS in cardiac diseases. The chromosome of iNOS, located within the immune and the cardiovascular system, acts as major immune defence against pathogens. The chromosome of eNOS, located within the endothelium of the coronary vessels and in cardiac myocytes, causes vasodilation and decreases the blood pressure and cardiac load.

The mechanisms of cardioprotective action of flavonoids in CH at cellular and molecular levels are mainly due to (Tilak-Jain and Devasagayam 2006):

- Modification of cell membrane properties.
- Modulation of ion channels.
- Receptor perspective.
- Transporter mechanism.
- Antioxidant approach.
- Inhibition of enzymatic activity.

9.14 MODIFICATION OF CELL MEMBRANE PROPERTIES

Phytochemicals, flavonoids, terpenoids, stilbenoids, capsaicinoids, phloroglucinols, naphthodian-thrones, organosulfur compounds, alkaloids, anthraquinonoids, ginsenosides, pentacyclic triterpene acids and curcuminoids are presumed to regulate membrane proteins, lipid bilayers and stabilize the physical and chemical properties of the extracellular and intracellular membrane. Plant flavonoids are reported to decrease the membrane fluidity by altering the inner part of liposomal cell membranes comprising of POPC, POPE, POPS and cholesterol (Hironori Tsuchiya 2015).

A membrane interactivity study suggested that 3-hydroxylation of the C ring, non-modification or 3',4'-dihydroxylation of the B ring and 5,7-dihydroxylation of the A ring is essential in flavonoids for good membrane interaction to rigidify membranes.

9.15 MODULATION OF ION CHANNELS

Cardiac action potential expresses the progressive activation and inactivation of inflex (Na^+ and Ca^{2+}) at extracellular ion channel and efflex K^+ at intracellular ion channels. Discrete action potential waves produced in different parts of the heart, due to difference in expression and activation of ion channels that contribute to modification in propagation and generation of normal and altered cardiac functions (Nerbonne and Kass 2005).

Quercetin can encourage vasodilatory action via attenuation of endothelin-1 receptor, which can enhance the vascular NO release, thereby activating the conductivity of Ca^{2+} activated K^+ channels which can suppress the recurrence of calcium entry. Such versatile actions of quercetin potentially deal with the ischemia/reperfusion injury (Zhang, Zhang, and Wang 2020). Further, quercetin can ameliorate the post-traumatic cardiac dysfunction by suppressing apoptosis process through the downregulation of TNF-α, ROS and Ca^{2+} release in cardiomyocytes which demonstrates better preventive therapy for mechanical trauma-induced secondary cardiac injury (Jing et al. 2016).

Apigenin primarily regulates small and large conductance Ca^{2+} activated K^+ channels, leading to hyperpolarization followed by Ca^{2+} influx. The increased Ca^{2+} responsible for the activation NO production thereby mediates the anti-angiogenic effect via AKT mediated dephosphorylation pathway (Erdogan et al. 2007).

9.16 RECEPTOR PERSPECTIVE

Apigenin shows cardioprotective activity by attenuating the adrenergic β receptor-induced myocardial injury with the escalation of antioxidant defense mechanism (Buwa et al. 2016). Apigenin also increases the expression of myocardial PPARα and decreases the expression of PPAR-γ receptors that could improve hypertensive cardiac hypertrophy through the downregulation of myocardial HIF-1α gene expression (Zhu et al. 2016).

Quercetin ameliorates the Angiotensin II receptor mediated atrial natriuretic factor and β-myosin-induced cardiac hypertrophic responses (Chen et al. 2021). Further quercetin activates muscarinic (M2) receptor associated NO release which induces vasodilation and inhibition of Ca^{+2} influx in anti-hypertensive condition (Umme Salma et al. 2018). Evidence from the echocardiographic investigation of rutin significantly improved the heart function through alleviation of cardiac fibrosis and cell apoptosis via inhibition of overt autophagy reaction and by regulating the AKT receptor pathway (Yanyan et al. 2017). Luteolin effectively regulates the cardiac function through NO release along with the inhibition of Kim-1/NF-κB/Nrf2 pathway and cardiac troponin release (Oyagbemi et al. 2021).

9.17 TRANSPORTER MECHANISM

Apigenin decreases the expression of myocardial glucose transporter (GLUT)-4 proteins by this means and ameliorates the irregular myocardial glucose-lipid metabolic pathway (Zhu et al. 2016). Epigallocatechin potentially inhibits the sodium-dependent glucose transporter 1 (SGLT1) activity in cardiomyopathic condition, which would prevent the systemic glucose uptake (Othman et al. 2017). Luteolin effectively ameliorates the abnormal glucose and lipid metabolism of Angiotensin II/hypoxia-induced hypertrophic myocardial cells via inhibiting GLUT-4 transporter (Wang et al. 2019). Moreover, luteolin regulates the sarcoplasmic and endoplasmic reticulum of Ca^{2+} ATPase 2a (SERCA2a) to maintain myocardial systolic-diastolic pressure during the ischemic condition through the initiation of Sp1 signaling (Hu et al. 2020).

9.18 ANTIOXIDANT APPROACH

Oxidative stress process is mainly due to increase in ROS production that leads to alteration in cellular and molecular functions, eventually resulting in cardiac dysfunction. Owing to the existence of potent antioxidants like flavonoids, glycosides, tannins and saponins, CH counteracts free radicals. Particularly, the presence of flavonoids in aerial parts of CH is considered as a potential source for the treatment of oxidative stress. CH extract in 40% ethanol is reported to reduce free radical and NO generation in RAW 264.7 macrophage cells and N9 microglial cells in *in vitro* study, thereby exerting its action against oxidative stress (Merighi et al. 2021). Flavonoids of CH extract potentially regulates the enzymatic and non-enzymatic antioxidant markers (viz. SOD, GSH, CAT, GPx, MDA and GSH). Rutin potentially suppresses the oxidative stress pathway and cardiac inflammatory process by reducing SOD, CAT, GSH and CRP levels through stimulating Nrf2 and by downregulating the NF-κB signaling mechanism (Oluranti et al. 2021). Luteolin significantly improves the oxidative stress condition in cardiac myocytes and inhibits apoptotic markers such as Bcl-2, BAX and caspase-3 via downregulating PHLPP1 activity and triggering the AKT/Bcl-2 signaling mechanism (Zhang, Zhang, Wang 2020).

9.19 INHIBITION OF ENZYMATIC ACTIVITY

Decrease in activity of enzymes (viz. xanthine oxidase, NADPH oxidase and lipoxygenase (involving reactive oxygen species production)) may mainly be due to the flavonoids present in CH. Flavonoids suppressing the inflammation on the blood vessel walls by the inhibition of leucocyte infiltration is considered to be a therapeutic approach for the anti-arteriosclerotic action. Flavonoids are reported to decrease in activity of enzymes like 15-LOX and cyclooxygenase that cause reduction in the release of PGE2, LB4 and TA2, thus suppress the inflammation and platelet aggregation, thereby regulating the capillary pressure back to normal.

HMG-CoA enzyme chiefly involves the formation of secondary active metabolite cholesterol from the cell membrane, where flavonoids are reported to inhibit HMG-CoA activity, lower intracellular cholesterol concentrations and augment the availability of extracellular membrane LDL receptors, thereby increasing the cellular uptake of lipoproteins and elimination of cholesterol from the blood circulation (Zeka 2017).

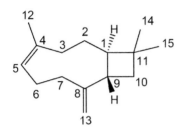

METABOLITE 1

[(1R,9S,Z)-4,11,11-trimethyl-8-methylenebicyclo[7.2.0]undec-4-ene]

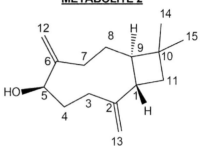

METABOLITE 2

[(1S,5R,9R)-10,10-dimethyl-2,6-dimethylenebicyclo[7.2.0]undecan-5-ol]

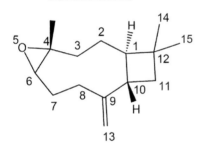

METABOLITE 3

[(1R,4R,10S)-4,12,12-trimethyl-9-methylene-5-oxatricyclo[8.2.0.0 4,6]dodecane]

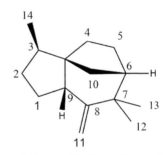

METABOLITE 4

[(3S,3aS,6R,9S)-3,7,7-trimethyl-8-methyleneoctahydro-3a,6-methanoazulene]

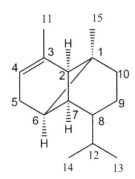

METABOLITE 5

[(1R,2S,6S,7S)-8-isopropyl-1,3-dimethyltricyclo[4.4.0.02,7]dec-3-ene]

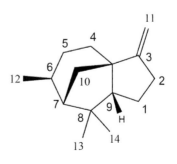

METABOLITE 6

[(3aR,6R,7S,9S)-6,8,8-trimethyl-3-methyleneoctahydro-3a,7-methanoazulene]

FIGURE 9.4 Metabolites reported in the entire plant of *Cardiospermum canescens* Wall.

9.20 METABOLIC ASPECTS

Metabolites of the whole plant or parts of CH were not reported in the literature. Ketha et al. (2020) identified six known metabolites (Figure 9.4) from the entire plant (methanol extract) of *Cardiospermum canescens* (*Cardiospermum corindum*) using chromatographic and spectral techniques.

Among the six metabolites, authors claimed that metabolites 2 and 3 are highly responsible for antioxidant, anti-inflammatory, and anticancer activities of methanol extract of the whole plant *Cardiospermum canescens* Wall.

Phytoflavonoids luteolin and apigenin in CH undergo metabolism mainly by conjugation with UGTs and SULTs. The enzyme COMT is recognized for the metabolism of luteolin, where it catalyzes flavonoids containing catechol moiety in ring B, mainly the 3'-OH group to methylated metabolites. This biotransformation (Figure 9.5) causes the formation of two methylated metabolites, namely 4', 5, 7-trihydroxy-3'-methoxyflavone and 3', 5, 7-trihydroxy-4'-methoxyflavone (Chen et al. 2011).

9.21 TOXICITY AND CAUTIONARY NOTES

CH is reported to be safe and nontoxic up to a dose of 800 mg/kg leaves, 500 mg/kg whole plant (in mice); 40 mg/kg in rats (Santhakumari et al 1981). Study reports confirmed that the prolonged use of CH extracts was found to be tolerable and safe (Ferrara 2018).

CH is toxic due to the presence of cyanolipids that causes the release of hydrocyanic acid. One mg/kg of HCN is permitted in European Union for food stuffs, where CH was reported to contain less than this limit (The European Agency, 1999).

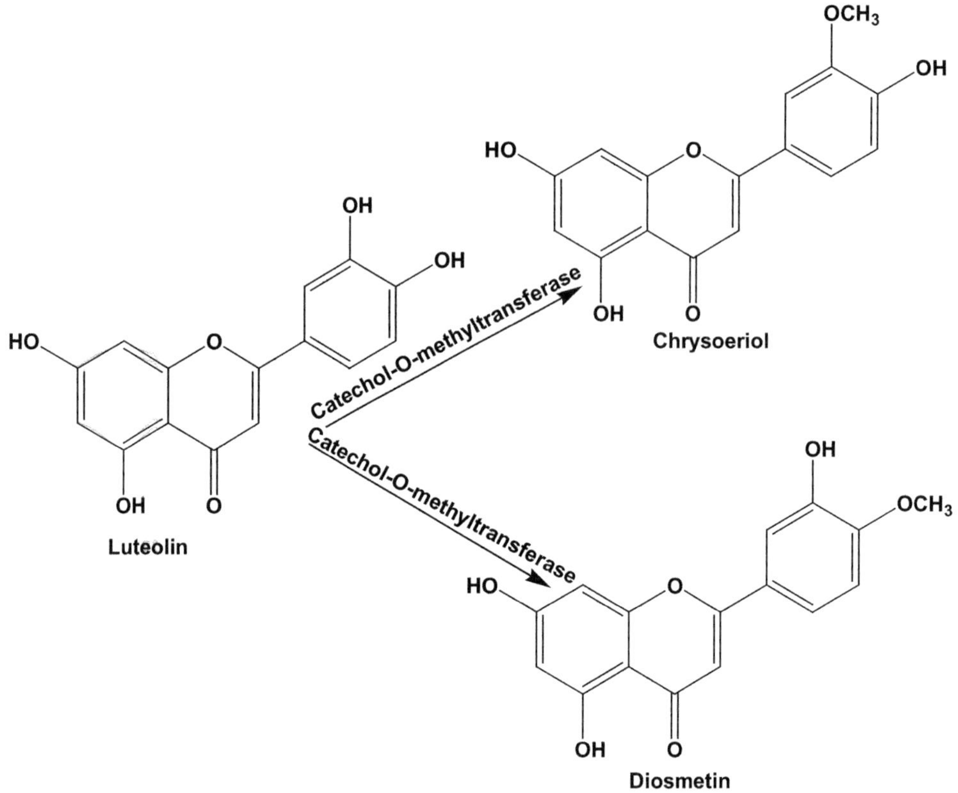

FIGURE 9.5 Biotransformation pathway of luteolin by Catechol-O-methyltransferase.

9.22 SUMMARY POINTS

This chapter focuses on the plant *Cardiospermum halicacabum* L.

- *Cardiospermum halicacabum* L. is clinically used for rheumatism, fever, ear ache and chronic bronchitis by the Siddha practitioners.
- Various formulations of CH as gel, cream, shampoo and spray are therapeutically used in the treatment of dry itchy skin.
- In rural parts of Tamil Nadu, India, it is harvested and sold in urban and local markets as a green vegetable as a source of revenue for low-income families.
- CH may exerts its cardioprotective action by modifying cell membrane properties, by modulating ion channels, through receptors and transporters, by antioxidant approach and by inhibiting enzyme activity.
- Beneficial effects of CH on human health may be due to the presence of a rich amount of flavonoids.

REFERENCES

An, M., Kim, M. 2015. Protective effects of kaempferol against cardiac sinus node dysfunction via CaMKII deoxidization. Anatomy and Cell Biology 48(4):235–243.

Atrahimovich, D., Vaya, J., Khatib, S. 2013. The effects and mechanism of flavonoid – rePON1 interactions: Structure – activity relationship study. Bioorganic & Medicinal Chemistry 21(11):3348–3355.

Awaad, A. A., El-Meligy, R. M., Zain, G. M., Safhi, A. A. Al Qurain, N. A., Almoqren, S. S., Zain, Y. M., Sesh Adri, V. D., Al-Saikhan, F. I. 2018. Experimental and clinical antihypertensive activity of *Matricaria chamomilla* extracts and their angiotensin-converting enzyme inhibitory activity. Phytotherapy Research 32(8):1564–1573.

Bopana, N., Saxena, S. 2007. Asparagus racemosus ethnopharmacological evaluation and conservation needs. Journal of Ethnopharmacology 110(1):1–15.

Brighenti, A. M., Voll, E., Gazziero, D. L. P. 2003. Biology and management of *Cardiospermum halicacabum*. Planta Daninda 21:229–237.

Buwa, C. C., Mahajan, U. B., Patil, C. R., Goyal, S. N. 2016. Apigenin attenuates β-receptor-stimulated myocardial injury via safeguarding cardiac functions and escalation of antioxidant defence system. Cardiovascular Toxicology 16(3):286–297.

Cha, B. Y., Shi, W. L., Yonezawa, T., Teruya, T., Nagai, K., Woo, J. T. 2009. An inhibitory effect of chrysoeriol on platelet-derived growth factor (PDGF)-induced proliferation and PDGF receptor signaling in human aortic smooth muscle cells. Journal of Pharmacological Sciences 110(1):105–110.

Chen, W. J., Cheng, Y., Li, W., Dong, X. K., Wei, J. L., Yang, C. H., Jiang, Y. H. 2021. Quercetin attenuates cardiac hypertrophy by inhibiting mitochondrial dysfunction through SIRT3/PARP-1 pathway. Frontiers in Pharmacology 12:739615.

Chen, Z., Chen, M., Pan, H., Sun, S., Li, L., Zeng, S. 2011. Role of catechol-O-methyltransferase in the disposition of luteolin in rats. Drug Metabolism & Disposition 39:667–674.

Cheng, H. L., Zhang, L. J., Liang, Y. H., Hsu, Y. W., Lee, I. J., Liaw, C. C., Hwang, S. Y., Kuo, Y. H. 2013. Antiinflammatory and antioxidant flavonoids and phenols from *Cardiospermum halicacabum*. Journal of Traditional and Complementary Medicine 3(1):33–40.

Chisholm, M. J., Hopkins, C. Y. 1958. Fatty acids of the seed oil of *Cardiospermum halicacabum*. Canadian Journal of Chemistry 36:1537–1540.

Chopra, R. N., Nayar, S. L., Chopra, I. C. 1986. Glossary of Indian medicinal plants. Council for Scientific and Industrial Research, New Delhi.

Dass, A. K. 1966. Chemical examination of *Cardiospermum halicacabum Linn*. Bulletin Botanical Survey of India 8:357–358.

Dec, G. W. 2003. Digoxin remains useful in the management of chronic heart failure. Medicina Clínica 87(2):317–337.

Devi Sampath, P., Vijayaraghavan, K. 2007. Cardioprotective effect of a-mangostin, a xanthone derivative from mangosteen on tissue defense system against isoproterenol-induced myocardial infarction in rats. Journal of Biochemical and Molecular Toxicology 21(6):336–339.

Eman, M. E.-S., El-azeem, A. S. A., Afify, A. A., Shabana, M. H., Ahmed, H. H. 2011. Cardioprotective effects of Curcuma longa L. Extracts against doxorubicin induced cardiotoxicity in rats. Journal of Medicinal Plants Research 5(17):4049–4058.

Erdogan, A., Most, A., Wienecke, B., Fehsecke, A., Leckband, C., Voss, R., Grebe, M. T. Schaefer, C. A., Kuhlmann, C. R. W. 2007. Apigenin-induced nitric oxide production involves calcium-activated potassium channels and is responsible for antiangiogenic effects. Journal of Thrombosis and Haemostasis 5:1774–1781.

Esakkimuthu, S., Mutheeswaran, S., Elankani, P., Pandikumar, P., Ignacimuthu, S. 2021. Quantitative analysis of medicinal plants used to treat musculoskeletal ailments by non-institutionally trained siddha practitioners of Virudhunagar district, Tamil Nadu, India. Journal of Ayurveda Integrative Medicine 12(1):58–64.

The European Agency for the Evaluation of Medicinal Products. 1999. *Cardiospermum halicacabum* summary report. Committee for veterinary medicinal products. Veterinary Medicines Evaluation Unit, Canary Wharf, London, UK.

Fai, D., Fai, C., Di Vito, M., Martini, C., Zilio, G., De Togni, H. 2020. *Cardiospermum halicacabum* in atopic dermatitis: Clinical evidence based on phytotherapic approach. Dermatology Therapy 33(6):e14519.

Ferrara, L. *Cardiospermum halicacabum Linn*. 2018. Food and drug. International Journal of Medical Reviews 5(4):146–150.

Forstermann, U., Kleinert, H., Gath, I., Schwarz, P., Closs, E. I., Dun, N. J. 1995. Expression and expressional control of nitric oxide synthases in various cell types. Advances in Pharmacology 34:171–186.

Gao, J. Y., Wymore, R. S., Wang, Y. L., Gaudette, G. R., Krukenkamp, I. B., Cohen, I. S., Mathias, R. T. 2002. Isoform-specific stimulation of cardiac Na+/K+ pumps by nanomolar concentrations of glycosides. Journal of General Physiology 119:297–312.

Hironori Tsuchiya. 2015. Membrane interactions of phytochemicals as their molecular mechanism applicable to the discovery of drug leads from plants. Molecules 20(10):18923–18966.

Hong, F., Cao, J., Zhang, G., Wang, Y. 2017. Kaempferol attenuates cardiac hypertrophy via regulation of ASK1/MAPK signalling pathway and oxidative stress. Planta Medica 83(10):837–845.

Hu, Y., Zhang, C., Zhu, H., Wang, S., Zhou, Y., Zhao, J., Xia, Y., Li, D. 2020. Luteolin modulates SERCA2a via Sp1 upregulation to attenuate myocardial ischemia/reperfusion injury in mice. Scientific Reports 10(1):15407.

Huang, C., La, Y. 2016. Chinese herbal medicine on cardiovascular diseases and the mechanisms of action. Frontiers in Pharmacology 7:469.

Huang, Y., Yao, X. Q., Tsang, S. Y., Lau, C. W., Chen, Z. Y. 2000. Role of endothelium/nitric oxide in vascular response to flavonoids and epicatechin. Acta Pharmacologica Sinica 21:1119–1124.

Hung, L. M., Chen, J. K., Huang, S. S., Lee, R. S., Su, M. J. 2000. Cardioprotective effect of resveratrol, a natural antioxidant derived from grapes. Cardiovascular Research 47(3):549–555.

Jabeen, Q., Bashir, S., Lyoussi, B., Gilani, A. H. 2009. Coriander fruit exhibits gut modulatory, blood pressure lowering and diuretic activities. Journal of Ethnopharmacology 122:123–130.

Jing, Z., Wang, Z., Li, X. 2016. Protective effect of quercetin on posttraumatic cardiac injury. Science Report 6:30812.

Joshi, S. K., Sharma, B. D., Bhatia, C. R., Singh, R. V., Thakur, R. S. 1992. The wealth of India. Raw Materials (Revised) Vol. III, Council of Scientific and Industrial Research Publication, New Delhi.

Kapil, S., Malik, S., Gamad, N., Malhotra, R. K., Goyal, S. N., Chaudhary, U., Bhatia, J., Arya, S. O. D. S. 2016. Kaempferol attenuates myocardial ischemic injury *via* inhibition of MAPK signalling pathway in experimental model of myocardial ischemia-reperfusion injury. Oxidative Medicine and Cellular Longevity 7580731.

Ketha, A., Vedula, G. S., Sastry, A. V. S. 2020. *In vitro* antioxidant, anti-inflammatory, and anticancer activities of methanolic extract and its metabolites of whole plant *Cardiospermum canescens* Wall. Future Journal of Pharmaceutical Sciences 6(1):1–10.

Khan, M. S. Y., Arya, M., Javed, K., Khan, M. H. 1990. Chemical examination of *Cardiospermum halicacabum* Linn. Indian Drugs 27:257–258.

Khare, C. P. 2007. Indian Medicinal Plants: An Illustrated Dictionary. Springer.

Kirtikar, K. R., Basu, B. D. 1984. Indian Medicinal Plants. 2nd Ed. Lalit Mohan Basu, Allahabad, India.

Kuppusamy Mudaliar, K. N. 1987. Kuruthi Azhal, Siddha Maruthuvam. Tamil Nadu Siddha Maruthuva Variyam, 201–210.

Liu, R., Heiss, E. H., Sider, N., Schinkovitz, A., Groblacher, B., Guo, D., Bucar, F., Bauer, R., Dirsch, V. M., Atanasov, A. G. 2015. Identification and characterization of 6-shogaol from ginger as inhibitor of vascular smooth muscle cell proliferation. Molecular Nutrition & Food Research 59:843–852.

Luo, Y., Pingping, S., Dongye, L. 2017. Luteolin a flavonoid that has multiple cardioprotective effects and its molecular mechanisms. Frontiers in Pharmacology 8:692.

Marijan-Jankovic, N. 1957. Effect of luteolin on the heart and vascular system in animals. Arzneimittelforschung 7:442–445.

Merighi, S., Travagli, A., Tedeschi, P., Marchetti, N., Gessi, S. 2021. Antioxidant and antiinflammatory effects of *Epilobium parviflorum*, *Melilotus officinalis* and *Cardiospermum halicacabum* plant extracts in macrophage and microglial cells. Cells 10(10):2691.

Muthu, C., Ayyanar, M., Raja, N., Ignacimuthu, S. 2006. Medicinal plants used by traditional healers in Kanchipuram district of Tamil Nadu, India. Journal of Ethnobiology and Ethnomedicine 2:43–46.

Nadkarni, K. M. 1976. Indian Materia Medica. Popular Prakashan, Mumbai.

Naik, V. K., Babu, K. S., Latha, J., Prabakar, V. 2014. A review on its ethnobotany, phytochemical and pharmacological profile of *Cardiospermum halicacabum* Linn. International Journal of Pharmaceutical Research Bioscience 3(Suppl 6):392–402.

Navjot, K., Nusrat, S., Harish, N. A. P. Srinivas, R. Harpreet, K. Neelima, C. Samir, M. 2014. Terminalia arjuna in chronic stable angina: Systematic review and meta-analysis. Cardiology Research and Practice 14:7.

Nerbonne, J. M., Kass, R. S. 2005. Molecular physiology of cardiac repolarization. Physiological Reviews 85(4):1205–1253.

Oluranti, O. I., Alabi, B. A., Michael, O. S., Ojo, A. O., Fatokun, B. P. 2021. Rutin prevents cardiac oxidative stress and inflammation induced by bisphenol A and dibutyl phthalate exposure via NRF-2/NF-κB pathway. Life Sciences 284(1):119878.

Othman, A. I., El-Sawi, M. R., El-Missiry, M. A., Abukhalil, M. H. 2017. Epigallocatechin-3-gallate protects against diabetic cardiomyopathy through modulating the cardiometabolic risk factors, oxidative stress, inflammation, cell death and fibrosis in streptozotocin-nicotinamide-induced diabetic rats. Biomedicine and Pharmacotherapy 94:362–373.

Oyagbemi, A. A., Adejumobi, O. A., Ajibade, T. O., Asenuga, E. R., Afolabi, J. M., Ogunpolu, B. S., Falayi, O. O., Hassan, F. O., Nabofa, E. W., Olutayo, O. T., Ola-Davies, O. E., Saba, A. B., Adedapo, A. A., Oguntibeju, O. O., Yakubu, M. A. 2021. Luteolin attenuates glycerol-induced acute renal failure and cardiac complications through modulation of kim-1/NF-κB/Nrf2 signaling pathways. Journal of Dietary Supplements 18(5):543–565.

Patel, R. V., Mistry, B. M., Shinde, S. K., Syed, R., Singh, V., Shin, H.-S. 2018. Therapeutic potential of quercetin as a cardiovascular agent. European Journal of Medicinal Chemistry 155:889–904.

Pavek, P., Dvorak, Z. 2008. Xenobiotic-induced transcriptional regulation of xenobiotic metabolizing enzymes of the cytochrome P450 superfamily in human extrahepatic tissues. *Current Drug Metabolism* 9:129–143.

Pieroni, A., Nebel, S., Quave, C., Münz, H., Heinrich, M. 2012. Ethnopharmacology of liakra: Traditional weedy vegetables of the Arbëreshë of the Vulture area in southern Italy. Journal of Ethnopharmacology 81(2):165–185.

Pogula, B. K., Maharajan, M. K., Oddepalli, D. R., Boini, L., Arella, M., Sabarimuthu, D. Q. 2012. Morin protects heart from beta-adrenergic stimulated myocardial infarction: An electrocardiographic, biochemical, and histological study in rats. Journal of Physiology and Biochemistry 68(3):433–446.

Ragupathy, S., Newmaster, S. G., Gopinadhan, P., Newmaster, C. B. 2007. Exploring ethnobiological classifications for novel alternative medicine: A case study of *Cardiospermum halicacabum* L. ('Modakathon', balloon vine) as a traditional herb for treating rheumatoid arthritis. Ethnobotany 19(1–2):1–16.

Ramanathan, P. (2002). Mooligai seyal thokuppu action of herbs, Ezhalai Mahathma Atchagam.

Ren, K., Jiang, T., Zhou, H. F., Liang, Y., Zhao, G. J. 2018. Apigenin retards atherogenesis by promoting ABCA1-mediated cholesterol efflux and suppressing inflammation. Cell Physiology and Biochemistry 47:2170–2184.

Riley, D. S. 2018. Cardiospermum halicacabum. In: Materia Medica of New and Old Homeopathic Medicines. Springer, Berlin, Heidelberg.

Santhakumari, G., Pillai, N. R., Nair, R. B. 1981. Diuretic activity of *Cardiospermum halicacabum* Linn in rats. Journal of Scientific Research in Plant Medicine 2(1):32–34.

Saravanan, G., Ponmurugan, P. M., Sathiyavathi, M., Vadivukkarasi, S., Sengottuvelu, S. 2013. Cardioprotective activity of Amaranthus viridis Linn: Effect on serum marker enzymes, cardiac troponin and antioxidant system in experimental myocardial infarcted rats. International Journal of Cardiology 165(3): 494–498.

Shareef, H. R., Mahmood, G., Khursheed, S., Hina, R. Z. 2012. *In vitro* antimicrobial and phytochemical analysis of *Cardiospermum halicacabum* L. Pakistan Journal of Botany 44:1677–1680.

Sharma, M., Kishore, K., Gupta, S. K., Joshi, S., Arya, D. S. 2001. Cardioprotective potential of Ocimum sanctum in isoproterenol induced myocardial infarction in rats. Molecular and Cellular Biochemistry 225(1–2):75–78.

Sheeba, M. S., Asha, V. V. 2009. *Cardiospermum halicacabum* ethanol extract inhibits LPS induced COX-2, TNF-alpha and iNOS expression, which is mediated by NF-kappa B regulation, in RAW264.7 cells. Journal of Ethnopharmacology 124:39–44.

Soni, R., Jaiswal, S., Bara, J. K., Saksena, P. 2016. The use of Rauwolfia serpentina in hypertensive patients. Journal of Biochemistry and Biotechnology 2(5):28–32.

Srinivas, K., Choudary, K. A., Rao, S. S., Satyanarayana, T., Krishna Rao, R. V. 1998. Phytochemical examination of *Cardiospermum halicacabum* Linn. Indian Journal of Natural Products 14:24–27.

Subramanyam, R., Newmaster, S. G., Paliyath, G., Newmaster, C. B. 2007. Exploring ethnobiological classifications for novel alternative medicine: A case study of *Cardiospermum halicacabum* L. (*Modakathon*, Balloon Vine) as a traditional herb for treating rheumatoid arthritis. Ethnobotany 19:1–18.

Tilak-Jain, J. A., Devasagayam, T. P. 2006. Cardioprotective and other beneficial effects of some Indian medicinal Plants. Journal of Clinical Biochemistry and Nutrition 38:9–18.

Umme, S., Taous, K., Abdul Jabbar, S. 2018. Antihypertensive effect of the methanolic extract from Eruca sativa Mill., (Brassicaceae) in rats: Muscarinic receptor-linked vasorelaxant and cardiotonic effects. Journal of Ethnopharmacology 224:409–420.

Van Dam, R. M., Naidoo, N., Landberg, R. 2013. Dietary flavonoids and the development of type 2 diabetes and cardiovascular diseases: Review of recent findings. Current Opinion Lipidology 24:25–33.

Venkatesh Babu, K. C., Krishnakumari, S. 2006. *Cardiospermum halicacabum* suppresses the production of TNF-α and NO by human peripheral blood mononuclear cells. African Journal of Biomedical Research 9:95–99.

Vimal, V., Devaki, T. 2004. Linear furanocoumarin protects rat myocardium against lipid peroxidation and membrane damage during experimental myocardial injury. Biomedical Pharmacotherapy 58(6–7):3 93–400.

Wai-Jo, J., Chan Andrew, J., McLachlan Edward, J., Luca Joanna, E. H. 2020. Garlic (*Allium sativum* L.) in the management of hypertension and dyslipidemia: A systematic review. Journal of Herbal Medicine 19:10029.

Wang, J., Gao, T., Wang, F., Xue, J., Ye, H., Xie, M. 2019. Luteolin improves myocardial cell glucolipid metabolism by inhibiting hypoxia inducible factor-1α expression in angiotensin II/hypoxia-induced hypertrophic H9c2 cells. Nutrition Research 65:63–70.

Yanyan, M. L., Jipeng, Y., Linhe, M., Xiaowu, L., Wang, J. R., Jian, Y. 2017. Rutin attenuates doxorubicin-induced cardiotoxicity via regulating autophagy and apoptosis. Biochimica Biophysica Acta 1863 (8):1904–1911.

Zeka, K., Ruparelia, K., Arroo, R. R. J., Budriesi, R., Micucci, M. 2017. Flavonoids and their metabolites: Prevention in cardiovascular diseases and diabetes. Diseases 5(3):19.

Zhang, C. Y., Tan, B. K. 1996. Hypotensive activity of aqueous extract of *Andrographis paniculata* in rats. Clinical and Experimental Pharmacology and Physiology 23:675–678.

Zhang, Y. M., C., Liu, C., Wei, F. 2020. Luteolin attenuates doxorubicin-induced cardiotoxicity by modulating the PHLPP1/AKT/Bcl-2 signalling pathway. Peer J 11(8):e8845.

Zhang, Y. M., Zhang, Z. Y., Wang, R. X. 2020. Protective mechanisms of quercetin against myocardial ischemia reperfusion injury. Frontiers in Physiology 11:956.

Zhu, Z. Y., Gao, T., Huang, Y., Xue, J., Xie, M. L. 2016. Apigenin ameliorates hypertension-induced cardiac hypertrophy and down-regulates cardiac hypoxia inducible factor-1α in rats. Food and Function 7(4):1992–1998.

10 Black Cumin (*Nigella sativa*)
Biological Activities and Molecular Aspects in Relation to Cardiovascular Disease

Maryam Moradi Binabaj and Fereshteh Asgharzadeh

CONTENTS

10.1 Introduction 146
    10.1.1 Cardiovascular Disease 146
10.2 *Nigella sativa* 146
    10.2.1 Plant Morphology 146
    10.2.2 Chemical Composition and Bioactive Constituents 146
    10.2.3 Therapeutic Potential of *NS* 148
10.3 Cardio-Protective Effects 148
    10.3.1 Anti-Inflammatory Effects of *NS* in CVD.. 148
    10.3.2 Antioxidative Effects of *NS* in CVD 149
    10.3.3 Anti-Apoptotic Effects of *NS* in CVD 151
    10.3.4 Anti-Fibrotic Effects of *NS* in CVD 152
    10.3.5 Other Foods, Herbs, Spices and Botanicals Used in
            Cardiovascular Health and Disease 154
    10.3.6 Toxicity and Cautionary Notes 154
    10.3.7 Conclusion 154
10.4 Summary Points 155
References.. 155

LIST OF ABBREVIATIONS

ACE	Angiotensin-converting enzyme
ATII	Angiotensin II
BP	Blood pressure
CVD	Cardiovascular disease
DEP	Diesel exhaust particles
EGF	Epidermal growth factor
FGF	Fibroblast growth factors
HGF	Hepatocyte growth factor
HO-1	Heme oxygenase-1
hs-CRP	High-sensitivity C-reactive protein
IGF-1	Insulin-like growth factor 1
IL	Interleukins
I/R	Ischemia/Reperfusion
LPS	Lipopolysaccharide
MI	Myocardial infarction

DOI: 10.1201/9781003220329-12

MPTP	Mitochondrial permeability transition pore
mtDNA	Mitochondrial DNA
NO	Nitric oxide
NRG-1	Neuregulin 1
NS	*Nigella sativa*
ROS	Reactive oxygen species
TGF-β	Transforming growth factor beta
TNF-α	Tumor necrosis factor alpha
TQ	Thymoquinone
VEGF	Vascular endothelial growth factor

10.1 INTRODUCTION

10.1.1 CARDIOVASCULAR DISEASE

Cardiovascular disease (CVD) is one of the major causes of death globally (Einarson et al. 2018) and it is estimated that each year more than 17 million people are dying in consequence of such disorders and it is predicted that CVD mortality will reach 23.3 million in future years until 2030 (Shaito et al. 2020; Suroowan and Mahomoodally 2015). CVD is a class of disorders affecting the heart and blood vessels function and it could result in hypertension and coronary heart failure (Mayakrishnan et al. 2013; Olorunnisola, Bradley, and Afolayan 2011). Atherosclerosis is an important clinical problem and is associated with artery lesions due to plaque formation which leads to cardiovascular disease (Libby, Ridker, and Hansson 2011). The exact molecular mechanisms underlying the pathophysiology of cardiovascular disease is not elucidated yet, but there are numerous factors which are associated with CVD pathogenesis, including metabolic abnormalities, oxidative stress, autophagy, apoptosis, activation of metalloproteinases and inflammation (Haffner 2003; Chistiakov et al. 2018; Lüscher and Vanhoutte 2020). There are different treatment modalities for CVD, including diuretics, vasodilators, anticoagulants, antiplatelet therapy and β-blockers, but due to the low efficiency, high price of medication and undesirable side effects, there is a need to find alternative treatments to optimize and maximize therapeutic effects and outcomes (Jahan and Ali 2012; Shoaib 2010; Panda and Naik 2009; Zheng et al. 2013).

10.2 *NIGELLA SATIVA*

10.2.1 PLANT MORPHOLOGY

Nigella sativa (black cumin or black seed) is an annual herbaceous and bushy, self-branching plant from the Ranunculaceae family, which can grow to 90 cm tall (Figure 10.1).

Leaves are divided into a number of linear segments and are separated on both sides of the stem. Branches produce flowers at the terminals and flowers vary naturally in color (Goreja 2003; Chevallier 1996). It commonly grows in different places including the Mediterranean, the Middle East, the eastern region of Europe and western Asia. Its seeds have an angular pattern, are typically small in size, are characterized by grey or black color, are a little bitter in taste and have a crispy texture (Ahmad et al. 2013; Cheikh-Rouhou et al. 2007; Al-Gaby 1998).

10.2.2 CHEMICAL COMPOSITION AND BIOACTIVE CONSTITUENTS

The number of *NS* chemical compositions depends on crop varieties, regional location, storage conditions and the nature of extraction method. The seeds of *NS* contain fixed oils; heavier molecules that do not vaporize readily including ω-9 fatty acid, oleic and palmitic acid, thymoquinone (TQ), flavonoids, alkaloids and saponin. TQ is the major component of its essential oil (Table 10.1) (Kazemi 2014; Ali and Blunden 2003; Cheikh-Rouhou et al. 2007).

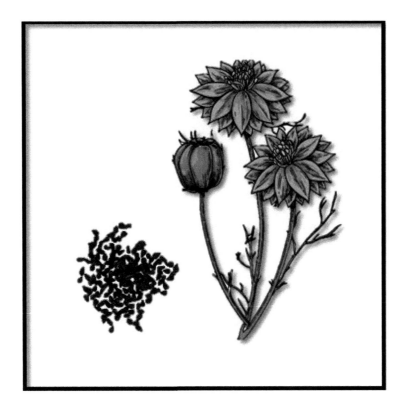

FIGURE 10.1 The schematic of *NS* flowers and its seeds.

TABLE 10.1
Analyzing *NS* Essential Oil with Gas Chromatography-Mass Spectrometry

No	Compound	Concentration
1	Alpha-thujene, origanene, or 3-thujene	13.60
2	Alpha-pinene	2.20
3	Beta-pinene	2.18
4	1,2,4-Trimethylbenzene or pseudocumene, Psi-cumene	1.30
5	Beta-cymene	37.76
6	Gamma-terpinene	0.69
7	Lilac aldehyde	0.55
8	2-Cyclohexen-1-ol, 2-methyl-5-(1-methylethyl)-, (1S-cis)	2.19
9	Thymoquinone	5.69

There are studies showing that TQ is the major active ingredient of *NS* seeds and is accountable for its observed biological actions (Fadishei et al. 2021; Khazdair, Ghafari, and Sadeghi 2021; Tabassum and Ahmad 2021; Jangjo-Borazjani et al. 2021). Moreover, the seeds are rich in carotene, carbohydrates (glucose, xylose, arabinose and rhamnose), fiber, amino acids and minerals including zinc, potassium, phosphor, copper, iron and calcium (Al-Jassir 1992; Tembhurne et al. 2014).

10.2.3 Therapeutic Potential of *NS*

NS, with established health benefits, has a different role in human nutrition and health. In *The Canon of Medicine*, one of the famous references of Avicenna, he describes black seed as a regulator of human body energy homeostasis which is useful for recovery from fatigue (Yarnell and Abascal 2011). It has been prescribed in domestic medicine for many years for the treatment of different disease in respiratory system and skin (Aboutabl, El-Azzouny, and Hammerschmidt 2019; Merfort et al. 1997). It also prescribed as a diuretic, lactagogue, carminative and vermifuge agent and preservative and spice in many foods (Burits and Bucar 2000). Recently, many studies and researches revealed that *NS* exerts anti-diabetic (Qidwai et al. 2009), anti-cancer (Zhang, Du, et al. 2018), antiseizure (Seghatoleslam et al. 2016) and anti-allergic (Günel et al. 2017) effects. Table 10.2 shows the effect of *NS* against toxicities induced by natural toxins and chemicals in different tissues.

Numerous studies have been conducted using various scientific techniques on *NS* extracts or its active compounds and its pharmacological actions, particularly in the past few decades. The following is to address and discuss the therapeutic potential of this herbal plant in terms of molecular and cellular properties for the treatment of CVD.

10.3 CARDIO-PROTECTIVE EFFECTS

10.3.1 Anti-Inflammatory Effects of *NS* in CVD

Chronic inflammation may cause plaque formation, which contributes to many thrombotic features and complications of atherosclerosis (Libby, Ridker, and Maseri 2002). Therefore, agents with anti-inflammatory properties may reflect preventative or therapeutic action and may affect risk of CVD (Moubayed, Heinonen, and Tardif 2007). There are studies showing that TQ, one of the important constituents of *NS*, exerts anti-inflammatory properties, especially in the context of the CVD. It has been found that TQ decreased the level of inflammatory markers like IL-1β, TNF-α, hs-CRP, interlukine-6 and hyperlipidemia-induced cardiac damage in rats (Pei et al. 2020). *NS* administration significantly decreased the level of IL-6 and TNF-α in comparison to the mice treated with lipopolysaccharide (LPS), which is used to induce inflammatory response. Moreover, *NS* has inhibitory effects against inflammatory cell infiltration and is contributed to fibrosis through the process of inflammation (Norouzi et al. 2017). *NS* extract in human endothelial vascular cell-line decreased the level of different mediators of inflammation which are associated with atherosclerosis (Amartey

---

TABLE 10.2
NS Protects against the Toxicities Induced by Chemicals and Natural Toxins

Chemical-Induced Toxicity	Hepatotoxicity	Metals (e.g. Cd, Al, Pb)
		Antibiotics: Isoniazid, Oxytetracycline
		Anticancer: Cisplatin, Cyclophosphamide, Tamoxifen
		Chemical agents: ethanol, BPA, NaF
	Nephrotoxicity	Antibiotics (Amikacin), anti-cancers (Doxorubicin), metals (Pb)
	Neurotoxicity	Metals (Pb, Al), Gentamicin, Ethanol, Toluene
	Reproductive toxicity	Metals, anti-cancers, pesticides, Toluene
	Cardiotoxicity	Anti-cancers: Isoproterenol, diesel exhaust particles
	Gastrointestinal toxicity	Ethanol, Methotrexate, Fenitrothion
	Pulmonary toxicity	Sulfur mustard, toluene, Bleomycin
	Hepatotoxicity	Metals (Cd, Al), Cisplatin, CCL4, Acetaminophen

et al. 2019). Recent evidence also highlights the involvement of TQ on ameliorating cardiac damage caused by hyperlipidemia. For instance, the level of TNF-α and IL-6 expression was decreased after TQ administration in mice (Xu et al. 2018). TQ supplementation downregulated the TNF-α and IL-6 gene expression in rats with diabetes mellitus. These findings are in line with the aforementioned studies showing the cardio-protective and anti-inflammatory properties of TQ and *NS*. TQ also exerts cardio-protective effects against diesel exhaust particles (DEP) as an air pollutant. TQ improved adverse effects of DEP on cardiopulmonary via decreasing inflammatory marker, IL-6 level and inflammatory cells (Nemmar et al. 2011). In addition, it was observed that *NS* oil could prevent cardiotoxicity in relation to lead exposure in albino adult rats. This effect is mediated through reduction in concentration of inflammatory factors including IL-6 and hs-CRP (Ahmed and Hassanein 2013).

These findings indicated that *NS* and its main constituent TQ exerts preventive and therapeutic action against cardiovascular events via decreasing inflammatory mediators, which accelerate initiation and progression of atherosclerotic plaques formation (Figure 10.2).

10.3.2 Antioxidative Effects of *NS* in CVD

Antioxidants aid to combat reactive oxygen species (ROS) and unstable free radicals, which cause cell damage and contribute to a variety of diseases (Wajid et al. 2014). In the pathophysiology of CVDs like atherosclerosis, heart failure, hypertension, cardiac hypertrophy, and ischemia-reperfusion, increased oxidative stress plays a significant role (Kurian et al. 2016).

Cardiomyocytes have a large number of mitochondria to assist them with their high energy demands, but mitochondrial malfunction will impair heart function (Shokolenko et al. 2009). Circular mitochondrial DNA (mtDNA) is very vulnerable to damage from excessive ROS production (Shokolenko et al. 2009). Because of its proximity to the inner mitochondrial membrane and

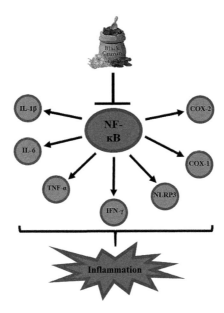

FIGURE 10.2 *NS* has anti-inflammatory potentials. *NS* was shown to diminish nuclear translocation and the DNA binding of Nuclear Factor-Kappa-B (NF-κB) via the blockade of phosphorylation and subsequent degradation of IκBα. As a result, decreased Interleukin 1 beta (IL-1β), Interleukin 6 (IL-6), Tumor necrosis factor alpha (TNF-α), Interferon gamma (IFN-γ), NLR Family Pyrin Domain Containing 3 (NLRP3), Cyclooxygenase (COX-1), Cyclooxygenase (COX-2) levels.

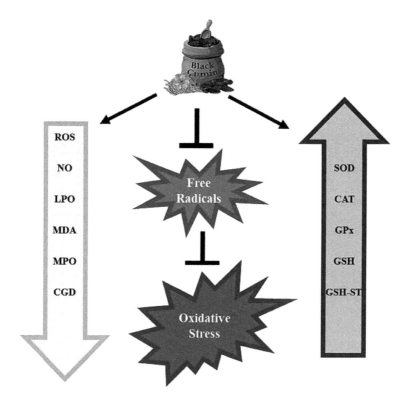

FIGURE 10.3 *NS* effectively increased the antioxidant parameters including superoxide dismutase (SOD), catalase (CAT), glutathione peroxidase (GPx), glutathione (GSH), Glutathione-S-transferase (GSH-ST) and decreased oxidant parameters, reactive oxygen species (ROS), nitric oxide (NO), lipid peroxidase (LPO), malondialdehyde (MDA), Myeloperoxidase (MPO), conjugated diene (CGD).

the lack of repair pathways, mtDNA is extremely vulnerable. Furthermore, oxidative stress damage to mtDNA causes a continual loop of increased ROS production, exacerbating oxidative stress damage and further mitochondrial dysfunction (Shokolenko et al. 2009). Consequently, mtDNA released into the bloodstream, serves as pro-inflammatory chemicals, exacerbating the inflammation (Qin et al. 2017; Siasos et al. 2018).

Antioxidants derived from plants have been known for prevention of the aging process. TQ revealed antioxidant or pro-oxidant properties (Wajid et al. 2014). *NS* may act as an antioxidant agent by scavenging ROS (Figure 10.3). It has the ability to reduce ischemic reperfusion injury and ROS levels in the heart tissue (Wajid et al. 2014).

Ischemic reperfusion in the heart induces the release of ROS, which leads to the opening of the mitochondrial permeability transition pore (MPTP) and consequently cardio-myocyte death. *NS* treatment resulted in a significant recovery of cardiac functions, maybe due to the inhibition of MPTP opening, which improved cardiovascular risk factors and reduced ROS (Seif 2013). Ischemic myocardium results in a variety of negative effects, including myocardial damage and potentially fatal ventricular arrhythmias. ROS products release following reperfusion of the ischemic myocardium, causing the formation of fatal ventricular arrhythmias, and tissue injury. TQ decreases arrhythmia scores, ventricular tachycardia, and the incidence of ventricular fibrillation. TQ appears to be beneficial in preventing deadly ventricular arrhythmias caused by IRI in rats (Gonca and Kurt 2015; Tappia et al. 2001; Tullio et al. 2013). It has been established that antioxidants result in myocardial dysfunction prevention and decrease the progression of myocardial infarction (MI) (Agrawal et al. 2014; Goyal et al. 2010). TQ has the potential to decrease MI, increasing influencing

Black Cumin (*Nigella sativa*)

antioxidant status, lowering ROS levels, decreasing heart rate and blood pressure and exertion protective effect (Gonca and Kurt 2015). Moreover, TQ has cardiovascular protective activity through modulating arterial force and rate of constriction by blocking voltage-gated Ca^{+2} channels (Ghayur, Gilani, and Janssen 2012; Xiao et al. 2018; Frank et al. 2012). In another study, after Ischemia/Reperfusion (I/R) injury, TQ decreased enhanced oxidative state, suggesting that antioxidants may play a role in TQ's cardio-protective action in I/R (Xiao et al. 2018).

In addition, development of hypertension is linked to oxidative stress. Excessive ROS generation reduces nitric oxide (NO) availability and this causes endothelial dysfunction, which leads to a rise in total peripheral resistance.

The volatile oil of *NS* and TQ have been shown to lower arterial blood pressure (BP) and heart rate (Leong, Rais Mustafa, and Jaarin 2013), as well as reduce the risk of stroke, coronary artery disease, heart failure, and peripheral vascular disease. To control hypertension and avoid its consequent health problems, patients with hypertension must take medications for the rest of their lives. Some of these medications are expensive and have different side effects. As a result, this is a good time to look into complementary therapies that are more effective and have fewer side effects. A cardiac depressive impact, calcium channel blocking property and diuretic action are only a few of the mechanisms. The effect of cardiac depression with *NS* administration appears to be mediated by central pathways involving the medulla's vasomotor center and sympathetic output to the periphery rather than NO or eicosanoid (Leong, Rais Mustafa, and Jaarin 2013), which include stroke, coronary artery disease, heart failure and peripheral vascular disease.

Thymol, one of the active chemicals in *NS*, is primarily responsible for calcium channel blockage. Thymol relaxes vascular smooth muscle cells via decreasing Ca^{2+} currents through L-type Ca^{2+} channels. Thymol has also been found to have a negative inotropic effect (Szentandrássy et al. 2004). Finally, *NS* has been shown to increase the excretion of Na^+, K^+ and Cl^- (Zaoui et al. 2000). *NS* may affect the vascular wall and disrupt blood vessels' functionality and structure. TQ boosts endothelial function by lowering oxidative stress and increasing eNOS expression (Ahmad et al. 2013). NOS has also been shown to have an anti-hypertensive effect by lowering the activity of the angiotensin-converting enzyme (ACE), while increasing the activity of the heme oxygenase-1 (HO-1). ACE not only increases the formation of angiotensin II (AT II), which has a direct vasoconstrictor effect on the arteries, but also induces the generation of ROS, which exacerbates vascular damage, whereas HO-1 decreases AT II activity (Jaarin et al. 2015).

10.3.3 Anti-Apoptotic Effects of *NS* in CVD

Apoptosis or programmed cell death is a type of cell death which is mediated by both extrinsic and intrinsic pathways. The intrinsic pathway stimulates apoptosis in response to pro-apoptotic proteins such as Bax and Bak and anti-apoptotic proteins such as Bcl-2, which alters mitochondrial membrane permeability, and leads to changes in membrane potential, cytochrome c release and caspase (Cas)-3 formation due to the overproduction of free radicals (Tibaut, Mekis, and Petrovic 2016).

TQ exerts anti-apoptotic characteristics, serves as an excellent cardio-protective agent for ischemic heart conditions such as MI via modulating oxidative stress parameters, inflammatory markers, apoptotic indicators and myocardial content of mtDNA (Hassan et al. 2017; Ojha et al. 2015; Khalifa, Rashad, and El-Hadidy 2021). TQ also reduces cell death and helps the heart tissue cope with its dynamic character by keeping heart mtDNA content, which regulates energy generation in the myocytes (Khalifa, Rashad, and El-Hadidy 2021).

TQ dramatically reduces apoptosis through lowering Cas-3 levels in cardiac tissue (Khalifa, Rashad, and El-Hadidy 2021). There is also a substantial negative association between Cas-3 level and cardiac mtDNA content, indicating that TQ reduces Cas-3 activation, inhibiting apoptosis and conserving cardiac mtDNA content. These findings are in agreement with other previous studies (Galaly, Ahmed, and Mahmoud 2014; Xiao et al. 2018).

Apoptosis is the most common cause of cardio-myocyte cell death in the peri-infarct zone (Zepeda et al. 2014). Many studies have shown that cellular oxidative stress, specially in MI, activates Bax (pro-apoptotic protein) and triggers apoptosis (Redza-Dutordoir and Averill-Bates 2016). Investigations revealed that when TQ is given before or after another drug, the level of Bax protein is reduced considerably. TQ also inhibited the Bax expression in various ischemia scenarios (El-Ghany et al. 2009; Xiao et al. 2018). During the apoptotic process, both Bax and Bak oligomerize to form mitochondrial outer membrane permeabilization (MOMP) pores in the outer membrane of the mitochondria (Westphal et al. 2011). The substantial negative association between cardiac mtDNA content and Bax level is supported by this sequential evidence. While TQ prevented mitochondrial-induced apoptosis and reduced Bax levels, it protected mtDNA content (Westphal et al. 2011). Bcl2, an anti-apoptotic protein, is vital for cardio-protection in ischemic conditions (Xu et al. 2014). In the Khalifa et al. study, ISP-induced MI resulted in a substantial decrease in Bcl2 levels when compared to the control group, but ISP-induced MI resulted in a significant increase in Bcl2 levels when compared to the TQ-treated group (Zhang, Zhang, et al. 2018). The Bcl2 level and cardiac mtDNA content were found to have a substantial positive association. Bcl-2 proteins are located on the outer mitochondrial membrane and suppress the activation of the pro-apoptotic family members Bax and Bak, preventing apoptosis and mtDNA release (Lindsay, Degli Esposti, and Gilmore 2011). As a result, elevated Bcl2 levels caused by TQ play an important role in cardiac mtDNA content preservation.

Autophagy, a type of apoptosis in which the cell undergoes dynamic morphological changes, plays a vital part in the myocardial apoptosis process, which is known to be a critical mechanism for cardiac damage and dysfunction in the I/R heart tissue (Ma et al. 2012; Xiao et al. 2018). Lack of autophagy leads to cardio-myocytes apoptosis (Ma et al. 2012). In the Xiao et al. study, when myocardial I/R damage occurred, cell apoptosis was apparently elevated (Xiao et al. 2018), which decreased in the TQ group and indicates an autophagy inhibitory effect of TQ. Infarction aggravation, myocardial dysfunction, arrhythmia and myocyte death can all be triggered by reperfusion (Wo et al. 2008; Lei et al. 2012). The induction of autophagy is one of the main mechanisms of action by which TQ exerts cardio-protective effects (Xiao et al. 2018). LC3 conversion (LC3II/LC3I) and p62 immunoblotting are two commonly used types of autophagy flow assessment (Tang, Ellis, and Lovat 2016).

The TQ pretreatment group had higher levels of LC3II and lower expression of p62, indicating that autophagy was substantially activated (Xiao et al. 2018). However, in the presence of CQ, the effects of TQ on myocardial autophagy were largely reversed, suggesting that autophagy may play a role in TQ-mediated cardio-protection. Their findings revealed that following I/R injury, Cas-3 and apoptosis rose, but this effect was prevented by TQ therapy. Cell autophagy was reduced with CQ to further establish TQ's underpinning mechanism. TQ could improve heart function, reduce myocardial infarction size, lower myocardial enzyme activities and prevent oxidative stress (Xiao et al. 2018).

10.3.4 Anti-Fibrotic Effects of *NS* in CVD

Fibrosis is a well-known cause of mortality and morbidity (Hinderer and Schenke-Layland 2019). The most prevalent cause of cardiac fibrosis is myocardial infarction. Despite the human body's outstanding self-healing capacity, not all defects can regenerate effectively (Hinderer and Schenke-Layland 2019). When cardiac fibroblasts create collagenous connective tissue, it causes myocardial fibrosis, which impairs the myocardium's ability to receive oxygen and nutrients (El-Kerdasy, Badr Eldeen, and Ali 2021). Ischemia, arrhythmias and heart failure are all possible outcomes of myocardial fibrosis (El-Kerdasy, Badr Eldeen, and Ali 2021; Hinderer and Schenke-Layland 2019). As a result of increased fibrosis and heart failure, excessive collagen by fibrocytes affects the ventricular wall structures and interferes with normal function of the heart (Asgharzadeh et al. 2018). A fibrotic scar is said to be caused by the buildup of collagens following the maturation process. With increasing crosslinking density, the tensile strength of such scars increases (Brauchle et al. 2018). As a result, cardiac contractility and relaxation suffer, and heart function disrupts (Hinderer and Schenke-Layland 2019). Electric coupling is also affected by excessive collagen deposition in the heart muscle, which acts as electrical insulators (Rog-Zielinska et al. 2016). As shown by Norouzi et al. (Norouzi et al. 2017) and Asgharzadeh et al. (Asgharzadeh et al. 2018), treatment with *NS* and TQ reduced collagen deposition through suppressing chronic inflammation and improved oxidative stress status. This process may be useful in the treatment of cardiac fibrosis. TQ also has the potential to prevent cardiac fibrosis (Pei et al. 2018).

Inflammation has been identified as a risk factor for heart fibrosis in studies. It further said that ROS activation could result in heart fibrosis (Asgharzadeh et al. 2018). Moreover, persistent inflammation generated by LPS resulted in cardiac fibrosis (as demonstrated by higher collagen content) (Asgharzadeh et al. 2018). TQ improved perivascular fibrosis and left ventricular wall fibrosis in a dose-dependent manner (Asgharzadeh et al. 2018). TQ possesses anti-inflammatory and antioxidant action in both in vitro and in vivo settings, and its effects on cardiovascular health have been studied (Gholamnezhad, Havakhah, and Boskabady 2016). It has been claimed that NF-κB activation causes the production of inflammatory markers and fibrotic factors, and that TQ may inhibit this pathway, resulting in TQ's anti-fibrotic and antioxidant properties (Figure 10.4) (Fiordelisi et al. 2019).

Although fibrotic reactions, including fibroblast recruitment and activation, can result in scar formation, these activities are also necessary for normal wound healing (Groeber et al. 2011; Rog-Zielinska et al. 2016). As a result, in order to establish new therapeutic targets or methods, it is vital to comprehend the specifics of the events that contribute to physiological or pathological tissue remodeling. The heart tissue has been encouraged to develop "better" and more useful scars by modifying scar characteristics (Rog-Zielinska et al. 2016). The therapeutic strategy of heart fibrosis is the application of growth factors and cytokines such as VEGF, IGF-1, HGF, NRG-1, EGF, FGF and TGF-β to induce cardiac repair (Lewis, Kumar, and Ellison-Hughes 2018). This method can be used to target resident cells in the heart and affect cell activities such as survival, migration, proliferation and differentiation (Lewis, Kumar, and Ellison-Hughes 2018). Several studies demonstrated

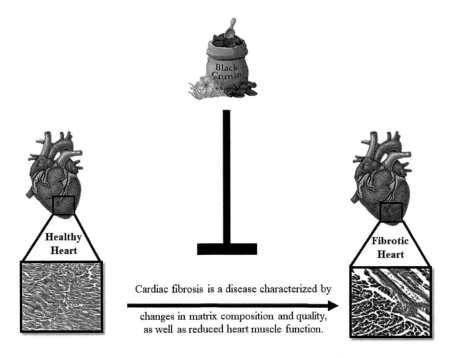

FIGURE 10.4 *NS* improved myocardial fibrosis.

that *NS* could increase growth factors (VEGF, FGF and IGF-1) (Al Asoom 2017; Al-Asoom et al. 2014) and decrease TGF-β in heart tissue (Pei et al. 2018). As a result, it appears that *NS* and its active components can help to reduce cardiac fibrosis by lowering inflammation and oxidative stress while enhancing growth factors.

10.3.5 OTHER FOODS, HERBS, SPICES AND BOTANICALS USED IN CARDIOVASCULAR HEALTH AND DISEASE

Herbal and natural medicine is increasingly getting widespread popularity and medical professionals' acceptance, with respect to the progress in the current explanation of the underlying biological actions, which results in overall improvement of health and quality of life. Based on the World Health Organization (WHO) report, around 80% of the people all around the world depend mostly on natural products from herbal plants for their health care (Suroowan and Mahomoodally 2015). Regarding the therapeutic potential of medicinal plants, there is growing attention in the world toward the consumption of these products for prevention and treatment of cardiovascular disease (Fathiazad et al. 2012; Ojha et al. 2011).

Medicinal plants are rich in bioactive secondary metabolites, which have therapeutic properties and these metabolites (known as phytochemicals) could have a beneficial effect on human health (Hasler 1998). Following several decades of research and development, numerous plant-derived drugs have developed, or have been used in preparation of commercial drugs (Suroowan and Mahomoodally 2015).

Nearly, more than 2000 plants are recorded in the list of traditional medicine (herbal/alternative) and they have been shown to provide adequate relief for patients with cardiovascular disease in the clinical setting and have been shown to improve patient care outcomes (Rajalakshmy, Pydi, and Kavimani 2011).

There are so many herbs, plants and food supplements for treatment of cardiovascular disease like ginger, garlic, green tea (Tachjian, Maria, and Jahangir 2010).

To alleviate the adverse effects of cardiovascular disease, there is need to further investigate the cardioprotective effects of bioactive components in food and plant sources.

10.3.6 TOXICITY AND CAUTIONARY NOTES

To determine the safety of *NS*, researchers have investigated its toxicity and tolerability over the years. The results of these studies, including clinical trials, have shown a high degree of safety. In vivo studies have been shown that long-term administration of *NS* was not associated with organ damage or decreasing leukocyte and platelet counts less than the normal limits. In another study, chronic supplementation of rats with fixed or volatile oils extracted from black seed demonstrates no detrimental effects (Zaoui et al. 2002; Sultan, Butt, and Anjum 2009). The results of another research study, conducted by Dollah et al. revealed that *NS* has no toxic side effects on hepatic function and no abnormalities were observed in liver enzymes (Dollah et al. 2013).

In addition, Mashhadian et al. have been shown that different forms of *NS* extract, which are prepared based on aqueous, methanol and chloroform solutions, exert no significant toxicity effects (Vahdati-Mashhadian, Rakhshandeh, and Omidi 2005).

10.3.7 CONCLUSION

In conclusion, *NS* can improve cardiac function, decrease myocardial infarct size and reduce myocardial enzyme activity. Because of its antioxidative, anti-inflammatory, anti-fibrotic and anti-apoptotic properties including autophagy regulation, *NS* has a wide spectrum of therapeutic potential, notably in cardiovascular illnesses. Long-term human trials are also needed to prove the therapeutic usefulness of this old alternative medicine.

Black Cumin (*Nigella sativa*) 155

10.4 SUMMARY POINTS

- An overview of the effect of black cumin (*Nigella sativa*) molecular mechanisms underlying cardiovascular diseases is presented in this chapter.
- *Nigella sativa* is a plant with very few side effects, without substantial toxicity.
- The beneficial effects of *Nigella sativa* are attributable to its anti-inflammatory, antioxidant, anti-apoptotic and anti-fibrotic properties.
- Several constituents of *Nigella sativa* show therapeutic potential in cardiovascular disorders.
- Bioactive secondary metabolites found in medicinal plants act therapeutically.

REFERENCES

Aboutabl, EA, AA El-Azzouny, and F-J Hammerschmidt. 2019. "Aroma volatiles of Nigella sativa L. seeds." In *Progress in Essential Oil Research*, 49–56. de Gruyter.

Agrawal, Yogeeta O, Pankaj Kumar Sharma, Birendra Shrivastava, Shreesh Ojha, Harshita M Upadhya, Dharamvir Singh Arya, and Sameer N Goyal. 2014. "Hesperidin produces cardioprotective activity via PPAR-γ pathway in ischemic heart disease model in diabetic rats." *PloS One* 9 (11):e111212.

Ahmad, Aftab, Asif Husain, Mohd Mujeeb, Shah Alam Khan, Abul Kalam Najmi, Nasir Ali Siddique, Zoheir A Damanhouri, and Firoz Anwar. 2013. "A review on therapeutic potential of Nigella sativa: A miracle herb." *Asian Pacific Journal of Tropical Biomedicine* 3 (5):337–352.

Ahmed, Marwa A, and Khaled MA Hassanein. 2013. "Cardio protective effects of Nigella sativa oil on lead induced cardio toxicity: Anti inflammatory and antioxidant mechanism." *Journal of Physiology and Pathophysiology* 4 (5):72–80.

Al Asoom, LI. 2017. "Coronary angiogenic effect of long-term administration of Nigella sativa." *BMC Complementary and Alternative Medicine* 17 (1):1–7.

Al-Asoom, LI, BA Al-Shaikh, AO Bamosa, and MN El-Bahai. 2014. "Effect of Nigella sativa supplementation to exercise training in a novel model of physiological cardiac hypertrophy." *Cardiovascular Toxicology* 14 (3):243–250.

Al-Gaby, AMA. 1998. "Amino acid composition and biological effects of supplementing broad bean and corn proteins with Nigella sativa (black cumin) cake protein." *Food/Nahrung* 42 (05):290–294.

Ali, BH, and Gerald Blunden. 2003. "Pharmacological and toxicological properties of Nigella sativa." *Phytotherapy Research: An International Journal Devoted to Pharmacological and Toxicological Evaluation of Natural Product Derivatives* 17 (4):299–305.

Al-Jassir, M Saleh. 1992. "Chemical composition and microflora of black cumin (Nigella sativa L.) seeds growing in Saudi Arabia." *Food Chemistry* 45 (4):239–242.

Amartey, Jason, Samuel Gapper, Nurudeen Hussein, Keith Morris, and Cathryn E Withycombe. 2019. "Nigella sativa extract and thymoquinone regulate inflammatory cytokine and TET-2 expression in endothelial cells." *Artery Research* 25 (3–4):157–163.

Asgharzadeh, Fereshteh, Rahimeh Bargi, Farimah Beheshti, Mahmoud Hosseini, Mehdi Farzadnia, and Majid Khazaei. 2018. "Thymoquinone prevents myocardial and perivascular fibrosis induced by chronic lipopolysaccharide exposure in male rats:-thymoquinone and cardiac fibrosis." *Journal of Pharmacopuncture* 21 (4):284.

Brauchle, Eva, Jana Kasper, Ruben Daum, Nicolas Schierbaum, Claudius Falch, Andreas Kirschniak, Tilman E Schäffer, and Katja Schenke-Layland. 2018. "Biomechanical and biomolecular characterization of extracellular matrix structures in human colon carcinomas." *Matrix Biology* 68:180–193.

Burits, M, and F Bucar. 2000. "Antioxidant activity of Nigella sativa essential oil." *Phytotherapy Research* 14 (5):323–328.

Cheikh-Rouhou, Salma, Souhail Besbes, Basma Hentati, Christophe Blecker, Claude Deroanne, and Hamadi Attia. 2007. "Nigella sativa L.: Chemical composition and physicochemical characteristics of lipid fraction." *Food chemistry* 101 (2):673–681.

Chevallier, Andrew. 1996. "The encyclopedia of medicinal plants."

Chistiakov, Dimitry A, Tatiana P Shkurat, Alexandra A Melnichenko, Andrey V Grechko, and Alexander N Orekhov. 2018. "The role of mitochondrial dysfunction in cardiovascular disease: A brief review." *Annals of Medicine* 50 (2):121–127.

Dollah, Mohammad Aziz, Saadat Parhizkar, Latiffah Abdul Latiff, and Mohammad Hafanizam Bin Hassan. 2013. "Toxicity effect of Nigella sativa on the liver function of rats." *Advanced Pharmaceutical Bulletin* 3 (1):97.

Einarson, Thomas R, Annabel Acs, Craig Ludwig, and Ulrik H Panton. 2018. "Prevalence of cardiovascular disease in type 2 diabetes: A systematic literature review of scientific evidence from across the world in 2007–2017." *Cardiovascular Diabetology* 17 (1):1–19.

El-Ghany, Abd, M Ragwa, Nadia M Sharaf, Lobna A Kassem, Laila G Mahran, and Ola A Heikal. 2009. "Thymoquinone triggers anti-apoptotic signaling targeting death ligand and apoptotic regulators in a model of hepatic ischemia reperfusion injury." *Drug Discoveries & Therapeutics* 3 (6).

El-Kerdasy, Hanan, Bodour Badr Eldeen, and Ali Ali. 2021. "Effect of Nigella sativa and Angiotensin converting enzyme inhibitor on myocardial fibrosis induced by lipopolysaccharide." *Benha Medical Journal* 38 (Academic issue):30–46.

Fadishei, Masoumeh, Mahboobeh Ghasemzadeh Rahbardar, Mohsen Imenshahidi, Ahmad Mohajeri, Bibi Marjan Razavi, and Hossein Hosseinzadeh. 2021. "Effects of Nigella sativa oil and thymoquinone against bisphenol A-induced metabolic disorder in rats." *Phytotherapy Research* 35 (4):2005–2024.

Fathiazad, Fatemeh, Amin Matlobi, Arash Khorrami, Sanaz Hamedeyazdan, Hamid Soraya, Mojtaba Hammami, Nasrin Maleki-Dizaji, and Alireza Garjani. 2012. "Phytochemical screening and evaluation of cardioprotective activity of ethanolic extract of Ocimum basilicum L. (basil) against isoproterenol induced myocardial infarction in rats." *DARU Journal of Pharmaceutical Sciences* 20 (1):1–10.

Fiordelisi, Antonella, Guido Iaccarino, Carmine Morisco, Enrico Coscioni, and Daniela Sorriento. 2019. "NFkappaB is a key player in the crosstalk between inflammation and cardiovascular diseases." *International Journal of Molecular Sciences* 20 (7):1599.

Frank, Anja, Megan Bonney, Stephanie Bonney, Lindsay Weitzel, Michael Koeppen, and Tobias Eckle. 2012. "Myocardial ischemia reperfusion injury: From basic science to clinical bedside." Seminars in cardiothoracic and vascular anesthesia.

Galaly, SR, OM Ahmed, and AM Mahmoud. 2014. "Thymoquinone and curcumin prevent gentamicin-induced liver injury by attenuating oxidative stress, inflammation and apoptosis." *J Physiol Pharmacol* 65 (6):823–832.

Ghayur, Muhammad Nabeel, Anwarul Hassan Gilani, and Luke Jeffrey Janssen. 2012. "Intestinal, airway, and cardiovascular relaxant activities of thymoquinone." *Evidence-Based Complementary and Alternative Medicine.*

Gholamnezhad, Zahra, Shahrzad Havakhah, and Mohammad Hossein Boskabady. 2016. "Preclinical and clinical effects of Nigella sativa and its constituent, thymoquinone: A review." *Journal of Ethnopharmacology* 190:372–386.

Gonca, Ersöz, and Çağla Kurt. 2015. "Cardioprotective effect of Thymoquinone: A constituent of Nigella sativa L., against myocardial ischemia/reperfusion injury and ventricular arrhythmias in anaesthetized rats." *Pakistan Journal of Pharmaceutical Sciences* 28 (4).

Goreja, WG. 2003. *Black Seed: Nature's Miracle Remedy*: Karger Publishers.

Goyal, Sameer, Sachin Arora, Tarun Kumar Bhatt, Prasenjit Das, Amit Sharma, Santosh Kumari, and Dharamvir Singh Arya. 2010. "Modulation of PPAR-γ by telmisartan protects the heart against myocardial infarction in experimental diabetes." *Chemico-Biological Interactions* 185 (3):271–280.

Groeber, Florian, Monika Holeiter, Martina Hampel, Svenja Hinderer, and Katja Schenke-Layland. 2011. "Skin tissue engineering: In vivo and in vitro applications." *Advanced Drug Delivery Reviews* 63 (4–5):352–366.

Günel, Ceren, Buket Demirci, İbrahim Meteoğlu, Mustafa Yılmaz, İmran Kurt Ömürlü, and Tolga Kocatürk. 2017. "The anti-inflammatory effects of thymoquinone in a rat model of allergic rhinitis." *J Ear Nose Throat* 27:226–232.

Haffner, Steven M. 2003. "Pre-diabetes, insulin resistance, inflammation and CVD risk." *Diabetes Research and Clinical Practice* 61:S9–S18.

Hasler, Clare M. 1998. "Functional foods: Their role in disease prevention and health promotion." *Food Technology-Champaign Then Chicago* 52:63–147.

Hassan, Md Quamrul, Mohd Akhtar, Sayeed Ahmed, Aftab Ahmad, and Abul Kalam Najmi. 2017. "Nigella sativa protects against isoproterenol-induced myocardial infarction by alleviating oxidative stress, biochemical alterations and histological damage." *Asian Pacific Journal of Tropical Biomedicine* 7 (4):294–299.

Hinderer, Svenja, and Katja Schenke-Layland. 2019. "Cardiac fibrosis: A short review of causes and therapeutic strategies." *Advanced Drug Delivery Reviews* 146:77–82.

Jaarin, Kamsiah, Wai Dic Foong, Min Hui Yeoh, Zaman Yusoff Nik Kamarul, Haji Mohd Saad Qodriyah, Abdullah Azman, Japar Sidik Fadhlullah Zuhair, Abdul Hamid Juliana, and Yusof Kamisah. 2015. "Mechanisms of the antihypertensive effects of Nigella sativa oil in L-NAME-induced hypertensive rats." *Clinics* 70:751–757.

Jahan, Nazish, and Shoukat Ali. 2012. "Cardioprotective and antilipidemic potential of Cyperus rotundus in chemically induced cardiotoxicity." *International Journal of Agriculture and Biology* 14 (6).

Jangjo-Borazjani, Soheila, Maryam Dastgheib, Efat Kiyamarsi, Roghayeh Jamshidi, Saleh Rahmati-Ahmadabad, Masoumeh Helalizadeh, Roya Iraji, Stephen M Cornish, Shiva Mohammadi-Darestani, and Zohreh Khojasteh. 2021. "Effects of resistance training and nigella sativa on type 2 diabetes: Implications for metabolic markers, low-grade inflammation and liver enzyme production." *Archives of Physiology and Biochemistry*:1–9.

Kazemi, Mohsen. 2014. "Phytochemical composition, antioxidant, anti-inflammatory and antimicrobial activity of Nigella sativa L. essential oil." *Journal of Essential Oil Bearing Plants* 17 (5):1002–1011.

Khalifa, Asmaa A, Radwa M Rashad, and Wessam F El-Hadidy. 2021. "Thymoquinone protects against cardiac mitochondrial DNA loss, oxidative stress, inflammation and apoptosis in isoproterenol-induced myocardial infarction in rats." *Heliyon* 7 (7):e07561.

Khazdair, Mohammad Reza, Shoukouh Ghafari, and Mahmood Sadeghi. 2021. "Possible therapeutic effects of Nigella sativa and its thymoquinone on COVID-19." *Pharmaceutical Biology* 59 (1):696–703.

Kurian, Gino A, Rashmi Rajagopal, Srinivasan Vedantham, and Mohanraj Rajesh. 2016. "The role of oxidative stress in myocardial ischemia and reperfusion injury and remodeling: Revisited." *Oxidative Medicine and Cellular Longevity*.

Lei, Xiaofei, Xiaoguang Lv, Meng Liu, Zirong Yang, Mengyao Ji, Xufeng Guo, and Weiguo Dong. 2012. "Thymoquinone inhibits growth and augments 5-fluorouracil-induced apoptosis in gastric cancer cells both in vitro and in vivo." *Biochemical and Biophysical Research Communications* 417 (2):864–868.

Leong, Xin-Fang, Mohd Rais Mustafa, and Kamsiah Jaarin. 2013. "Nigella sativa and its protective role in oxidative stress and hypertension." *Evidence-Based Complementary and Alternative Medicine*.

Lewis, Fiona C, Siri Deva Kumar, and Georgina M Ellison-Hughes. 2018. "Non-invasive strategies for stimulating endogenous repair and regeneration mechanisms in the damaged heart." *Pharmacological Research* 127:33–40.

Libby, Peter, Paul M Ridker, and Göran K Hansson. 2011. "Progress and challenges in translating the biology of atherosclerosis." *Nature* 473 (7347):317–325.

Libby, Peter, Paul M Ridker, and Attilio Maseri. 2002. "Inflammation and atherosclerosis." *Circulation* 105 (9):1135–1143.

Lindsay, Jennefer, Mauro Degli Esposti, and Andrew P Gilmore. 2011. "Bcl-2 proteins and mitochondria: Specificity in membrane targeting for death." *Biochimica et Biophysica Acta (BBA)-Molecular Cell Research* 1813 (4):532–539.

Lüscher, Thomas F, and Paul M Vanhoutte. 2020. *The Endothelium: Modulator of Cardiovascular Function: Modulator of Cardiovascular Function*: CRC press.

Ma, Xiucui, Haiyan Liu, Sarah R Foyil, Rebecca J Godar, Carla J Weinheimer, Joseph A Hill, and Abhinav Diwan. 2012. "Impaired autophagosome clearance contributes to cardiomyocyte death in ischemia/reperfusion injury." *Circulation* 125 (25):3170–3181.

Mayakrishnan, Vijayakumar, Priya Kannappan, Noorlidah Abdullah, and Abdul Bakrudeen Ali Ahmed. 2013. "Cardioprotective activity of polysaccharides derived from marine algae: An overview." *Trends in Food Science & Technology* 30 (2):98–104.

Merfort, I, V Wray, HH Barakat, SAM Hussein, MAM Nawwar, and G Willuhn. 1997. "Flavonol triglycosides from seeds of Nigella sativa." *Phytochemistry* 46 (2):359–363.

Moubayed, Sami P, Therese M Heinonen, and Jean-Claude Tardif. 2007. "Anti-inflammatory drugs and atherosclerosis." *Current Opinion in Lipidology* 18 (6):638–644.

Nemmar, Abderrahim, Suhail Al-Salam, Shaheen Zia, Fatima Marzouqi, Amna Al-Dhaheri, Deepa Subramaniyan, Subramanian Dhanasekaran, Javed Yasin, Badreldin H Ali, and Elsadig E Kazzam. 2011. "Contrasting actions of diesel exhaust particles on the pulmonary and cardiovascular systems and the effects of thymoquinone." *British Journal of Pharmacology* 164 (7):1871–1882.

Norouzi, Fatemeh, Azam Abareshi, Fereshteh Asgharzadeh, Farimah Beheshti, Mahmoud Hosseini, Mehdi Farzadnia, and Majid Khazaei. 2017. "The effect of Nigella sativa on inflammation-induced myocardial fibrosis in male rats." *Research in Pharmaceutical Sciences* 12 (1):74.

Ojha, Shreesh, Sheikh Azimullah, Rajesh Mohanraj, Charu Sharma, Javed Yasin, Dharamvir S Arya, and Abdu Adem. 2015. "Thymoquinone protects against myocardial ischemic injury by mitigating oxidative stress and inflammation." *Evidence-Based Complementary and Alternative Medicine*.

Ojha, Shreesh, Saurabh Bharti, Ashok K Sharma, Neha Rani, Jagriti Bhatia, Santosh Kumari, and Dharamvir Singh Arya. 2011. "Effect of Inula racemosa root extract on cardiac function and oxidative stress against isoproterenol-induced myocardial infarction."

Olorunnisola, OS, G Bradley, and AJ Afolayan. 2011. "Ethnobotanical information on plants used for the management of cardiovascular diseases in Nkonkobe Municipality, South Africa." *Journal of Medicinal Plants Research* 5 (17):4256–4260.

Panda, Vandana S, and Suresh R Naik. 2009. "Evaluation of cardioprotective activity of Ginkgo biloba and Ocimum sanctum in rodents." *Alternative Medicine Review* 14 (2):161.

Pei, Zuo-Wei, Ying Guo, Huo-Lan Zhu, Min Dong, Qian Zhang, and Fang Wang. 2020. "Thymoquinone protects against hyperlipidemia-induced cardiac damage in Low-Density Lipoprotein Receptor-Deficient (LDL-R-/-) mice via its anti-inflammatory and antipyroptotic effects." *BioMed Research International.*

Pei, Zuowei, Jiahui Hu, Qianru Bai, Baiting Liu, Dong Cheng, Hainiang Liu, Rongmei Na, and Qin Yu. 2018. "Thymoquinone protects against cardiac damage from doxorubicin-induced heart failure in Sprague-Dawley rats." *RSC Advances* 8 (26):14633–14639.

Qidwai, Waris, Hasan Bin Hamza, Riaz Qureshi, and Anwar Gilani. 2009. "Effectiveness, safety, and tolerability of powdered Nigella sativa (kalonji) seed in capsules on serum lipid levels, blood sugar, blood pressure, and body weight in adults: Results of a randomized, double-blind controlled trial." *The Journal of Alternative and Complementary Medicine* 15 (6):639–644.

Qin, Chao-Yi, Hong-Wei Zhang, Jun Gu, Fei Xu, Huai-Min Liang, Kang-Jun Fan, Jia-Yu Shen, Zheng-Hua Xiao, Er-Yong Zhang, and Jia Hu. 2017. "Mitochondrial DNA-induced inflammatory damage contributes to myocardial ischemia reperfusion injury in rats: Cardioprotective role of epigallocatechin." *Molecular Medicine Reports* 16 (5):7569–7576.

Rajalakshmy, I, R Pydi, and S Kavimani. 2011. "Cardioprotective medicinal plants: A review." *International Journal of Pharmaceutical Science Invention* 1:24–41.

Redza-Dutordoir, Maureen, and Diana A Averill-Bates. 2016. "Activation of apoptosis signalling pathways by reactive oxygen species." *Biochimica et Biophysica Acta (BBA)-Molecular Cell Research* 1863 (12):2977–2992.

Rog-Zielinska, Eva A, Russell A Norris, Peter Kohl, and Roger Markwald. 2016. "The living scar: Cardiac fibroblasts and the injured heart." *Trends in Molecular Medicine* 22 (2):99–114.

Seghatoleslam, Masoumeh, Fatemeh Alipour, Reihaneh Shafieian, Zahra Hassanzadeh, Mohammad Amin Edalatmanesh, Hamid Reza Sadeghnia, and Mahmoud Hosseini. 2016. "The effects of Nigella sativa on neural damage after pentylenetetrazole induced seizures in rats." *Journal of Traditional and Complementary Medicine* 6 (3):262–268.

Seif, Ansam Aly. 2013. "Nigella sativa attenuates myocardial ischemic reperfusion injury in rats." *Journal of Physiology and Biochemistry* 69 (4):937–944.

Shaito, Abdullah, Duong Thi Bich Thuan, Hoa Thi Phu, Thi Hieu Dung Nguyen, Hiba Hasan, Sarah Halabi, Samar Abdelhady, Gheyath K Nasrallah, Ali H Eid, and Gianfranco Pintus. 2020. "Herbal medicine for cardiovascular diseases: Efficacy, mechanisms, and safety." *Frontiers in Pharmacology* 11:422.

Shoaib, Samia. 2010. "Cardioprotective effect of gemmotherapeutically treated withania somnifera against chemically induced myocardial." *Pak. J. Bot* 42 (2):1487–1499.

Shokolenko, Inna, Natalia Venediktova, Alexandra Bochkareva, Glenn L Wilson, and Mikhail F Alexeyev. 2009. "Oxidative stress induces degradation of mitochondrial DNA." *Nucleic Acids Research* 37 (8):2539–2548.

Siasos, Gerasimos, Vasiliki Tsigkou, Marinos Kosmopoulos, Dimosthenis Theodosiadis, Spyridon Simantiris, Nikoletta Maria Tagkou, Athina Tsimpiktsioglou, Panagiota K Stampouloglou, Evangelos Oikonomou, and Konstantinos Mourouzis. 2018. "Mitochondria and cardiovascular diseases: From pathophysiology to treatment." *Annals of Translational Medicine* 6 (12).

Sultan, M Tauseef, Masood Sadiq Butt, and Faqir Muhammad Anjum. 2009. "Safety assessment of black cumin fixed and essential oil in normal Sprague Dawley rats: Serological and hematological indices." *Food and Chemical Toxicology* 47 (11):2768–2775.

Suroowan, Shanoo, and Fawzi Mahomoodally. 2015. "Common phyto-remedies used against cardiovascular diseases and their potential to induce adverse events in cardiovascular patients." *Clinical Phytoscience* 1 (1):1–13.

Szentandrássy, Norbert, Gyula Szigeti, Csaba Szegedi, Sándor Sárközi, János Magyar, Tamás Bányász, László Csernoch, László Kovács, Péter P Nánási, and István Jóna. 2004. "Effect of thymol on calcium handling in mammalian ventricular myocardium." *Life Sciences* 74 (7):909–921.

Tabassum, Heena, and Iffat Z Ahmad. 2021. "Molecular docking and dynamics simulation analysis of thymoquinone and thymol compounds from Nigella sativa L. that inhibit cag A and Vac A oncoprotein of helicobacter pylori: Probable treatment of H. pylori Infections." *Medicinal Chemistry* 17 (2):146–157.

Tachjian, Ara, Viqar Maria, and Arshad Jahangir. 2010. "Use of herbal products and potential interactions in patients with cardiovascular diseases." *Journal of the American College of Cardiology* 55 (6):515–525.

Tang, Diana YL, Robert A Ellis, and Penny E Lovat. 2016. "Prognostic impact of autophagy biomarkers for cutaneous melanoma." *Frontiers in Oncology* 6:236.

Tappia, Paramjit S, Tomoji Hata, Lena Hozaima, Manjot S Sandhu, Vincenzo Panagia, and Naranjan S Dhalla. 2001. "Role of oxidative stress in catecholamine-induced changes in cardiac sarcolemmal Ca2+ transport." *Archives of Biochemistry and Biophysics* 387 (1):85–92.

Tembhurne, SV, S Feroz, BH More, and DM Sakarkar. 2014. "A review on therapeutic potential of Nigella sativa (kalonji) seeds." *Journal of Medicinal Plants Research* 8 (3):167–177.

Tibaut, Miha, Dusan Mekis, and Daniel Petrovic. 2016. "Pathophysiology of myocardial infarction and acute management strategies." *Cardiovascular & Hematological Agents in Medicinal Chemistry (Formerly Current Medicinal Chemistry-Cardiovascular & Hematological Agents)* 14 (3):150–159.

Tullio, Francesca, Carmelina Angotti, Maria-Giulia Perrelli, Claudia Penna, and Pasquale Pagliaro. 2013. "Redox balance and cardioprotection." *Basic Research in Cardiology* 108 (6):392.

Vahdati-Mashhadian, N, H Rakhshandeh, and A Omidi. 2005. "An investigation on LD50 and subacute hepatic toxicity of Nigella sativa seed extracts in mice." *Die Pharmazie-An International Journal of Pharmaceutical Sciences* 60 (7):544–547.

Wajid, Nadia, Fatima Ali, Muhammad Tahir, Abdul Rehman, and Azib Ali. 2014. "Dual properties of Nigella Sativa: Anti-oxidant and pro-oxidant." *Advancements in Life Sciences* 1 (2):79–88.

Westphal, Dana, Grant Dewson, Peter E Czabotar, and Ruth M Kluck. 2011. "Molecular biology of Bax and Bak activation and action." *Biochimica et Biophysica Acta (BBA)-Molecular Cell Research* 1813 (4):521–531.

Wo, Yan-bo, Dan-yan Zhu, Ying Hu, Zhi-Qiang Wang, Jian Liu, and Yi-Jia Lou. 2008. "Reactive oxygen species involved in prenylflavonoids, icariin and icaritin, initiating cardiac differentiation of mouse embryonic stem cells." *Journal of Cellular Biochemistry* 103 (5):1536–1550.

Xiao, Junhui, Zun-Ping Ke, Yan Shi, Qiutang Zeng, and Zhe Cao. 2018. "The cardioprotective effect of thymoquinone on ischemia-reperfusion injury in isolated rat heart via regulation of apoptosis and autophagy." *Journal of Cellular Biochemistry* 119 (9):7212–7217.

Xu, Jingyi, Liyue Zhu, Hongyang Liu, Mengye Li, Yingshu Liu, Fan Yang, and Zuowei Pei. 2018. "Thymoquinone reduces cardiac damage caused by hypercholesterolemia in apolipoprotein E-deficient mice." *Lipids in Health and Disease* 17 (1):1–9.

Xu, Tongda, Xin Wu, Qiuping Chen, Shasha Zhu, Yang Liu, Defeng Pan, Xiaohu Chen, and Dongye Li. 2014. "The anti-apoptotic and cardioprotective effects of salvianolic acid a on rat cardiomyocytes following ischemia/reperfusion by DUSP-mediated regulation of the ERK1/2/JNK pathway." *PloS One* 9 (7):e102292.

Yarnell, Eric, and Kathy Abascal. 2011. "Nigella sativa: Holy herb of the Middle East." *Alternative and Complementary Therapies* 17 (2):99–105.

Zaoui, A, Y Cherrah, MA Lacaille-Dubois, A Settaf, H Amarouch, and M Hassar. 2000. "Diuretic and hypotensive effects of Nigella sativa in the spontaneously hypertensive rat." *Therapie* 55 (3):379–382.

Zaoui, A, Y Cherrah, N Mahassini, K Alaoui, H Amarouch, and M Hassar. 2002. "Acute and chronic toxicity of Nigella sativa fixed oil." *Phytomedicine* 9 (1):69–74.

Zepeda, Ramiro, Jovan Kuzmicic, Valentina Parra, Rodrigo Troncoso, Christian Pennanen, Jaime A Riquelme, Zully Pedrozo, Mario Chiong, Gina Sánchez, and Sergio Lavandero. 2014. "Drp1 loss-of-function reduces cardiomyocyte oxygen dependence protecting the heart from ischemia-reperfusion injury." *Journal of Cardiovascular Pharmacology* 63 (6):477–487.

Zhang, Hui-Hui, Ying Zhang, Yan-Na Cheng, Fu-Lian Gong, Zhan-Qi Cao, Lu-Gang Yu, and Xiu-Li Guo. 2018. "Metformin in combination with curcumin inhibits the growth, metastasis, and angiogenesis of hepatocellular carcinoma in vitro and in vivo." *Molecular Carcinogenesis* 57 (1):44–56.

Zhang, Mengzhao, Hongxia Du, Zhixin Huang, Pu Zhang, Yangyang Yue, Weiyi Wang, Wei Liu, Jin Zeng, Jianbin Ma, and Guanqiu Chen. 2018. "Thymoquinone induces apoptosis in bladder cancer cell via endoplasmic reticulum stress-dependent mitochondrial pathway." *Chemico-Biological Interactions* 292:65–75.

Zheng, Chun-Song, Xiao-Jie Xu, Hong-Zhi Ye, Guang-Wen Wu, Hui-Feng Xu, Xi-Hai Li, Su-Ping Huang, and Xian-Xiang Liu. 2013. "Computational pharmacological comparison of Salvia miltiorrhiza and Panax notoginseng used in the therapy of cardiovascular diseases." *Experimental and Therapeutic Medicine* 6 (5):1163–1168.

11 Date Palm (*Phoenix dactylifera*) and Cardiovascular Protection
Molecular, Cellular and Physiological Aspects

Heba Abd Elghany Sahyon

CONTENTS

11.1   Introduction 162
11.2   Background 162
11.3   Date Palm Fruit Antioxidant Activity 163
11.4   Date Palm Phenolic Composition 163
11.5   Date Palm Polyphenols-Related Cardioprotection Activity 164
11.6   Date Palm Composition and Health Promotion 164
11.7   Therapeutic Properties of Date Fruit 165
11.8   Edible Date Palm Parts in Experimental Research 165
11.9   Date Palm Fruit and Cardiovascular Protection 168
11.10 Date Palm Fruit and Lipids Metabolism 168
11.11 Date Palm Fibers and Lipid Metabolism 169
11.12 Date Pollen Cardioprotective Effect 169
11.13 Date Fruit Cardiovascular Protection Molecular Mechanisms 169
11.14 Other Foods, Herbs, Spices, and Botanicals Used in Cardiovascular
       Health and Disease 171
11.15 Toxicity and Cautionary Notes 171
11.16 Summary Points 171
References 172

LIST OF ABBREVIATIONS

ALT   Alanine transaminase
AST   Aspartate transaminase
CPK   Creatine phosphokinase
CVD   Cardiovascular disease
GPx   Glutathione peroxidase
GSH   Glutathione reductase
HDL   High-density lipoprotein
IFN-γ Interferon gamma
IL-1β Interleukin-1 beta
IL-2   Interleukin-2
IL-6   Interleukin-6
IL-12   Interleukin-12
LDH   Lactate dehydrogenase
LDL   Low-density lipoprotein

DOI: 10.1201/9781003220329-13

NF-κB	Nuclear factor kappa
NO	Nitric oxide
PD-1	Programmed cell death protein-1
ROS	Reactive oxygen species
SOD	Superoxide dismutase
TBARS	Thiobarbituric acid reactive compounds
TG	Triglycerides
TNF-α	Tumor necrose factor α
VLDL	Very low-density lipoprotein

11.1 INTRODUCTION

The date palm tree is the oldest fruit-bearing tree in Southwest Asia, North America, Australia, Africa, and the Arab regions. Its botanical name is *Phoenix dactylifera L.*, and it belongs to the *Palmaceae* family (Hussain, Farooq, and Syed 2020). The word "finger-bearing" in the species name, Dactylifera, refers to the clusters structure of the date fruits. Dactylifera is a combination of the Latin term ferous, which means "bearing," and the Greek word dactylus, which means "finger." The fruits, pollen, and head of the date palm (*Phoenix dactylifera L.*) were among the edible portions that were used as food and, in some countries, as medicine (Daoud et al. 2017). Date seeds were also used to make coffee and as a component of animal feed due to their high protein content. Date seeds also contain selenium, in very small quantities, and the selenium is a potent anticancer component because of its high antioxidant activity in addition to its ability to detoxify toxicants (Al-Farsi and Lee 2011).

The date palm's non-edible parts, including clusters, leaves, and skin, have a noticeable amount of polyphenolic constituents, but they were not frequently used as the other palm parts in traditional medicine (Farag, Otify, and Baky 2021). The date palm's fruit, or date, is the most widely consumed part. Dates come in more than 5000 varieties, with different shapes, sizes, and weights. Some varieties of date fruit are spherical, although most are oblong and oval. Among the most famous varieties are Ajwa, Dhakki, Aseel, Zaghlool, Majdool, Mabrook, Hyany, and Halawi. Iran and Iraq have the most date varieties, between 370 and 400 kinds. According to FAO, around 75% of the world's dates are produced in Arab nations. Saudi Arabia and Egypt produced 17% and 21% of the world's production of date fruit, with a high quality date in Saudi Arabia (Food and Agriculture Organisation (FAO) 2020).

11.2 BACKGROUND

The date palm (*P. dactylifera*) is a multifunctional, valuable tree with a richness of nutritional, medicinal, financial, and environmental qualities. The date fruit has been used in several cultures around the world as an essential food crop and in traditional medicine since an earlier period. The fruits of the date palm are currently a crucial economic crop in the world and are consumed on a large worldwide scale. Dates provide therapeutic benefits in the management of diseases due to their antioxidant, antidiabetic, anti-tumor, and anti-inflammatory potentials. Additionally, they have demonstrated antibacterial, antifungal, antiviral, and hepatoprotective properties (Zihad et al. 2021). It has been demonstrated that date fruit consumption as suspension or extract have enhanced DNA and sperm quality in males as well as regulation of female sex hormones (Shehzad et al. 2021). The date fruit has long been used in traditional medicine to cure a variety of illnesses across the Middle East, Africa, and Persia. Mostly in Arabic countries, it is particularly famous for its widespread use in treating hepatic disease and malaria (Bagherzadeh Karimi et al. 2020). Boiling date pulp in milk has been demonstrated to have positive health effects on pregnancy and breastfeeding women. According to historical records, dates were used to treat diabetes and hypertension in southern Morocco (Tahraoui et al. 2007).

Dates have reportedly been proposed to aid in the hardness of baby gum. When cooked with cardamom and black pepper, dates can also help to lessen a dry cough, a slight fever, headaches, and lethargy. Date consumption was advised in traditional medicine for pregnant women and those with jaundice disease. Date fruit eating has been associated with demulcent, diuretic, expectorant, and restorative qualities (Echegaray et al. 2020). Although it is well known that there was not as much scientific research available in the past to empirically demonstrate the therapeutic properties of date palms, recent studies are starting to validate these claims and demonstrate their therapeutic mechanisms.

Recent *in vivo* studies have linked the fruit of the palm date with additional health benefits, including anti-inflammatory, anti-hyperlipidemic, and antioxidant actions (Silabdi et al. 2021; Al-Shwyeh 2019). Consuming 50 g of date palm fruit daily resulted in an expansion in stool motility, decreased ammonia concentration in stool, and a reduction in genotoxicity (Eid et al. 2015). The aphrodisiac benefits of date palm pollen have historically been established.

Furthermore, *P. dactylifera*'s other parts have been used for centuries in traditional medicine to cure hypertension, memory problems, diabetes, fever, paralysis, atherosclerosis, and nervous system abnormalities (Hussain, Farooq, and Syed 2020). Due to their high polyphenol content, many edible portions of the *Phoenix dactylifera L.* have been tested in medical and therapeutic researches (Gad El-Hak et al. 2022; Abdelaziz, Ali, and Mostafa 2015).

Regarding possible health impacts of date palm *P. dactylifera*, several biological activities have been described. These activities were primarily based on clinical trials and animal models, and to a lesser extent, the *in vitro* studies. These include anti-inflammatory and gastroprotective benefits, support for antioxidant protection, and cardioprotective activities (Bouhlali et al. 2020). A thorough analysis of date palm edible parts and their potential role in maintaining vascular health is necessary because of the increasing incidence of cardiovascular disease (CVD) around the globe. Here, we concentrate on how date palm *P. dactylifera* guides of cardiovascular function, paying close attention to their positive effects on people.

11.3 DATE PALM FRUIT ANTIOXIDANT ACTIVITY

Dietary antioxidants, such as phenolic chemicals found in dates, may protect the body from a variety of degenerative diseases by reducing oxidative stress. Additionally, they support the stimulation of antioxidant systems that are both enzymatic and non-enzymatic. Date extracts have powerful antioxidant abilities that can both be seen *in vitro* and *in vivo*, as well as the ability to scavenge free radicals (Al-Shwyeh 2019; Trabzuni 2019; Trabzuni 2019; Mohamed and Al-Okabi 2004). They work to prevent oxidative damage to lipids, nucleic acids, and proteins and are mostly attributed to their phenolic component (Al-Shwyeh 2019).

11.4 DATE PALM PHENOLIC COMPOSITION

The polyphenolic composition of dates is mostly determined by the date's variety and degree of ripening. Dates undergo a considerable chemical and functional transformation during the ripening process, with sugar levels rising and vitamin, mineral, and fiber levels declining steadily in correlation to the date fruit weight. As demonstrated by Ajwa dates, ripening decreases the concentration of phenolic acids (such as hydroxybenzoic acids and hydroxycinnamic acids) and flavonoids (such as flavonoid glycosides, catechin flavanol, and anthocyanidins).

The antioxidant and antiatherogenic potential of phenolic acid and flavonol fractions extracted from Amari and Halawi dates at the tamer stage were tested *in vitro* via TBARS and lipid peroxide assays. The two fractions showed varying capacity to decrease ferric ions, scavenge radicals, and suppress low-density lipoprotein (LDL) oxidation, with the flavonol fractions having the largest effects. Only the flavonol components encouraged macrophages to remove cholesterol, and that could suggest the hypolipidemic activity of the date fruit. Amari dates were significantly higher in

TABLE 11.1

Phenolic and Flavonoid Components of Edible Parts of the Date Palm

P. dactylifera Part	Highest Phenolic and Flavonoids Ratios	References
Fruit	quercetin, apigenin, luteolin, kaempferol glycosides, and malonyl derivatives. Ferulic acid, protocatechuic, caffeic acid, chlorogenic acid, gallic acid. Anthocyanidins, flavones, flavonols, hydroxycinnamates, chrysoeriol.	(Abu-Reidah et al. 2017; Zihad et al. 2021; Hussain, Farooq, and Syed 2020; Khatib et al. 2022)
Pollen	quercetin derivatives, isorhamnetin derivatives, apigenin derivative, steroidal saponins	(Abu-Reidah et al. 2017; Mrabet et al. 2016; Abdul-Hamid et al. 2020; Otify et al. 2019)
Heart of the palm	Gallic acid, caffeic acid, ctechin, kaempferol, and rutin	(Sahyon and Al-Harbi 2020; Hameed et al. 2021)

Note: This table lists the highest phenolic and flavonoid levels that have been tested in date fruit, pollen, and heart of the palm, which have therapeutic potentials.

phenolic acids than Halawi dates by around 3.5- to 10-fold. Other studies that listed the phenolic and flavonoid composition in different date varieties were listed in Table 11.1.

11.5 DATE PALM POLYPHENOLS-RELATED CARDIOPROTECTION ACTIVITY

Edible parts of the *P. dactylifera* tree have high contents of flavonoids, terpenoids, and polyphenolic compounds. According to recent investigations using HPLC, UPLC-MS, GC-MS, mass spectrometry, and NMR, the polyphenols contained in the fruit, pollen, and heart of the palm of *P. dactylifera* trees are listed in Table 11.1. Numerous cardiovascular parameters have been studied in relation to the action of date polyphenols. Potent flavonoids that can be detected in both pollen and fruit of the date palm are quercetin and rutin glycoside, which have antioxidant activities and potential effects on cardiac muscle protection. Kaempferol was recently detected in some date fruit varieties and is also found in the heart of the palm, and has anti-inflammatory and cardioprotective activities (Tram et al. 2017). Ferulic acid and protocatechuic acid that are detected in the date fruit could protect the cardiac muscle from oxidative stress and prevent cardiac hypertrophy through several signaling pathways (Aswar et al. 2019; Bai et al. 2021).

Date palm fruit and pollen prevent oxidative heart damage in diabetic rats by acting as reactive oxygen species (ROS) scavengers and cardioprotective agents in response to isoproterenol induction (Daoud et al. 2017; Al-Yahya et al. 2016). Date palm's hepatoprotective, cardioprotective, and anti-inflammatory activities were proven by date palm fruit supplementation (Abdeen et al. 2021). Date fruit flesh contains a variety of phenolic acids and flavonoids (catechin and rutin) that make them effective health-promoting agents for preventing cardiovascular disease (CVD) (Topal et al. 2018).

11.6 DATE PALM COMPOSITION AND HEALTH PROMOTION

Date palm fruit was tested, in many studies, for their nutrients. It was found that date fruit has a wide range of carbohydrate levels ranging from 81.4–71.2% according to the date variety. Also, the date fruit crude protein contents were found to be in the range of 2.5–4.73 g per 100 gram date weight (Hussain, Farooq, and Syed 2020). High levels of essential amino acids were also found in the date fruit such as aspartic acid, glutamic acid glutamine, asparagine, histidine, glycine, alanine, and proline with a minimal amount of cysteine. In addition, minimum levels of nonessential amino acids lysine and tryptophane were also detected (Abdul-Hamid et al. 2020). Another date fruit component is the dietary fibers such as lignin and cellulose that are found in high amounts in all date varieties and can improve gut movement as well as its ability to generate short-chain fatty acids (George et al. 2020). The high insoluble fiber content in the date fruit causes satiety and has a laxative effect due to increased stool weight. Therefore, it might contribute to a reduction in the risk of diverticular illness and bowel cancer.

Date fruits have been shown to contain high levels of macro-minerals such as magnesium which reaches 64.2 mg per 100 g date weight. Magnesium has several health benefits such as contributing to several enzyme processes, modulating the immune system, regulating blood pressure, preventing cardiovascular disease, and assisting with muscle and nerve function. Some micro-minerals also exist in date fruits, such as zinc and iron, which improve the immune system's performance and help to combat fatigue, respectively. Sodium is also detected in a trace amount and is necessary for respiration. Additionally, dates include various amounts of vitamins such as carotenoids (vitamin A), thiamine, folic acid, ascorbic acid, riboflavin, and retinol. These vitamins can improve vision as in vitamin A, regulate metabolism, improve liver and heart function, and promote the immune system.

11.7 THERAPEUTIC PROPERTIES OF DATE FRUIT

Date fruit is a rich source of a wide range of phytochemicals that gives the fruit unique therapeutic properties (Figure 11.1). Using botanical extracts as antimicrobial agents is very useful as they are high in safety and more favorable than synthetic ones for patients. Different varieties of date fruit extracts have confirmed their antibacterial and antifungal activities against resistance organisms.

Polyphenols and flavonoids act as antioxidant agents by scavenging ROS, preventing membrane lipid peroxidation, and maintaining the function of vital organs such as the liver, kidney, and heart. ROS is also generated by some synthetic drugs that can damage the vital organs as a side effect of that drug. Date extract has a large quantity of phenolic acids, which can act as antioxidant agents for scavenging the ROS released from normal metabolism, bacterial infection, toxicants, and synthetic drugs. Recent animal studies confirmed the antioxidant and hepatoprotective potential of date fruit extract against several toxicants (CCl_4, dichloroacetic acid) (Echegaray et al. 2020), and against anticancer drugs (doxorubicin and cisplatin) that induce cardiotoxicity and hepatotoxicity (Gad El-Hak et al. 2022).

In many *in vitro* studies, the anti-tumor effect of date fruit extract against human cancer cell lines (Colo-205, MCF7, PC3, and T47D) was confirmed by different date varieties. However, no human trials have been conducted to demonstrate its anticancer effect.

The antidiabetic properties of date fruit extract were also established by experimental studies (Abdelaziz, Ali, and Mostafa 2015), but there were no clinical studies to confirm that effect.

11.8 EDIBLE DATE PALM PARTS IN EXPERIMENTAL RESEARCH

Many experimental models have been established to test the antioxidant, anti-inflammatory, and cardioprotective properties of edible parts of date palm. As listed in Table 11.2, date fruit has been the subject of most experimental studies as it is rich in polyphenols and flavonoids that give it several therapeutic, hepatoprotective, and cardioprotective properties. This antioxidant property results in the scavenging of ROS produced by various carcinogens, anticancer drugs, antibiotics, and toxicants, which can prevent oxidative damage and protect the vital organs. Furthermore, the ability of date fruit supplementation to increase the antioxidant enzyme system can reduce oxidative stress caused by increased ROS and thus protect vital organs.

In addition to the reduction of lipoproteins and cholesterol levels and inhibition of inflammation by a reduction in inflammatory cytokines (IL-2, IL-12, and IL-6), date fruit also prevents organ damage by inhibiting the severe immune response to inflammation. That decreased inflammatory response appears in decreasing foot swelling in the arthritis mouse model. On the other hand, the anticancer, antiapoptotic, and antioxidant activities of the date fruit extract were clearly

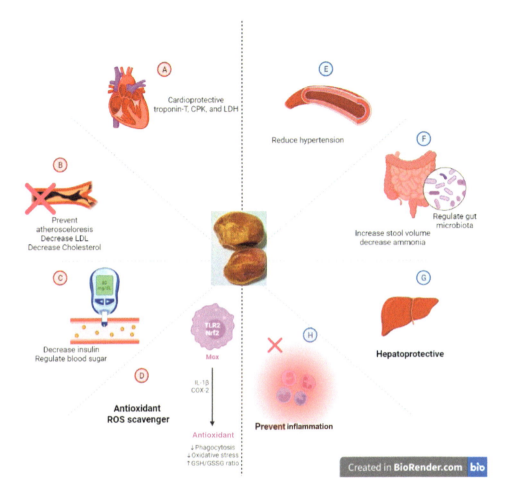

FIGURE 11.1 Date palm fruit health benefits.

Note: An illustration of all the studies that have used the date palm fruit for health benefits in human and animal studies.

demonstrated by the inhibition of liver cancer in a rat model. From all these animal studies, we can conclude that oral supplementation of date fruit could markedly prevent lipid peroxidation, neutralize the ROS released from different toxicants, activate the antioxidant system, and inhibit the inflammatory response, which could protect the liver and heart.

Date palm pollen oral supplementation also has a diversity of phenolic and flavonoid compositions (Table 11.1). Those compounds give it antioxidant properties, but the studies were more validated in increasing fertility, testosterone level, and sperm count as the pollen has a steroid-like substance that is absent in the date fruit. A study was conducted by Elblehi et al. 2021, which used date pollen to prevent heart tissue oxidative damage by doxorubicin injection in a rat model. In this study, pollen supplementation successfully prevented cardiotoxicity by increasing the antioxidant enzymes, lipid peroxidation, and regulating the serum cardiac markers. Also, decreasing the inflammatory cytokines along with regulating TGF-β1 led to apoptotic inhibition by downregulating both caspase-3 and Bax gene expression.

A study by Sahyon and Al-Harbi (2020) confirmed the antioxidant activity of *P. dactylifera* palm heart, making it an excellent supplement for scavenging free radicals caused by doxorubicin injection. In addition, the heart of the palm extract supplementation increased antioxidant enzymes

TABLE 11.2
Experimental Studies of *P. dactylifera* Edible Parts

P. dactylifera Part	Animal Model	Response	References
Fruit	• Rat model (gentamicin-induced liver and kidney injury) • Rat arthritis model (chronic inflammation) • Rabbit model of liver injury (CCl4 induction) • Rat model (isoproterenol-induced myocardial infarction) • Rat hepatotoxicity and oxidative damage (dimethoate induction) • Mice model • Rat liver damage model (dichloroacetic acid induction) • Rat liver cancer model (diethyl nitrosamine induction) • Rat • Female rat	▼ALT, AST, and creatinine ▲Albumin, ▼MDA, ▲catalase, ▼iNOS. Inhibited liver fibrosis ▼Arthritis (foot swelling) ▼MDA ▼ALT, AST, and TBARS ▼ALT, AST, ALP, GGT, LDH, and CK ▲SOD, catalase, and NO ▼ MDA, NP-SH, MPO, and lipoproteins ▼ALT, AST, ALP, GGT, and LDH ▲SOD, GPx, and catalase Stimulation of the immune response (▲IFN-γ⁺CD4⁺, IFN-γ⁺CD49b⁺ and IL-12⁺CD11b⁺ cells) ▼ALT, AST, ALP, and LDH. ▼Hepatic TBARS ▲SOD, catalase, and GPx ▼ALT, AST, ALP. ▲SOD, GSH, catalase and GPx. ▲Anti-tumor cytokines (IL-2, IL-12). ▼AFP and IL-6 ▼Cholesterol, TG, and LDL. ▲HDL ▼Troponin-I, TG, LDL, and cholesterol. ▲HDL ▼Cardiac risk ratio	(Abdeen et al. 2021) (Mohamed and Al-Okabi 2004) (Al-Shoaibi et al. 2012) (Al-Yahya et al. 2016) (Saafi et al. 2011) (Karasawa et al. 2011) (El Arem et al. 2014) (Khan et al. 2017) (Silabdi et al. 2021) (Mubarak et al. 2018)
Pollen	• Male rats • Rat model injected with testosterone (atypical prostatic hyperplasia) • Male diabetic rats • Rat cardiotoxicity model (Doxorubicin induction)	▲Sperm count, motility, morphology, and testis weights ▼Cytokine expression (IL-6, IL-8, TNF-α, IGF-1) ▲Testosterone level ▼LDH, CK-MB, cTnI, cTnT, NT-pro BNP, and cytosolic calcium. ▼NO, lipid peroxidation and GPx, SOD, and catalase. ▼Inflammation (▼NF-κB, p65, TNF-α, IL-1β, and IL-6). ▼TGF-β1, casp-3 and Bax, Bcl-2	(Bahmanpour et al. 2006) (Elberry et al. 2011) (Kazeminia, Kalaee, and Nasri 2014) (Elblehi et al. 2021)
Heart of the Palm	• Rat model cardiotoxicity and nephrotoxicity (Doxorubicin induction) • Rat • Male rat	▼LDH, CK-MB ▼Apoptosis, casp-3, and COX-2. ▲Catalase, TAC, and GSH ▼ MDA and apoptosis ▲PD-1 ▲SOD, GPx, and CAT ▼Insulin and leptin ▼Cholesterol, VLDL, and TG. ▲HDL. ▼T3 and T4. ▲TSH	(Sahyon and Al-Harbi 2020) (Trabzuni 2019) (Trabzuni 2019)

Note: This table lists all the animal studies that used the edible parts of the date palm and their effects on the enzymes or cytokines of the specific organ.

and decreased both the cardiac and kidney parameters along with inhibiting apoptosis percentage in both the heart and kidney by decreasing caspase-3 and cyclooxygenase-2 levels. Heart of palm supplementation improves histopathological images of both heart and kidney tissues by preventing inflammatory responses and decreasing the programmed cell death protein-1 (PD-1), which suppresses activated T-lymphocytes and regulates the activated immune response.

Other studies on normal rats supplemented with the heart of the palm have confirmed the decrease in insulin, leptin, cholesterol, VLDL, and TG along with elevations in antioxidant enzymes and HDL, which also prove the ability of that extract to improve liver and heart functions (Table 11.2).

11.9 DATE PALM FRUIT AND CARDIOVASCULAR PROTECTION

Numerous chronic diseases, such as cardiovascular disease (CVD), diabetes, and several malignancies, can be made more likely by lifestyle decisions, including diet and exercise. Due to higher health care costs and decreased productivity, chronic diseases are expected to rise gradually, resulting in a cumulative global economic loss worldwide. To lessen this burden, prevention and hazard-reducing approaches are essential. Focusing on healthy nutrients that support modern nutritional policies is essential for the avoidance and management of many chronic conditions, especially CVDs, in addition to recommendations on what to avoid.

According to worldwide population statistics, cardiovascular disease killed about 17.8 million lives globally in 2017 and is predicted to kill more than 22.2 million people by the year 2030 (*Circulation* 2020). For both sexes, age-homogenous occurrence levels of CVDs per 100,000 people range from around 7066 to more than 9266 in North Africa and the Middle East, Central Asia, and North America. The emergence and spread of CVD are correlated with several risk factors. While nutritive behaviors associated with hypertension, hypercholesterolemia, diabetes, obesity, laziness, and smoking can be adjusted, they can have a major impact on cardiovascular health in contrast to unalterable risk factors such as family history, age, and sex.

Cardiovascular disease associated with atherosclerosis is a long-term inflammatory condition and disturbance of lipid metabolism caused by atherogenesis and injury, which is facilitated by immune-related strategies that engage platelets, leukocytes, and LDL to trigger the spread of lesions in the arteries. Cellular mediators such as nitric oxide (NO), and vasoconstrictors including thromboxane and endothelin-1 (ET-1) help to regulate platelet activation, inflammation, and smooth muscle cell growth. Endothelial dysfunction typically results from a breakdown of the equilibrium and regulating function between substances that relax and contract vascular smooth muscle, promote and inhibit growth, and are pro- and antiatherogenic.

Most of the animal studies on the vascular effects of date palm has been on lipid and cholesterol management, as well as induced oxidant defense and reduced inflammatory responses. However, rodents have a different metabolism, absorption, distribution, and excretion profile for lipids than humans do; these observations, although promising, should be taken with caution.

11.10 DATE PALM FRUIT AND LIPIDS METABOLISM

In a clinical trial on healthy volunteers who consume date fruit daily, it was found to cause an increase in para-oxonase 1 (PON1) activity, and no change in lipoprotein (Rock et al. 2009). However, diabetic patients who daily consume three date fruits have lower cholesterol levels and elevated HDL (Alalwan et al. 2020). The decreased cholesterol could modulate the blood pressure in the pulmonary circulation and prevent CVD. The *in vivo* animal investigations have provided additional support for the findings of the *in vitro* antioxidant defense experiments mentioned before. Recent animal studies showed protective effects of different date varieties against several toxins that cause the production of free radicals (CCl_4, ISO, cadmium, and streptozotocin) (Table 11.2). The improved antioxidant defense enzymes like CAT, SOD, GPx, GSH, and glutathione S-transferase, as well as a considerable decline in MDA levels, were attributed to dates' protective effects against oxidative stress. Limited antioxidant enzyme levels in the heart muscles cause ROS produced by various toxins to accumulate quickly, increasing oxidative stress, which in turn causes lipid peroxidation and mitochondrial membrane damage, leading to myocardial ischemia (Alkuraishy, Al-gareeb, and Al-hussaniy 2017). The high polyphenol content in the date palm protects the limited cardiac antioxidant enzymes from depletion besides neutralizing the excess ROS, protecting the heart muscles.

11.11 DATE PALM FIBERS AND LIPID METABOLISM

Dietary fibers, which are known to decrease cholesterol, have been linked to some of the cardioprotective properties of dates. Dates have a large portion of insoluble fiber. Rats given 100 g/kg of dietary fiber had significantly decreased serum triacylglycerol, total cholesterol, and LDL levels. As a result of these fibers' high affinity to bind cholesterol and triacylglycerols in the colon and facilitate their elimination, circulating cholesterol levels are reduced (George et al. 2020). Less lipoprotein is consequently prone to oxidation, which lessens the effect on atherogenesis. Additionally, diets high in fiber can encourage the growth of helpful gut flora while inhibiting the growth of known pathogenic organisms.

11.12 DATE POLLEN CARDIOPROTECTIVE EFFECT

Date fruit and pollen supplementation have also been shown to reduce oxidative damage, inflammation, and apoptosis in the heart tissue of rats receiving ISO treatment. Pre-co-treatment with date pollen extract has markedly reverse the myocardial necrosis induced by ISO. The date pollen extract-treated rats resulted in a significant decline in the myocardial damage markers (ALT, troponin-T, CPK, and LDH). Also, the plasma angiotensin-converting enzyme activity was also decreased by date pollen co-treatment indicating the protection of cardiac muscles injury (Daoud et al. 2017). Another study of lyophilized Ajwa date extract (250 and 500 mg/kg body weight) was administered orally to demonstrate the anti-inflammatory and antiapoptotic ability of dates against ISO-induced cardiac damage. The data extract treatment has reduced the expression of interleukin (IL-6 and -10), and tumor necrosis factor-alpha as well as caspase-3 and Bax with the elevation Bcl-2 in Wistar rat heart tissue (Al-Yahya et al. 2016). These data can prove the cardioprotective potential of the date fruit by its antiapoptotic and antioxidant abilities through regulation of proinflammatory cytokines through inhibited caspase-3 and elevated the antiapoptotic protein.

A study of the extracts of four different varieties of dates (Berhi, Khalase, Reziz, and Khenizi) found that they had positive effects on preventing and repairing tissue damage through antioxidant defense activities and mobilization of circulating progenitor cells from bone marrow and peripheral circulation in a rodent model of myocardial infarction (MI) caused by either ISO or temporary ligation of the left anterior descending coronary artery (Alhaider et al. 2017). All four date varieties have high concentrations of phenolics and flavonoids. As compared to the control group, the state of MI was considerably improved by oral pre-treatment with date extracts for a period of 28 days prior to ISO injection. Rat heart tissue showed increased levels of GSH, SOD, and catalase and decreased levels of thiobarbituric acid reactive compounds (TBARS). Interestingly, date extracts have markedly raised the circulation levels of CD34 and CD133 positive progenitor cells, which are involved in tissue repair.

11.13 DATE FRUIT CARDIOVASCULAR PROTECTION MOLECULAR MECHANISMS

The mechanism by which the date palm could protect the cardiovascular system was mainly through the decreased cholesterol and LDL as well as clearing the free radicals produced by drug toxicity. Date palm could act through several molecular mechanisms to protect the cardiovascular system from injury (Figure 11.2). Elblehi et al. (2021) discovered the antiapoptotic and anti-inflammatory

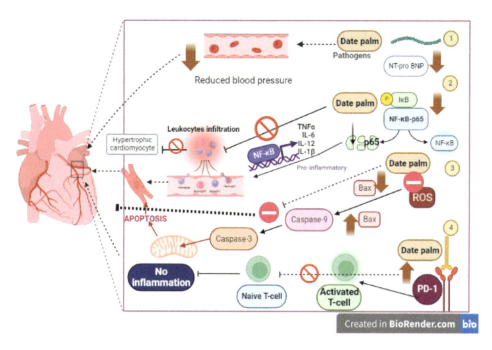

FIGURE 11.2 Date palm cardioprotective activity (molecular mechanism).

Note: An illustration of all the suggested molecular mechanisms for the date palm's edible parts as a cardioprotective supplement.

pathways of the cardioprotective potential of the date palm. One of the mechanisms is through reduced N-terminal pro-brain natriuretic peptide (NT-pro BNP), a peptide designed to control blood pressure and fluid equilibrium. It is released from the heart after ventricular volume expansion and/or increased pressure. A significant proportion of NT-pro BNP is released into the bloodstream during cardiac injury, severely damaging cardiomyocytes. The decreased NT-pro BNP release could decrease the blood pressure and protect the cardiac muscles from injury, and this could be a good explanation for the clinical studies that correlate the date palm supplementation with the decreased blood pressure (Husaidah, Ikhtiar, and Nurlinda 2019).

It is well known that increasing levels of ROS production, together with lipid peroxidation, speed up the production of inflammatory cytokines, which in turn promote the inflammatory response in the heart tissue. A transcription factor called NF-kB is implicated in immunological responses, inflammation, and cell sustainability. The NF-kB-p65 is a form of NF-kB that binds to the p65 subunit during B-cell activation by any stimuli. When NF-kB-p65 is elevated and diffused to the nucleus, the pro-inflammatory cytokines (IL-1β, TNF-α, and IL-6) are more effectively produced (Figure 11.2). They then increase inflammation and cause infiltration of inflammatory cells, especially leukocytes, into the cardiac muscles. Date palm was established to have anti-inflammatory action through decreasing the NF-kB-p65 expression, which in turn inhibited the production of the pro-inflammatory cytokines (IL-1β, TNF-α, and IL-6), preventing the leukocyte infiltration into the cardiomyocytes and preventing cardiac injury (Elblehi et al. 2021).

Another molecular mechanism for the protective mechanism of the date palm is through its antiapoptotic effect. It was discovered that date palm could decrease the pro-apoptotic proteins along with increasing the antiapoptotic proteins in cardiomyocytes, leading to protection of mitochondria from damage (Elblehi et al. 2021). Bcl-2 family members, which include antiapoptotic (Bcl-2) and pro-apoptotic (Bax, caspase-3) proteins, are the main regulators of apoptosis. Bcl-2 expression decreases during apoptosis, whereas Bax and caspase-3 levels increase. Bax activation promotes cell death by creating gaps in the mitochondrial membrane and causing mitochondrial cytochrome-c to be generated. In the meantime, Bcl-2 prevents apoptosis in cardiac tissue by preventing the disturbance in the membrane permeability, preserving the structure and functionality of the mitochondria. As part of the apoptotic process, caspases are crucial. The release of mitochondrial cytochrome-c is caused by opened mitochondrial membrane pores, and the death of cells is brought on by activated caspase-3. Date palm supplementation has been shown to protect cardiomyocytes from apoptosis caused by toxins or drugs by inhibiting Bax expression and decreasing caspase-3 cleavage while stimulating Bcl-2 expression (Elblehi et al. 2021).

The last molecular mechanism of date palm was revealed by Sahyon and Al-Harbi (2020), where date palm cardioprotective potential is enhanced through improvement of PD-1 protein. Activated T-lymphocytes, as a result of inflammatory response, are suppressed by the immune checkpoint membrane protein PD-1, which helps the cardiac tissues regain equilibrium by resolving aggressive immune response cascades and preventing subsequent tissue injury. Cardiac PD-1 can resolve cardiomyocyte inflammation; conversely, PD-1 suppression results in cardiac muscle injury. Elevated PD-1 by date palm supplementation resolved the cardiomocyte inflammation and hence protected the cardiac muscles from severe damage (Figure 11.2).

11.14 OTHER FOODS, HERBS, SPICES, AND BOTANICALS USED IN CARDIOVASCULAR HEALTH AND DISEASE

Extensive scientific research on the bioactivity, nutritive qualities, and health advantages of fruits has been conducted nowadays. Research findings suggest a noticeable synergistic relationship between consuming plenty of fruits and vegetables and a decline in the death rate from heart disease and other degenerative illnesses (Michaëlsson et al. 2017). This was connected to dietary fiber and polyphenols that they have.

Currently recommended eating patterns include lots of fruits, vegetables, nuts and seeds, legumes, whole grains, seafood, yogurt, and vegetable oils, while consuming little to no red meat, processed foods, and sugar. Berries, citrus, apples, and green leafy vegetables are just a few examples of fruits and vegetables that are abundant in various bioactive compounds like polyphenols and carotenoids, which are critical nutrients that can help prevent many chronic diseases. Nutritional guidelines encourage consuming five to nine servings of a variety of fruits and vegetables daily, which are rich in vitamins (C, A, and folate), minerals (potassium, calcium, and magnesium), and fiber. Elevated polyphenol consumption, especially flavonoids, has been linked to a lower risk of cardiovascular disease by enhancing vascular function, leading to lower blood pressure and LDL, as well as inhibiting platelet aggregation.

11.15 TOXICITY AND CAUTIONARY NOTES

According to recent investigations, pollen and dates might cause hypersensitivity or allergic reactions (Kwaasi et al. 1999). Additionally, caution must be taken by some date varieties' high selenium levels, which are linked to the soil's high selenium content (Al-Farsi and Lee 2011). Furthermore, a study of the date palm fruits in Oman that were cultivated near industrial areas detected heavy metal levels (Zn, Pb, Ni, and Cd) but no study on human consumption of those date fruits has been conducted. Also, another study of the date fruit in Riyadh found lead and cadmium in the skin of some varieties but when washed the metal concentration lowered to the safe limits. However, there are no published studies that document toxic effects of the heart of the date palm.

11.16 SUMMARY POINTS

- This chapter focuses on the therapeutic use of the date palm *Phoenix dactylifera L.*
- *P. dactylifera L.* fruit was used in folk medicine to treat liver disease and malaria.

- *P. dactylifera L.* is characterized by high phenolic acids and flavonoids.
- Date palm edible parts have obvious antioxidant and cardioprotective properties.
- Date extract's molecular mechanism is via pro-inflammatory cytokine depletion.

REFERENCES

Abdeen, Ahmed, Amira Samir, Ashraf Elkomy, Mohamed Aboubaker, Ola A. Habotta, Ahmed Gaber, Walaa F. Alsanie, et al. 2021. "The Potential Antioxidant Bioactivity of Date Palm Fruit against Gentamicin-Mediated Hepato-Renal Injury in Male Albino Rats." *Biomedicine & Pharmacotherapy = Biomedecine & Pharmacotherapie* 143 (November): 112154. doi:10.1016/j.biopha.2021.112154.

Abdelaziz, Dalia H. A., Sahar A. Ali, and Mahmoud M. A. Mostafa. 2015. "Phoenix Dactylifera Seeds Ameliorate Early Diabetic Complications in Streptozotocin-Induced Diabetic Rats." *Pharmaceutical Biology* 53 (6): 792–799. doi:10.3109/13880209.2014.942790.

Abdul-Hamid, Nur Ashikin, Nur Hafizah Mustaffer, M. Maulidiani, Ahmed Mediani, Intan Safinar Ismail, Chau Ling Tham, Khalid Shadid, and Faridah Abas. 2020. "Quality Evaluation of the Physical Properties, Phytochemicals, Biological Activities and Proximate Analysis of Nine Saudi Date Palm Fruit Varieties." *Journal of the Saudi Society of Agricultural Sciences* 19 (2): 151–160. doi:10.1016/j. jssas.2018.08.004.

Abu-Reidah, Ibrahim M., Ángel Gil-Izquierdo, Sonia Medina, and Federico Ferreres. 2017. "Phenolic Composition Profiling of Different Edible Parts and By-Products of Date Palm (Phoenix Dactylifera L.) by Using HPLC-DAD-ESI/MSn." *Food Research International* 100 (October): 494–500. doi:10.1016/j. foodres.2016.10.018.

Alalwan, Tariq A., Simone Perna, Qaher A. Mandeel, Aalaa Abdulhadi, Adel Salman Alsayyad, Giuseppe D'Antona, Massimo Negro, et al. 2020. "Effects of Daily Low-Dose Date Consumption on Glycemic Control, Lipid Profile, and Quality of Life in Adults with Pre- and Type 2 Diabetes: A Randomized Controlled Trial." *Nutrients* 12 (1): 217. doi:10.3390/nu12010217.

Al-Farsi, Mohamed Ali, and Chang Young Lee. 2011. "Usage of Date (Phoenix Dactylifera L.) Seeds in Human Health and Animal Feed." In *Nuts and Seeds in Health and Disease Prevention*, 447–452. Elsevier. doi:10.1016/B978-0-12-375688-6.100532.

Alhaider, Ibrahim A., Maged E. Mohamed, K. K. M. Ahmed, and Arun H. S. Kumar. 2017. "Date Palm (Phoenix Dactylifera) Fruits as a Potential Cardioprotective Agent: The Role of Circulating Progenitor Cells." *Frontiers in Pharmacology* 8 (September). doi:10.3389/fphar.2017.00592.

Alkuraishy, Hayder M., Ali I. Al-gareeb, and Hany Akeel Al-hussainy. 2017. "Doxorubicin-Induced Cardiotoxicity: Molecular Mechanism and Protection by Conventional Drugs and Natural Products." *International Journal of Clinical Oncology and Cancer Research* 2 (2): 31–44. doi:10.11648/j.ijcocr.20170202.12.

Al-Shoaibi, Zakaria, Mohamed A. Al-Mamary, Molham A. Al-Habori, Adel S. Al-Zubairi, and Siddig I. Abdelwahab. 2012. "In Vivo Antioxidative and Hepatoprotective Effects of Palm Date Fruits (Phoenix Dactylifera)." *International Journal of Pharmacology* 8 (3): 185–191. doi:10.3923/ijp.2012.185.191.

Al-Shwyeh, Hussah A. 2019. "Date Palm (Phoenix Dactylifera L.) Fruit as Potential Antioxidant and Antimicrobial Agents." *Journal of Pharmacy And Bioallied Sciences* 11 (1): 1. doi:10.4103/JPBS. JPBS_168_18.

Al-Yahya, Mohammed, Mohammad Raish, Mansour S. AlSaid, Ajaz Ahmad, Ramzi A. Mothana, Mohammed Al-Sohaibani, Mohammed S. Al-Dosari, Mohammad K. Parvez, and Syed Rafatullah. 2016. "'Ajwa' Dates (Phoenix Dactylifera L.) Extract Ameliorates Isoproterenol-Induced Cardiomyopathy through Downregulation of Oxidative, Inflammatory and Apoptotic Molecules in Rodent Model." *Phytomedicine: International Journal of Phytotherapy and Phytopharmacology* 23 (11): 1240–1248. doi:10.1016/j.phymed.2015.10.019.

Aswar, Urmila, Umesh Mahajan, Amit Kandhare, and Manoj Aswar. 2019. "Ferulic Acid Ameliorates Doxorubicin-Induced Cardiac Toxicity in Rats." *Naunyn-Schmiedeberg's Archives of Pharmacology* 392 (6): 659–668. doi:10.1007/s00210-019-01623-4.

Bagherzadeh Karimi, Alireza, Asghar Elmi, Arman Zargaran, Mojgan Mirghafourvand, Seyed Mohammad Bagher Fazljou, Mostafa Araj-Khodaei, and Roghayeh Bagvand Navid. 2020. "Clinical Effects of Date Palm (Phoenix Dactylifera L.): A Systematic Review on Clinical Trials." *Complementary Therapies in Medicine* 51 (June): 102429. doi:10.1016/j.ctim.2020.102429.

Bahmanpour, Soghra, T. Talaei, Z. Vojdani, M. R. Panjehshahin, A. Poostpasand, S. Zareei, and M. Ghaeminia. 2006. "Effect of Phoenix Dactylifera Pollen on Sperm Parameters and Reproductive System of Adult Male Rats." *Iranian Journal of Medical Sciences* 31 (4): 208–212.

Bai, Liyan, Hae Jin Kee, Xiongyi Han, Tingwei Zhao, Seung-Jung Kee, and Myung Ho Jeong. 2021. "Protocatechuic Acid Attenuates Isoproterenol-Induced Cardiac Hypertrophy via Downregulation of ROCK1 – Sp1 – PKCγ Axis." *Scientific Reports* 11 (1): 17343. doi:10.1038/s41598-021-96761-2.

Benjamin, E. J., P. Muntner, A. Alonso, M. S. Bittencourt, C. W. Callaway, A. P. Carson, A. M. Chamberlain, A. R. Chang, S. Cheng, S. R. Das, F. N. Delling, L. Djousse, M. S. V. Elkind, J. F. Ferguson, M. Fornage, L. C. Jordan, S. S. Khan, B. M. Kissela, K. L. Knutson, T. W. Kwan, . . . American Heart Association Council on Epidemiology and Prevention Statistics Committee and Stroke Statistics Subcommittee. (2019). Heart Disease and Stroke Statistics—2019 Update: A Report From the American Heart Ass ociation. *Circulation*, *139*(10), e56–e528. https://doi.org/10.1161/CIR.0000000000000659 [Published erratum in Circulation 2020;141(2), e33. https://doi.org/10.1161/CIR.0000000000000746.

Bouhlali, Eimad dine Tariq, Abdelbasset Hmidani, Bouchra Bourkhis, Tarik Khouya, Mhamed Ramchoun, Younes Filali-Zegzouti, and Chakib Alem. 2020. "Phenolic Profile and Anti-Inflammatory Activity of Four Moroccan Date (Phoenix Dactylifera L.) Seed Varieties." *Heliyon* 6 (2): e03436. doi:10.1016/j.heliyon.2020.e03436.

Daoud, Amal, Fedia Ben mefteh, Kais Mnafgui, Mouna Turki, Salwa Jmal, Rawdha Ben amar, Fatma Ayadi, et al. 2017. "Cardiopreventive Effect of Ethanolic Extract of Date Palm Pollen against Isoproterenol Induced Myocardial Infarction in Rats through the Inhibition of the Angiotensin-Converting Enzyme." *Experimental and Toxicologic Pathology* 69 (8): 656–665. doi:10.1016/j.etp.2017.06.004.

Echegaray, Noemí, Mirian Pateiro, Beatriz Gullón, Ryszard Amarowicz, Jane M. Misihairabgwi, and José M. Lorenzo. 2020. "Phoenix Dactylifera Products in Human Health: A Review." *Trends in Food Science & Technology* 105 (November): 238–250. doi:10.1016/j.tifs.2020.09.017.

Eid, Noura, Hristina Osmanova, Cecile Natchez, Gemma Walton, Adele Costabile, Glenn Gibson, Ian Rowland, and Jeremy P. E. Spencer. 2015. "Impact of Palm Date Consumption on Microbiota Growth and Large Intestinal Health: A Randomised, Controlled, Cross-over, Human Intervention Study." *British Journal of Nutrition*. doi:10.1017/S0007114515002780.

El Arem, Amira, Fatma Ghrairi, Lamia Lahouar, Amira Thouri, Emna Behija Saafi, Amel Ayed, Mouna Zekri, et al. 2014. "Hepatoprotective Activity of Date Fruit Extracts against Dichloroacetic Acid-Induced Liver Damage in Rats." *Journal of Functional Foods* 9 (1): 119–130. doi:10.1016/j.jff.2014.04.018.

Elberry, Ahmed A., Shagufta T. Mufti, Jaudah A. Al-Maghrabi, Essam A. Abdel-Sattar, Osama M. Ashour, Salah A. Ghareib, and Hisham A. Mosli. 2011. "Anti-Inflammatory and Antiproliferative Activities of Date Palm Pollen (Phoenix Dactylifera) on Experimentally-Induced Atypical Prostatic Hyperplasia in Rats." *Journal of Inflammation*. doi:10.1186/1476-9255-8-40.

Elblehi, Samar S., Yasser S. El-Sayed, Mohamed Mohamed Soliman, and Mustafa Shukry. 2021. "Date Palm Pollen Extract Avert Doxorubicin-Induced Cardiomyopathy Fibrosis and Associated Oxidative/ Nitrosative Stress, Inflammatory Cascade, and Apoptosis-Targeting Bax/Bcl-2 and Caspase-3 Signaling Pathways." *Animals* 11 (3): 886. doi:10.3390/ani11030886.

Farag, Mohamed A., Asmaa Otify, and Mostafa H. Baky. 2021. "Phoenix Dactylifera L. Date Fruit By-Products Outgoing and Potential Novel Trends of Phytochemical, Nutritive and Medicinal Merits." *Food Reviews International*, May, 1–23. doi:10.1080/87559129.2021.1918148.

Food and Agriculture Organisation (FAO). 2020. "FAOSTAT: Statistical Database." *FAOSTAT: Statistical Database*.

Gad El-Hak, Heba Nageh, Hany Salah Mahmoud, Eman A. Ahmed, Heba M. Elnegris, Tahany Saleh Aldayel, Heba M. A. Abdelrazek, Mohamed T. A. Soliman, and Menna Allah I. El-Menyawy. 2022. "Methanolic Phoenix Dactylifera L. Extract Ameliorates Cisplatin-Induced Hepatic Injury in Male Rats." *Nutrients* 14 (5): 1025. doi:10.3390/nu14051025.

George, Navomy, Annica A. M. Andersson, Roger Andersson, and Afaf Kamal-Eldin. 2020. "Lignin Is the Main Determinant of Total Dietary Fiber Differences between Date Fruit (Phoenix Dactylifera L.) Varieties." *NFS Journal*. doi:10.1016/j.nfs.2020.08.002.

Hameed, Mustafa, Ihsan Mkashaf, Ali A. A. Al-Shawi, and Kawkab Hussein. 2021. "Antioxidant and Anticancer Activities of Heart Components Extracted from Iraqi Phoneix Dactylifera Chick." *Asian Pacific Journal of Cancer Prevention* 22 (11): 3533–3541. doi:10.31557/APJCP.2021.22.11.3533.

Husaidah, Siti, Muhammad Ikhtiar, and Andi Nurlinda. 2019. "The Effect of Giving Date Palm (Phoenix Dactylifera L) toward Changes in Blood Pressure on Pregnant Women Getting Hypertension." *Window of Health: Jurnal Kesehatan* 2 (1): 34–43. http://jurnal.fkmumi.ac.id/index.php/woh/article/view/woh2105.

Hussain, M. Iftikhar, Muhammad Farooq, and Qamar Abbas Syed. 2020. "Nutritional and Biological Characteristics of the Date Palm Fruit (Phoenix Dactylifera L.): A Review." *Food Bioscience*. doi:10.1016/j.fbio.2019.100509.

Karasawa, Koji, Yuji Uzuhashi, Mitsuru Hirota, and Hajime Otani. 2011. "A Matured Fruit Extract of Date Palm Tree (Phoenix Dactylifera L.) Stimulates the Cellular Immune System in Mice." *Journal of Agricultural and Food Chemistry* 59 (20): 11287–11293. doi:10.1021/jf2029225.

Kazeminia, Seyed Mohammad, Soheila Ebrahimi Vosta Kalaee, and Sima Nasri. 2014. "Effect of Dietary Intake Alcoholic Extract of Palm Pollen (L. Phoenix Dactylifera) on Pituitary-Testicular Axis in Male Diabetic Rats." *Journal of Mazandaran University of Medical Sciences* 24: 166–175.

Khan, Fazal, Tariq Jamal Khan, Gauthaman Kalamegam, Peter Natesan Pushparaj, Adeel Chaudhary, Adel Abuzenadah, Taha Kumosani, Elie Barbour, and Mohammed Al-Qahtani. 2017. "Anti-Cancer Effects of Ajwa Dates (Phoenix Dactylifera L.) in Diethylnitrosamine Induced Hepatocellular Carcinoma in Wistar Rats." *BMC Complementary and Alternative Medicine* 17 (1): 418. doi:10.1186/s12906-017-1926-6.

Khatib, Mohamad, Amal Al-tamimi, Lorenzo Cecchi, Alessandra Adessi, Marzia Innocenti, Diletta Balli, and Nadia Mulinacci. 2022. "Phenolic Compounds and Polysaccharides in the Date Fruit (Phoenix Dactylifera L.): Comparative Study on Five Widely Consumed Arabian Varieties." *Food Chemistry* 395 (November 2021). Elsevier Ltd: 133591. doi:10.1016/j.foodchem.2022.133591.

Kwaasi, A. A., H. A. Harfi, R. S. Parhar, S. T. Al-Sedairy, K. S. Collison, R. C. Panzani, and F. A. Al-Mohanna. 1999. "Allergy to Date Fruits: Characterization of Antigens and Allergens of Fruits of the Date Palm (Phoenix Dactylifera L.)." *Allergy* 54 (12): 1270–1277. doi:10.1034/j.1398-9995.1999.00116.x.

Michaëlsson, Karl, Alicja Wolk, Håkan Melhus, and Liisa Byberg. 2017. "Milk, Fruit and Vegetable, and Total Antioxidant Intakes in Relation to Mortality Rates: Cohort Studies in Women and Men." *American Journal of Epidemiology* 185 (5): 345–361. doi:10.1093/aje/kww124.

Mohamed, D. A., and S. Al-Okabi. 2004. "In Vivo Evaluation of Antioxidant and Anti-Inflammatory Activity of Different Extracts of Date Fruits in Adjuvant Arthritis." *Pol J Food Nutr Sci.* 13 (4): 397–402.

Mrabet, Abdessalem, Ana Jiménez-Araujo, Juan Fernández-Bolaños, Fátima Rubio-Senent, Antonio Lama-Muñoz, Marianne Sindic, and Guillermo Rodríguez-Gutiérrez. 2016. "Antioxidant Phenolic Extracts Obtained from Secondary Tunisian Date Varieties (Phoenix Dactylifera L.) by Hydrothermal Treatments." *Food Chemistry* 196 (April): 917–924. doi:10.1016/j.foodchem.2015.10.026.

Mubarak, Shimaa, Shadia Abdel Hamid, Abdel Razik Farrag, Nahla Samir, and Jihan Seid Hussein. 2018. "Atherogenic Coefficient and Atherogenic Index in Doxorubicin-Induced Cardiotoxicity: Impact of Date Palm Extract." *Comparative Clinical Pathology* 27 (6): 1515–1522. doi:10.1007/s00580-018-2766-6.

Otify, Asmaa M., Aly M. El-Sayed, Camilia G. Michel, and Mohamed A. Farag. 2019. "Metabolites Profiling of Date Palm (Phoenix Dactylifera L.) Commercial by-Products (Pits and Pollen) in Relation to Its Antioxidant Effect: A Multiplex Approach of MS and NMR Metabolomics." *Metabolomics* 15 (9): 119. doi:10.1007/s11306-019-1581-7.

Rock, Wasseem, Mira Rosenblat, Hamutal Borochov-Neori, Nina Volkova, Sylvie Judeinstein, Mazen Elias, and Michael Aviram. 2009. "Effects of Date (Phoenix Dactylifera L., Medjool or Hallawi Variety) Consumption by Healthy Subjects on Serum Glucose and Lipid Levels and on Serum Oxidative Status: A Pilot Study." *Journal of Agricultural and Food Chemistry* 57 (17): 8010–8017. doi:10.1021/jf901559a.

Saafi, Emna Behija, Mouna Louedi, Abdelfattah Elfeki, Abdelfattah Zakhama, Mohamed Fadhel Najjar, Mohamed Hammami, and Lotfi Achour. 2011. "Protective Effect of Date Palm Fruit Extract (Phoenix Dactylifera L.) on Dimethoate Induced-Oxidative Stress in Rat Liver." *Experimental and Toxicologic Pathology: Official Journal of the Gesellschaft Fur Toxikologische Pathologie* 63 (5): 433–441. doi:10.1016/j.etp.2010.03.002.

Sahyon, Heba A., and Sami A. Al-Harbi. 2020. "Chemoprotective Role of an Extract of the Heart of the Phoenix Dactylifera Tree on Adriamycin-Induced Cardiotoxicity and Nephrotoxicity by Regulating Apoptosis, Oxidative Stress and PD-1 Suppression." *Food and Chemical Toxicology* 135 (January): 111045. doi:10.1016/j.fct.2019.111045.

Shehzad, Maham, Hina Rasheed, Summar A. Naqvi, Jameel M. Al-Khayri, Jose Manuel Lorenzo, Mohammed Abdulrazzaq Alaghbari, Muhammad Faisal Manzoor, and Rana Muhammad Aadil. 2021. "Therapeutic Potential of Date Palm against Human Infertility: A Review." *Metabolites* 11 (6): 408. doi:10.3390/metabo11060408.

Silabdi, Selma, Mustapha Khali, Gian Carlo Tenore, Paola Stiuso, Daniela Vanacore, and Ettore Novellino. 2021. "Phoenix Dactylifera Polyphenols Improve Plasma Lipid Profile in Hyperlipidemic Rats and Oxidative Stress on HepG2 Cells." *Journal of Herbs, Spices & Medicinal Plants* 27 (2): 161–176. doi:1 0.1080/10496475.2021.1891175.

Tahraoui, A., J. El-Hilaly, Z. H. Israili, and B. Lyoussi. 2007. "Ethnopharmacological Survey of Plants Used in the Traditional Treatment of Hypertension and Diabetes in South-Eastern Morocco (Errachidia Province)." *Journal of Ethnopharmacology* 110 (1): 105–117. doi:10.1016/j.jep.2006.09.011.

Topal, İsmail, Aslı Özbek Bilgin, Ferda Keskin Çimen, Nezahat Kurt, Zeynep Süleyman, Yasin Bilgin, Adalet Özçiçek, and Durdu Altuner. 2018. "The Effect of Rutin on Cisplatin-Induced Oxidative Cardiac Damage in Rats." *Anatolian Journal of Cardiology* 20 (3): 136–142. doi:10.14744/AnatolJCardiol.2018.32708.

Trabzuni, Dina. 2019. "In Vivo Evaluation of Therapeutic Potential of Heart of Date Palm Extract on Lipid Profile and Thyroid Hormones in Normal Male Wistar Rats." *Progress in Nutrition*. doi:10.23751/pn.v21i1.7836.

Trabzuni, Dina Mohammed. 2019. "Effect of the Heart of Date Palm Aqueous Extract Administration on Antioxidant Enzymes and Obesity-Related Hormones Levels in Rats." *Progress in Nutrition*. doi:10.23751/pn.v21i4.8926.

Tram, Nguyen Cong Thuy, Ninh The Son, Nguyen Thi Nga, Vu Thi Thu Phuong, Nguyen Thi Cuc, Do Thi Phuong, Gilles Truan, Nguyen Manh Cuong, and Do Thi Thao. 2017. "The Hepatoprotective Activity of a New Derivative Kaempferol Glycoside from the Leaves of Vietnamese Phyllanthus Acidus (L.) Skeels." *Medicinal Chemistry Research* 26 (9): 2057–2064. doi:10.1007/s00044-017-1914-x.

Zihad, S. M. Neamul Kabir, Shaikh Jamal Uddin, Nazifa Sifat, Farhana Lovely, Razina Rouf, Jamil A. Shilpi, Bassem Yousef Sheikh, and Ulf Göransson. 2021. "Antioxidant Properties and Phenolic Profiling by UPLC-QTOF-MS of Ajwah, Safawy and Sukkari Cultivars of Date Palm." *Biochemistry and Biophysics Reports* 25 (March): 100909. doi:10.1016/j.bbrep.2021.100909.

12 The Beneficial Action of *Artemisia* Genus on the Cardiovascular System

Smail Amtaghri and Mohamed Eddouks

CONTENTS

12.1 Introduction 177
12.2 Background... 177
12.3 The Main Pharmacological Activities of the *Artemisia* Genus............................ 179
12.4 Phytochemical Compounds Isolated from the *Artemisia* Genus.......................... 180
12.5 *Artemisia* and Hypertension 184
12.6 Toxicological Assessment of *Artemisia* Genus... 187
12.7 Conclusion 187
12.8 Summary Points 188
12.9 Funding... 188
References.. 188

LIST OF ABBREVIATIONS

A.	*Artemisia*
ACE	Angiotensin-converting enzyme
RAS	Renin-angiotensin system
VOCC	Voltage-operated calcium channels
WHO	World Health Organization

12.1 INTRODUCTION

Early humans have long used plants for therapeutic purposes. It's an old myth that plants have medicinal properties, and throughout history, humans have relied on nature for food, housing, medicine, clothes, and transportation (Ahmad et al. 2006). Currently, medicinal plants are employed as traditional home treatments in both developed and developing nations worldwide. Given their crucial role in traditional medicine, natural resources including plants and animals are prospective agents for the development of new drugs (Ahmad et al. 2015). According to the WHO, traditional medicines are used by approximately 80% of the population in developing countries (Calixto 2005). Several studies have been conducted in different areas of Morocco over the last decade to describe the main medicinal plants used in the cardiovascular system pharmacopoeia (Eddouks et al. 2002).

12.2 BACKGROUND

Artemisia is a genus of small herbs and shrubs native to northern temperate regions. It is a member of the Asteraceae family, which is one of the most diverse botanical taxa, with over 1000 genera and over 20,000 species. It is one of the largest and most widely distributed genera of the approximately 60 genera in the Anthemideae tribe. It contains hundreds (approximately 500) of different

DOI: 10.1201/9781003220329-14

177

species, but its systematic classification is still debated. In general, five subtaxa are considered. Its genetic "polymorphism," or more specifically, the ploidy levels sought as the promoter mechanism for evolution and ecological adaption, was the source of this complexity (Abdelfattah et al. 2012). The majority of *Artemisia* herbs are perennials that thrive in the northern hemisphere. They are widely used for a variety of purposes, including medicine, food, spices, and ornaments (Zeggwagh et al. 2014).

The genus *Artemisia* was named after the Greek goddess of hunting. *Artemisia*'s etymology has revealed another source of the name. A mausoleum tomb was built by Queen Artemisia, the wife of the Greek/Persian King Mausolus, who was a famous medical and botanical researcher. *Artemisia* herbs have a wide range of medicinal effects, including cell protection from peptic ulcers, liver protection, antimalarial, antitumor, and antidiabetic properties (Moufid and Eddouks 2012; Zeggwagh et al. 2014).

The genus *Artemisia* is indigenous to North America (particularly the United States and Canada), Asia, and Europe (mostly in arid and semi-arid areas); additionally, it is found in South America (primarily Brazil), Australia, and Southeast Asia. It is found all over the world (Figure 12.1) and has drawn attention due to its significant economic importance, particularly for its therapeutic uses. These plants were rationally utilized throughout history for their anticancer, antidepressant, antiseptic, antivenom, anthelminthic, diuretic, hypoglycemia, antispasmodic, etc. properties. They also underwent rigorous testing (Coopoosamy 2015).

Artemisia species have traditionally been used to treat a wide range of feverish illnesses, including malaria, the treatment of colds, infections, parasites, liver inflammations, as well as dyspepsia, diabetes, hypertension, and a host of other ailments (Yazdiniapour et al. 2021). Many *Artemisia* (*A.*) plants, such as *A. herba-alba*, *A. santonicum*, and *A. pallens*, have been reported to be beneficial for laboratory animals or people with diabetes (Moufid and Eddouks 2012). Since ancient times, the people of Morocco have employed herbs to heal a range of ailments. *A. herba-alba Asso*, also known as desert wormwood (known in Arabic as *shih*), has been used in folk medicine by many cultures since antiquity, and it is used in Moroccan pharmacopoeia to treat high blood pressure and/or diabetes (Zeggwagh et al. 2008). The plant *A. vestita* has long been used in traditional medicine to treat inflammatory conditions including rheumatoid arthritis (Sun et al. 2006). In addition, *A. dracunculus* has been utilized orally as an antiepileptic in those with anticonvulsant potential (Sayyah et al. 2004).

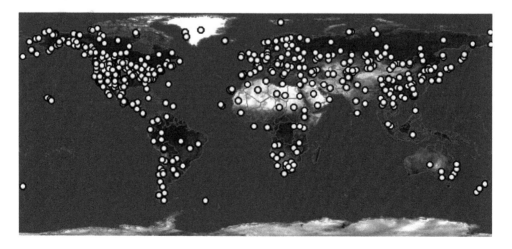

FIGURE 12.1 Schematic map of *Artemisia* genus distribution across the world.

Source: www.discoverlife.org/mp/20m?&kind=Artemisia.

12.3 THE MAIN PHARMACOLOGICAL ACTIVITIES OF THE *ARTEMISIA* GENUS

According to experimental research, numerous studies have demonstrated the significance and therapeutic efficacy of diverse *Artemisia* species, notably as antihypertensive, antibacterial, cytotoxic, antimalarial, anti-inflammatory, antioxidant, antitumoral, immunomodulatory, hepatoprotective, antispasmodic, and antiseptic and anticancer agents. The *Artemisia* genus contains a lot of pharmacological properties involving some bioactive compounds, mostly artemisinin (Figure 12.2, Table 12.1), which exhibits antimalarial activity and profound cytotoxicity against tumor cells, and arglabin, which is used in the former USSR to treat certain types of cancer (Wong and Brown 2002). *A. annua* was the original source of the sesquiterpene lactone artemisinin, which was later found in *A. vulgaris* and other species of *Artemisia* (Iqbal et al. 2010).

A. vulgaris has a wide range of therapeutic properties, including antimalarial, anti-inflammatory, antihypertensive, antioxidant, antitumoral, immunomodulatory, hepatoprotective, antispasmodic, and antiseptic activities (Abiri et al. 2018).

Several substances from this genus have previously been reported to have antimalarial, antiulcerogenic, antitumoral, antihemorrhagic, antipyretic, anticoagulant, antioxidant, antiviral, anti-hepatitis, antispasmodic, antidepressant, anticomplementary, and interferon-inducing activities (Mahmoudi et al. 2009). The extract of *A. kermanensis* has been claimed to have antibacterial and antioxidant properties (Yazdiniapour et al. 2021).

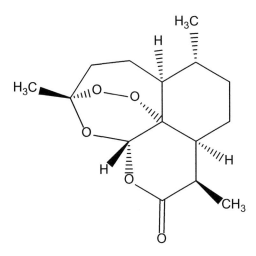

FIGURE 12.2 Chemical structure of artemisinin.

TABLE 12.1
The Main Pharmacological Activities of the *Artemisia* Genus

Activity	Species	Plant Part	Model	Mechanism of Action	Reference
Antidiabetic	*Artemisia dracunculus*	Leaves frozen	*In vivo* *in vitro*	Inhibits phosphoenolpyruvate carboxykinase	(Bower et al. 2016)
Antimalarial Anticancer Antioxidant	*Artemisia annua*	Whole plant	*In vivo* *In vitro* *In silico*	Inhibits angiogensis	(Kadioglu et al. 2021)

(Continued)

TABLE 12.1 *(Continued)*

The Main Pharmacological Activities of the *Artemisia* Genus

Activity	Species	Plant Part	Model	Mechanism of Action	Reference
Anti-inflammatory Antidepressant	*Artemisia vulgaris*	Whole parts	*In vivo* *In vitro*	Inhaling moxa smoke has a depressant effect on the human body	(Zhao et al. 2011)
Cytotoxic	*Artemisia sacrorum*	Aerial part	*In vitro*	Inhibits glucose production via the AMPK-glycogen synthase kinase-cAMP response element binding protein signaling pathway in HepG2 cells	(Yuan et al. 2016)
Antisepsis, Anti-inflammatory	*Artemisia vestita*	Whole plant	*In vivo* *In vitro*	Inhibits TNF-alpha release from macrophages by suppressing MAPK and NF-kappaB signaling	(Sun et al. 2006)
Antidiabetic, Antioxidant	*Artemisia juncea*	Aerial parts	*In vitro*	Inhibitory effect on amylase and glucosidase was observed in eupatilin	(Okhundedaev et al. 2019)
Antioxidant, Antiplatelet	*Artemisia campestris*	Aerial parts	*In vitro*	Inhibits aggregation triggered by thrombin	(Dib, Fauconnier et al. 2017)
Anti-inflammatory, antinociceptive	*Artemisia copa*	Aerial parts	*In vitro*	*A. copa* was able to prevent the production of proinflammatory mediators, specially those related with cyclooxygenase and lipoxygenase pathway	(Mino et al. 2004)

12.4 PHYTOCHEMICAL COMPOUNDS ISOLATED FROM THE *ARTEMISIA* GENUS

Numerous studies have demonstrated the traditional usage of *Artemisia* species' flowers, stems, roots, leaves, aerial parts, and whole plants in the treatment of a variety of ailments. The primary pharmacological effects of the *Artemisia* genus are listed in Table 12.2. *Artemisia* species contain principally terpenoids, flavonoids, coumarins, caffeoylquinic acids, sterols, and acetylenes. They contain a high content of bioactive compounds such as apigenin, hesperetin, kaempferol, luteolin, quercetin, 1,8-cineole, alpha and beta thujone, camphor, borneol, and many others (Ben-Nasr et al. 2013). Many secondary metabolites, including terpenoids, flavonoids, coumarins, caffeoylquinic acids, sterols, and acetylenes, have been identified in the *Artemisia* genus so far (Koul et al. 2017). A number of flavonoids, as well as flavonoid glycosides, are present in apigenin, luteolin, chrysoeriol, kaempferol, rhamnocitrin, quercetin, tamarixetin, mikanin, casticin, cirsineol, eupatin, mearnsetin, and chrysosplenol E (Lee et al. 2002). In addition, the compound scoparone, isolated from *Artemisia*, has an antianginal action (Yamahara et al. 1989a; Yamahara et al. 1989b).

As studied previously, *A. kermanensis* contains two pharmacologically active flavone compounds, eupatilin and its hydroxylated form, with a wide range of biological activity. Eupatilin is well known for its anticancer activity (Son et al. 2013).

Luteolin and its derivatives have been reported to have several intriguing pharmacological activities, including antitumoral, antioxidant, anti-inflammatory, and analgesic properties (Kotanidou et al. 2002). Moreover, a new flavone glucoside known as 40,5-dihydroxy-30,50,6-trimethoxyflavone7-O-b-D-glucoside was isolated from aerial parts of *A. juncea*, together with the well-known flavone, eupatilin (5,7-dihydroxy30,40,6-trimethoxyflavone) (Okhundedaev et al. 2019).

The Beneficial Action of *Artemisia* Genus

TABLE 12.2
Phytochemical Compounds Isolated from the *Artemisia* Genus

Species	Plant Part	Compounds	Reference
Artemisia dracunculus	Whole parts Leaves frozen	Chalcones davidigenin. Sakuranetin. 20,40-dihydroxy-4-methoxydihydrochalcone Pinene, Myrcene, Limonene, Caryophyllene, Methyl chavicol, Anethole	(Bower et al. 2016)
	Aerial parts (essential oils)	Trans-anethole, Alpha-trans-ocimene, Limonene, Alpha-pinene, Allo ocimene, Methyl eugenol, Beta-pinene, Alpha-terpinolene, Bornyl acetate, Bicyclogermacrene	(Sayyah et al. 2004)
Artemisia annua	Crude extract, volatile, hydrosol	Artesunate (derived artemisinin) Flavonoids Flavonol Flavone Coumarins Artemisia ketone, Trans-caryophyllene, 1,8-cineole, Camphor, Germacrene D, β-selinene. Camphor, 1,8-cineole, Artemisia ketone, Trans-pinocarveol, Yomogi alcohol	(Kadioglu et al. 2021)
Artemisia capillaris	Aerial parts	Scoparone	(Yamahara et al. 1989a; Yamahara et al. 1989b)
Artemisia vulgaris	Whole parts	Yomogin. Sesquiterpene lactone Jaceosidine, Eupafolin, Luteolin, Quercetin, Apigenine, Aesculetin, Esculetin-6-methylether, Scopoletin	(Lee et al. 2000)

(Continued)

TABLE 12.2 *(Continued)*
Phytochemical Compounds Isolated from the *Artemisia* Genus

Species	Plant Part	Compounds	Reference
Artemisia herba-alba	Aerial parts	Chrysanthenyl acetate, Chrysantheno, Acetophenone xanthocyclin, 1,8-cineole as the major compound, Thujone, Terpinen-4-ol, Camphor, Borneol.	(Aziz et al. 2012)
Artemisia kermanensis	Whole parts	5,7-dihydroxy-3',4', 6-trimethoxyflavone (eupatilin). 5,7,3'-Trihydroxy-6,4', 5'-trimethoxyflavone	(Yazdiniapour et al. 2021)
Artemisia selengensis	Aerial parts	1',3'-propanediol,2'-amino-1'-(1,3-benzodioxol-5-yl). Artanomaloide. Canin. Eupatilin. Quercetin-3-O-β-D-glucoside-7-O-α-L-rhamnoside. 1,3-di-O-caffeoylquinic acid. Isoquercitrin. Pinoresinol-4-O-β-D-glucoside. Scopolin. Isofraxidin-7-O-β-D-glucopyranoside.	(Kim et al. 2015)
Artemisia aucheri Boiss	Aerial parts	Verbenone, Camphor, 1,8-cineole, Trans-verbenol.	(Sefidkon et al. 2002)
Artemisia santolina Schrenk	Aerial parts	Neryl acetate, Bornyl acetate, Trans-verbenol, Lavendulol, Linalool, 1,8-cineole	(Sefidkon et al. 2002)
Artemisia sieberi Besser	Aerial parts	Camphor, 1,8-cineole, Bornyl acetate.	(Sefidkon et al. 2002)
Artemisia afra	Steam-distilled essential oils	Artemisia ketone, 1,8-cineole, α-copaene/camphor, Santolina alcohol.	(Chagonda et al. 1999)
	Oil for fresh and semi-dried herb	α-copaene/camphor, 1,8-cineole, Santolina alcohol, 1,8-cineole, α-copaene/camphor, Borneol, Camphene, Bornyl acetate, β-caryophyllene, Sabinene, γ-terpinene, p-cymene.	

TABLE 12.2 *(Continued)*
Phytochemical Compounds Isolated from the *Artemisia* Genus

Species	Plant Part	Compounds	Reference
Artemisia fragrans	Stem, leaf, flower (essential oils)	Camphor, 1, 8-cineole. α-cadinol τ-muurolol Phytol. Chrysanthenon, 1, 8-cineole, Beta-caryophyllene, p-cymene, Filifolide-A, Filifolone.	(Farghadan et al. 2016)
Artemisia juncea	Aerial parts	40,5-Dihydroxy-30,50,6trimethoxyflavone-7-O-b-D-glucoside, Eupatilin (5,7-dihydroxy-30,40,6-trimethoxyflavone)	(Okhundedaev et al. 2019)
Artemisia campestris	Aerial parts (essential oil)	Spathulenol, ß-eudesmol, p-cymene, δ-cadinene, ß-pinene, Caryophyllene oxide, Salvial-4(14)-en-1-one, Chlorogenic acid, Isochlorogenic acid, Vicenin-2.	(Dib, Fauconnier et al. 2017)
Artemisia scoparia	Aerial parts	Scopariachromane, Coumarins, Flavonoids, Sterols, Sesquiterpene lactones Scoparanolide, Estafiatone, 3β,4α-dihydroxyguaia-11(13),10(14)-dien-6α,12-olide, Estafiatin, Preeupatundin, 3β-hydroxycostunolide, Ludovicin B, Scopoletin, Scoparone, Isofraxidin	(Cho et al. 2016)
Artemisia asiatica	Aerial parts	Eupatilin, Jaceosidin, Hispidulin, 5,7,4',5'-tetrahydroxy-6,3'-dimethoxy-flavone, 6-methoxytricin, Cirsilineol, Chrysosplenetin.	(Hajdú et al. 2014)

12.5 *ARTEMISIA* AND HYPERTENSION

Cardiovascular disease is the primary reason for the high mortality rate in developed countries, as well as the collapse of economies due to hypertensive patients bearing high health care costs (Hiepen et al. 2020). Hypertension is a common disease to which everyone is susceptible, and it affects millions of people worldwide. Because of its asymptomatic nature, hypertension is a high risk factor for cardiovascular, cerebrovascular, and renal diseases (World Health Organization 2003). Many organs are affected by hypertension, including the eyes, heart, brain, and kidney, which gradually deteriorate and eventually fail. As a result, treatment is postponed. It gets worse when people lack individual awareness and poor drug adherence when it comes to controlled hypertension (Zakaria et al. 2009). There are several medications available to treat hypertension, such as beta blockers, angiotensin-II receptor blockers, calcium channel blockers, diuretics, and angiotensin-converting enzyme inhibitors. Due to the prolonged drug treatment, these medications are very expensive (World Health Organization 2003).

The renin-angiotensin system (RAS) regulates body fluids, but one of its enzymes, angiotensin-converting enzyme (ACE), causes hypertension indirectly by constricting blood vessels. Autoimmune diseases are associated with an increased risk of hypertension and cardiovascular disease (Shahid et al. 2022). Angiotensin I is converted to angiotensin II by angiotensin-converting enzymes in the RAS system, which narrows blood vessels and results in hypertension. Numerous antihypertensive medications, including captopril, lisinopril, and aliskiren, have been found to block ACE. These medications have positive advantages, but they also have harmful side effects, including low potassium levels, taste loss, and dizziness. Several medications are needed to achieve the best results because antihypertensive medications are only effective at a level of 40–60% (Chen et al. 2020). A deficit of potassium, angioedema, sexual dysfunction, depression, sleeplessness, psychosis, cough, and fetal abnormalities were among the side effects of antihypertensive medications (Zakaria et al. 2009). As a result, it has become a difficult responsibility for centuries to find a safe and effective way to manage hypertension. Worldwide, the long-used practice of using herbal therapy is making a resurgence. This is due to its minimal adverse effects and effective therapeutic results (Table 12.3) (Maghrani et al. 2005). In addition, many *Artemisia* plants have shown significant and beneficial effects against hypertension, as shown in Figure 12.3.

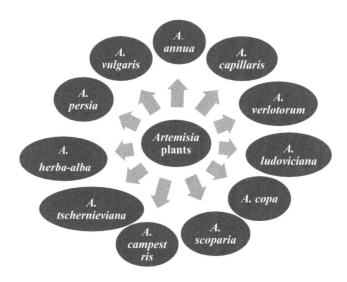

FIGURE 12.3 *Artemisia* species that exert antihypertensive activity.

TABLE 12.3
Antihypertensive Activity of *Artemisia* Species

Species	Extract	Model	Activity	Mechanism of Action	Reference
Artemisia verlotorum	Aqueous dried	*In vivo, in vitro*	Transient hypotension in mesentery.	Release of endothelial nitric oxide and to the nitric oxide-guanosine 3′ – 5′-cyclic monophosphate (cGMP) pathway	(Calderone et al. 1999)
Artemisia capillaris	Acetone	*In vitro*	Enhances coronary flow and heart rate. Inhibition of the ST wave (antianginal action). No influence on cardiac output and left ventricular performance.	Inhibitory effect on the contractions induced by norepinephrine	(Yamahara et al. 1989a; Yamahara et al. 1989b)
Artemisia annua	Water	*In vivo, in vitro*	Inhibits angiogensis. Enhances the acetylcholine-induced endothelial-dependent relaxation of aorta.	Suppression of CYP450 enzymes responsible for altering the absorption and metabolism of artemisinin in the body	(Dell'Eva et al. 2004)
		In vivo, in vitro	Artemisinin decreases the heart rate and basal vascular tension and improves attenuated endothelium-dependent vascular relaxation.	Inhibition of NAD(P)H oxidase activity derived-ROS generation and increasing eNOS activation NO release by endothelial cells	(Liu et al. 2021)
Artemisia persia	Methanolic and water	*In vivo, in vitro*	Reduces heart rate and systolic blood pressure.	Inhibitory effect on myocardial contractility and vascular dilatory action of *Artemisia*	(Esmaeli et al. 2012; Yamahara et al. 1989a)
Artemisia herba-alba	Aqueous	*In vivo, in vitro*	Potent acute hypotensive. Affects renal function to increase urine and electrolytes excretion.	Inhibition of renal Na$^+$-K$^+$ pump. Elevation of diuresis and electrolytes excretion may reduce arterial blood pressure.	(Zeggwagh et al. 2014; Zeggwagh et al. 2008)
		In vitro	Vasorelaxant.	Activation of NO/cGMP pathway and KATP channels	(Skiker et al. 2010)
Artemisia tschernieviana	Hexane, ethyl acetate, aqueous	*In vivo*	Antihemolytic, antioxidant.	Inhibition of hemoglobin-induced linoleic acid peroxidation. Inhibition of lipid peroxidation by antioxidants may be due to their free radical scavenging activities.	(Naqinezhad et al. 2012)

(Continued)

TABLE 12.3 *(Continued)*
Antihypertensive Activity of *Artemisia* Species

Species	Extract	Model	Activity	Mechanism of Action	Reference
Artemisia campestris	Essential oil	*In vitro*	Vasorelaxant.	Inhibition of L-type Ca^{2+} channels and the activation of SERCA pumps of reticulum plasma	(Dib, Fauconnier et al. 2017)
Artemisia copa	Aqueous	*In vitro*	Vasorelaxant and hypotensive.	Inhibition of Ca^{2+} influx via membranous calcium channels and intracellular stores	(Gorzalczany 2013)
Artemisia ludoviciana	Hexan, dichloromethan, methanolic	*In vitro*	Vasorelaxant.	Possible muscarinic receptor antagonism and calcium channel blockade in tracheal rings. Also, the vasorelaxant activity by dichloromethane is partially endothelium-dependent.	(Estrada-Soto et al. 2012)

The aerial part of *Artemisia herba-alba* has yielded a number of secondary metabolites, the most significant of which are sesquiterpene lactones, and flavonoids (Skiker et al. 2010). Numerous polyphenolic substances, such as flavonoids, which are well known for their circulatory properties, including vasodilator and antioxidant activities, may be responsible for the vasodilator effect of *Artemisia herba-alba*. The study *in vitro* shows that the vasorelaxant effects of *A. herba-alba* aqueous extract are dependent on the integrity of functional endothelium but unrelated to endothelial muscarinic receptor activation. In addition, activation of KATP is also implicated in the mediation of *A. herba-alba*-induced vasodilatory effects in vascular smooth muscle, in addition to the involvement of endothelial eNOS/cGMP pathway (Skiker et al. 2010).

Another study reported that aqueous extract of *A. herba-alba* produced a significant reduction in heart rate, implying that *A. herba-alba* may reduce arterial pressure by reducing heart rate (Zeggwagh et al. 2008). However, it is not ruled out that *A. herba-alba* could reduce vascular tone via the adrenergic system (Zeggwagh et al. 2008).

The rapid decrease in arterial pressure prompts us to hypothesize that the sympathic or cholinergic systems are likely involved in the hypotensive action of the aqueous extract of *A. herba-alba*. Normal rats' blood pressure is tightly regulated by a sophisticated neurological and hormonal system. The observed drop in arterial blood pressure demonstrates that the aqueous extract of *A. herba-alba* has a potent hypotensive action (Zeggwagh et al. 2014).

According to evidence on the effects of *Artemisia* on cardiovascular events, scoparone, a coumarin derivative isolated from the Chinese crude drug *Artemisia capillaries*, could increase coronary flow and heart rate but not cardiac output or left ventricular function in isolated perfuse rat hearts (Yamahara et al. 1989a; Yamahara et al. 1989b).

Additionally, *A. annua* or artemisinin has a hypotensive effect. Some studies claim that artesunate, a semi-synthetic derivative of artemisinin derived from the plant *A. annua*, can suppress angiogenesis both *in vitro* and *in vivo* (Anfosso et al. 2006).

A study conducted *in vitro* found that the aqueous extract of *A. copa* has vasorelaxing and hypotensive effects via blocking Ca^{2+} influx through intracellular storage and membrane calcium channels. On isolated aortic rings, luteolin, chrysoeriol, and p-coumaric acid had a vasorelaxant effect. They could be responsible for this vasorelaxant activity, at least in part (Gorzalczany 2013).

The model of ischemia reperfusion injury in the rat intestine mesentery according to Tigno and Gumila has shown that extracts from *A. vulgaris* have no impact on mean arterial blood pressure and heart rate (Tigno and Gumila 2000). Instead, administration of *A. vulgaris* aqueous extract fractions was extremely successful in counteracting the hypertensive action brought on by norepinephrine, and had no discernible impact on heart rate in either the normotensive or hypertension states (Yamahara et al. 1989a). Similar hypotensive effects have been noticed in other *Artemisia* plants, for example, *A. herba-alba* (Zeggwagh et al. 2008; Skiker et al. 2010), or *A. Persia* (Esmaeili et al. 2009), or *A. copa* in Argentina (Gorzalczany 2013).

Using an animal model, Esmaeili et al. (2009) have proved that *A. Persia* extracts reversed epinephrine-induced hypertension much more than enalapril, a conventional antihypertensive drug. However, the actual mechanisms of these effects are still unclear. This difference could be due to variability in quantitative and qualitative chemical composition, as discussed previously. In fact, many *Artemisia* derivatives could modulate cardiac and vascular function, directly or indirectly, through the control of cardiovascular endocrine and/or nervous regulations (Haze et al. 2002).

A. campestris aqueous extract appears to be mostly made up of phenolic compounds (chlorogenic and isochlorogenic acids as well as vicenin-2) that may be primarily responsible for the vasodilator effect, according to the chemical components of the extract. This investigation demonstrated the powerful hypotensive, antihypertensive, and vasorelaxant effects of this plant. The vasorelaxant effect of *A. campestris* appears to be due to muscarinic receptor activation and stimulation of the calmodulin-NO-sGC-PK pathway. Another mechanism of action of *A. campestris* is the activation of the SERCA pump and the inhibition of VOCC channels (Dib, Tits et al. 2017).

12.6 TOXICOLOGICAL ASSESSMENT OF *ARTEMISIA* GENUS

According to toxicological research, *Artemisia* plants are either non- or low-toxic when used sparingly and for a brief period of time. A high dose of 3 g/kg for a longer period of time, on the other hand, can have hazardous effects such fast breathing, neurotoxicity, reproductive toxicity, etc. (Bisht et al. 2021). Besides that, there were no discernible toxicological patterns in the *Artemisia* extracts, which is essential for pharmaceutical application (Ben-Nasr et al. 2013). Clearly, *Artemisia* extracts powerfully scavenge free radicals which are common features of many diseases (Higdon et al. 2012). However, there have been some debates about the effects of *Artemisia* extracts on cardiovascular system regulation (Ben-Nasr et al. 2013). In contrast, *A. absinthium* essential oil used over an extended period of time may result in physical and mental issues in people, with symptoms like convulsions, insomnia, and hallucinations (Batiha et al. 2020).

12.7 CONCLUSION

Various research studies have suggested that *Artemisia* plants have antihypertensive properties. There were no concise experimental or clinical papers describing its true mechanisms and the substances involved, though. However, as entire *Artemisia* extracts integrated numerous biological activities that are efficient in concurrently treating various disorders, employing them could better address cardiovascular disorders. The effects of these plant extracts on blood pressure are thought to be primarily due to inhibition of adenylyl cyclase and stimulation of cGMP enzymes. As a result, the energetic machinery required for vascular constriction will be dampened. To explain the value of entire *Artemisia* extracts against cardiovascular diseases, perspective systemic works are necessary. Our comprehension of these effects will inevitably be improved by a pharmaceutical model that targets the antihypertensive and cardiovascular protective actions of *Artemisia* extracts, defining the plants' usefulness in this sector.

12.8 SUMMARY POINTS

- This chapter focuses on the pharmacological uses of Artemisia genus.
- *Artemisia* possesses a variety of biologically significant properties, including, antihypertensive, antimalarial, anti-ulcerogenic, antitumoral, antihemorrhagic, antipyretic, anticoagulant, antioxidant, antiviral, anti-hepatitis, antispasmodic, antidepressant, anticomplementary, and interferon-inducing activities.
- Terpenoids, flavonoids, coumarins, caffeoylquinic acids, sterols, and acetylenes are the most abundant constituents of *Artemisia* species.
- Bioactive compounds found in the *Artemisia* shrub include apigenin, hesperetin, kaempferol, luteolin, quercetin, 1,8-cineole, alpha and beta thujone, camphor, borneol, and many others.
- Toxicological studies revealed that the plants are non- or low-toxic at low doses and for short periods of time.

12.9 FUNDING

This study was supported by CNRST under grant number PPR/2015/35.

REFERENCES

Abdelfattah, B., Wafaa, M., Sahar, A., Sahar, S., and Amal, S. 2012. Genetic diversity in Artemisia monosperma and Artemisia judaica populations in Egypt based on morphological, karyological and molecular variations. Journal of Medicinal Plants Research 6(1), 66–78.

Abiri, R., Silva, A.L.M., de Mesquita, L.S.S., de Mesquita, J.W.C., Atabaki, N., de Almeida Jr, E.B., and Malik, S. 2018. Towards a better understanding of Artemisia vulgaris: Botany, phytochemistry, pharmacological and biotechnological potential. Food Research International 109, 403–415.

Ahmad, I., Aqil, F., and Owais, M. (Eds.). 2006. Modern phytomedicine: Turning medicinal plants into drugs. John Wiley & Sons.

Ahmad, L., Semotiuk, A., Zafar, M., Ahmad, M., Sultana, S., Liu, Q. R., . . . Yaseen, G. 2015. Ethnopharmacological documentation of medicinal plants used for hypertension among the local communities of DIR Lower, Pakistan. Journal of Ethnopharmacology 175, 138–146.

Anfosso, L., Efferth, T., Albini, A., and Pfeffer, U. 2006. Microarray expression profiles of angiogenesis-related genes predict tumor cell response to artemisinins. The Pharmacogenomics Journal 6(4), 269–278.

Aziz, M., Karim, A., El Ouariachi, E.M., Bouyanzer, A., Amrani, S., Mekhfi, H., . . . Legssyer, A. 2012. Relaxant effect of essential oil of Artemisia herba-alba Asso. on rodent jejunum contractions. Scientia Pharmaceutica 80(2), 457–468.

Batiha, G.E.S., Olatunde, A., El-Mleeh, A., Hetta, H.F., Al-Rejaie, S., Alghamdi, S., and Rivero-Perez, N. 2020. Bioactive compounds, pharmacological actions, and pharmacokinetics of wormwood (Artemisia absinthium). Antibiotics 9(6), 353.

Ben-Nasr, H., Abderrahim, M.A.B., Salama, M., Ksouda, K., and Zeghal, K.M. 2013. Potential phytotherapy use of Artemisia plants: Insight for anti-hypertension. Journal of Applied Pharmaceutical Science 3(5), 120–125.

Bisht, D., Kumar, D., Kumar, D., Dua, K., and Chellappan, D.K. 2021. Phytochemistry and pharmacological activity of the genus artemisia. Archives of Pharmacal Research 44(5), 439–474.

Bower, A., Marquez, S., de Mejia, E.G. 2016. The health benefits of selected culinary herbs and spices found in the traditional Mediterranean diet. Crit Rev Food Sci Nutr 56(16):2728–2746.

Calderone, V., Martinotti, E., Baragatti, B., Cristina Breschi, M., and Morelli, I. 1999. Vascular effects of aqueous crude extracts of Artemisia verlotorum Lamotte (Compositae): In vivo and in vitro pharmacological studies in rats. Phytotherapy Research: An International Journal Devoted to Pharmacological and Toxicological Evaluation of Natural Product Derivatives 13(8), 645–648.

Calixto, J.B. 2005. Twenty-five years of research on medicinal plants in Latin America: A personal view. Journal of Ethnopharmacology 100(1–2), 131–134.

Chagonda, L.S., Makanda, C., and Chalchat, J.C. 1999. The essential oil of cultivated Artemisia afra (Jacq.) from Zimbabwe. Flavour and Fragrance Journal 14(2), 140–142.

The Beneficial Action of *Artemisia* Genus

Chen, J., Ryu, B., Zhang, Y., Liang, P., Li, C., Zhou, C. et al. 2020. Comparison of an angiotensin-I-converting enzyme inhibitory peptide from tilapia (Oreochromis niloticus) with captopril: Inhibition kinetics, in vivo effect, simulated gastrointestinal digestion and a molecular docking study. Journal of the Science of Food and Agriculture 100(1), 315–324.

Cho, J.Y., Jeong, S.J., Lee, H.L., Park, K.H., Hwang, D.Y., Park, S. Y., et al. 2016. Sesquiterpene lactones and scopoletins from Artemisia scoparia Waldst. & Kit. and their angiotensin I-converting enzyme inhibitory activities. Food Science and Biotechnology 25(6), 1701–1708.

Coopoosamy, S.O.O.R.M. 2015. Preliminary studies on the antibacterial and antioxidative potentials of hydroalcoholic extract from the whole parts of Artemisia vulgaris L. Int J Pharm 11, 561–569.

Dell'Eva, R., Pfeffer, U., Vené, R., Anfosso, L., Forlani, A., Albini, A., and Efferth, T. 2004. Inhibition of angiogenesis in vivo and growth of Kaposi's sarcoma xenograft tumors by the anti-malarial artesunate. Biochemical Pharmacology 68(12), 2359–2366.

Dib, I., Fauconnier, M.L., Sindic, M., Belmekki, F., Assaidi, A., Berrabah, M., . . . Ziyyat, A. 2017. Chemical composition, vasorelaxant, antioxidant and antiplatelet effects of essential oil of Artemisia campestris L. from Oriental Morocco. BMC Complementary and Alternative Medicine 17(1), 1–15.

Dib, I., Tits, M., Angenot, L., Wauters, J.N., Assaidi, A., Mekhfi, H., . . . Ziyyat, A. 2017. Antihypertensive and vasorelaxant effects of aqueous extract of Artemisia campestris L. from Eastern Morocco. Journal of Ethnopharmacology 206, 224–235.

Eddouks, M., Maghrani, M., Lemhadri, A., Ouahidi, M.L., and Jouad, H. 2002. Ethnopharmacological survey of medicinal plants used for the treatment of diabetes mellitus, hypertension and cardiac diseases in the south-east region of Morocco (Tafilalet). Journal of Ethnopharmacology 82(2–3), 97–103.

Esmaeili, F., Sepehri, G., Moshtaghi-Kashanian, G.R., Khaksari, M., Salari, N., and Sepehri, E. 2009. The effect of acute administration of Artemisia persia extracts on arterial blood pressure and heart rate in rats. American Journal of Applied Sciences 6(5), 843.

Esmaeli, F., Sepehri, G., Joneidi, H., Daneshvar, S., and Hasannejad, M. 2012. Cardiac effects of subacute administration of Artemisia persia extract in normotensive and hypertensive rats. Ann Biol Res 3(7), 34043–3409.

Estrada-Soto, S., Sánchez-Recillas, A., Navarrete-Vázquez, G., Castillo-España, P., Villalobos-Molina, R., and Ibarra-Barajas, M. 2012. Relaxant effects of Artemisia ludoviciana on isolated rat smooth muscle tissues. Journal of Ethnopharmacology 139(2), 513–518.

Farghadan, M., Ghafoori, H., Vakhshiteh, F., Fazeli, S.A.S., Farzaneh, P., and Kokhaei, P. 2016. The effect of artemisia fragrans willd: Essential oil on inducible nitric oxide synthase gene expression and nitric oxide production in lipopolysaccharide-stimulated murine macrophage cell line. Iranian Journal of Allergy, Asthma and Immunology, 515–524.

Gorzalczany, S., Moscatelli, V., and Ferraro, G. 2013. Artemisia copa aqueous extract as vasorelaxant and hypotensive agent. Journal of Ethnopharmacology 148(1), 56–61.

Hajdú, Z., Martins, A., Orbán-Gyapai, O., Forgo, P., Jedlinszki, N., Máthé, I., and Hohmann, J. 2014. Xanthine oxidase-inhibitory activity and antioxidant properties of the methanol extract and flavonoids of Artemisia asiatica. Rec Nat Prod 8(3), 299–302.

Haze, S., Sakai, K., and Gozu, Y. 2002. Effects of fragrance inhalation on sympathetic activity in normal adults. Japanese Journal of Pharmacology 90(3), 247–253.

Hiepen, C., Jatzlau, J., and Knaus, P. 2020. Biomechanical stress provides a second hit in the establishment of BMP/TGFβ-related vascular disorders. Cell Stress 4(2), 44.

Higdon, A., Diers, A.R., Oh, J.Y., Landar, A., and Darley-Usmar, V.M. 2012. Cell signalling by reactive lipid species: New concepts and molecular mechanisms. Biochemical Journal 442(3), 453–464.

Iqbal, H., Khan, F.U., Lajber, K., Sultan, A., and Khan, I.U. 2010. Analysis of artemisinin in Artemesia species using high performance liquid chromatography. World Applied Sciences Journal 10(6), 632–636.

Kadioglu, O., Klauck, S.M., Fleischer, E., Shan, L., and Efferth, T. 2021. Selection of safe artemisinin derivatives using a machine learning-based cardiotoxicity platform and in vitro and in vivo validation. Archives of Toxicology 95(7), 2485–2495.

Kim, A.R., Ko, H.J., Chowdhury, M.A., Chang, Y.S., Woo, E.R. 2015. Chemical constituents on the aerial parts of Artemisia selengensis and their IL-6 inhibitory activity. Arch Pharm Res 38(6):1059–1065.

Kotanidou, A., Xagorari, A., Bagli, E., Kitsanta, P., Fotsis, T., Papapetropoulos, A., and Roussos, C. 2002. Luteolin reduces lipopolysaccharide-induced lethal toxicity and expression of proinflammatory molecules in mice. American Journal of Respiratory and Critical Care Medicine 165(6), 818–823.

Koul, B., Taak, P., Kumar, A., Khatri, T., and Sanyal, I. 2017. The artemisia genus: A review on traditional uses, phytochemical constituents, pharmacological properties and germplasm conservation. J Glycomics Lipidomics 7(1), 142.

Lee, J.Y., Chang, E.J., Kim, H.J., Park, J.H., and Choi, S.W. 2002. Antioxidative flavonoids from leaves of Carthamus tinctorius. Archives of Pharmacal Research 25(3), 313–319.

Lee, S.J., Chung, H.Y., Lee, I.K., Oh, S.U., and Yoo, I.D. 2000. Phenolics with inhibitory activity on mouse brain monoamine oxidase (MAO) from whole parts of Artemisia vulgaris L (Mugwort). Food Science and Biotechnology 9(3), 179–182.

Liu, X., Wang, X., Pan, Y., Zhao, L., Sun, S., Luo, A., . . . Han, Y. 2021. Artemisinin improves acetylcholine-induced vasodilatation in rats with primary hypertension. Drug Design, Development and Therapy 15, 4489.

Maghrani, M., Zeggwagh, N.A., Michel, J.B., and Eddouks, M. 2005. Antihypertensive effect of Lepidium sativum L. in spontaneously hypertensive rats. Journal of Ethnopharmacology 100(1–2), 193–197.

Mahmoudi, M., Ebrahimzadeh, M.A., Ansaroudi, F., Nabavi, S.F., and Nabavi, S.M. 2009. Antidepressant and antioxidant activities of Artemisia absinthium L. at flowering stage. African Journal of Biotechnology 8(24).

Mino, J., Moscatelli, V., Hnatyszyn, O., Gorzalczany, S., Acevedo, C., and Ferraro, G. 2004. Antinociceptive and antiinflammatory activities of Artemisia copa extracts. Pharmacological Research 50(1), 59–63.

Moufid, A., and Eddouks, M. 2012. Artemisia herba alba: A popular plant with potential medicinal properties. Pakistan Journal of Biological Sciences: PJBS 15(24), 1152–1159.

Naqinezhad, A., Nabavi, S.M., Nabavi, S.F., and Ebrahimzadeh, M.A. 2012. Antioxidant and antihemolytic activities of flavonoid rich fractions of Artemisia tschemieviana Besser. European Review for Medical and Pharmacological Sciences 16, 88–94.

Okhundedaev, B.S., Bacher, M., Mukhamatkhanova, R.F., Shamyanov, I.J., Zengin, G., Böhmdorfer, S., . . . Rosenau, T. 2019. Flavone glucosides from Artemisia juncea. Natural Product Research 33(15), 2169–2175.

Sayyah, M., Nadjafnia, L., and Kamalinejad, M. 2004. Anticonvulsant activity and chemical composition of Artemisia dracunculus L. essential oil. Journal of Ethnopharmacology 94(2–3), 283–287.

Sefidkon, F., Jalili, A., and Mirhaji, T. 2002. Essential oil composition of three Artemisia spp. from Iran. Flavour and Fragrance Journal 17(2), 150–152.

Shahid, M.N., Zawar, M., Jamal, A., Mohamed, B.B., Khalid, S., and Bahwerth, F.S. 2022. Exploration of ACE-inhibiting peptides encrypted in *Artemisia annua* using in silico approach. BioMed Research International 2022(May 23), 5367125. doi: 10.1155/2022/5367125.

Skiker, M., Mekhfi, H., Aziz, M., Haloui, B., Lahlou, S., Legssyer, A., . . . Ziyyat, A. 2010. Artemisia herba-alba Asso relaxes the rat aorta through activation of NO/cGMP pathway and KATP channels. Journal of Smooth Muscle Research 46(3), 165–174.

Son, J.E., Lee, E., Seo, S.G., Lee, J., Kim, J.E., Kim, J., . . . Lee, H.J. 2013. Eupatilin, a major flavonoid of Artemisia, attenuates aortic smooth muscle cell proliferation and migration by inhibiting PI3K, MKK3/6, and MKK4 activities. Planta Medica 79(12), 1009–1016.

Sun, Y., Li, Y.H., Wu, X.X., Zheng, W., Guo, Z.H., Li, Y., . . . Xu, Q. 2006. Ethanol extract from Artemisia vestita, a traditional Tibetan medicine, exerts anti-sepsis action through down-regulating the MAPK and NF-κB pathways. International Journal of Molecular Medicine 17(5), 957–962.

Tigno, X.T., and Gumila, E. 2000. In vivo microvascular actions of Artemisia vulgaris L. in a model of isch-emia-reperfusion injury in the rat intestinal mesentery. Clinical Hemorheology and Microcirculation 23(2, 3, 4), 159–165.

Wong, H.F., and Brown, G.D. 2002. Germacranolides from Artemisia myriantha and their conformation. Phytochemistry 59(5), 529–536.

World Health Organization, and International Society of Hypertension Writing Group. 2003. 2003 World Health Organization (WHO)/International Society of Hypertension (ISH) statement on management of hypertension. Journal of Hypertension 21(11), 1983–1992.

Yamahara, J., Kobayashi, G., Matsuda, H., Katayama, T., and Fujimura, H. 1989a. Vascular dilatory action of Artemisia capillaris bud extracts and their active constituent. Journal of Ethnopharmacology 26(2), 129–136.

Yamahara, J., Kobayashi, G., Matsuda, H., Katayama, T., and Fujimura, H. 1989b. The effect of scoparone, a coumarin derivative isolated from the Chinese crude drug Artemisiae capillaris flos, on the heart. Chemical and Pharmaceutical Bulletin 37(5), 1297–1299.

Yazdiniapour, Z., Yegdaneh, A., and Akbari, S. 2021. Isolation and characterization of methylated flavones from Artemisia kermanensis. Advanced Biomedical Research 10.

Yuan, H., Lu, X., Ma, Q., Li, D., Xu, G., and Piao, G. 2016. Flavonoids from Artemisia sacrorum Ledeb and their cytotoxic activities against human cancer cell lines. Experimental and Therapeutic Medicine 12(3), 1873–1878.

Zakaria, Z., Baharudin, A., and Razali, R. 2009. The effect of depressive disorders on compliance among hypertensive patients undergoing pharmacotherapy. ASEAN Journal of Psychiatry 10(1), 89–99.

Zeggwagh, N.A., Farid, O., Michel, J.B., and Eddouks, M. 2008. Cardiovascular effect of Artemisia herba alba aqueous extract in spontaneously hypertensive rats. Methods and Findings in Experimental and Clinical Pharmacology 30(5), 375–381.

Zeggwagh, N.A., Michel, J.B., and Eddouks, M. 2014. Acute hypotensive and diuretic activities of Artemisia herba alba aqueous extract in normal rats. Asian Pacific Journal of Tropical Biomedicine 4, S644–S648.

Zhao, B., Litscher, G., Li, J., Wang, L., Cui, Y., Huang, C., and Liu, P. 2011. Effects of moxa (Artemisia vulgaris) smoke inhalation on heart rate and its variability. Chinese Medicine 2(2), 53.

13 Kalmegh (*Andrographis paniculata*) and Cardioprotective Mechanisms

Vuanghao Lim, Jun Jie Tan and Yoke Keong Yong

CONTENTS

13.1 Introduction 194
13.2 Background.. 196
13.3 Phytoconstituents 197
13.4 Direct Cardioprotective Mechanism of Action 197
     13.4.1 Cardioprotective Effects of *Andrographis paniculata* and Its Derivatives 197
     13.4.2 Myocarditis.. 198
     13.4.3 Myocardial Infarction and Cardiotoxic Drug-Induced Cardiac Injuries 204
     13.4.4 Pressure Overload and High Fat Diet-Induced Cardiac Hypertrophy 204
     13.4.5 The Effects of Andrographolide on Cardiac Ion Channels.................................. 204
13.5 Indirect Cardioprotective Mechanism of Action.. 205
     13.5.1 Antioxidant Effect... 205
     13.5.2 Anti-Inflammatory Effect... 205
     13.5.3 Endothelial Protective Effect 206
     13.5.4 Vasorelaxant Effect 206
     13.5.5 Anti-Platelet Aggregation Effect... 207
     13.5.6 Reduction of Smooth Muscle Cell Migration and Proliferation......................... 207
13.6 Other Foods, Herbs, Spices and Botanicals Used in Cardiovascular Health and Disease 208
13.7 Toxicity and Cautionary Notes 210
13.8 Summary Points 210
13.9 Acknowledgment 210
References.. 210

LIST OF ABBREVIATIONS

Ach — Acetylcholine
A.D. — Anno Domini (in the year of the Lord)
APD — Action potential duration
ATP — Adenosine triphosphate
Bax — Bcl-2 associated X-protein
Bax-xL — B-cell lymphoma-extra large
Bcl-2 — B-cell lymphoma-2
CAT — Catalase
CD4 — Cluster of differentiation 4
cGMP — Cyclic guanosine monophosphate
COX-2 — Cyclooxygenase-2
eNOS — Endothelial nitric oxide synthase

DOI: 10.1201/9781003220329-15

ERK1/2	Extracellular signal-regulated kinase 1/2
ET-1	Endothelin-1
GPx	Glutathione peroxidase
GSH	Glutathione
GST	Glutathione S-transferase
H_2O_2	Hydrogen peroxide
HFD	High fat diet
HIV	Human immunodeficiency virus
HMGB1	High-mobility group box chromosomal protein 1
hs-CRP	High-sensitive C-reactive protein
HUVECs	Human umbilical vein endothelial cells
ICAM-1	Intercellular adhesion molecule-1
IL-1	Interleukin-1
IL-1β	Interleukin-1 beta
IL-6	Interleukin-6
ISO	Isoproterenol
LAD	Left anterior descending
LD50	Lethal dose 50%
LDH	Lactate dehydrogenase
LPS	Lipopolysaccharide
LTCC	L-type calcium channel
MAPK	Mitogen-activated protein kinase
MCP-1	Monocyte chemoattractant protein-1
MI	Myocardial infarction
MPO	Myeloperoxidase
NADPH	Nicotinamide adenine dinucleotide phosphate
NE	Noradrenaline
NF-κB	Nuclear factor kappa B
NO	Nitric oxide
Nrf2	Nuclear factor erythroid 2-related factor 2
PAF	Platelet-activating factor
PCNA	Proliferating cell nuclear antigen
PDGF	Platelet-derived growth factor
PGI2	Prostaglandin I2
PI3K/Akt	Phosphatidylinositol 3-kinase/protein kinase B
P-IκBα	Phospho-nuclear factor of kappa light polypeptide gene enhancer in B-cells inhibitor, alpha
PP2A	Protein phosphatase 2
PPAR-α	Peroxisome proliferator-activated receptor-alpha
ROS	Reactive oxygen species
SOD	Superoxide dismutase
TNF-α	Tumor necrosis factor-α
VSMC	Vascular smooth muscle cell
WHO	World Health Organization

13.1 INTRODUCTION

The King of Bitters, *Andrographis paniculata*, is a member of the Acanthaceae family. It is native to China and India; however, it is found abundantly across the tropical and sub-tropical regions, and Southeast Asia. Locally, it is named "Hempedu Bumi" (bile of earth, due to its extremely bitter taste) in Malaysia while the other vernacular names of AP include "Chuan Xin Lian" in Chinese,

Kalmegh (*Andrographis paniculata*)

"Sambiroto" or "Sambiloto" in Indonesian, "Nilavembu" in Tamil, "The Create" in English (Hossain et al. 2014), "Kalmegh" in India and Fah Talai Jone in Thailand. *A paniculata* is commonly used to treat various illnesses, such as fevers, snake bites and skin diseases (Hossain et al. 2021; Kumar, Singh, and Bajpai 2021). It has been known to cure various diseases caused by insects and diseases. This plant is widely recognized in various traditional Indian and Chinese medicines. It is also used in Thailand for the treatment of respiratory diseases. *A paniculata* is a widely used herb for its annual flowering. It thrives in moist woodland, farm, roadsides and hedgerows. This herb is also

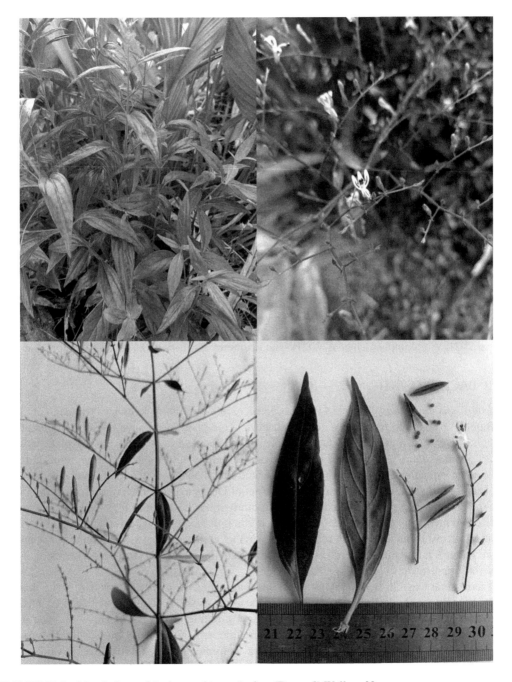

FIGURE 13.1 Morphology of *Andrographis paniculate* (Burm. f.) Wall. ex Nees.

TABLE 13.1

Taxonomic Hierarchy of *Androgaphis paniculata* (Burm. f.) Wall. ex Nees from Kingdom to Species

Kingdom	Plantae
Subkingdom	Viridiplantae
Infrakingdom	Streptophyta
Superdivision	Embryophyta
Division	Tracheophyta
Subdivision	Spermatophytina
Class	Magnoliopsida
Superorder	Asteranae
Order	Lamiales
Family	Acanthaceae
Genus	Andrographis
Species	paniculata

Source: "Integrated Taxonomic Information System – Report" (n.d.).

known to grow in hill slopes and woodland. This plant can be grown in moist and shady areas. It is also well suited to forests and wastelands. It is a salt-sensitive species, and its growth is limited under stress. This plant has a central stem that can reach a height of 30 to 110 cm. It has a narrow, quadrangular, green, central stalk that has longitudinal furrows and wings. The leaves are dark green, with a pale green outer layer and a venation pinnate. They are 2 to 12 cm long and have a broad, almost lanceolate shape. The flowers are small, have a narrow tube and a rose-purple spot on the petals. They are usually flowering and fruiting during December to April. The fruits are small capsules that are 2 to 5 mm long. They have a bitter taste and are filled with seeds. The leaf is linear-oblong and has sub-quadrate seeds (Figure 13.1) (Hossain et al. 2021; Kumar, Singh, and Bajpai 2021; Worakunphanich et al. 2021). The taxonomy for *A. paniculata* is shown in Table 13.1.

13.2 BACKGROUND

Andrographis paniculata (Burm. f.) Wall. ex Nees, or also commonly known as Kalmegh or "King of Bitters," belongs to the family of Acanthaceae. This plant has a short lifespan of about one year; however it is high in reproductive capacity which could become an enemy plant in some places. *A. paniculata* has been used for centuries as a traditional medicine in China, India and Java. It has been officially documented in the Ayurvedic Pharmacopoeia, while in Thailand this plant has been included in "The National List of Essential Drugs a.d. 1999" by the Ministry of Public Health (Pholphana et al., 2004) and more importantly it has been selected as "WHO monographs on selected medicinal plants" (WHO 2002). According to the literature, different parts of the plant are used to treat different types of illness; however, due to the main active compounds presented in the aerial part, it is commonly used as a folklore remedy for a wide spectrum of ailments or also as an herbal supplement to promote health.

There are at least 26 Ayurvedic formulations that include *A. paniculata* as one of the ingredients, according to the Indian Pharmacopoeia (Varma et al. 2011). This shows that *A. paniculata* played an important role in treating illnesses and promoting health in ancient India. The whole plant is consumed orally or applied locally as an antidote against snake bites, while the juice of the leaf alone or in combination with other natural ingredients is used to treat digestive disorders among children, including griping, irregular stools, loss of appetite, flatulence and diarrhea in the southern region of India (Subramaniam et al. 2012). On the other hand, infusion of whole plant or leaves is used to treat fever, neuralgia, dysentery as well as used as a blood purifier (Subramaniam et al. 2012) in the eastern region of India. Based on traditional Chinese medicine, this plant exhibits a "cold property," where it functions to eliminate or neutralize the "heat" and dispose toxins from the body. Thus, it was prescribed by ancient Chinese physicians to especially treat cold and fever, laryngitis and other inflammatory conditions (Huang and Wu 2002). Similarly, this plant was consumed for the prevention and relief of cold and sore throat in Scandinavian countries (Subramaniam et al. 2012). According to the Forestry Department of Peninsular Malaysia (2021), this plant has been used traditionally to relieve pain, as a laxative, expectorant and for digestive disorders such as stomach ache. Apart from these, it is also used to treat other illnesses including diabetes, fever, worm infections, chronic bronchitis, leprosy, flatulence, colic, dysentery and skin disease such as burns, wounds and ulcers. It is also a good remedy for neutralizing snakebite and female-related disorders.

13.3 PHYTOCONSTITUENTS

Bioassay-guided studies revealed that compounds found in *A. paniculata* can dilate coronary vessels and reduce blood pressure. These compounds might be useful in the treatment of coronary artery disease and high blood pressure. The phytoconstituents, 14-deoxyandrographolide (3) and 14-deoxy-11,12-didehydroandrographolide (5) (Yoopan et al. 2007) augmented the flow of blood to the coronary vessels by decreasing the size of the aortic rings. Both phytoconstituents exert vasorelaxant activity by releasing nitric oxide. They also activate the guanylate cyclase signaling pathway and the calcium (Ca^{2+}) influx blockade (Awang et al. 2012). Andrographolide (1) exerts antiproliferative effects on human umbilical vein endothelial cell lines that have been induced by growth factors deprivation. Both (1) and (5) also decreased the platelet aggregation *in vitro*. The anti-platelet activity of certain flavonoids can be linked to the ERK1/2 pathway. Some of these flavonoids (13–20, 28) inhibit collagen and promote platelet aggregation. Studies also revealed that andrographolide (1) can protect the heart without causing significant liver damage. It was able to lower the levels of various hypolipidemic effects in rats and mice (Jayakumar et al. 2013). The neoandrographolide (2) treatment significantly suppressed the infarct size, cell infiltration, inflammatory cell death and the number of inflammatory cytokines in the cell. It also cleaved caspase-3 and P-Iκ-B protein expressions. (5) could be developed to treat patients with heart failure due to their condition. It has been shown that suppressing the activation of the Bcl-2 and NF-κB signaling pathways could help prevent the development of heart failure (Liu et al. 2021). Some other compounds were also found to be effective as cardioprotectives and are listed in Figure 13.2.

13.4 DIRECT CARDIOPROTECTIVE MECHANISM OF ACTION

13.4.1 CARDIOPROTECTIVE EFFECTS OF *ANDROGRAPHIS PANICULATA* AND ITS DERIVATIVES

Heart disease is the world's most common cause of morbidity and mortality. The damaged hearts are prone to fibrosis and hypertrophic remodeling, and the altered architecture renders the heart to deteriorate over time and eventually cease to function. *A. paniculata* has also been tested for treating heart injuries, and several previous studies have shown that *A. paniculata* does exert cardioprotective effects. Andrographolides were the most extensively tested in different types of myocardial injuries in animals, ranging from the left anterior descending coronary artery (LAD) ligation-induced ischemic cardiomyopathy (Xie et al. 2020), aortic banding-induced (Wu et al. 2017) or high fat diet (HFD)-induced cardiac hypertrophy (Lin et al. 2020), isoproterenol (ISO) (Elasoru et al. 2021) or lipopolysaccharide (LPS)-induced cardiac injury (Zhang et al. 2015), aconitine-induced arrhythmias (Zeng et al. 2017) and viral myocarditis (Zhao et al. 2018). Here, the effects of *A. paniculata* are discussed according to the nature of cardiac injury each tested model represents, and the mechanisms underlying observed effects (Table 13.2).

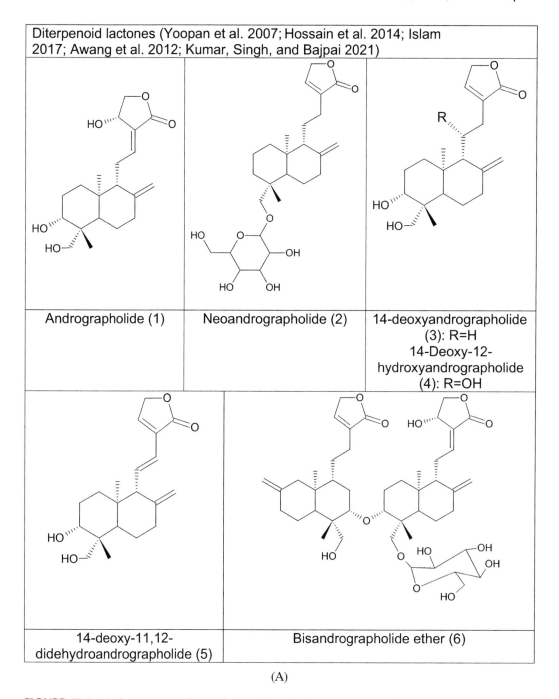

FIGURE 13.2 Active phytoconstituents isolated from *Andrographis paniculata* (Burm. f.) Wall. ex Nees which exhibit cardioprotective effects.

13.4.2 Myocarditis

Myocarditis is an inflammatory disease of the myocardium which can be a result of infections, a drug response or an immune response. It can cause sudden cardiac death and extensive fibrosis that stimulate ventricular remodeling and dilated cardiomyopathy. Andrographolide has previously

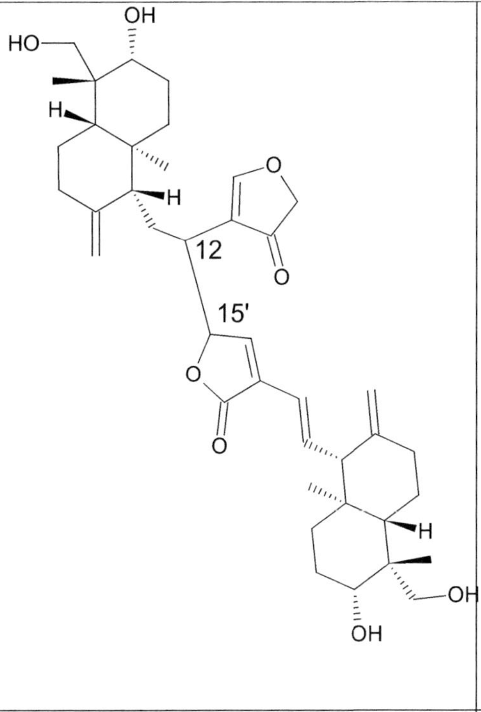

Kalmegh (*Andrographis paniculata*) 199

Bisandrographolide B (7): 12S/15'R
Bisandrographolide C (8): 12R/15'S
Bisandrographolide D (9): 12R/15'R

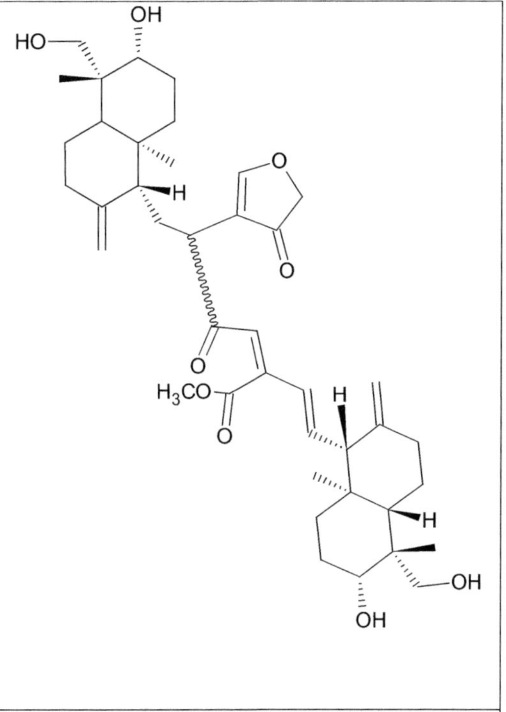

Bisandrographolide E (10)

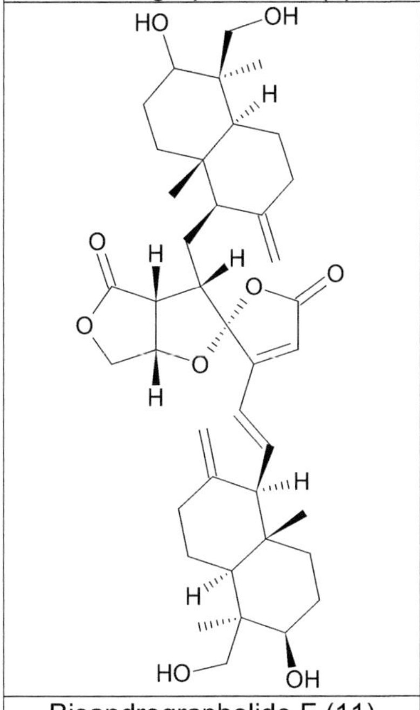

Bisandrographolide F (11)

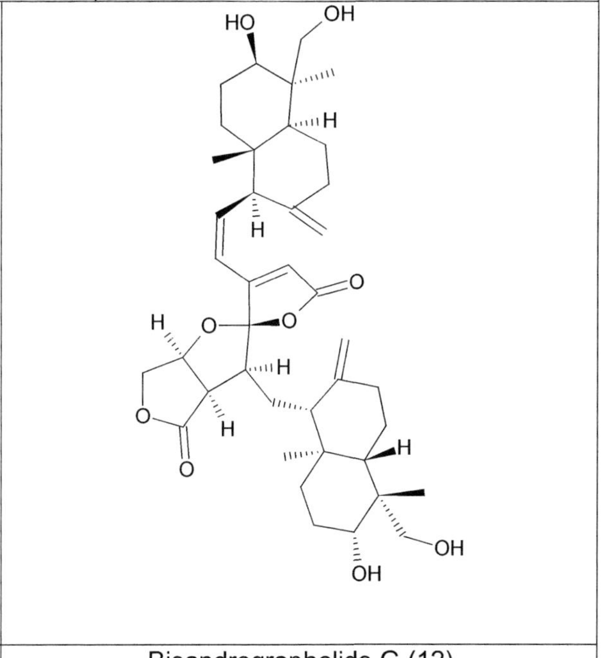

Bisandrographolide G (12)

(B)

FIGURE 13.2 (*Continued*)

Flavones (Kumar, Singh, and Bajpai 2021)							
	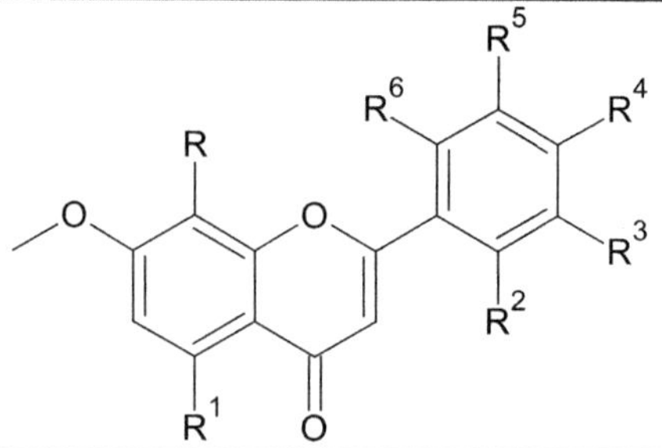 R	R¹	R²	R³	R⁴	R⁵	R⁶
Andropaniculosin A (13)	OCH_3	OH	OCH_3	H	H	OH	H
5,2′,6′-Trihydroxy-7-methoxyflavone (14)	H	OH	OH	H	H	H	OH
Andropaniculoside A (15)	OCH_3	Oglc	OH	H	H	H	H
Andrographidine B (16)	OCH_3	OH	H	H	H	Oglc	OH
Andrographidine D (17)	OCH_3	Oglc	H	H	H	OCH_3	OCH_3
Andrographidine E (18)	OCH_3	Oglc	OCH_3	H	H	H	H
5,2′,6′-Trihydroxy-7-methoxyflavone 2′-Oglucoside (19)	H	OH	OH	H	H	H	Oglc

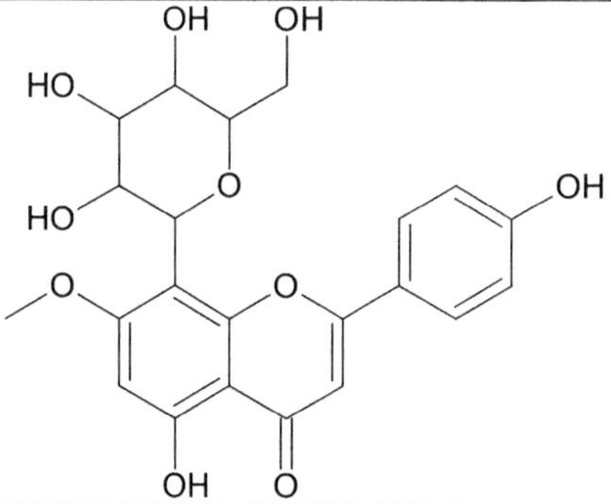

Isoswertisin (20)

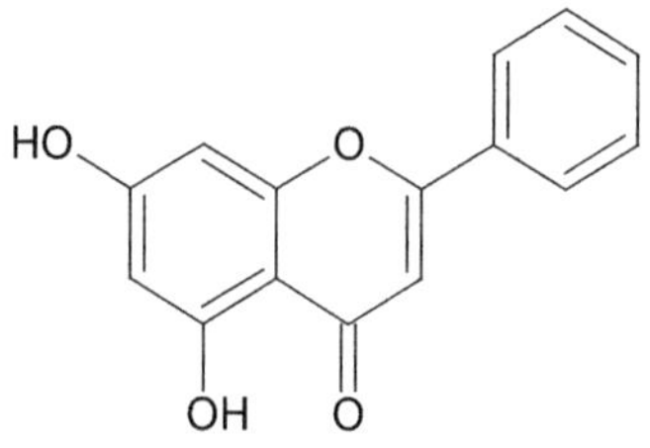

Apigenin (21)

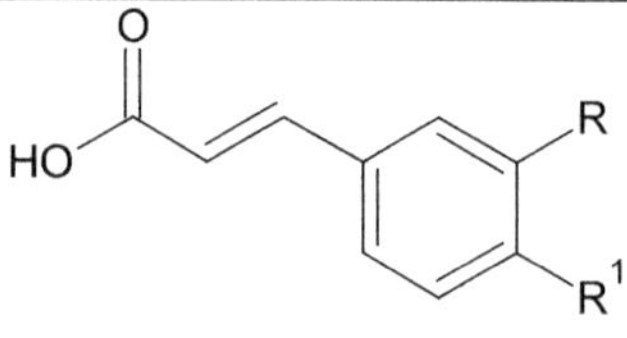

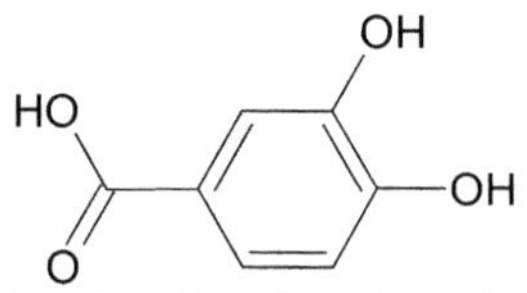

(C)

FIGURE 13.2 (*Continued*)

Kalmegh (*Andrographis paniculata*)

Caffeic acid (22): R=OH; R^1=OH Ferulic acid (23): R=OH; R^1=OCH$_3$	Protocatechuic acid (24)
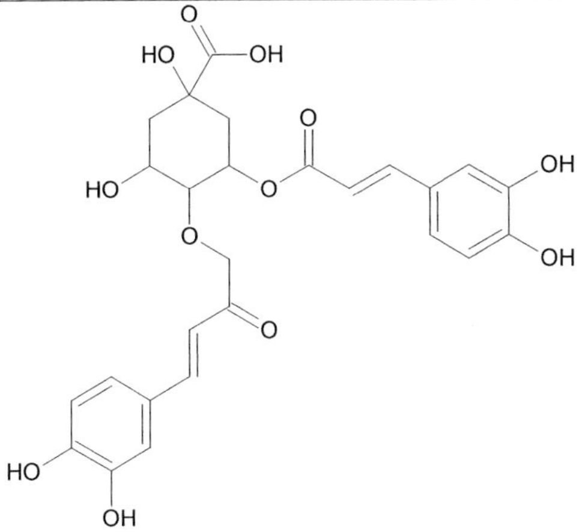 3,4-dicaffeoylquinic acid (25)	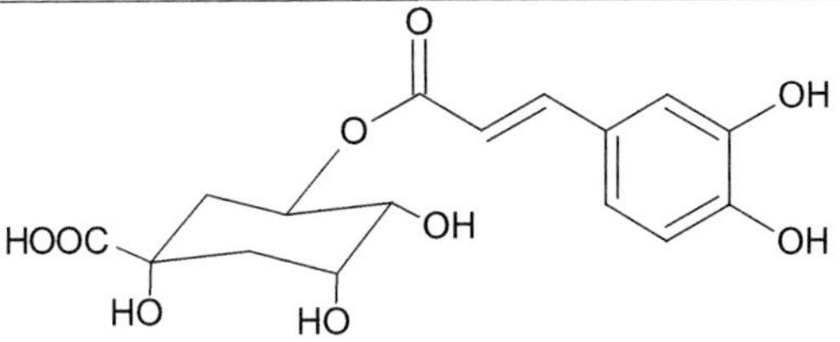 Chlorogenic acid (26)
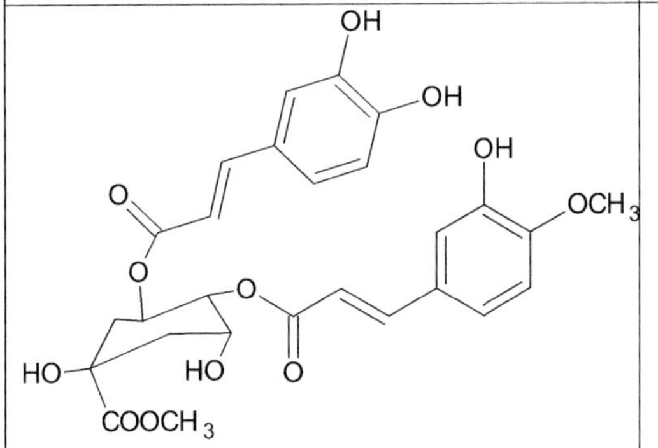 Methyl-3,4-dicaffeoylquinate (27)	
Flavanones (Hossain et al. 2014)(Kumar, Singh, and Bajpai 2021)	
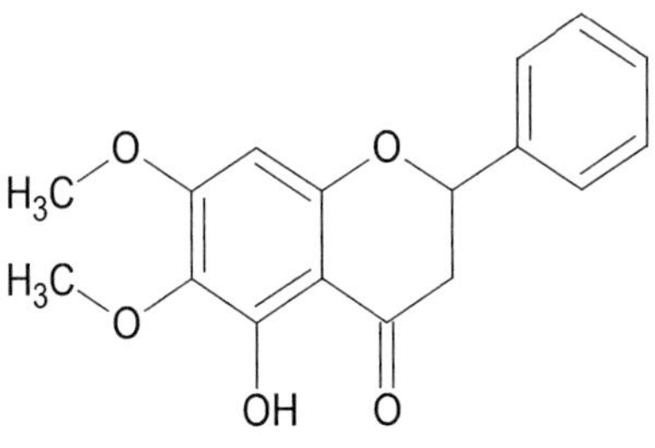 Onysilin (28)	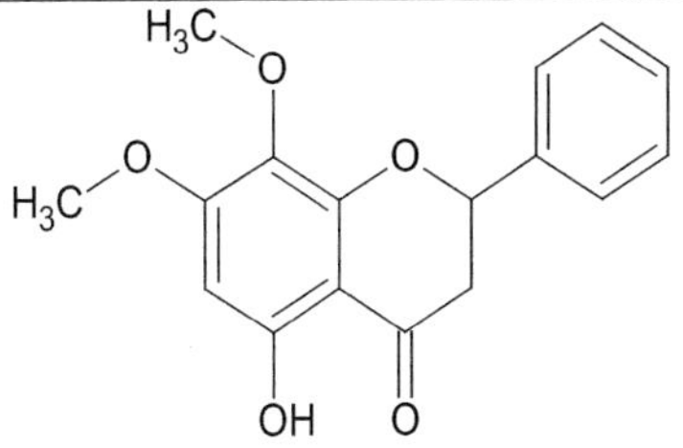 7-O-methyl-dihydrowogonin (29)

(D)

FIGURE 13.2 (*Continued*)

TABLE 13.2

Direct Cardioprotective Effects of *Andrographis paniculate*

vp No.	AP or Its Derivatives (Dose)	Types of Heart Injury (Time Used in Inducing Injury)	Subject (Age)	Observed Effects on the Heart	References
1	Andrographolide (25 mg/kg/day, daily for 14 days)	Myocardial ischemia-induced by LAD coronary ligation (injury was established for 7 days prior to andrographolide treatment for 14 days)	C57/BL6 mice (eight to ten weeks old)	Improved survival rate and cardiac function following myocardial infarction. Attenuated progression to cardiac hypertrophy and ventricular dilatation. Reduced cardiac fibrosis and inflammation.	Xie et al. 2020
2	Andrographolide (20 mg/kg/day, for 21 days)	Isoproterenol-induced myocardial injury (2 days on 80 mg/kg/day isoproterenol, applied after 19 days of andrographolide)	Male Wistar rats (six weeks old, 250–300 g)	Attenuated isoproterenol-induced cardiac remodeling. Reduced infarct size. Increased heart rate, contractility and cardiac antioxidant enzymes catalase and GPx.	Elasoru et al. 2021
3	Hydroalcoholic lyophilized AP extract (200 and 400 mg/kg, for 31 days)	Isoproterenol-induced myocardial injury (85 mg/kg, for 2 days, applied after 29 days of AP treatment)	Male Wister rats (ten–twelve weeks old)	Alleviated isoproterenol-depressed mean arterial blood pressure, heart rate, LV dP/dt. Reversed isoproterenol-induced increased in LVEDP. Increased glutathione (GSH) content and restored myocardial antioxidant enzymes SOD, CAT and GPx.	Ojha et al. 2012
4	Andrographolide (30 or 50 mg/kg/day for 5 days	Carbon tetrachloride-induced oxidative damage (1 ml/kg for 24 and 48 h after 5 days of andrographolide treatment)	Sprague Dawley rats (seven weeks old)	Increased antioxidant enzymes catalase, superoxide dismutase, GSH peroxidase, GSH reductase, GSH S-transferase.	Chen et al. 2014
4	Andrographolide (50 mg/kg, daily for 1 week after a week of acclimatization)	High fat diet-induced obesity (on high fat diet for 10 months)	C57/BL6 mice (four weeks old)	Inhibited cardiac cell apoptosis. Reduced effects of cardiac remodeling.	Lin et al. 2020
5	Andrographolide (25 mg/kg body weight/day, daily for 8 weeks)	Aortic banding-induced cardiac hypertrophy (1 week)	Male C57/BL6 mice (eight to ten weeks old)	Attenuated further deterioration of cardiac dysfunction. Reduced cardiac fibrosis and hypertrophic response to angiotensin II.	Wu et al. 2017

6	Andrographolide (10 mg/kg, daily for 7 days)	Lipopolysaccharide-induced cardiac malfunctions (LPS from Escherichia coli 055:B5, (20 mg/kg, 0.2 mL/10 g body weight, 7 days after andrographolide)	Male BALB/c mice (six to eight weeks old, 22–25 g)	Attenuated LPS-induced left ventricular systolic dysfunction, with improved EF, FS and E/A ratio. Reduced cardiac cell apoptosis.	Zhang et al. 2015
7	Andrographolide (1 mg/kg, administered 7 days before viral induction)	Coxsackie B3m-induced viral myocarditis $(1 \times 10^6$ PFU in 0.2 PBS)	BALB/c mice (four–six weeks old)	Ameliorated cardiac dysfunction and attenuated progression to remodeling.	Zhao et al. 2018
8	Andrographolide (10 ml andrographolide, 10 mg/kg in 5 min prior to aconitine induction)	Aconitine-induced arrythmias (2 µg/kg/min, flow rate: 80 µl/min	Adult New Zealand white rabbits	Reduced incidence of VT and VF.	Zeng et al. 2017
9	Crude AP water extract, semi-purified butanol fraction and aqueous fraction	Normal heart under general anesthesia (Inactin and sodium pentobarbital)	Male Sprague Dawley rats (250–300 g)	All AP extracts demonstrated hypotension. 1.4% of n-butanol fraction caused hypotension, with a fall in mean arterial pressure, through the α-adrenoceptors, autonomic ganglion and histaminergic receptors.	Zhang et al. 1997
10	AP water extract (2 g/kg/day, for a week)	High fat diet-induced obesity	C57/BL6 mice (four weeks old)	Reduced cardiac inflammation. Attenuated progression to cardiac hypertrophy. Suppressed cardiac fibrosis. Inhibited cardiac cell apoptosis via IGF1R signaling.	Hsieh et al. 2016
11	Andrographolide (dose not mentioned) and AP aqueous extract (AE, 250 mg/kg body weight/day)	Nicotine-induced oxidative stress (1.0 mg/kg/day, 7 days)	Male Wistar rats (120–140 g)	AE suppressed MDA activity following nicotine toxicity. Both andrographolide and AE were able to elevate the glutathione expression and enhance the antioxidant capacity in the nicotine-intoxicated heart.	Neogy et al. 2008

Note: This table shows the cardioprotective effects of *Andrographis paniculate* or its derivatives on the heart in response to anesthesia, drugs or viral-induced injury.

known for its anti-inflammatory properties. In bacteria endotoxin LPS or Coxsackie B3 m virus-induced myocarditis and cardiac dysfunction mice models, andrographolide showed significant suppressive effects on the pro-inflammatory cytokine tumor necrosis factor-α (TNF-α) and NF-κB signaling (Zhang et al. 2015; Zhao et al. 2018). This suggests that andrographolide protects the heart from myocarditis and is able to reverse myocardial dysfunction following the endotoxin or viral insults via its anti-inflammatory property. Noteworthy, both experiments had included a long andrographolide "priming" phase (7 days) prior to introducing LPS- or virus-induced cardiac injury. Hence, evidence to elucidate whether andrographolide could demonstrate the similar therapeutic effects to salvage the established myocarditis is still lacking.

13.4.3 MYOCARDIAL INFARCTION AND CARDIOTOXIC DRUG-INDUCED CARDIAC INJURIES

Myocardial infarction (MI) is manifested as the myocardial damage and cell death as a result of ischemia or drug-induced toxicity. Infarct expansion and myocardial cell death are the major contributors to detrimental ventricular remodeling. In a study by Xie et al. (2020), they showed that LAD-ligated MI mice manifested typical cardiac remodeling features with hypertrophy, elevated oxidative stress and extensive fibrosis after three weeks, all of which were demonstrated to have been attenuated by andrographolide. They attributed the observed cardioprotective effect to the antioxidative capability of andrographolide (Xie et al. 2020), which stimulated the significant upregulation of nuclear factor E2-related factor 2/heme-oxigease-1 signaling, the regulators of cellular response to oxidative stress. In *in vitro* modeling of the myocardial ischemia using neonatal rat cardiac fibroblast in hypoxia for 24 h, the increased in smooth muscle actin expression indicative of myofibroblast differentiation and proliferation were both blunted by andrographolide treatment through transforming growth factor β and smad3 inhibitions.

Coincides with this observation, myocardial injuries induced by ISO, carbon tetrachloride or nicotine (Elasoru et al. 2021; Neogy et al. 2008) were also be attenuated by andrographolide treatment through the increase in endogenous antioxidant enzyme glutathione (GSH), superoxide dismutase (SOD), catalase (CAT) and glutathione peroxidase (GPx) activities. The similar antioxidative effects have also resulted in reduced infarct size, cardiac fibrosis and remodeling.

13.4.4 PRESSURE OVERLOAD AND HIGH FAT DIET-INDUCED CARDIAC HYPERTROPHY

Excessive fat consumption is a common contributor of cardiac metabolic disease and dysfunction. Two studies were published by Huang and colleagues who examined the effects of *A. paniculata* extract and andrographolide in rats after 10 months of high fat diets which developed increased body weight and cardiac hypertrophy (Lin et al. 2020; Hsieh et al. 2016). Cardiac inflammation as evidenced by the upregulation of COX-2, p-IκBα and NF-κB pro-inflammatory markers in the high fat-fed mice were significant reduced by *A. paniculata* extract and andrographolide, which also resulted in reduced cellular apoptosis in the heart (Lin et al. 2020), with significant reduction in collagen deposition and cardiac cell apoptosis via the upregulation of pro-survival signaling proteins such as Bcl-2, Bax-xL and insulin-like growth factor-1 receptor (Hsieh et al. 2016). Likewise in the model of pressure overload-induced concentric, hypertrophic cardiomyopathy model using aortic banding method, andrographolide was found to, again, exert anti-inflammatory, antifibrotic and anti-apoptotic effects (Wu et al. 2017). The mechanisms underlying the cardioprotective effects were found to be the simultaneous suppression of angiotensin II-induced cardiomyocyte hypertrophy and the inhibition of mitogen-activated protein kinase-induced activation of cardiac fibroblasts.

13.4.5 THE EFFECTS OF ANDROGRAPHOLIDE ON CARDIAC ION CHANNELS

To date, two independent studies by Zeng et al. (2017) and Elasoru et al. (2021) suggested that andrographolide treatment has a profound effect on cardiac LTCC current ($I_{Ca,L}$). Changes in L-type calcium channel (LTCC) may cause remodeling of intracellular calcium signaling and action potential duration (APD). Isoproterenol is known to induce prolonged APD, indicative of depressed excitation and contraction coupling in the isolated rat cardiomyocytes, which has been associated with the increased LTCC density (Elasoru et al. 2021; Ito et al. 2019). Both Zeng and Elasoru have found that treatment with andrographolide was found to suppress ISO-induced increase of $I_{Ca,L}{}^{+}$ while Elasoru and his team also showed the increased the cardiac transient outward K^{+} current in rats (Elasoru et al. 2021) but not sodium channel current as shown by Zeng in rabbit, possibly attributed to species differences used in their studies (Zeng et al. 2017). Additionally, Zeng (2017) also concluded that andrographolide is effective against iconitine-induced arrhythmia *in vivo*.

13.5 INDIRECT CARDIOPROTECTIVE MECHANISM OF ACTION

13.5.1 ANTIOXIDANT EFFECT

Our body maintains homeostasis through multiple regulation processes including balance between oxidant and antioxidants. Oxidants such as reactive oxygen species (ROS) are essential for the preservation of cellular homeostasis; however excessive production of ROS may lead to oxidative stress which can result in cell damage and eventually diseases states. Despite an established endogenous antioxidant and repair mechanisms, oxidative stress and damage remains an unavoidable consequence owing to high-calorie diet, drugs, environmental factors and other xenobiotics that spontaneously produce ROS. Cardiovascular diseases are multifaceted entities with many pathophysiologic processes, and overproduction of ROS has been suggested as one of the commonest etiologies (Steven et al. 2019). Excessive ROS generation causes decreased nitric oxide availability, arrhythmia, trigger atherosclerosis formation and even heart failure (Steven et al. 2019). Due to this, more personalized redox medicine is required to prevent cardiovascular diseases as mentioned earlier. *A. paniculata* has been showed to possess antioxidant properties by three main mechanisms: elimination of ROS, suppression of ROS generation, and enhanced endogenous antioxidant systems (Mussard et al. 2019). A number of studies documented that extract of *A. paniculata* and its bioactive compounds, particularly andrographolide, exhibited significant antioxidative activity. Extract of *A. paniculata* and andrographolide is found to significantly scavenge free radicals such as hydroxyl radicals, superoxide, lipid peroxidation and nitric oxide in an *in vitro* and *in vivo* model (Mussard et al. 2019). Moreover, *A. paniculata* exhibited its antioxidative properties via protecting mitochondria (Mussard et al. 2019). Mitochondria are crucial organelles which function to generate energy in terms of ATP for the maintenance of cell viability. Excessive generation of mitochondrial ROS, on the other hand, is detrimental to cells. Furthermore, evidence also proved that andrographolide is capable of blocking free radical-producing enzymes activities such as NADPH oxidase and xanthine oxidase while, at the same time, enhancing the endogenous antioxidant systems, for instance SOD, CAT and GPx (Woo et al. 2008). This can also be seen from the study done by Adedapo et al. (2019) where data showed that *A. paniculata* significantly decreased blood serum oxidant level (MDA level, MPO and H_2O_2 production) while increasing antioxidant defense systems, including SOD, GPx, GST and GSH in isoproterenol induced-myocardial infarction rats (Adedapo et al. 2019). Collectively, cardioprotective effect of *A. paniculata* is highly contributed by its antioxidant activities and this activity might be associated with the Nrf2 signaling pathway where this signaling molecule plays a critical role in protecting cells from oxidative and electrophilic damage (Mussard et al. 2019).

13.5.2 ANTI-INFLAMMATORY EFFECT

Inflammation is multifaceted and highly associated with complex and multiple series of molecular and cellular processes. Undeniably, inflammation is a protective response to restoring tissue homeostasis by removing the toxic agents or foreign bodies from entering the host of an organism at the site of an injury. However, persistently triggered and maintained inflammation may be maladaptive, resulting in increasing tissue damage and decreased survival (Golia et al. 2014). It is firmly established that inflammation has a crucial role in the initiation, development, progression and presentation of cardiovascular diseases (Golia et al. 2014). In experimental models, targeting inflammatory pathways has been shown to be effective in decreasing myocardial and vascular damage, slowing disease progression, as well as encouraging recovery although using targeted medicines to safely modulate inflammation remains to be difficult. Chen and his team (2011) successfully demonstrated that andrographolide exhibited anti-inflammatory activity against TNF-α-induced inflammation on HUVECs. Andrographolide significantly decreased monocyte adhesion on HUVECs after being stimulated with TNF-α or high-mobility group box chromosomal protein 1 (HMGB1) by reducing ICAM-1 protein expression or TNF-α production (Chen et al. 2011; Lee et al. 2014). This activity showed by andrographolide may be attributed to suppression of the PI3K/Akt signaling cascade, NF-κB activity and ERK1/2 (Chen et al. 2011; Lee et al. 2014). TNF-α and HMGB1 both are pro-inflammatory cytokines which are capable of activating vascular endothelial cells and promoting inflammation via recruitment of leucocytes. Inhibiting both cytokines will help in preventing cardiovascular diseases. Moreover, andrographolide significantly reduced IL-1β, IL-6, LDH and MDA levels in inflammatory vascular endothelial cells induced by high glucose (Duan et al. 2019). A more recent study documented that mice treated with andrographolides caused TNF-α, MCP-1, hs-CRP and IL-1 levels to decrease by changing the macrophage phenotype, and endothelial dysfunction was improved by raising serum levels of ET-1 and TAX2 while reducing NO and PGI2 levels (Shu et al. 2020). Taken together, *A. paniculata* and its active compounds, andrographolide, exhibited a cardiovascular protective effect, probably due to its strong anti-inflammatory activities which was mainly mediated via NF-κB signaling pathways.

13.5.3 ENDOTHELIAL PROTECTIVE EFFECT

Vascular endothelial cells cover the entire circulatory system, including lymph vessels, and play a critical role in cardiovascular homeostasis by regulating vascular tone and growth, hemostasis, as well as leukocyte interaction via release of regulatory substances (Sun et al. 2020). Furthermore, vascular endothelial cells also acts as a barrier to restrict the movement of blood cells and solutes. Excessive production of reactive oxygen species, pro-inflammatory mediators, imbalance between vasoconstrictor and vasodilator factors and the lack of nitric oxide bioavailability are the major factors contributed to endothelial dysfunction (Sun et al. 2020) where it is known as one of the cardiovascular disease's hallmarks. In addition, apoptosis of endothelial cells contributes to destabilizing the barrier function thus leading to cardiovascular diseases, especially atherosclerosis. Interestingly, andrographolide-induced activation of PI3K/Akt, an event that in turn results in inhibition of endothelial apoptosis (Chen et al. 2004). Recently, andrographolide also has been shown to protect endothelial dysfunction by increasing NO bioavailability via suppression of PI3K-Akt-eNOS signaling pathway against high glucose as well as cisplatin *in vitro* (Duan et al. 2019; Bodiga et al. 2020). Other than *in vitro*, andrographolide also significantly mitigated endothelial dysfunction in rat models via blocking the activation of PPAR-α/NF-κB axis (Shu et al. 2020).

13.5.4 VASORELAXANT EFFECT

Vascular muscle tone plays an important role in the regulation of blood pressure. Increased vascular tone or contraction which is triggered by an increase in intracellular calcium concentration is highly associated with the development of hypertension which eventually leads to stroke, heart failure or ischemia. Vasodilator or vasorelaxant is known as one of the regimens to reduce the vascular tone by promoting vasorelaxation or vasodilatation, and it is an important intervention in the management and/or treatment of high blood pressure. 14-deoxyandrographolide, a diterpenoid from *A. paniculata*, demonstrated the vasodilator effect in rat isolated thoracic aorta by activating endothelium-dependent

NO synthase (Zhang and Tan 1998). NO stimulates a vasorelaxing effect via activation of guanidyl cyclase signaling pathway. Furthermore, 14-deoxyandrographolide showed to block calcium ion influx via voltage- and receptor-operated calcium channels, thus leading to vasodilatation (Zhang and Tan 1998). In addition, *A. paniculata* extract exerts a vasorelaxant effect by changing alpha-adrenoceptor and muscarinic responses to NE and Ach, respectively in VSMC (Yoopan et al. 2007). Calcium ions (Ca^{2+}), either extracellular or intracellular, play an important role in the smooth muscle contraction. Thus, therapeutic agents which are capable of suppressing either or both sources of Ca^{2+} have become a strategy treatment to cause vasodilation. Interestingly, diterpene lactones from *A. paniculata* have been found to cause vasorelaxation by suppressing the calcium influx (Sriramaneni et al. 2010), and thus indirectly contributing to the protection of the cardiovascular system.

13.5.5 Anti-Platelet Aggregation Effect

Platelets are one of the specialized blood cells that play an essential role in the hemostasis as well as wound healing processes, even extending to inflammation and immunity. Activated platelets are capable of adhering to the site of vascular injury, assisting the wound-healing process. Moreover, it also stimulates the production of thrombin which is known as an endogenous potent enzyme involved in the coagulation process (Vélez and García 2015). Due to this, abnormal platelet count could lead to a number of disorders, for instance hemorrhage and prolonged bleeding time in thrombocytopenia (low platelet count), while formation of clots in the blood vessels (thrombosis), stroke and heart attack could happen in thrombocytosis (high platelet count) (Vélez and García 2015). Platelet aggregation, although is an essential mechanism in normal hemostasis, still has the possibility to increase the risks for cardiovascular disease by forming the thrombus. Due to this, it is a need to explore a therapeutic agent which can block thromboembolic diseases in order to prevent further cardiovascular diseases. Extensive studies have been carried out to determine the anti-platelet aggregation activity on *A. paniculata* extract as well as its active compounds. Hot water extract of *A. paniculata* and its active diterpenoids, including andrographolide and 14-deoxy-11, 12-didehydroandrographolide, significantly inhibited washed platelets of rats' aggregation in concentration- and time-dependent manners (Jayakumar et al. 2013). However, neoandrographolide showed no significant difference compared to the control in the same study (Jayakumar et al. 2013). On the other hand, andrographolide showed successfully inhibited human platelet aggregation against platelet-activating factor (PAF) (Jayakumar et al. 2013). Due to *A. paniculata* and its active compounds showing anti-platelet activities in an *in vitro* model, Sirikarin and his team (2018) further investigate this activity on human subjects. Data indicated that individuals who consumed the *A. paniculata* powder showed variability in the platelet activity and this could be due to multifactorial mechanisms of platelet aggregation as it was tested in whole organisms (Sirikarin et al. 2018). The anti-platelet aggregation activity of *A. paniculata* and its active compounds might involve the activation of the eNOS-NO-cGMP signaling cascade (Jayakumar et al. 2013).

13.5.6 Reduction of Smooth Muscle Cell Migration and Proliferation

Vascular smooth muscle cells (VSMC) provide structural integrity and regulate the blood vessels' diameter by contracting and relaxing dynamically in response to vasoactive stimuli under physiological conditions. Moreover, it also secretes and releases vascular regulatory substances in order to maintain a proper vascular function. However, a phenotype of VSMC will change from quiescent "contractile" to active "synthetic" state, being stimulated by inflammatory mediators which are released from endothelium, platelets and inflammatory cells during vascular injury. Thus, abnormal proliferation and migration of VSMC from media to intima in response to vascular injury is one of the important hallmarks for the pathogenesis of cardiovascular diseases such as atherosclerosis and hypertension. Hence, inhibiting VSMC proliferation and migration might be a potential treatment of cardiovascular diseases. Evidence showed that andrographolide, an active compound isolated

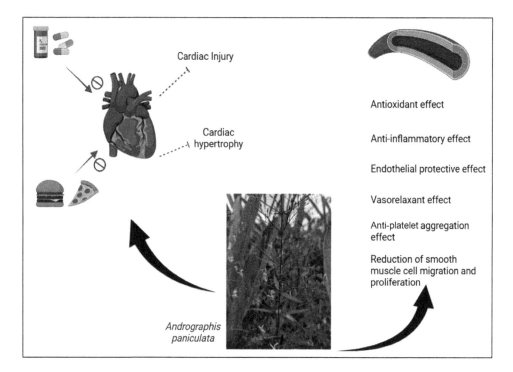

FIGURE 13.3 Cardioprotective effects of *Andrographis paniculate* exhibited *in vitro* and *in vivo*.

from *A. paniculata*, induced VSMC apoptosis via ceramide-p47phox-ROS signaling cascade (Chen et al. 2013). Platelet-derived growth factor (PDGF) suppressed VSMC apoptosis in the atherosclerosis (Bennett and Joseph 1998), therefore andrographolide might be a potential pro-apoptotic agent against PDGF which in turn could conceivably ameliorate cardiovascular disease. Apart from this, PDGF also promotes vascular smooth muscle cells proliferation and migration via overlapping complex signaling cascade. Interestingly, andrographolide significantly attenuated PDGF-BB-induced proliferation by blocking ERK1/2 and PCNA expressions in VSMC (Chang et al. 2014). On top of that, andrographolide is capable of inducing mitochondrial dysfunction by activating the PP2A-p38MAPK-p53-Bax cascade and SHP-1-dependent mechanism which eventually leads to apoptosis of VSMC (Chen et al. 2014). Taken all these, *A. paniculata* might be a potential treatment of cardiovascular diseases.

13.6 OTHER FOODS, HERBS, SPICES AND BOTANICALS USED IN CARDIOVASCULAR HEALTH AND DISEASE

Herbal remedies play an important part in the health care of a substantial proportion of the world's population, and they have long been recognized as an important component of the cultural legacy of many tribes across the world. Due to being rich in secondary metabolites and essential oils which might contribute to therapeutic importance, medicinal plants, vegetables and fruits are being considered as significant potential sources of drugs. The trend for the usage of medicinal plants against various ailments is increasing and this could be due to the availability, economy, effectiveness as well as safety compared to modern medicine. On top of that, because of their ability to treat or prevent a number of diseases, the bioactive compounds from natural sources have gained vital relevance in the current system of medicine. Numerous plants and their bioactive phytoconstituents are well known for their low toxicity, suggesting that they may offer an alternative treatment option for cardiovascular disorders. Table 13.3 summarizes some of the plants which are found in Malaysia and Southeast Asia which possess cardioprotective potentials.

TABLE 13.3

Plants Used in Cardiovascular Health and Diseases and Found in Malaysia

Scientific Name	Family	Common Name/ Local Name	Origin	Part Used	In Vivo /In Vitro / Ex Vivo	Cardioprotective Effects	Ref.
Eurycoma longifolia Jack	Simaroubaceae	Tongkat Ali	Southeast Asia	Roots	*In vitro*	Vasodilatory effect	Tee et al. 2016
					In vivo	Vasodilatory effect; anti-hypertensive	Mokhtar et al. 2014
					In vivo	Anti-atherosclerosis	Al-Joufi et al. 2016
Labisia pumila var. *alata*	Myrsinaceae	Kacip Fatimah	Malaysia	Whole plant	*In vivo*	Protection from myocardial infarction; antioxidant	Dianita et al. 2015
Momordica charantia	Cucurbitaceae	Bitter melon, bitter gourd	Tropical and sub-tropical regions	Fruits	*In vivo*	Protection from myocardial infarction; improved blood circulation following ischemia- reperfusion injury	Czompa et al. 2017
				Fruits	*In vivo*	Prevent cardiac fibrosis; enhanced antioxidant properties; decreased collagen deposition	Abas et al. 2014
				Fresh leaves and stems	*In vivo*	Prevent degeneration of myocardium and aortic tissues; decreased LDL-cholesterol level	Innih et al. 2021
Zingiber officinale Roscoe	Zingiberaceae	Ginger	Tropical and sub-tropical	Rhizomes	*In vivo* and *in vitro*	Antioxidant; anti-inflammation; anti-atherosclerosis; reduced low-density lipoprotein peroxidation; prevents platelet aggregation; antithrombotic, protection against myocardial ischemic-reperfusion injury	Amran et al. 2015

13.7 TOXICITY AND CAUTIONARY NOTES

Numerous independent studies from different laboratories have shown that *A. paniculata or* andrographolide has an extremely safe pharmacological profile which suggests that they are nontoxic in nature even at high doses. No apparent toxicity was found in testicle, liver, kidney heart or spleen in rodents or rabbits, and no death was reported with oral *A. paniculata* extract consumption up to a daily dose of 10 g/kg for 7 days in mice (Jayakumar et al. 2013). The LD50 of the standardized ethanolic *A. paniculata* extract was reported to be more than 5 g/kg body weight in mice with no adverse effects (Worasuttayangkurn et al. 2019).

Nonetheless, in a published safety review of AP by the Therapeutic Goods Administration (TGA) of Australian Government Department of Health in 2015 indicated that the major side effects from consuming *A. paniculata* at a large dose may cause gastric discomfort, emesis and anorexia (Therapeutic Goods Administration, Health Safety Regulation 2015). They also advised against the use of andrographidis (dried aerial region of *A. paniculata*) during pregnancy and lactation, as well as administration of crude extract due to the potential anaphylactic reactions. The anaphylactic effect has also been previously reported in a human trial involving HIV patients who were treated with an escalating dose from 5 mg/kg to 10 mg/kg (thrice a day, each dose for 3 weeks), albeit with a rise in CD4 cells after *A. paniculata* administration at 10 mg/kg.

13.8 SUMMARY POINTS

- This chapter focuses on the possible cardioprotective effects of *Andrographis paniculate* which is commonly known as King of Bitter.
- It is native to China and India but widely distributed in Southeast Asian countries.
- The main active compound, andrographolide, exhibits an extraordinarily wide range of pharmacological activities.
- The plant, mainly consumed in whole or via its leaves, promotes health and treats different type of diseases including cardiovascular diseases.
- Andrographolide exhibits direct cardioprotective effects by preventing cardiotoxic drug-induced cardiac injuries through antioxidant capability.
- Extract of *Andrographis paniculata* and andrographolide showed to prevent high fat diet-induced cardiac hypertrophy.
- Indirect cardioprotective mechanism of action possessed by *Andrographis paniculata* includes antioxidant, anti-inflammatory effects, and promotes good health in blood vessels.

13.9 ACKNOWLEDGMENT

The authors would like to thank Mr. Izlamira Roslan and Mr. Mohd Zulkhairi Azid for providing images of the plants.

REFERENCES

Abas, R., Othman, F. and Thent, Z.C., 2014. Protective effect of Momordica charantia fruit extract on hyperglycaemia-induced cardiac fibrosis. Oxidative Medicine and Cellular Longevity: 429060.

Adedapo, A.D., Adedapo, A.A., Ayodele, A.E., Adeoye, B.O., Ajibade, T.O., Oyagbemi, A.A., Omobowale, T.O. and Yakubu, M.A., 2019. Cardioprotective effects and antioxidant status of Andrographis paniculata in isoproterenol-induced myocardial infarction in rats. Journal of Medicinal Plants for Economic Development, 3: 1–12.

Al-Joufi, F., Al-Ani, I.M., Saxena, A.K., Talib, N.A., Mokhtar, R.H. and Ku-Zaifah, N., 2016. Assessment of anti-atherosclerotic effect of Eurycoma longifolia extract on high-fat diet model in rats. I: Histological study. European Journal of Anatomy, 20: 131–136.

Amran, A.Z., Jantan, I., Dianita, R. and Buang, F., 2015. Protective effects of the standardized extract of Zingiber officinale on myocardium against isoproterenol-induced biochemical and histopathological alterations in rats. Pharmaceutical Biology, 53: 1795–1802.

Australian Government, Department of Health, Therapeutic Goods Administration, 2015. Safety review of Andrographis paniculate and anaphylactic/allergic reactions. www.tga.gov.au/sites/default/files/safety-review-andrographis.pdf.

Awang, K., Abdullah, N.H., Hadi, A.H.A. and Su Fong, Y., 2012. Cardiovascular activity of labdane diterpenes from Andrographis paniculata in isolated rat hearts. Journal of Biomedicine and Biotechnology: 876458.

Bennett, M.R. and Boyle, J.J., 1998. Apoptosis of vascular smooth muscle cells in atherosclerosis. Atherosclerosis, 138: 3–9.

Bodiga, V.L., Bathula, J., Kudle, M.R., Vemuri, P.K. and Bodiga, S., 2020. Andrographolide suppresses cis-platin-induced endothelial hyperpermeability through activation of PI3K/Akt and eNOS: Derived nitric oxide. Bioorganic & Medicinal Chemistry, 28: 115809.

Chang, C.C., Duann, Y.F., Yen, T.L., Chen, Y.Y., Jayakumar, T., Ong, E.T. and Sheu, J.R., 2014. Andrographolide, a novel NF-κB inhibitor, inhibits vascular smooth muscle cell proliferation and cerebral endothelial cell inflammation. Acta Cardiologica Sinica, 30: 308–315.

Chen, H.W., Huang, C.S., Li, C.C., Lin, A.H., Huang, Y.J., Wang, T.S., Yao, H.T. and Lii, C.K., 2014. Bioavailability of andrographolide and protection against carbon tetrachloride-induced oxidative damage in rats. Toxicology and Applied Pharmacology, 280: 1–9.

Chen, H.W., Lin, A.H., Chu, H.C., Li, C.C., Tsai, C.W., Chao, C.Y., Wang, C.J., Lii, C.K. and Liu, K.L., 2011. Inhibition of TNF-α-induced inflammation by andrographolide via down-regulation of the PI3K/Akt signaling pathway. Journal of Natural Products, 74: 2408–2413.

Chen, J.H., Hsiao, G., Lee, A.R., Wu, C.C. and Yen, M.H., 2004. Andrographolide suppresses endothelial cell apoptosis via activation of phosphatidyl inositol-3-kinase/Akt pathway. Biochemical Pharmacology, 67: 1337–1345.

Chen, Y.Y., Hsieh, C.Y., Jayakumar, T., Lin, K.H., Chou, D.S., Lu, W.J., Hsu, M.J. and Sheu, J.R., 2014. Andrographolide induces vascular smooth muscle cell apoptosis through a SHP-1-PP2A-p38MAPK-p53 cascade. Scientific Reports, 4: 5651.

Chen, Y.Y., Hsu, M.J., Sheu, J.R., Lee, L.W. and Hsieh, C.Y., 2013. Andrographolide, a novel NF-κB inhibitor, induces vascular smooth muscle cell apoptosis via a ceramide-p47phox-ROS signaling cascade. Evidence-Based Complementary and Alternative Medicine: 821813.

Czompa, A., Gyongyosi, A., Szoke, K., Bak, I., Csepanyi, E., Haines, D.D., Tosaki, A. and Lekli, I., 2017. Effects of Momordica charantia (Bitter Melon) on ischemic diabetic myocardium. Molecules, 22: 488.

Dianita, R., Jantan, I., Amran, A.Z. and Jalil, J., 2015. Protective effects of Labisia pumila var. alata on biochemical and histopathological alterations of cardiac muscle cells in isoproterenol-induced myocardial infarction rats. Molecules, 20: 4746–4763.

Duan, M.X., Zhou, H., Wu, Q.Q., Liu, C., Xiao, Y., Deng, W. and Tang, Q.Z., 2019. Andrographolide protects against HG-induced inflammation, apoptosis, migration, and impairment of angiogenesis via PI3K/AKT-eNOS signalling in HUVECs. Mediators of Inflammation: 6168340.

Elasoru, S.E., Rhana, P., de Oliveira Barreto, T., de Souza, D.L.N., de Menezes-Filho, J.E.R., de Souza, D.S., Moreira, M.V.L., Campos, M.T.G., Adedosu, O.T., Roman-Campos, D. and Melo, M.M., 2021. Andrographolide protects against isoproterenol-induced myocardial infarction in rats through inhibition of L-type Ca2+ and increase of cardiac transient outward K+ currents. European Journal of Pharmacology, 906: 174194.

Forestry Department of Peninsular Malaysia. 2022. Hempedu Bumi. www.forestry.gov.my/en/tumbuhan-ubatan/item/hempedu-bumi (accessed November 15, 2021).

Golia, E., Limongelli, G., Natale, F., Fimiani, F., Maddaloni, V., Pariggiano, I., Bianchi, R., Crisci, M., D'Acierno, L., Giordano, R. and Di Palma, G., 2014. Inflammation and cardiovascular disease: From pathogenesis to therapeutic target. Current Atherosclerosis Reports, 16: 435.

Hossain, M.D., Urbi, Z., Sule, A., and Rahman, K.M. 2014. Andrographis paniculata (Burm. f.) Wall. ex Nees: A review of ethnobotany, phytochemistry, and pharmacology. The Scientific World Journal: 274905.

Hossain, S., Urbi, Z., Karuniawati, H., Mohiuddin, R.B., Moh Qrimida, A., Allzrag, A.M.M., Ming, L.C., Pagano, E. and Capasso, R., 2021. Andrographis paniculata (Burm. f.) Wall. ex Nees: An updated review of phytochemistry, antimicrobial pharmacology, and clinical safety and efficacy. Life, 11: 348.

Hsieh, Y.L., Shibu, M.A., Lii, C.K., Viswanadha, V.P., Lin, Y.L., Lai, C.H., Chen, Y.F., Lin, K.H., Kuo, W.W. and Huang, C.Y., 2016. Andrographis paniculata extract attenuates pathological cardiac hypertrophy and apoptosis in high-fat diet fed mice. Journal of Ethnopharmacology, 192: 170–177.

Huang, C.J. and Wu, M.C., 2002. Differential effects of foods traditionally regarded as 'heating' and 'cooling' on prostaglandin E2 production by a macrophage cell line. Journal of Biomedical Science, 9: 596–606.

Innih, S.O., Eze, I.G. and Omage, K., 2021. Cardiovascular benefits of Momordica charantia in cholesterol-fed Wistar rats. Clinical Phytoscience, 7: 65.

Ito, D.W., Hannigan, K.I., Ghosh, D., Xu, B., Del Villar, S.G., Xiang, Y.K., Dickson, E.J., Navedo, M.F. and Dixon, R.E., 2019. β-adrenergic-mediated dynamic augmentation of sarcolemmal CaV1. 2 clustering and co-operativity in ventricular myocytes. The Journal of Physiology, 597: 2139–2162.

Jayakumar, T., Hsieh, C.Y., Lee, J.J. and Sheu, J.R., 2013. Experimental and clinical pharmacology of Andrographis paniculata and its major bioactive phytoconstituent andrographolide. Evidence-Based Complementary and Alternative Medicine: 846740.

Kumar, S., Singh, B. and Bajpai, V., 2021. Andrographis paniculata (Burm. f.) Nees: Traditional uses, phytochemistry, pharmacological properties and quality control/quality assurance. Journal of Ethnopharmacology, 275: 114054.

Lee, W., Ku, S., Yoo, H., Song, K. and Bae, J., 2014. Andrographolide inhibits HMGB 1-induced inflammatory responses in human umbilical vein endothelial cells and in murine polymicrobial sepsis. Acta Physiologica, 211: 176–187.

Lin, K.H., Marthandam Asokan, S., Kuo, W.W., Hsieh, Y.L., Lii, C.K., Viswanadha, V., Lin, Y.L., Wang, S., Yang, C. and Huang, C.Y., 2020. Andrographolide mitigates cardiac apoptosis to provide cardioprotection in high-fat-diet-induced obese mice. Environmental Toxicology, 35: 707–713.

Liu, Y., Liu, Y., Zhang, H.L., Yu, F.F., Yin, X.R., Zhao, Y.F., Ye, F. and Wu, X.Q., 2021. Amelioratory effect of neoandrographolide on myocardial ischemic-reperfusion injury by its anti-inflammatory and anti-apoptotic activities. Environmental Toxicology, 36: 2367–2379.

Mokhtar, R.H., Abdullah, N. and Ayob, A., 2014. Effects of Eurycoma longifolia extract on the isolated rat heart. IIUM Medical Journal Malaysia, 13: 25–34.

Mussard, E., Cesaro, A., Lespessailles, E., Legrain, B., Berteina-Raboin, S. and Toumi, H., 2019. Andrographolide, a natural antioxidant: An update. Antioxidants, 8: 571.

Neogy, S., Das, S., Mahapatra, S.K., Mandal, N. and Roy, S., 2008. Amelioratory effect of Andrographis paniculata Nees on liver, kidney, heart, lung and spleen during nicotine induced oxidative stress. Environmental Toxicology and Pharmacology, 25: 321–328.

Ojha, S., Bharti, S., Golechha, M., Sharma, A.K., Rani, N., Kumari, S. and Arya, D.S., 2012. Andrographis paniculata extract protect against isoproterenol-induced myocardial injury by mitigating cardiac dysfunction and oxidative injury in rats. Acta Poloniae Pharmaceutica, 69: 269–278.

Pholphana, N., Rangkadilok, N., Thongnest, S., Ruchirawat, S., Ruchirawat, M. and Satayavivad, J., 2004. Determination and variation of three active diterpenoids in Andrographis paniculata (Burm. f.) Nees. Phytochemical Analysis: An International Journal of Plant Chemical and Biochemical Techniques, 15: 365–371.

Shu, J., Huang, R., Tian, Y., Liu, Y., Zhu, R. and Shi, G., 2020. Andrographolide protects against endothelial dysfunction and inflammatory response in rats with coronary heart disease by regulating PPAR and NF-κB signaling pathways. Annals of Palliative Medicine, 9: 1965–1975.

Sirikarin, T., Palo, T., Chotewuttakorn, S., Chandranipapongse, W., Limsuvan, S. and Akarasereenont, P., 2018. The effects of Andrographis paniculata on platelet activity in healthy Thai volunteers. Evidence-Based Complementary and Alternative Medicine: 2458281.

Sriramaneni, R.N., Omar, A.Z., Ibrahim, S.M., Amirin, S. and Zaini, A.M., 2010. Vasorelaxant effect of diterpenoid lactones from Andrographis paniculata chloroform extract on rat aortic rings. Pharmacognosy Research, 2: 242–246.

Steven, S., Frenis, K., Oelze, M., Kalinovic, S., Kuntic, M., Bayo Jimenez, M.T., Vujacic-Mirski, K., Helmstädter, J., Kröller-Schön, S., Münzel, T. and Daiber, A., 2019. Vascular inflammation and oxidative stress: Major triggers for cardiovascular disease. Oxidative Medicine and Cellular Longevity: 7092151.

Subramanian, R., Asmawi, M.Z. and Sadikun, A., 2012. A bitter plant with a sweet future? A comprehensive review of an oriental medicinal plant: Andrographis paniculata. Phytochemistry Reviews, 11: 39–75.

Sun, H.J., Wu, Z.Y., Nie, X.W. and Bian, J.S., 2020. Role of endothelial dysfunction in cardiovascular diseases: The link between inflammation and hydrogen sulfide. Frontiers in Pharmacology, 10: 1568.

Tee, B.H., Hoe, S.Z., Cheah, S.H. and Lam, S.K., 2016. First report of Eurycoma longifolia Jack root extract causing relaxation of aortic rings in rats. BioMed Research International: 1361508.

Therapeutic Goods Administration, Health Safety Regulation, 2015. Safety Review of Andrographis Paniculata and Anaphylactic/Allergic Reactions. Australian Government Department of Health.

Varma, A., Padh, H. and Shrivastava, N., 2011. Andrographolide: A new plant-derived antineoplastic entity on horizon. Evidence-Based Complementary and Alternative Medicine: 815390.

Vélez, P. and García, Á., 2015. Platelet proteomics in cardiovascular diseases. Translational Proteomics, 7: 15–29.

WHO Geneva, 2002. WHO monographs on selected medicinal plants, 2: 12–24. Geneva: World Health Organization.

Woo, A.Y., Waye, M.M., Tsui, S.K., Yeung, S.T. and Cheng, C.H., 2008. Andrographolide up-regulates cellular-reduced glutathione level and protects cardiomyocytes against hypoxia/reoxygenation injury. Journal of Pharmacology and Experimental Therapeutics, 325: 226–235.

Worakunphanich, W., Thavorncharoensap, M., Youngkong, S., Thadanipon, K. and Thakkinstian, A., 2021. Safety of Andrographis paniculata: A systematic review and meta-analysis. Pharmacoepidemiology and Drug Safety, 30: 727–739.

Worasuttayangkurn, L., Nakareangrit, W., Kwangjai, J., Sritangos, P., Pholphana, N., Watcharasit, P., Rangkadilok, N., Thiantanawat, A. and Satayavivad, J., 2019. Acute oral toxicity evaluation of Andrographis paniculata-standardized first true leaf ethanolic extract. Toxicology Reports, 6: 426–430.

Wu, Q.Q., Ni, J., Zhang, N., Liao, H.H., Tang, Q.Z. and Deng, W., 2017. Andrographolide protects against aortic banding-induced experimental cardiac hypertrophy by inhibiting MAPKs signaling. Frontiers in Pharmacology, 8: 808.

Xie, S., Deng, W., Chen, J., Wu, Q.Q., Li, H., Wang, J., Wei, L., Liu, C., Duan, M., Cai, Z. and Xie, Q., 2020. Andrographolide protects against adverse cardiac remodeling after myocardial infarction through enhancing Nrf2 signaling pathway. International Journal of Biological Sciences, 16: 12–26.

Yoopan, N., Thisoda, P., Rangkadilok, N., Sahasitiwat, S., Pholphana, N., Ruchirawat, S. and Satayavivad, J., 2007. Cardiovascular effects of 14-deoxy-11, 12-didehydroandrographolide and Andrographis paniculata extracts. Planta Medica, 73: 503–511.

Zeng, M., Jiang, W., Tian, Y., Hao, J., Cao, Z., Liu, Z., Fu, C., Zhang, P. and Ma, J., 2017. Andrographolide inhibits arrhythmias and is cardioprotective in rabbits. Oncotarget, 8: 61226–61238.

Zhang, C.Y. and Tan, B.K.H., 1997. Mechanisms of cardiovascular activity of Andrographis paniculata in the anaesthetized rat. Journal of Ethnopharmacology, 56: 97–101.

Zhang, C.Y. and Tan, B.K.H., 1998. Vasorelaxation of rat thoracic aorta caused by 14-deoxyandrographolide. Clinical and Experimental Pharmacology and Physiology, 25: 424–429.

Zhang, J., Zhu, D., Wang, Y. and Ju, Y., 2015. Andrographolide attenuates LPS-induced cardiac malfunctions through inhibition of IκB phosphorylation and apoptosis in mice. Cellular Physiology and Biochemistry, 37: 1619–1628.

Zhao, Y., Wang, M., Li, Y. and Dong, W., 2018. Andrographolide attenuates viral myocarditis through interactions with the IL-10/STAT3 and P13K/AKT/NF-κβ signaling pathways. Experimental and Therapeutic Medicine, 16: 2138–2143.

14 Ka'á Jaguá (*Aloysia polystachya* (Griseb.) Moldenke (Verbenaceae))

From Traditional Use to Pharmacological Investigations in Relation to Cardiovascular Disease

Jane Manfron, Karyne Garcia Tafarelo Moreno, Vanessa Samudio Santos Zanuncio, Denise Brentan Silva and Arquimedes Gasparotto Junior

CONTENTS

14.1 Introduction 215
    14.1.1 Pharmacobotany and Traditional Use 216
    14.1.2 Pharmacological Investigations 219
    14.1.3 Safety Evaluations 220
    14.1.4 Chemical Constituents 220
    14.1.5 Other Foods, Herbs, Spices and Botanicals Used in
        Cardiovascular Health and Disease 224
14.2 Summary Points 227
References 227

LIST OF ABBREVIATIONS

$GABA_A$	γ-Aminobutyric acid type A
GC-MS	Gas chromatography coupled to mass spectrometry
HAM-A	Hamilton Anxiety Rating Scale
IC50	Half maximal inhibitory concentration
LC-MS	Liquid chromatography coupled to mass spectrometry
NCI	National Cancer Institute
SHR	Spontaneous hypertensive rats
TROLOX	6-hydroxy-2,5, 7, 8-tetramethyl-chroman-carboxylic acid
VO	Volatile oil

14.1 INTRODUCTION

The genus *Aloysia* Paláu belongs to the family Verbenaceae and comprises 46 species. The genus occurs in subtropical and temperate South America extending from the southern region of United States and Mexico to Chile and Central Argentina. In South America, it is represented by 28 species

DOI: 10.1201/9781003220329-16

and six varieties (O'Leary et al. 2016; O'Leary and Moroni 2020). Species of *Aloysia* are aromatic, with an intense lemon-like aroma. They are economically and medically significant due to their essential oils with biological activities (Mohammadhosseini et al. 2021).

One of the most important species of the genus is *Aloysia polystachya* (Griseb.) Moldenke (synonym *Lippia polystachya* Griseb.) and it is native to the southern region of Bolivia and northern region of Argentina (O'Leary et al. 2016; Royal Botanic Gardens 2021). It is also commonly cultivated as an ornamental and medicinal plant. *Aloysia polystachya* is commonly known as *ka'á jaguá, burrito, té-burro, poleo-riojano, poleo-de-castilla, aloisia* or *erva-serrana* (mountain grass). The generic name *Aloysia* was in honor of María Luisa de Parma (1751–1819), King Carlos IV's wife from Spain (Alonso and Desmarchelier 2006). The specific epithet *polystachya* means "many-branches", due to the plant having many branches.

14.1.1 Pharmacobotany and Traditional Use

Aloysia polystachya (Figure 14.1) is a shrub and its height is 0.5–1.5 m. The stems have short internodes and are glabrous when mature. The leaves are alternate, narrowly lanceolate-elliptic, 1–5 × 0.3–1 cm, subsessile, entire along margins, acute to obtuse at the apex, and acute to attenuate at

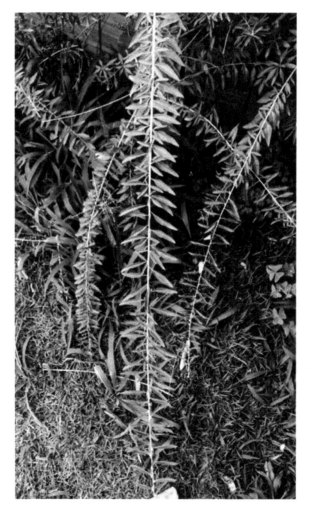

FIGURE 14.1 *Aloysia polystachya* (Griseb.) Moldenke.

Source: Image courtesy of Aline Aparecida Macedo Marques.

Ka'á Jaguá (*Aloysia polystachya* (Griseb.))

the base. The phyllotaxy, the size and shape of the leaves make it easy to differentiate this species from other *Aloysia* species. In comparison, *Aloysia salsoloides* (Griseb.) Lu-Irving & N. O'Leary is the only other species in the genus having alternate leaves, and smaller leaves, less than 0.5 cm. The inflorescences are axillary, solitary or sometimes fasciculate, densely flowered, 0.5–3 cm long. The flowers are small, white; calyx 1–1.5 mm, with two to four unequal triangular teeth; corolla four-lobed, tube about 2 mm long. The fruits are dry schizocarps, obovoid, 1–1.2 mm, glabrous, dividing into two one-seeded mericarps (O'Leary et al. 2016).

Considering microscopic characteristics, the adaxial leaf epidermis in surface view has wavy anticlinal walls, while the abaxial epidermis has sinuous walls. Striate cuticle covers the unilayered epidermis. The leaves are amphistomatic with a few anomocytic stomata (Figure 14.2a). Four types of trichomes are present: 1) non-glandular trichomes, 1–2 celled, conical, thick-walled, verrucose and cystolithic (Figure 14.2b, d), localized on the adaxial side; 2) non-glandular

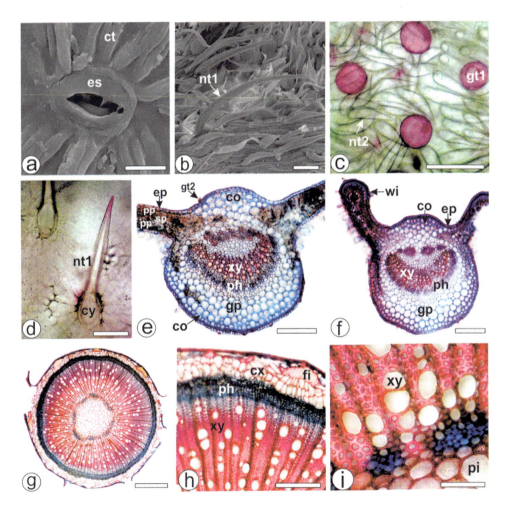

FIGURE 14.2 Microscopy of leaves and stems of *Aloysia polystachya* (Griseb.) Moldenke.

Note: Microscopy of leaves and stems of *Aloysia polystachya* (Griseb.) Moldenke. (a, b) Scanning electron microscopy; (c–i) light microscopy; (c, d) leaf in surface view; (e) midrib, (f) petiole and (g–i) stem in cross-section. (co, collenchyma; ct, cuticle; cx, cortex; cy, cystolith; ep, epidermis; fi, fiber; gp, ground parenchyma; gt1, stalk and big head glandular trichome; gt2, small head glandular trichome; nt1, conical non-glandular trichome; nt2, simple and short non-glandular trichome; ph, phloem; pi, pith; pp, palisade parenchyma; sp, spongy parenchyma; st, stomata; xy, xylem). Scale bar: a = 10 cm; g = 500 μm; f = 300 μm; e = 100 μm; b–d, i = 50 μm; h = 25 μm.

Source: Images courtesy of Lislaine Maria Klider.

trichomes, 1–2 celled, simple, short, thickened, cystolithic (Figure 14.2c, d), occurring numerously on abaxial surface; 3) glandular trichomes with a simple or compound base, 1–2 celled stalk and big and unicellular head (Figure 14.2c), more abundant on abaxial side; 4) glandular trichomes with a simple base, small and unicellular head, found on both epidermises (Michetti et al. 2019; Marques et al. 2021).

In cross-section, the leaf mesophyll is isobilateral. The midrib has a biconvex shape with collateral vascular bundles arranged in an open arc (Figure 14.2e). A parenchymatous sheath surrounds the vascular bundles. The petiole is biconvex in shape and conspicuously winged. The vascular system is represented by a collateral vascular bundle in an open arc (Figure 14.2f). The stem is a circular shape (Figure 14.2g), and the cortical parenchyma has large groups of fibers (Figure 14.2h). Small calcium oxalate crystals are present in the pith. Phenolic compounds are located in the xylem and phloem of midrib, petiole and stem, as well as in the leaf mesophyll (Marques et al. 2021).

The leaves of *A. polystachya* were found to be adulterated to herbal tea mixtures marketed in Argentina (Michetti et al. 2019). The anatomical markers used to identify the species include 1) the conical cystolithic non-glandular trichomes, 2) 1–2 celled, conical, non-glandular trichomes, and 3) glandular trichomes with a unicellular head and a 1–2-celled stalk.

Latin American countries have rich medicinal flora and have a tradition of using medicinal plants to treat various illnesses. Therefore, leaves, inflorescences and stems of *A. polystachya* are widely used in folk medicine in Argentina, Bolivia, Brazil and Paraguay (Gonzáles et al. 2014; Mohammadhosseini et al. 2021). In Central Chaco Argentina, the leaves of *A. polystachya* are used for respiratory and gastrointestinal disorders in the Pilagá traditional medicine (Filipov 1994). In the Northwest of Corrientes of Argentina, *A. polystachya* leaves are used as an antiemetic (Martinez-Crovetto 1981). In San Luis, in the Midwest region of Argentina, this species is used in the popular medicine as digestive and sedative remedies (Del Vitto et al. 1997). The indigenous communities of Quilmes in the northwestern region of Argentina use leaf infusion in traditional medicine to treat stomachache and liver diseases (Scarpa 2002; Ceballos and Perea 2014). It is also used for the same purposes in criollo's folk medicine in the Northwestern Chaco of Argentina (Scarpa 2002). In the Rioplatense wetlands of Buenos Aires, Argentina, the leaves of *A. polystachya* are used in folk medicine as digestive, hepatic and antidermatotic (Hernández et al. 2019).

Leaf infusion is traditionally used in the Grande Dourados region of Mato Grosso do Sul, Brazil, to treat digestive and cardiovascular disorders. In Midwest Brazil, it is frequently used as a traditional drink named *tereré*, which has a minty and refreshing flavor (Coelho et al. 2019). Despite the frequent use of *A. polystachya* in Argentinian folk medicine, this species is not included in the Argentinian Pharmacopoeia. However, it is included in the recently published *Brazilian Pharmacopoeia Herbal Medicines Form*, 2nd edition (ANVISA 2021), in which *A. polystachya* is indicated to treat dyspeptic symptoms, such as cramping and bloating and as a weak anxiolytic.

In the Luque District, Paraguay, *A. polystachya* is known as a tonic for nerves and is used in folk medicine to treat neurological disorders (Hellión-Ibarrola et al. 2006). In this country, *A. polystachya* is part of the herbal mixture containing *yerba mate* (*Ilex paraguariensis* A.St.-Hil.) (Arrúa et al. 2011).

Aloysia polystachya is commonly used as digestive, hepatic, anti-hypertensive, analgesic and sedative (Paredes et al. 2009). Its carminative and dyspeptic activities have been attributed to carvone and limonene, the major compounds present in the essential oil (Mohammadhosseini et al. 2021). Based on an ethnobotanical investigation in Brazil, Coelho et al. (2019) have found that *A. polystachya* leaf infusion has been widely prescribed by local healers for the treatment of various ailments, including digestive and cardiovascular disorders.

Considering the chemical profile and medicinal potential, *A. polystachya* presents significant economic importance. Specific chemotypes of *A. polystachya* have been developed with essential oils containing a high percentage of carvone, a volatile compound with antispasmodic activity (Werdin-Gonzalez et al. 2010), and a low quantity of α-thujone, which exhibits neurotoxicity

(Pina et al. 2012). Burdyn et al. (2006) performed micropropagation of *A. polystachya* plants using adventitious bud regeneration from leaf and internode explants. The authors observed that the essential oil extracts from these plants had carvone as the major compound, while thujone was not detected.

14.1.2 PHARMACOLOGICAL INVESTIGATIONS

Several biological activities have been described for *Aloysia polystachya*. Most studies of these effects are focused on validating ethnopharmacological uses of the species. Table 14.1 summarizes the biological effects of *A. polystachya* preparations.

Hellión-Ibarrola et al. (2006) found an anxiolytic-like effect for the hydro-ethanolic extract of *A. polystachya* due to increasing the duration of sleeping time induced by 30 mg/kg of sodium pentobarbital intraperitoneally. The authors suggest that the anxiolytic activity is probably mediated by another mechanism than the benzodiazepine binding site modulation at the $GABA_A$ receptors. In 2008, the antidepressant-like profile of the same extract and some components of the ethyl-acetate fraction was related to a significant reduction of the immobility time of male mice in the forced swimming test (Hellión-Ibarrola et al. 2008).

A behavioral study evaluated the effects of intraperitoneal administration of the hydro-alcoholic extract from leaves of *A. polystachya* in female Sprague-Dawley rats. All extract doses increased the exploration in the elevated plus-maze open arms similarly to diazepam. In the forced swimming test, the extract was as effective as fluoxetine and imipramine, reducing immobility. Authors suggest that thujone and carvone, among others, may have sedative, anxiolytic and antidepressant-like properties (Mora et al. 2005).

Other activities in the nervous system of a hydro-ethanolic extract of *A. polystachya* were observed in a study with fishes. The anxiolytic activity was tested through the scototaxis (light-dark box) test using caffeine (100 mg/kg) as an anxiogenic. Moreover, the authors used 1% ethanol to induce chronic stress and social isolation. The *A. polystachya* extract was also able to reverse the anxiogenic activity of caffeine in the fishes, without harming their locomotion. Moreover, the treatment caused antidepressant activity similar to fluoxetine, which is probably due to its main compound, acteoside (Melo et al. 2019).

To confirm the data obtained in the pre-clinical studies, a randomized, double-blind, placebo-controlled, phase-2 clinical trial was performed with 54 patients that were adult. The hydro-alcoholic extract of *A. polystachya* was encapsulated, and maltodextrin was used as a placebo. Participants were instructed to take one capsule (300 mg) twice a day, for eight weeks. The anxiety symptoms were assessed by Hamilton Anxiety Rating Scale (HAM-A). Results demonstrated a statistically significant decrease in HAM-A scores after four and eight weeks of treatment, indicating a significant anxiolytic effect for the *A. polystachya* extract (Carmona et al. 2019).

An ethanol-soluble fraction originating from *A. polystachya* infusion was administered in spontaneously hypertensive rats (SHR) (30, 100, and 300 mg/kg) to investigate the cardioprotective effects of the species orally in a 28-day treatment. The results suggest that the prolonged treatment normalized renal, electrocardiographic, and hemodynamic changes induced by hypertension, and modulated the mesenteric and renal arterial reactivity, evidencing a significant cardioprotective effect (Marques et al. 2021).

An *in vitro* study assessed the antioxidant activity of the *A. polystachya* hydro-alcoholic extract using the TROLOX equivalent antioxidant capacity assay. The authors showed that each milliliter of the extract has a total antioxidant activity equivalent to approximately 0.83 mg of TROLOX (Aguado et al. 2013). Another *in vitro* study identified the antitumor activity of hydro-alcoholic extract of the *A. polystachya* in human HCT116 and murine CT26 colorectal cancer cells. The results show that the extract was able to induce apoptosis of colorectal cancer cells and eliminated 5-Fluorouracil resistant cancer cells, inhibiting tumor growth at nontoxic doses (Machado et al. 2020).

Moller et al. (2020) evaluated in the same study the antioxidant and anti-proliferative activities of volatile oil from leaves of *A. polystachya*. Antioxidant tests showed significant antioxidant activity when compared to the controls. Moreover, the VO showed significant anti-proliferative effects against three lineages of cancer cells, with IC50 values of 5.85 ± 0.39, 6.74 ± 0.03 and 9.53 ± 0.45 µg/mL. According to National Cancer Institute (NCI) Plant Screening Program, a medicinal plant extract is considered to have potential if *in vitro* study reports an IC50 value of less than 20 µg/mL.

The antibacterial activity of *A. polystachya* was also evaluated. The VO from *A. polystachya* showed bactericide activity against *Escherichia coli* ATCC 35218, as well as clinical isolates of *Enterobacter cloacae*, *Klebsiella pneumoniae*, *Staphylococcus aureus* ATCC 29212, *S. aureus* ATCC 25923 and *S. aureus* methicillin-susceptible (Pérez et al. 2016). Moreover, the hydro-alcoholic extract also showed bactericidal activity against *Staphylococcus* strains (Aguado et al. 2016).

14.1.3 SAFETY EVALUATIONS

Marques et al. (2021) evaluated the toxicity of an ethanol-soluble fraction obtained from *A. polystachya* leaves and stem. A dosage of 2000 mg/kg was orally given to female Wistar rats in a single dose. The animals were observed periodically over two weeks. No signs of acute toxicity nor lethality were observed. Similarly, Hellión-Ibarrola et al. (2006) using the aerial parts from *A. polystachya* produced a hydro-ethanolic extract by conventional reflux. The doses of 30, 100, 300, 600 and 1000 mg/kg were used intraperitoneally, and the doses of 100, 300, 600, 1000, 2000 and 3000 mg/kg were orally given to Swiss albino male mice. Animals were observed periodically over two weeks. No evidence of toxicity was observed in all tested doses.

14.1.4 CHEMICAL CONSTITUENTS

A. polystachya was chemically studied of extracts obtained of leaves, stems and aerial parts. The chemical data are described in Tables 14.2 and 14.3 and they show the constituents from polar and non-polar (volatile) compounds from *A. polystachya* species showing the parts of the plant used to prepare the extracts, the type of solvents used for the extraction of the compounds, the chemical class of the compounds and the main compounds annotated from gas chromatography coupled to mass spectrometry (GC-MS) and liquid chromatography coupled to mass spectrometry (LC-MS) by electrospray ionization. In addition, the activities of these extracts were also reported together with the chemical compounds identified.

The studies performed by GC-MS were applied from essential oils, which were acquired by hydrodistillation and the main compounds identified included monoterpenes and sesquiterpenes, such as the monoterpenes carvone, limonene and α-thujone (Figure 14.3) that were observed with higher relative percentage as highlighted by Mohammadhosseini et al. (2021).

The chemical studies performed by LC-MS are listed in Table 14.3. The main metabolites identified from *A. polystachya* preparations (leaves and aerial parts) were flavonoids and glycosylated phenylpropanoids, as well as iridoids and nucleosides.

The flavonoids presented in *A. polystachya* include glycosylated and non-glycosylated structures, and they are flavonols, flavones and flavan-3-ols. For example, the flavonols quercetin, kaempferol and isorhamnetin; the flavones apigenin and velutin; and the flavan-3-ols catechin and epigallocatechin (Figure 14.4). The flavonoids and other phenolic components are recognized by antioxidant properties and nitric oxide dependent control for vascular and blood pressure (Actis-Goretta et al. 2006).

In addition, glycosylated phenylpropanoids and other glycosides are commonly found in *A. polystachya* such as acteoside and rosidirin (Figure 14.5), which are constituents also related with potent antioxidant effects and several therapeutic properties (Marques et al. 2021; Carmona et al. 2019). Glycosylated iridoids are generally found in polar extracts of *A. polystachya*, including theveside.

TABLE 14.1

Aloysia polystachya: Biological Activities Reported in Literature

Plant Part/Extraction Method	Effect/Test Subject	Dosage/Concentration	Experimental Resumed Method	Positive Control	Key Findings	Reference
Aerial parts/Hydro-ethanolic extraction by conventional reflux	Anxiolytic/Swiss albino male mice	Single doses: 1.0, 10.0, 100.0 and 1000.0 mg/kg Single doses: 1.0, 10.0, 50.0, 150.0 and 300.0 mg/kg Single doses: 1.0, 10.0 and 100.0 mg/kg	Barbiturate-induced hypnosis: sodium pentobarbital (30.0 mg/kg, i.p.). Barbiturate-induced hypnosis: sub-hypnotic dose of sodium thiopental (35 mg/kg i.p.) Ether-induced hypnosis: ethyl ether (5 mL) saturated glass cage for 10 min	Diazepam (0.5 mg/kg i.p.)	Extract increased the duration of the sleeping time induced by 30.0 mg/kg i.p. of sodium pentobarbital. Significant increase in the percentage of both entries and the time spent in the open arms of the elevated plus maze.	Hellión-Ibarrola et al. 2006
Aerial parts/Hydro-ethanolic extraction by conventional reflux	Antidepressant/Swiss albino male mice	Single doses or 7 days treatment: 1.0, 10.0, 100.0 and 1000.0 mg/kg orally	Forced swim in the glass vessel	Imipramine i.p. (32 mg/kg)	Significant decrease of the immobility time	Hellión-Ibarrola et al. 2008
Aerial parts/Hydro-ethanolic extraction by conventional reflux	Anxiolytic and antidepressant-like/Female Sprague-Dawley rats	Single doses 1.56, 6.25, 12.5, 25 and 50 mg/kg, i.p.	Elevated plus-maze test and forced swimming test	Diazepam (1 mg/kg), fluoxetine (10 mg/kg) and imipramine (12.5 mg/kg)	High doses of the extract caused a significant decrease in total motility, locomotion, rearing and grooming behavior. All doses increased the exploration of the elevated plus-maze test. In the forced swimming test, the extract was as effective as the control drugs.	Mora et al. 2005
Leaves and stems/Infusion treated with 3 volume ethanol	Cardioprotective/SHRs and Wistar-Kyoto female rats	30, 100, 300 mg/kg	28-day treatment followed by diuretic and heart's electrical system assays, hemodynamic parameter, vascular reactivity, biochemical analysis, histopathology and tissue redox status	Hydrochlorothiazide (25 mg/kg)	Treatment normalized renal, electrocardiographic and hemodynamic changes induced by hypertension and modulated the mesenteric and renal arterial reactivity	Marques et al. 2021

(Continued)

TABLE 14.1 (Continued)

Aloysia polystachya: Biological Activities Reported in Literature

Plant Part/Extraction Method	Effect/Test Subject	Dosage/Concentration	Experimental Resumed Method	Positive Control	Key Findings	Reference
Leaves/Hydro-ethanolic extraction by maceration over seven days	Anxiogenic and antidepressant/ Female fishes (*Danio rerio*, AB wild type)	Single dose of 10 mg/kg	Anxiogenic agent: caffeine at 100 mg/kg. Antidepressant agent: 2 μL/ animal of 1% ethanol. Each group was exposed to its respective compound over 60 min. Then, each fish was individually subjected to the tests.	Buspirone (25 mg/ kg) or fluoxetine (20 mg/kg)	Reversed anxiogenic activity of caffeine in the fishes, without impairing their locomotion. Antidepressant activity similar to fluoxetine.	Melo et al. 2019
Leaves/Hydro-alcoholic extraction by leaching for 24 hours	Antioxidant/None	Variable volumes (between 20 and 80 μl) of a dilution of the extract in EtOH 1:10	*In vitro* antioxidant activity quantified by spectrophotometry (DPPH method)	Trolox	Each milliliter of extract would have a total antioxidant activity equivalent to approximately 0.83 mg of Trolox	Aguado et al. 2013
Aerial parts/Hydro-alcoholic extraction by leaching for three weeks	Antitumor/None	233 ng/ml and 462 ng/ml	*In vitro* in human HCT116 and murine CT26 colorectal cancer cells. Extract was administrated alone or in combination with 5-Fluorouracile	5-Fluorouracile (combined effect)	Extract was capable to induce cytotoxicity in all the colorectal cancer cells analyzed, involving apoptosis as its mechanisms; and significantly increased the sensitivity to low concentrations of 5-Fluorouracile	Machado et al. 2020
Leaves/Aqueous extract by boiling dried leaves in distilled water for 20 min. The ethanolic tincture by maceration during eight to ten hours at 20% in 70° ethanol	Antispasmodic/ Sprague-Dawley rats	Concentrations from 0.0195 to 17.5 mmol/L	Dose-response curves to Ach and to $CaCl_2$, and dose relaxation curves of the extracts on rat isolated ileum and duodenum	Ach and $CaCl_2$	Extract relaxed the intestinal smooth muscle and non-competitively inhibited the dose-response curves to Ach. The tincture induced a higher antispasmodic effect than the aqueous extract.	Consolini et al. 2011
Leaves/Hydro-ethanolic extraction over seven days	Anxiolytic/ Humans	One capsule (300 mg) twice a day, for 8 weeks	Randomized, double-blind, placebo-controlled, phase-2 clinical trial	None	Statistically significant decrease in HAM-A scores up to week 4 in the intervention group. only patients receiving *A. polystachya* showed further improvement after week 4.	Carmona et al. 2019

Ka'á Jaguá (*Aloysia polystachya* (Griseb.))

Plant part / Extraction	Activity / Animal model	Concentration / Dose	Methodology	Controls	Results	References
Leaves/Essential oil extracted by hydrodistillation using a Clevenger-type apparatus	Anesthesia/Dusky grouper (*Epinephelus marginatus*)	50, 75, 100, 200, 300 or 400 µL L^{-1}	Fish were exposed to different concentrations of essential oil to evaluate time of induction and recovery from anesthesia	None	Essential oil concentrations above 100 µL L^{-1} were able to induce sedation and anesthesia	Fogliarini et al. 2017
Leaves/Essential oil was extracted from fresh leaves in a knife mill by steam distillation for 4 h	Antioxidant and anti-proliferative/None	0.001, 0.01, 0.1 and 1.0 mg/mL or 0.625–100 µg/mL	Antioxidant Assays: DPPH radical scavenging activity; ferric reducing antioxidant power and total reactive antioxidant potential. Anti-proliferative assay: three different tumor cell lines: human breast (MCF-7), prostate (PC-3) and colorectal (HT-29) adenocarcinoma	Butylated hydroxytoluene and gallic acid (antioxidant) and Daunorubicin and 5-Fluorouracil (anti-proliferative)	Antioxidant tests showed good antioxidant activity compared to commercial antioxidant controls. The oil showed pronounced effects against three cancer cells, with IC50 values of 5.85 ± 0.39, 6.74 ± 0.03 and 9.53 ± 0.45 µg/mL.	Moller et al. 2020
Aerial parts/Semipolar extract was extracted by maceration with EtOAc (99.8%) at room temperature for 48 h	Antichagasic/None	6 concentrations of extract from 100 µg/mL to 0.8 µg/mL for 72 h at 27°C	*In vitro* activity against *Trypanosoma cruzi* and *Trypanosoma brucei brucei* epimastigotes	Benznidazole and nifurtimox	Highly active and selective antitrypanosomal activity and significant inhibitory effects in the *T. cruzi* infection assay	Salm et al. 2021
N.i./Essential oil by steam distillation (hydrodistillation) using a Clevenger-type apparatus with a Dean Stark trap	Antibacterial/None	From 1.82 to 29.13 µL/mL	*In vitro*: agar disc diffusion method and microdilution method according to Clinical and Laboratory Standards Institute	Mueller Hinton Broth + Tween 80 + DMSO	The essential oil was bactericide against *Escherichia coli* ATCC 35218, clinical isolates of *Enterobacter cloacae*, *Klebsiella pneumoniae*, *Staphylococcus aureus* ATCC 29212, *S. aureus* ATCC 25923 and clinical strain of *S. aureus* methicillin susceptible	Pérez et al. 2016
Leaves/Hydro-alcoholic extract prepared by hydro-alcoholic simple percolation	Antioxidant and antibacterial/None	Antioxidant assay: plant extract dilutions (1:10)	Antioxidant assay: DPPH radical method. Antibacterial assay: agar microdilution and broth microdilution methods.	Ascorbic acid and Trolox	Extract showed antioxidant activity and bactericidal activity against *Staphylococcus* strains	Pérez et al. 2016

Note: Ach: Acetylcholine; DMSO: dimethylsulfoxide; DPPH: 2, 2-diphenyl-1-picrylhydrazyl; i.p: intraperitoneally; n.i: not informed; SHR: spontaneously hypertensive rats; TROLOX: 6-hydroxy-2,5, 7, 8-tetramethyl-chroman-carboxylic acid.

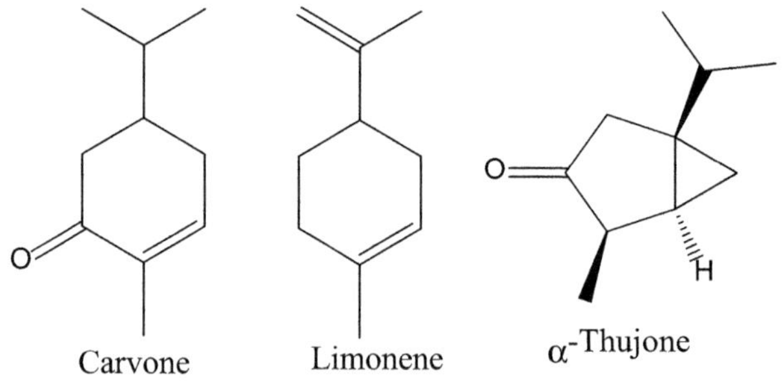

Carvone   Limonene   α-Thujone

FIGURE 14.3   Main monoterpenes identified from *A. polystachya* by GC-MS.

TABLE 14.2

Volatile Compounds Identified from *A. polystachya* Essential Oils by GC-MS and Their Biological Properties

Part	Metabolite Class	Main Compounds Identified (%)	Activity	Reference
Leaves and stems	Monoterpenes	Carvone (78.9%), Limonene (14.2%)	Antibacterial	Pérez et al. 2016
Leaves	Monoterpenes Sesquiterpenes	Carvone (91.0%), Limonene (4.1%), Dihydrocarvone (1.1%)	Antioxidant Anti-proliferative	Moller et al. 2021
Leaves	Monoterpenes	Carvone (83.5%), Limonene (16.5%)	Repellent effects	Werdin Gonzalez et al. 2010
Leaves	monoterpenes	Carvone (83.5%) Limonene (16.5%)	Repellent effects	Benzi et al. 2009
Leaves	Oxygenated monoterpenes	α-thujone, Carvone	-----	Cabanillas et al. 2003
Leaves	Monoterpenes	Carvone (58.8%), α-Limonene (33.7%)	Anesthetic effects	Fogliarini et al. 2017
Leaves	Monoterpenes	α-thujone (69.0%), Carvone (12.0%)	Repellent effects	Gleiser et al. 2011
Leaves	Monoterpenes	Carvone (38.2%), α-thujone (30.3%), Limonene (14.3%)	Antifungal	López et al. 2004
Leaves	Monoterpenes	Carvone (80.4%), Limonene (20.2%)	Antimicrobial	Pina et al. 2012
Leaves	Monoterpenes	Carvone (74–78%), α-thujone (60–74%)	------	Malizia et al. 1997

Note: %: relative percentage in the analyses.

14.1.5 OTHER FOODS, HERBS, SPICES AND BOTANICALS USED IN CARDIOVASCULAR HEALTH AND DISEASE

Brazilian biodiversity is one of the largest on the planet, distributed in six distinct biomes (tropical rainforest "Amazônia", tropical deciduous forest "Mata Atlantica", tropical grassland, and savannah "Cerrado", subtropical prairies or grasslands "Pampa", tropical scrub forest "Caatinga" and flooded grassland "Pantanal"). Thus, it is very common, in all regions of Brazil, to use several

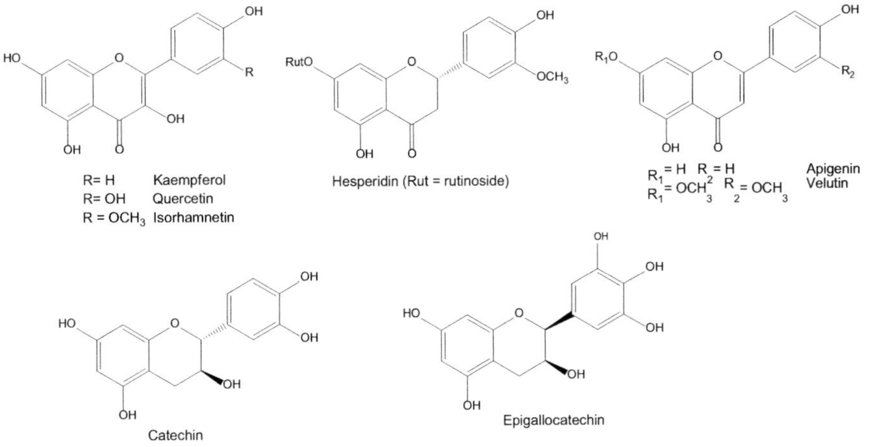

FIGURE 14.4 Flavonoids described from *A. polystachya* extracts.

TABLE 14.3
Compounds Annotated from *A. polystachya* by LC-MS or Isolated

Part	Extract	Metabolite Class	Compounds	Activity of Extract	Reference
Leaves	Ethanol-soluble fraction	Organic acids, nucleoside, methoxylated flavones, glycosylated phenolic acids, phenylpropanoids and iridoids	Epigallocatechin, O-hexosyl iridoid (theveside), Tuberonic acid hexoside or hydroxyjasmonic acid hexosideo, Rosiridol O-hexoside (rosiridin)	Cardioprotective effects	Marques et al. 2021
Leaves	Hydro-ethanolic	Glycosylated phenylpropanoid	Acteoside	Anxiolytic and antidepressant	Costa de Melo et al. 2019
Aerial parts	Hydro-ethanolic	Flavonoids	Kaemferol, Catechin, Quercetin	Anticancer	Soares Machado et al. 2020
Leaves	Hydro-ethanolic	Glycosylated phenylpropanoid	Acteoside	Anxiolytic	Carmona et al. 2019
Leaves	Methanolic extracts	Glycosylated phenylpropanoids	Forsytho-side A, plantainoside C, purpureaside D, martynoside	-----	Marchetti et al. 2019
Leaves	Ethyl acetate fractions	Flavonoids	Luteolin-O-glycoside, diosmetin diglycoside, chrysoeriol diglycoside, isorhamnetin-O-glycoside, isorhamnetin, apigenin, chrysoeriol/diosmetin, velutin	Antioxidant Antibacterial	Aguado et al. 2016
Leaves	Aqueous extracts	Monoterpenes, flavonoids	Quercetin, Hesperidin	Antispasmodic	Consolini et al. 2011

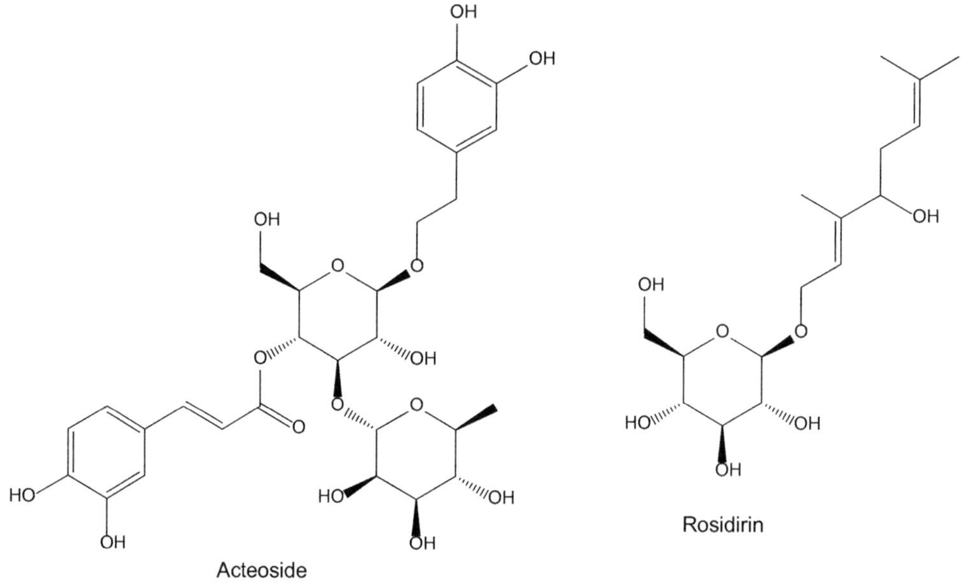

FIGURE 14.5 Glycosides described from *A. polystachya* extracts.

medicinal species to prepare traditional medicines employed in treating cardiovascular ailments. The parts of the plants used, and the ways of preparation are very varied and include decoction, infusion, juice, maceration, plaster, seat bath and tincture (Menetrier et al. 2020). Among these species, but not limited to, is *Rosmarinus officinalis* L., known as "alecrim". In Brazil, it is widely used as a cardiotonic, anti-hypertensive and lipid-lowering agent. Other species used as cardiotonic, or antiarrhythmic drugs are *Cecropia pachystachya* Trécul. ("embaúba"), *Viola odorata* L. ("voleta"), and *Vitex megapotamica* (Spreng.) Moldenke ("tarumã"). The lemon or "limão" (*Citrus limon* [L.] Osbeck), *Cuphea carthagenensis* (Jacq.) J.F. Macbr. ("sete-sangrias") and *Salvia officinalis* L., ("salvia") are used as anti-hypertensive and lipid-lowering drugs. The *Sechium edule* [Jacq.] Sw, ("chuchu"), *Lippia alba* [Mill.] N.E. Brown, ("cidreira"), *Chorisia glaziovii* (O. Kuntze) E. Santos ("barriguda-de-espinho" or "barriguda"), *Heliotropium indicum* L. ("crista-de-galo" or "fedegoso"), *Erythroxylum revolutum* Mart. ("araçá-brabo") and *Allamanda blanchetii* A.DC. ("sete-patacas-roxas" or "jasminho") are used as anti-hypertensive agents (Menetrier et al. 2020; de Albuquerque et al. 2007).

In the northeast region of Brazil, especially in the "Caatinga" biome, the *Equisetum hyemale* L. ("cavalinha"), *Aquarius grandiflorus* (Cham. & Schltdl.) Christenh. & Byng (syn. *Echinodorus grandiflorus* (Cham. & Schltdl.) Micheli ("chapéu-de-couro"), *Cynara cardunculus* subsp. *cardunculus* (syn. *Cynara scolymus* L. Baill.) ("alcachofra"), *Microgramma squamulosa* (Kaulf.) de la Sota ("cipó-cabeludo") and *Zingiber officinale* Roscoe ("gengibre") are used as diuretics (Menetrier et al. 2020; de Albuquerque et al. 2007). *Passiflora edulis* Sims. ("maracujá"), *Mentha* × *piperita* L. ("hortelã-da-folha-miúda"), *Annona montana* Macfad. (syn. *Anonna muricata* Vell.) ("graviola"), *Cymbopogon citratus* (DC.) Stapf ("capim-santo"), *Dysphania ambrosioides* (L.) Mosyakin & Clemants ("mentruz"), *Mandevilla tenuifolia* (J.C. Mikan) Woodson ("flor-de-santo-antonio"), *Tocoyena formosa* (Cham. & Schltdl.) K. Schum. ("genipapo") and *Baccharis trimera* (Less.) DC. ("carqueja") stands out (Cerqueira et al. 2020; da Costa Ferreira et al. 2021; de Albuquerque et al. 2007).

In the "Cerrado" biome of the state of Mato Grosso do Sul, local healers use, among others, *Monteverdia ilicifolia* (Mart. ex Reissek) Biral (syn. *Maytenus ilicifolia* Mart. ex Reissek ("espinheira-santa"), *Pelargonium graveolens* L'Hér. ("gerânio" or "malva-rosa"), *Verbena officinalis* L. ("gervão"), *Aloysia polystachya* ("burrito"), *Curcuma zerdoaria* (Christm.) Roscoe ("açafrão"),

Ka'á Jaguá (*Aloysia polystachya* (Griseb.))

Artemisia absinthium L. ("losna"), *Punica granatum* L. ("romã") and *Hibiscus sabdariffa* L. ("hibisco") (Coelho et al. 2019). In the "Amazon" biome it is common to use *Dipteryx odorata* (Aubl.) Forsyth f. ("cumaru"), *Paullinia cupana* Kunth ("guaraná"), *Lindernia diffusa* (L.) Wettst. ("caaataya", "mata-canna", "purga-de-joão-paez" or "orelha-de-rato"), *Phyllanthus brasiliensis* (Aubl.) Poir. ("conabi") and *Ertela trifolia* (L.) Kuntze ("alecrim-de-cobra") (Breitbach et al. 2013).

14.2 SUMMARY POINTS

- This chapter focuses on *Aloysia polystachya*.
- *A. polystachya* is native from the southern region of Bolivia up to the northern region of Argentina.
- *A. polystachya* is commonly known as *ka'á jaguá*, *burrito*, *té-burro*, *poleo-riojano*, *poleo-de-castilla*, *aloisia* or *erva-serrana* (mountain grass).
- *A. polystachya* is a shrub, the stems have short internodes and are glabrous when mature; leaves are alternate, narrowly lanceolate-elliptic, subsessile, entire along margins, acute to obtuse at apex and acute to attenuate at base.
- *A. polystachya* is used in folk medicine to treat respiratory, cardiovascular and gastrointestinal disorders, as digestive and sedative remedies.
- Previous studies demonstrated anxiolytic, antidepressant-like and cardioprotective effects, antitumor, anti-proliferative, antioxidant and antibacterial activities.
- No evidence of *A. polystachya* acute toxicity was observed in previous studies.
- Chemical compounds reported from *A. polystachya* essential oils are mainly monoterpenes, including limonene, carvone and α-thujone.
- The main constituents from *A. polystachya* polar extracts are flavonoids, iridoids and glycosylated phenylpropanoids.

REFERENCES

Actis-Goretta, L., Ottaviani, J. I., Fraga, C. G. 2006. Inhibition of angiotensin converting enzyme activity by flavanol-rich foods. *Journal of Agricultural and Food Chemistry* 54, 229–234.

Aguado, M. I., Dudik, N. H., Zamora, C. M. P., Torres, C. A., Nunez, M. B. 2016. Antioxidant and antibacterial activities of hydroalcoholic extracts from *Aloysia polystachy*a griseb moldenke and *Lippia turbinata* griseb (verbenaceae). *International Journal of Pharmacy and Pharmaceutical Sciences*, 393–395.

Aguado, M. I., Nuñez, M. B., Bela, A. J., Okulik, N. B., Bregni, C. 2013. Caracterización fisicoquímica y actividad antioxidante de un extracto etanólico de *Aloysia polystachya* (Griseb.) Mold. (Verbenaceae). *Revista mexicana de ciencias farmacéuticas* 44, 46–51.

Albuquerque, U. P. de, Medeiros, P. M. de, Almeida, A. L. S. de, Monteiro, J. M., Neto, E. M. de F. L., Melo, J. G. de, Santos, J. P. dos. 2007. Medicinal plants of the Caatinga (Semi-Arid) vegetation of NE Brazil: A quantitative approach. *Journal of Ethnopharmacology* 114 (3), 325–354. https://doi.org/10.1016/j.jep.2007.08.017.

Alonso, J., Desmarchelier, C. 2006. *Plantas medicinales autóctonas de la Argentina*. 2nd ed. Argentina: Ediciones Fitociencia. pp. 88, 89, 91.

ANVISA. 2021. *Agência Nacional de Vigilância Sanitária. Formulário de Fitoterápicos: Farmacopeia Brasileira*. 2nd ed. Brasília.

Arrúa, R. D. de, González, Y., de García, M. G. 2011. Análisis de la yerba mate elaborada completa, comercializadas em Asunción y Gran Asunción, Paraguay. *Rojasiana* 10, 81–91.

Benzi, V. S., Murray, A. P., Ferrero, A. A. 2009. Insecticidal and insect-repellent activities of essential oils from Verbenaceae and Anacardiaceae against *Rhizopertha dominica*. *Natural Product Communications* 4(9), 1934578X0900400926.

Breitbach, U. B., Niehues, M., Lopes, N. P., Faria, J. E. Q., Brandão, M. G. L. 2013. Amazonian Brazilian medicinal plants described by C.F.P. von Martius in the 19th century. *Journal of Ethnopharmacology* 147 (1), 180–189. https://doi.org/10.1016/j.jep.2013.02.030.

Burdyn, L., Luna, C., Tarraco, J., Sansberro, P., Dudit, N., Conzalez, A., Mrocinski, L. 2006. Direct shoot regeneration from leaf and internode explants of *Aloysia polystachya* [Gris.] Mold. (Verbenaceae). *In Vitro Cellular and Developmental Biology-Plant* 42, 235–239.

Cabanillas, C. M., Lopez, M. L., Daniele, G., Zygadlo, J. A. 2003. Essential oil composition of *Aloysia polystachya* (Griseb.) Moldenke under rust disease. *Flavour and Fragrance Journal* 18(5), 446–448.

Campos-Navarro, R., Scarpa, G. F. 2013. The cultural-bound disease "empacho" in Argentina: A comprehensive botanico-historical and ethnopharmacological review. *Journal of Ethnopharmacology* 148, 349–360. https://doi.org/10.1016/j.jep.2013.05.002

Carmona, F., Coneglian, F. S., Batista, P. A., Aragon, D. C., Angelucci, M. A., Martinez, E. Z., Pereira, A. M. S. 2019. *Aloysia polystachya* (Griseb.) Moldenke (Verbenaceae) powdered leaves are effective in treating anxiety symptoms: A phase-2, randomized, placebo-controlled clinical trial. *Journal of Ethnopharmacology* 242, 112060. https://doi.org/10.1016/j.jep.2019.112060

Ceballos, S. J., Perea, M. C. 2014. Plantas medicinales utilizadas por la comunidad indígena de Quilmes (Tucumán, Argentina). *Boletín Latinoamericano y del Caribe de Plantas Medicinales y Aromáticas* 13, 47–68.

Cerqueira, T. M. G., Correia, A. C. de C., Santos, R. V. dos, Lemos, R. P. L., Silva, A. A. S. da, Barreto, E. 2020. The use of medicinal plants in Maceió, Northeastern Brazil: An ethnobotanical survey. *Medicines* 7 (2): 7. https://doi.org/10.3390/medicines7020007.

Coelho, F. C., Tirloni, C. A. S., Marques, A. A. M., Gasparotto, F. M., Lívero, F. A. D. R., Gasparotto Junior, A. 2019. Traditional plants used by remaining healers from the region of Grande Dourados, Mato Grosso do Sul, Brazil. *Journal of Religion and Health* 58, 572–88. https://doi.org/10.1007/s10943-018-0713-0

Consolini, A. E. Berardi, A., Rosella, M. A., Volonté, M. 2011. Antispasmodic effects of *Aloysia polystachya* and *A. gratissima* tinctures and extracts are due to non-competitive inhibition of intestinal contractility induced by acethylcholine and calcium. *Revista brasileira de farmacognosia* 21, 889–900. https://doi.org/10.1590/S0102-695X2011005000137

Costa, F. E. da, Anselmo, M. da G. V., Guerra, N. M., Lucena, C. M. de, Felix, C. do M. P., Bussmann, R. W., Paniagua-Zambrana, N. Y., Lucena, R. F. P. de. 2021. Local knowledge and se of medicinal plants in a rural community in the Agreste of Paraíba, Northeast Brazil. *Evidence-Based Complementary and Alternative Medicine: eCAM*, 9944357. https://doi.org/10.1155/2021/9944357.

Costa de Melo, N., Sánchez-Ortiz, B. L., dos Santos Sampaio, T. I., Matias Pereira, A. C., Pinheiro da Silva Neto, F. L., Ribeiro da Silva, H., Tavares Carvalho, J. C. 2019. Anxiolytic and antidepressant effects of the hydroethanolic extract from the leaves of *Aloysia polystachya* (Griseb.) Moldenke: A study on zebrafish (Danio rerio). *Pharmaceuticals* 12(3), 106.

Del Vitto, L. A., Petenatti, E. M., Petenatti, M. E. 1997. Recursos Herbolarios de San Luis (República Argentina). Primera parte: Plantas Nativas. *Multequina* 6, 49–66.

Filipov, A. 1994. Medicinal plants of the Pilaga of Central Chaco. *Journal of Ethnopharmacology* 44, 181–193.

Fogliarini, C. O., Garlet, Q. I., Parodi, T. V., Becker, A. G., Garcia, L. O., Heinzmann, B. M., Pereira, A. M. S., Baldisserotto, B. 2017. Anesthesia of *Epinephelus marginatus* with essential oil of *Aloysia polystachya*: An approach on blood parameters. *Anais da Academia Brasileira de Ciências* 89, 445–456. https://doi.org/10.1590/0001-3765201720160457

Gleiser, R. M., Bonino, M. A., Zygadlo, J. A. 2011. Repellence of essential oils of aromatic plants growing in Argentina against Aedes aegypti (Diptera: Culicidae). *Parasitology Research* 108(1), 69–78.

González, Y., de Arrúa, R. D., de Rojas, G. D., de García, M. G. 2014. Etnofarmacobotánica foliar de "Burrito", *Aloysia polystachya* (Griseb) Moldenke (Verbenaceae), cultivado en Paraguay. *Rojasiana* 13, 31–41.

Hellión-Ibarrola, M. C., Ibarrola, D. A., Montalbetti, Y., Kennedy, M. L., Heinichen, O., Campuzano, M., Ferro, E. A., Alvarenga, N., Tortoriello, J., De Lima, T. C. M., Mora, S. 2008. The antidepressant-like effects of *Aloysia polystachya* (Griseb.) Moldenke (Verbenaceae) in mice. *Phytomedicine* 15, 478–483. https://doi.org/10.1016/j.phymed.2007.11.018

Hellión-Ibarrola, M. C., Ibarrola, D. A., Montalbetti, Y., Kennedy, M. L., Heinichen, O., Campuzano, M., Tortoriello, J., Fernández, S., Wasowski, C., Marder, M., De Lima, T. C. M., Mora, S. 2006. The anxiolytic-like effects of *Aloysia polystachya* (Griseb.) Moldenke (Verbenaceae) in mice. *Journal of Ethnopharmacology* 105, 400–408. https://doi.org/10.1016/j.jep.2005.11.013

Hernández, M. P., Calonge, F. S., Fernández, V. R., Sona, M. F., Hernández, M. V. 2019. Plantas usadas en medicina popular en el sector sur de los humedales rioplatenses de la Provincia de Buenos Aires, Argentina. *Revista da Faculdade de Agronomia* 118, 61–75.

López, A. G., Theumer, M. G., Zygadlo, J. A., Rubinstein, H. R. 2004. Aromatic plants essential oils activity on *Fusarium verticillioides* Fumonisin B 1 production in corn grain. *Mycopathologia*, 158(3), 343–349.

Machado, M. S., Palma, A., Panelo, L. C., Paz, L. A., Rosa, F., Lira, M. C., Azurmendi, P., Rubio, M. F., Lenz, G., Urtreger, A. J., Costas, M. A. 2020. Extract from *Aloysia polystachya* induces the cell death of colorectal cancer stem cells. *Nutrition and Cancer* 72, 1004–1017. https://doi.org/10.1080/01635581.2019.1669676

Malizia, R. A., Molli, J. S., Cardell, D. A., Grau, R. J. A., Zumelzu, G. 1997. Selection of material for cultivation in *Aloysia polystachya* (Gris.) Mold. *II WOCMAP Congress Medicinal and Aromatic Plants, Part 3: Agricultural Production, Post Harvest Techniques, Biotechnology* 502, 219–222.

Marchetti, L., Pellati, F., Graziosi, R., Brighenti, V., Pinetti, D., Bertelli, D. 2019. Identification and determination of bioactive phenylpropanoid glycosides of *Aloysia polystachya* (Griseb. et Moldenke) by HPLC-MS. *Journal of Pharmaceutical and Biomedical Analysis*, 166, 364–370.

Marques, A. A. M., Lorençone, B. R., Romão, P. V. M., Guarnier, L. P., Palozi, R. A. C., Moreno, K. G. T., Tirloni, C. A. S., dos Santos, A. C., Souza, R. I. C., Klider, L. M., Louurenço, E. L. B., Tolouei, S. E. L., Budel, J. M., Khan, S. I., Silva, D. B., Gasparotto Junior, A. 2021. Ethnopharmacological investigation of the cardiovascular effects of the ethanol-soluble fraction of *Aloysia polystachya* (Griseb.) Moldenke leaves in spontaneously hypertensive rats. *Journal of Ethnopharmacology* 274, 114077. https://doi.org/10.1016/j.jep.2021.114077

Martinez-Crovetto, R. 1981. *Plantas utilizadas en medicina en el Noroeste de Corrientes (República Argentina)*. Tucuman: Fundacion Miguel Lillo Miscelanea 69.

Melo, N. C. de, Sánchez-Ortiz, B. L., Sampaio, T. I., dos, S., Pereira, A. C. M., Neto, F. L. P., da, S., Silva, H. R. da, Cruz, R. A. S., Keita, H., Pereira, A. M. S., Tavares Carvalho, J. C. 2019. Anxiolytic and antidepressant effects of the hydroethanolic extract from the leaves of *Aloysia polystachya* (Griseb.) Moldenke: A study on Zebrafish (*Danio rerio*). *Pharmaceuticals (Basel)* 12, 106. https://doi.org/10.3390/ph12030106

Michetti, K. M., Cuadra, V. P., Cambi, V. N. 2019. Botanical quality control of digestive tisanes commercialized in an urban area (Bahía Blanca, Argentina). *Revista Brasileira de Farmacognosia* 29, 137–146. https://doi.org/10.1016/j.bjp.2019.01.002

Mohammadhosseini, M., Frezza, C., Venditti, A., Mahdavi, B. 2021: An overview of the genus *Aloysia* Paláu (Verbenaceae): Essential oil composition, ethnobotany and biological activities. *Natural Product Research*. DOI: 10.1080/14786419.2021.1907576

Moller, A. C., Parra, C., Said, B., Werner, E., Flores, S., Villena, J., Russo, A., Caro, N., Montenegro, I., Madrid, A. 2020. Antioxidant and anti-proliferative activity of essential oil and main components from leaves of *Aloysia polystachya* harvested in Central Chile. *Molecules* 26, 131. https://doi.org/10.3390/molecules26010131

Mora, S., Díaz-Véliz, G., Millán, R., Lungenstrass, H., Quirós, S., Coto-Morales, T., Hellión-Ibarrola, M. C. 2005. Anxiolytic and antidepressant-like effects of the hydroalcoholic extract from *Aloysia polystachya* in rats. *Pharmacology Biochemistry and Behavior* 82, 373–378. https://doi.org/10.1016/j.pbb.2005.09.007

O'Leary, N., Lu-irving, P., Moroni, P., Siedo, S. 2016. Taxonomic revision of *Aloysia* (Verbenaceae, Lantaneae) in South America. *Annals of the Missouri Botanical Garden* 101, 568–609.

O'Leary, N., Moroni, P. 2020. *Aloysia in* Flora do Brasil 2020. Jardim Botânico do Rio de Janeiro. Disponível em: <http://floradobrasil.jbrj.gov.br/reflora/floradobrasil/FB15122>. Acesso em: 24 nov. 2021.

Paredes, A., Benítez, A., Santacruz, P. 2009. *Guía para el cultivo y producción de diez plantas medicinales. Fundación Moisés Bertoni Fundación para la Conservación de la Naturaleza*. Assunción: Grafitec S.A.

Pérez, M. C., Torres, C., Aguado, M. I., Bela, A., Nuñez, M., Bregni, C. 2016. Antibacterial activity of essential oils of *Aloysia polystachya* and *Lippia turbinata* (Verbenaceae). *Latin American and Caribbean Bulletin of Medicinal and Aromatic Plants* 15, 199–215.

Pina, E. S., Coppede, J. da S., Sartoratto, A., Fachin, A. L., Bertoni, B. W., Franccedil, S. de C., Pereira, A. M. S. 2012. Antimicrobial activity and chemical composition of essential oils from *Aloysia polystachya* (Griseb.) Moldenke grown in Brazil. *Journal of Medicinal Plants Research* 6, 5412–5416.

Royal Botanic Gardens, Kew. 2021. Royal Botanic Gardens, Kew – Herbarium Specimens. Occurrence dataset https://doi.org/10.15468/ly60bx accessed via GBIF.org on 2021-11-29.

Salm, A., Krishnan, S. R., Collu, M., Danton, O., Hamburger, M., Leonti, M., Almanza, G., Gertsch, J. 2021. Phylobioactive hotspots in plant resources used to treat Chagas disease. *iScience* 24, 102310. https://doi.org/10.1016/j.isci.2021.102310

Scarpa, G. F. 2002. Plantas empleadas contra trastornos digestivos en la medicina tradicional criolla del Chaco Noroccidental. *Dominguezia* 18, 36–50.

Soares Machado, M., Palma, A., Panelo, L. C., Paz, L. A., Rosa, F., Lira, M. C., Costas, M. A. 2020. Extract from *Aloysia polystachya* induces the cell death of colorectal cancer stem cells. *Nutrition and Cancer* 72(6), 1004–1017.

Werdin-Gonzalez, J. O., Gutierrez, M. M., Murray, A. P., Ferrero, A. A. 2010. Biological activity of essential oils from *Aloysia polystachya* and *Aloysia citriodora* (Verbenaceae) against the soybean pest *Nezara viridula* (Hemiptera: Pentatomidae). *Natural Product Communications* 5, 301–306.

15 *Bridelia ferruginea* and Myocardial Protection in Mitochondrial Membrane Permeability

Oluwatoyin O. Ojo

CONTENTS

15.1 Introduction 232
15.2 Background 232
15.3 Isolated Metabolites of the Leaves, Roots, and Bark of *Bridelia ferruginea* and
 Their Importance in Diseases 236
15.4 The Importance of Some of the Active Components of *Bridelia ferruginea* in
 Cardiovascular Health 236
    15.4.1 Squalene 236
    15.4.2 Flavonoids 236
    15.4.3 Quercetin 236
    15.4.4 Vitamin E 237
15.5 Pharmacological Relevance of Other African Plants or Herbs
 in Cardiovascular Health 237
15.6 Cardiovascular Diseases 237
15.7 Global Epidemiology on Cardiovascular Disease 237
15.8 Pathophysiology of Myocardial Infarction 237
15.9 Myocardial Infarction in the Heart Mitochondria 238
15.10 The Mitochondrion Is the Determiner of Cell Survival and Death
 in Myocardial Infarction 239
15.11 The Mitochondrial Permeability Transition Pore in Myocardial Infarction 240
15.12 Cross-Talk between the Liver and Heart during Myocardial Infarction 240
15.13 Myocardial Protection by *Bridelia ferruginea* 240
15.14 Safety Concerns in the Use of *Bridelia ferruginea* 241
15.15 Future Perspectives for *Bridelia ferruginea* 241
15.16 Other Foods, Herbs, Spices Used in Cardiovascular Diseases in Africa 241
    15.16.1 *Artemisia herba-alba* 241
    15.16.2 *Aloe forex mill* 242
    15.16.3 *Aspalathus linearis* 242
    15.16.4 *Mondei white* 242
15.17 Toxicity and Cautionary Notes 242
15.18 Summary Points 242
References 243

DOI: 10.1201/9781003220329-17

LIST OF ABBREVIATIONS

ATP	Adenosine triphosphatase
BF	*Bridelia ferruginea*
CHD	Coronary heart disease
CVD	Cardiovascular diseases
IHD	Ischemic heart disease
LDL	Low-density lipoprotein
MI	Myocardial infarction
mPT	Mitochondrial permeability transition
ROS	Reactive oxygen species
SIRT	5 Sirtuin 5

15.1 INTRODUCTION

Traditional medicine is as old as human history and uses herbs as a form of medication to treat sicknesses or ailments. Herbs are any part of a plant or derived products of a plant used as a basis for drug formulations in traditional medicine (Shaito et al., 2020). Despite advances in cardiovascular disease (CVD) management and treatment, it has been shown to claim more lives than the combination of all cancer forms (Mozaffarian et al., 2015). Therefore, options for herbal remedies are warranted over expensive and unavailable synthetic drugs. There is a regained interest in herbs and medicinal plants because there must be treatment and management of diseases amid scarce socioeconomic resources. It has been shown that the biological activity and diversity of these natural products are unparalleled by any synthetic drug screening library. Notwithstanding, there is concern about the safety of herb-drug interactions of plant-derived products (Shaito et al., 2020). The use of traditional plants nonetheless continues to increase across the globe due to the awareness of their potential in the treatment of ailments or sicknesses (Ekor, 2014).

15.2 BACKGROUND

Bridelia ferruginea Benth (BF) is from the family Euphorbiaceae and was first described in 1806 as a genus. It has about 70 species, out of which BF has the highest medicinal properties (Alowanou et al., 2015; Mahomoodally et al., 2021). The plant is about 8 m tall but can grow up to 15 meters and can sometimes have spiny branches; it is predominant in the Savannah regions of West Africa, especially Nigeria, Benin Republic, Burkina Faso, and Ivory Coast (Figure 15.1).

The plant can also be found in India, Australia, the Pacific Ocean, and Southern Asia (Afolayan et al., 2018). The plant was named after the Swiss-German bryologist, Samuel Elisée Bridel-Brideri, with the leaves, stem, bark, and roots documented to be useful for medicinal purposes (Alowanou et al., 2015). Decoction from all parts of the plant is used in folklore medicine for the treatment of diabetes, arthritis (Olajide et al., 2012), as a purgative, vermifuge (Mbah et al., 2012), antipyretic, and analgesic (Akuodor et al., 2011), among others (Figure 15.2).

The crude extracts of the plant have also shown anti-proliferative, antibacterial, antimicrobial, and antioxidant activities (Akinsete et al., 2017; Mahomoodally et al., 2021). Active chemical components isolated from the leaves have been shown in Table 15.1 to contain rutin and quercetin, the bark has flavonoids (e.g. quercetin, quercitrin, ferrugin, myricetin-3-O-[beta]-glucoside, biflavonol (gallocatechin-4[4-O-7] epigallocatechin)), and the root has lignans.

These are significant in exerting biological and chemical effects when consumed (Alowanou et al., 2015; Mbah et al., 2012, Olajide et al., 2012). Recently, the extracts from the leaves of BF have been shown to be effective in inhibiting the complications arising from leishmanial pathogens, myocardial infarction, diabetes nephropathy among others (Afolayan et al., 2018; Ojo et al., 2019; Omoboyowa et al., 2020). Squalene, vitamin E, and alpha amyrin were found in the hexane fraction

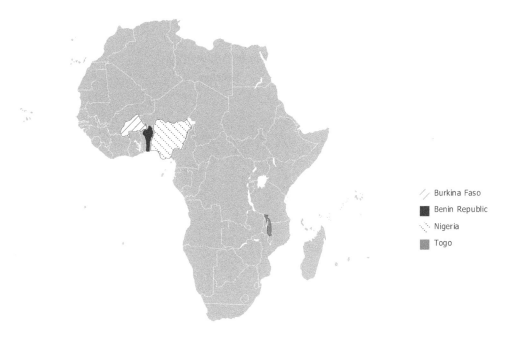

FIGURE 15.1 *Bridelia ferruginea* in the Savannah regions of West Africa.

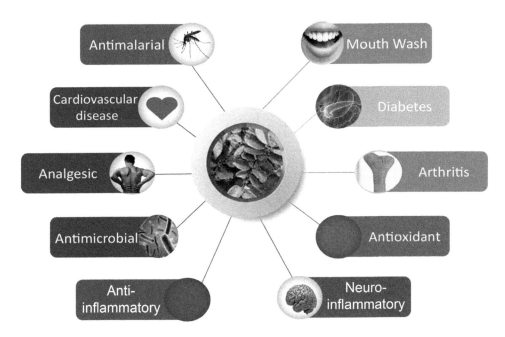

FIGURE 15.2 The important uses of *Bridelia ferruginea*.

of BF. These showed anti-trypanosoma activity against *Trypanasoma brucei* (Afolayan et al., 2020). More analytical work on the leaves of BF has shown the presence of tetradecanoic and hexadecanoic acids, which are critical antioxidant agents. Omega-3 fatty acid has also been identified in the leaves of the plant, and this is an important agent in the treatment of diabetes, arthritis, and cardiovascular complications, among others (Murthy et al., 2021).

TABLE 15.1
Certain Active Components Found in *Bridelia ferruginea*

S/N	Name of Active Component	Structure	Part of the Plant Found
1	2-O-β-D-glucosyl glycerol		Leaves
2	Corilagin		Leaves
3	Lutein		Leaves
4	Myricetin		Leaves
	Quercetin		Leaves
6	Rutin		Leaves
	Hydroxymethoxy rhamnosyl		Leaves
8	A-amyrin		Leaves

Bridelia ferruginea and Myocardial Protection

TABLE 15.1 *(Continued)*
Certain Active Components Found in *Bridelia ferruginea*

S/N	Name of Active Component	Structure	Part of the Plant Found
9	(+) gamma tocopherol		Leaves
10	Stigmastan 3,5-diene		Leaves
11	4, 8, 12, 16 tetramethylheptadecan-4-olide		Leaves
12	Squalene		Leaves
13	Apigenin		Leaves
14	Aloin (C-Glycoside)		Leaves
15	Rhein-8-Glycoside (O-Glycoside)		Leaves

15.3 ISOLATED METABOLITES OF THE LEAVES, ROOTS, AND BARK OF *BRIDELIA FERRUGINEA* AND THEIR IMPORTANCE IN DISEASES

Certain metabolites isolated from BF leaves have shown good antioxidant potentials. However, the procedure of extraction and the part of the plant used greatly influence this. The leaves obtained from the plant showed a higher content of flavonoid when extracted with methanol than with water or ethylacetate (Mahoomodally et al., 2021). Furthermore, the water and methanol extracts of the stem bark showed higher phenolic content than the ethylacetate extracts. The phenols and flavonoids have both shown good antioxidant characteristics in plants due to their redox potentials, chain breaking and free radical scavenging attributes (Mahomoodally et al., 2021). Using Nuclear Magnetic Resonance, Mass Spectroscopy and Gas Chromatography-Mass Spectroscopy analysis, Afolayan et al. (2018) showed that the methanolic extracts of BF leaves had 2-O-β-D-glycosylglycerol, stearic acid, 6-β-hydroxy-(2OR)-24-ethylcholest-4-en-3-one, corilagin, lutein, myricetin, isomyricetin, isoquercetin, myricitrin, quercitrin, and rutin among others (Afolayan et al., 2018). The crude methanol fraction was also shown to contain squalene, α-amyrin, stigmastan-3,5-diene, 8-formyl-6,7-bis[2-(methoxylcarbonyl)ethyl]-1,3,5-trimethyl-2,4-divinylporphyrin, vitamin E, (+) gamma tocopherol 4,8,12,16-tetramethylheptadecan-4-olide (Afolayan et al., 2018).

15.4 THE IMPORTANCE OF SOME OF THE ACTIVE COMPONENTS OF *BRIDELIA FERRUGINEA* IN CARDIOVASCULAR HEALTH

15.4.1 SQUALENE

This is one of the intermediates in phytosterol or cholesterol synthesis in plants and animals. Squalene decreases low-density lipoprotein (LDL) cholesterol levels, a factor in cardiovascular disease. In conditions of high cholesterol risk in the body, statins have been used as drugs to inhibit 3-hydroxy-3-methyl-glutaryl CoA synthase, a regulatory enzyme in cholesterol biosynthesis. The use of statin has shown serious complications in kidney and liver function. Studies by Strandberg et al. (1989) have shown the similarities between the action mechanism of statin and squalene, making it a natural substitute for synthetic statin. The presence of six double bonds in it has enabled it to act as a good antioxidant, therefore enhancing metabolic function. Squalene also improves immunity and acts as an anticancer, antisenescene, emollient, and moisturizer.

15.4.2 FLAVONOIDS

All parts of BF have been shown to consist of flavonoids, a good antioxidant that reduces the oxidation of LDL. Flavonoids have further shown relevance in the cardiovascular system by decreasing apoptotic processes in the endothelium and improving vasodilation. These flavonoids are generally present in fruits, vegetables, seeds, nuts, among others. They are consumed in our diets about 20 times more than vitamin E or C (Ciumărnean et al., 2020). Flavonoids like myricetin, quercetin, luteolin, and rutin are present at least in one part of the plant and have demonstrated antioxidant, anti-inflammatory, anticoagulant, vasorelaxation, hypolipidemic, and anti-atherosclerotic characteristics in the cardiovascular system (Ciumărnean et al., 2020). Specifically, these flavonoids are targeted against atherosclerosis, ischemic heart disease (ISH), hypertension, platelet hyperactivation, MI, and even stroke (Ciumărnean et al., 2020). While BF has not been thoroughly examined for all these conditions, it consists of an active component that could make it beneficial as adjuvant therapy in cardiovascular disorders.

15.4.3 QUERCETIN

This is an example of a flavonoid that acts as an anti-hypertensive agent by improving the function of the endothelial and modulating of the renin-angiotensis-aldosterone axis, thereby lowering blood pressure.

15.4.4 Vitamin E

This is another flavonoid found in BF and has been documented to be of relevance in IHD mortality. Huang et al. (2019) showed that high serum α-tocopherol reduced the risk of mortality in CVD. Vitamin E has also been reported to be important in reperfusion since there is a decrease in the serum level during myocardial infarction (MI) (Ziegler et al., 2020).

15.5 PHARMACOLOGICAL RELEVANCE OF OTHER AFRICAN PLANTS OR HERBS IN CARDIOVASCULAR HEALTH

Traditional African medicine is perhaps the oldest in Africa and is considered the cradle of all mankind. Africa has significant biodiversity resources; hence habitat for about 45,000 species of different plants and about 5,000 of these have shown medicinal properties (Mahomoodally, 2013). The location of the continent is the basis for the secondary metabolites present in these plants; they adjust to their environment through a mechanism of evolution that aims to survive a hostile habitat. Nonetheless, with the enormous resources on the continent, Africa has only few drugs that are globally commercialized (AAMPS). Plants native to Africa are used mostly by rural dwellers and traditional healers (Mahomoodally, 2013). These resources are important since about 80% of the world's population relies on traditional medicine (Chintamunnee and Mahomoodally, 2012).

15.6 CARDIOVASCULAR DISEASES

CVD accounts for ~30% of the annual 58 million global deaths, therefore is considered a socio-economic bane (Roth et al., 2020). The global burden disease has reported a decrease in the mortality in the Western world due to coronary heart disease (CHD); however, the incidence of hypertension, obesity, and diabetes mellitus is on the rise (Zhao, 2021). This is not unrelated to technological advancement in therapeutics and invasive intervention like cardiac resynchronization, use of beta blockers, corticoid receptor antagonists, among others (Schupp et al., 2021).

15.7 GLOBAL EPIDEMIOLOGY ON CARDIOVASCULAR DISEASE

Despite all these, there are still about 4 million deaths every year associated with CVD in Europe (Figure 15.3) (Roth et al., 2017; Townsend et al., 2016).

Reports have similarly been documented for the decline in the burden of CVD, CHD, and MI in the UK (Bhatnagar et al., 2016). In America, CVD is also a leading cause of death with about 850,000 deaths in 2016, creating a major socio-economic burden. However, a dramatic decline of about 18.6% in CVD and 31.8% in CHD has been shown between 2006–2019. In other countries like Latin America, Eastern Europe, South Asia, and others, the incidence of CVD has been on the rise, probably due to risk factors like diabetes, hypertension, or obesity (Jayaraj et al., 2018). Asia has documented a significant surge in mortality since westernization. In fact, in the Asian-Pacific region, with more than half of the world's population with acute coronary syndrome, a kind of MI accounts for 50% of the global burden (Chan et al., 2016). Furthermore, in Africa with a growing population of more than 1 billion people, data showed her as a contributor to the global burden of CVD (Figure 15.3) (Keates et al., 2017). Sub-Sahara regions of the continent recorded about 1 million mortality cases of CVD in 2013 alone, increasing the burden in Africa to about 38% of all non-communicable death in the continent (Mensah et al., 2015). This is a bane and a threat to the socio-economic status in the world's most vulnerable communities (Keates et al., 2017).

15.8 PATHOPHYSIOLOGY OF MYOCARDIAL INFARCTION

Myocardial infarction is the clinical manifestation of CHD, also called ISH (Frangogiannis, 2015). It is a cardiomyocytic death resulting from an ischemic insult due to the rupture of an atherosclerotic

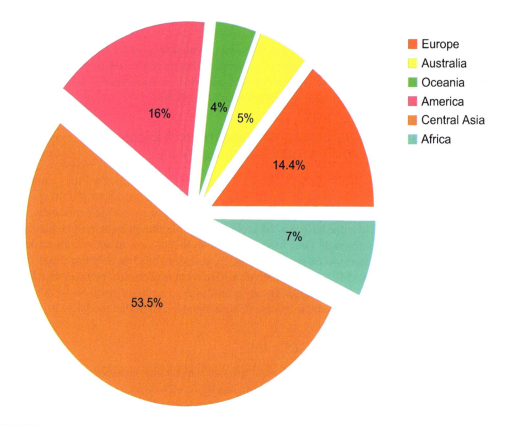

FIGURE 15.3 Incidence of ischemic heart disease in the world's continents.

plague causing thrombotic occlusion of the coronary artery (Heusch and Gersh, 2017). The size of the infarct scar is always dependent on the time and frequency of the coronary occlusion, ischemia area magnitude, and extent of residual collateral blood flow (Figure 15.4a) (Heusch and Gersh, 2017).

The occurrence of ischemia is a result of an imbalance in the oxygen demand and supply causing dysfunctional myocardium responsible for angina pectoris in MI. Angina pectoris is a pain in the chest region as a result of insufficient oxygen supply through the blood to the heart muscle. This event causes atherosclerosis, a super-imposed rupture of plaques called thrombosis which eventually leads to myocytic death in the affected region (Frangogiannis, 2015). The process of myocytic death ensues when the mitochondria receive injury caused by thrombosis.

15.9 MYOCARDIAL INFARCTION IN THE HEART MITOCHONDRIA

Mitochondria are critical organelles for energy production and respiration in cells; these are crucial in acute CHD and can thereby cause myocardial fibrosis when there is a dysfunction (Jiu et al., 2022). The mitochondria occupy about 30% of the total volume of the cardiomyocytes and they are said to produce approximately 30 kg adenosine triphosphate (ATP) daily (Yu and Miyamoto, 2021). It has been shown in several reports that mitochondrial dysfunction is implicated in CVD and is thereby involved in cardiomyocytic death (Jiu et al., 2022). Cardiomyocytic death is shown to be caused by casein kinase-2-α induced oxidative stress. This makes the mitochondria susceptible to injury, homeostatic imbalance and increased myocardial scar (Zhou et al., 2018). Similarly, findings from research have shown that casein kinase-2-α could phosphorylate fundci thereby inhibiting mitophagy, further potentiating mitochondrial permeability pore shift and then finally mitochondrial apoptosis (Figure 15.1c–e) (Zhou et al., 2018).

Bridelia ferruginea and Myocardial Protection 239

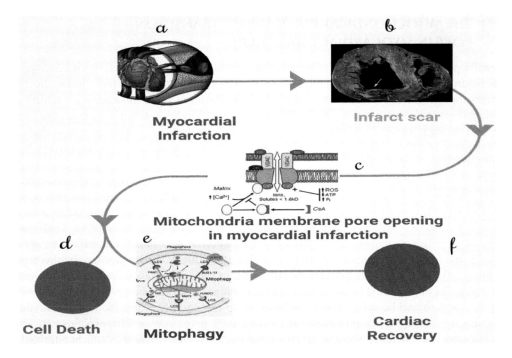

FIGURE 15.4 Mitochondrial dysfunction in ischemic heart disease. (a) Thrombosis occlusion in myocardial infarction. (b) Scar generated during myocardial infarction. (c) Mitochondrial permeability transition pore formation and opening in myocardial infarction. (d) Cardiomyocytic death in myocardial infarction. (e) Removal of damaged mitochondria by mitophagy. (f) Cardiac recovery by enhanced mitophagy.

15.10 THE MITOCHONDRION IS THE DETERMINER OF CELL SURVIVAL AND DEATH IN MYOCARDIAL INFARCTION

The heart mitochondrion generates ATP to sustain the contraction and other activities in the organelle (Ramachandra et al., 2020). Insufficient oxygen supply or hypoxia during MI has been revealed to trigger several biochemical activities in the heart cells thereby affecting the mitochondrial function (Hernandez-Resendiz et al., 2020). The mechanism of action involves accumulated proton induced pH decrease to less than 7 in MI. This occurs due to the reversal of oxidative phosphorylation in the mitochondria. Afterwards, anaerobic glycolysis ensues, resulting in increased lactate accumulation and decreased pH (Ramachandra et al., 2020). Accumulated lactate protons initiate the exchange of protons for Na^+ in the cell via the Na^+/H^+ ion exchanger. The event decreases the Na^+/K^+ ATPase activity causing Na^+ overload and subsequently altering the normal function of the Na^+/Ca^+ ion exchanger. All these culminate in mitochondria Ca^+ overload (Hernandez-Resendiz et al., 2020). Furthermore, other activities are altered in the mitochondria which include generation of reactive oxygen species, opening of the mitochondrial permeability transition (mPT) pore causing dysfunctional cardiomyocytes and eventually death (Hernandez-Resendiz et al., 2020). The mPT occurs as a result of opening of a pore on the inner mitochondrial membrane called the permeability transition pore. The pore formation leads to loss of ionic homeostasis, mitochondrial membrane swelling and eventual burst of the outer membrane, which can lead to cell death. Studies have shown that the cardiomyocytes have limited regenerative capacity due to their highly differentiated nature; hence the excessive death critically impacts ISH (Yu and Miyamoto, 2021).

15.11 THE MITOCHONDRIAL PERMEABILITY TRANSITION PORE IN MYOCARDIAL INFARCTION

The mPT pore is a crucial mediator of myocardial reperfusion injury, hence a target in cardioprotection. During the treatment of MI, findings have shown that within minutes of reperfusion, the infarct scar generated is about 50% of the total size, this is a significant value consequent upon mPT pore opening (Figure 15.1c) (Ong et al., 2015). The pore opening has been shown to be mediated by Ca^{2+} overload during ischemia; therefore protection would be by regulation of stress pathways that cause pore opening or intervention by mitochondria quality control mechanisms like mitophagy Figure 15.1d and e (Ong et al., 2015; Yu and Miyamoto, 2021).

In normal physiological conditions, the mPT pore remains intact and impermeable to molecules >1500 Da; however, ischemic insult induced the pore opening which is responsible for matrix swelling, apoptogenic cytochrome c release from the intermembrane space and irreversible activation of caspase 9 and 3 to induce cell death (Yu and Miyamoto, 2021). In the early 1990s, Griffiths and Halestrap (1993) recorded success in the use of cyclosporine A to inhibit the mPT pore opening sequel to the onset of ischemia and reperfusion (Ong et al., 2015). Further research by this team in the mid-1990s, showed that the pore opens only in the 2nd and 3rd minute of reperfusion. Revealing that during the index period of ischemia, the pore remains closed despite adverse conditions which may be due to the acidic environment (Griffiths and Halestrap, 1995). It is the rapid restoration of normalcy in reperfusion that precipitates the sudden mPT pore opening. This explains why a positive response was obtained with the MI treatment with BF, since it was a treatment administered before the onset of the disease. Therefore, the intactness of the pore was maintained, even during MI (Ojo et al., 2019). It is important to know that other mechanisms of cell death occur during MI that include necroptosis, ferroptosis, pyroptosis among others. These may be independent of the mPT pore pathways; however, using the mPT pore in cardioprotection during MI is highly dependent on the crucial time window. This suggests that the therapeutic regimen targeting this pathway should be either before the onset of or immediately after MI (Ruiz-Meana et al., 2011; Ong et al., 2015). Another form of mPT pore opening occurs in a non-pathological condition; this transiently and reversibly opens to allow the release of Ca^{2+} and reactive oxygen species (ROS) (Ong et al., 2015). This opening is important in cardioprotection because deleterious ROS and excess Ca^{2+} that could initiate cell death is released from the mitochondria.

15.12 CROSS-TALK BETWEEN THE LIVER AND HEART DURING MYOCARDIAL INFARCTION

The liver has been shown to be responsive to cardiac disorders, since about 25% of the cardiac output goes into the liver. It has been further shown that heart diseases could lead to cardio hepatopathy; however, there is limited information on its prognosy (Bannon et al., 2021). A cross-talk exists between the heart and liver in MI; however, the emphasis by different researchers varies. Tang et al. (2018) showed that the liver participates in interleukin-22 cardiac repair after MI, while Ojo et al. (2019) showed that inhibition of the liver mPT pore opening impacts the heart mPT pore. This demonstrates an inter-relationship between the organelles. Furthermore in 2021, Zhang and Fang established that there existed an interaction between the heart and liver in numerous diseases. Zhou et al. (2018) also identified the over-expression of hepatic sirtuin 5 (SIRT 5) in acute MI. This group showed that modulating SIRT 5 may demonstrate cardioprotection in MI, validating a cross-talk mechanism between the heart and liver. Extensive work on SIRT 5 has been done and this showed the importance of the protein in MI (Hershberget et al., 2018).

15.13 MYOCARDIAL PROTECTION BY *BRIDELIA FERRUGINEA*

There is limited information on the role of BF in MI; however, the aqueous extracts from the leaves of the plant showed important roles in decreasing the extent of infarct scar in the disease (Ojo et al.,

2019). Studies have shown that different parts of BF contain potent antioxidants, which is promising in preventing MI or probably decreasing the infarct scar in the disease. Furthermore, many researchers have explored the underlying potentials of BF in other diseases; however, Ojo et al. (2019) have reported that decrease in heart mitochondrial ATPase activity in MI could impact the mPT pore opening. This would lead to increased ATP hydrolysis instead of synthesis. Aqueous extract of BF was shown in the study to decrease the activity of mitochondrial adenosine triphosphatase. This enzyme is assumed to be a component of the mPT pore; however, there is still an ongoing debate on this (Alvian et al., 2014). Modulation of the enzyme activity by BF extracts is critical in mPT pore integrity. The findings suggest that extract from BF could regulate the mPT pore integrity under stress condition in MI. Furthermore, in the study, BF leaf extracts were shown to inhibit heart mitochondrial lipid peroxidation that increases the susceptibility of the mitochondrial pore opening to apoptogenic cytochrome c release, a prima facie for cell death. Other traditional plants have also been shown to be relevant in improving cardiovascular health and enhancing mitochondria quality (Ojo and Emoghwa, 2019).

15.14 SAFETY CONCERNS IN THE USE OF *BRIDELIA FERRUGINEA*

Acute and sub-acute toxicity studies performed on BF leaves have shown that the dose of up to 5000 mg/kg and 2500 mg/kg is safe for acute and sub-acute exposure respectively (Galalain and Aliyu, 2021). Irenee et al. (2020) also showed that the hydrochloric extracts of BF were safe up to 1000 mg/kg, while hydroethanolic extracts of BF showed no toxicity after acute and sub-chronic exposure. Investigating the possible cytotoxicity of certain components obtained from the methanolic extracts of the stem bark of BF, it was observed that using brine shrimp *A salina* lethality test, the LC_{50} value was less than 2 mg/mL, using about tenfold lower concentration (Mahomoodally et al., 2021). The extracts of BF were shown to be safe on the bacteria tested as documented by Mahomoodally et al. (2021) with the bacteriostatic effects at concentration lower than the compatibility limit.

15.15 FUTURE PERSPECTIVES FOR *BRIDELIA FERRUGINEA*

There is limited information on the effect of the secondary metabolite of BF on ailments, especially cardiovascular disorders. It is suggested that characterization of specific metabolites and investigation on animal studies and cell lines should be done to assist in drug design and development for CVD therapy. There should be provision of funds and collaboration with the continents where the plant is grown and cultivated. Researchers should investigate the pharmacological mechanism of BF in the human body as this would be relevant in attenuation, prevention, or delay of cardiovascular complications or probably the onset of the disease. The importance of BF for lipid modification, lowering of low-density lipoprotein in patients with CVD, should be investigated. Aside from the suggestion of rigorous scientific and clinical studies on BF in CVD, it is important to validate its safety in clinical trials. Physician-patient interaction should be encouraged to provide sufficient information on herb-drug interactions for appropriate counsel. It may be necessary to study the phenotypes and genotypes of cytochrome P450 enzyme family alleles in a different environment, so as to understand the effect of the plant on the enzyme activities. This can simply be achieved by in silico and computer-aided drug design studies and then the potentials of the plant can be translated from bench to bedside.

15.16 OTHER FOODS, HERBS, SPICES USED IN CARDIOVASCULAR DISEASES IN AFRICA

15.16.1 *ARTEMISIA HERBA-ALBA*

This is a plant distributed in Northern Africa, Western Asia, and the Arabian Peninsula (Mahomoodally, 2013). It is a perennial plant used in folklore medicine for the treatment of CVD, hypertension, diabetes mellitus, diarrhea, bacterial infections, among others. Metabolites isolated from this plant include carvone, piperitone, α-thujon e:camphor.

15.16.2 *ALOE FOREX MILL*

This is commonly found in South Africa and Lesotho. It is a plant used in ancient times by rural dwellers and even an export product in South Africa (Chen et al., 2012). The gel obtained from the plant is prominent in alleviating symptoms associated with cardiovascular disorders, neurodegenerative diseases, cancer therapy, among others. The sap from the plant is also used as health drinks and skin care products. Metabolites from *Aloe forex mill* include anthrone, anthraquinones, phenolic compounds, alkaloids, indoles among others.

15.16.3 *ASPALATHUS LINEARIS*

This plant is native to South Africa, commonly referred to as rooibos and used both as plant and food products. The plant possesses flavonoids, tannins, C-glycosides, dihydrochalcones, aspalathin among others. Aspalathus *linearis* has potent immune-modulatory effects and regular consumption could suppress the complications resulting from human immunodeficiency virus infection (Joubert and Beer, 2011). The plant has shown outstanding success in aging and CVD (Mahomoodally, 2013). Studies have shown the potency of rooibos tea in lowering blood pressure, and being a bronchodilator, among other properties.

15.16.4 *MONDEI WHITE*

This is a perennial plant of the Periplocaceae family used for the preparation of African dishes for the purpose of seasoning, taste enhancement, among others (Oludele et al., 2018). *Mondei white* is native to Eastern, Central, Southern and Western Africa and used in folklore medicine to treat fever, allergies, skin diseases, hypertension, and heart diseases (Chokwe et al., 2021). Secondary metabolites obtained from *Mondei white* include 2 hydroxy-4-methoxybenzaldehyde, 2,4,dihydroxy-6-methylbenzaldehyde, 3-hydroxy-6-methoxycoumarin, coumarin among others (Chokwe et al., 2021). These are responsible for the antimicrobial, anticoagulant, anti-inflammatory, antioxidant, and flavor enhancement characteristics.

15.17 TOXICITY AND CAUTIONARY NOTES

Despite the relevance of traditional foods, herbs, and plants used in the treatment of diseases, there are adverse effects that could even be life threatening (Tachjian et al., 2010). Some of these herbal products are known to directly or indirectly affect the cardiovascular system with serious consequences (Tachjian et al., 2010). BF has not been scientifically evaluated to determine its pharmacodynamics, pharmacokinetics nor its safety or efficacy. There is also a dearth of information on the randomized control trials to validate its safety. Furthermore, there is huge variation in the herbal sources and these could impact the active components present in the plant.

15.18 SUMMARY POINTS

- Coronary heart disease is clinically manifested as myocardial infarction.
- Myocardial infarction is caused by heart mitochondrial permeability transition pore opening during ischemic reperfusion injury.
- *Bridelia ferruginea* inhibits mitochondrial permeability transition pore opening in myocardial infarction.
- *Bridelia ferruginea*'s potential could be harnessed in treating ischemic reperfusion injuries.

REFERENCES

Afolayan, M., Srivedavyasasri, R., Asekun, O. T., Familoni, O. B., & Ross, S. A. (2018). Chemical and biological studies on Bridelia ferruginea grown in Nigeria. *Natural Product Research.* DOI: 10.1080/147 86419.2018.1440225

Afolayan, M. O., Asekun, O. T., & Familoni, O. (2020). Chemical constituents and biological evaluation of hexane fraction from *Bridelia ferruginea* (Benth.) leaves crude extract. *Nigerian Research Journal of Chemical Sciences*, 8(2), 252–264.

Akinsete, T. O., Adebayo-Tayo, B. C., & Adekanmbi, A. O. (2017). The phytochemical and antimicrobial potentials of the crude extracts of Bridelia ferruginea and the extracellular biosynthesized silver nanoparticles. *JAMPS*, 14(3), 1–13.

Akuodor, G. C., Mbah, C. C., Anyalewechi, N. A., TC, I. U. M. I., & Osunkwo, U. A. (2011). Pharmacological profile of aqueous extract of Bridelia ferruginea stem bark in the relief of pain and fever. *Journal of Medicinal Plants Research*, 5(22), 5366–5369.

Alowanou, G. G., Olounlade, A. P., Azando, E. V. B., Dedehou, V. F. G. N., & Daga, F. D., Adote, M. S. H. (2015). A review of *Bridelia ferruginea, Combretum glutinosum* and *Mitragina inermis* plants used in zootherapeutic remedies in West Africa: Historical origins, current uses and implications for conservation. *Journal of Applied Biosciences,* 87(1):8003. DOI: 10.4314/jab.v87i1.4

Alvian, K. N., Beutner, G., Lazrove, E., Sacchetti, S., Park, H. A., Licznerski, P., Li, H., Nabili, P., Hockensmith, K., Graham, M. et al. (2014). An uncoupling channel within the c-subunit ring of the F1F0-ATP synthase is the mitochondrial permeability transition pore. *Proc. Natl. Acad. Sci. USA.* DOI:111:10580–10585[PubMed:24979777].

Angelini, P., Angeles Flores, G. et al. (2021). Pharmacological potential and chemical characterization of Bridelia ferruginea Benth: A native tropical African medicinal plant. *Antibiotics*, 10, 223. https://doi.org/10.3390/antibiotics10020223

Association of African Medicinal Plants Standards (AAMPS). www.aamps.org/

Bannon, L., Merdler, I., Bar, N., Lupu, L., Banai, S., Jacob, G., & Shacham, Y. (2021). The cardio-hepatic relation in STEMI. *Journal of Personalized Medicine,* 11(12), 1241. DOI: 10.3390/jpm.11121241

Bhatnagar, P., Wickramasinghe, K., Wilkins, E., & Townsend, N. (2016). Trends in the epidemiology of cardiovascular disease in the UK. *Heart*, 102(24), 1945–1952.

Chan, M. Y., Du, X., Eccleston, D., Ma, C., Mohanan, P. P., Ogita, M., Shyu, K. G., Yan, B. P., & Jeong, Y. H. (2016, January 1). Acute coronary syndrome in the Asia-Pacific region. *Int J Cardiol.*, 202, 861–869. DOI:10.1016/j.ijcard.2015.04.073. Epub 2015 Apr 11. PMID: 26476044.

Chen, W., Van Wyk, B. E., Vermaak, I., & Viljoen, A. M. (2012). Cape aloes – a review of the phytochemistry, pharmacology and commercialisation of *Aloe ferox. Phytochemistry Letters.*

Chintamunnee, V., & Mahomoodally, M. F. (2012). Herbal medicine commonly used against infectious diseases in the tropical island of Mauritius. *Journal of Herbal Medicine*, 2, 113–125.

Chokwe, R. C., Dube, S., & Nindi, M. M. (2021). Development of a quantitative method for analysis of compounds found in Mondia whitei using HPLC-DAD. *Processes*, 9(11), 1864.

Ciumărnean, L., Milaciu, M. V., Runcan, O., Vesa, Ş. C., Răchişan, A. L., Negrean, V., Perné, M. G., Donca, V. I., Alexescu, T. G., Para, I., & Dogaru, G. (2020). The effects of flavonoids in cardiovascular diseases. *Molecules (Basel, Switzerland)*, 25(18), 4320. https://doi.org/10.3390/molecules25184320

Ekor, M. (2014). The growing use of herbal medicines: Issues relating to adverse reactions and challenges in monitoring safety. *Frontiers in Pharmacology*, 4, 177.

Frangogiannis, N. G. (2015). Pathophysiology of myocardial infarction. *Comprehensive Physiology*, 5(4), 1841–1875. DOI: 10.1002/cphy.c150006

Galalain, A. M., & Aliyu, B. S. (2021). Evaluation of the toxicity profile of Bridelia ferruginea methanol stem bark extract.

Griffiths, E. J., & Halestrap, A. P. (1993). Protection by Cyclosporin A of ischemia/reperfusion-induced damage in isolated rat hearts. *Journal of Molecular and Cellular Cardiology*, 25(12), 1461–1469.

Griffiths, E. J., & Halestrap, A. P. (1995). Mitochondrial non-specific pores remain closed during cardiac ischaemia, but open upon reperfusion. *Biochemical Journal*, 307(1), 93–98.

Hernandez-Resendiz, S., Prunier, F., Girao, H., Dorn, G., Hausenloy, D. J., & EU-CARDIOPROTECTION COST Action (CA16225). (2020). Targeting mitochondrial fusion and fission proteins for cardioprotection. *Journal of Cellular and Molecular Medicine*, 24(12), 6571–6585.

Hershberger, K. A., Abraham, D. M., Liu, J., Locasale, J. W., Grimsrud, P. A., & Hirschey, M. D. (2018, July 6). Ablation of *Sirtuin5* in the postnatal mouse heart results in protein succinylation and normal survival in response to chronic pressure overload. *J Biol Chem.*, 293(27), 10630–10645. DOI:10.1074/jbc. RA118.002187. Epub 2018 May 16. PMID: 29769314; PMCID: PMC6036188.

Heusch, G., & Gersh, B. J. (2017). The pathophysiology of acute myocardial infarction and strategies of protection beyond reperfusion: A continual challenge. *European Heart Journal, 38*(11), 774–784.

Huang, J., Weinstein, S. J., Yu, K., MänniStö, S., & Albanes, D. (2019, June 21). Relationship between Serum Alpha-Tocopherol and overall and cause-specific mortality. *Circ Res., 125*(1), 29–40. DOI:10.1161/CIRCRESAHA.119.314944. Epub 2019 May 6. PMID: 31219752; PMCID: PMC8555690.

Irénée, K. M. D., Dossou-Yovo, K. M., Diallo, A., Vovor, A., & Eklu-Gadegbeku, K. (2020). Sub-chronic (28-days) toxicity study of hydroalcohol stem bark extract of Bridelia ferruginea (Euphorbiaceae) on wistar rat. *J. Applied Sci.,* 20, 191–195.

Jayaraj, J. C., Davatyan, K., Subramanian, S., & Priya, J. (2018). Epidemiology of myocardial infarction. In (Ed.), Myocardial Infarction. *IntechOpen.* https://doi.org/10.5772/intechopen.74768

Jiu, H., Liu, X., Zhou, J., & Li, T. (2022). Mitochondrial DNA is a vital driving force in Ischemia reperfusion injury in cardiovascular diseases. *Oxidative Medicine and Cellular Longevity, 2022,* Article ID 6235747. DOI: 10.1155/2022/6235747

Joubert, E., & de Beer, D. (2011). Rooibos (*Aspalathus linearis*) beyond the farm gate: From herbal tea to potential phytopharmaceutical. *South African Journal of Botany, 77*(4), 869–886.

Keates, A. K., Mocumbi, A. O., Ntsekhe, M., Sliwa, K., & Stewart, S. (2017). Cardiovascular disease in Africa: Epidemiological profile and challenges. *Nature Reviews Cardiology, 14*(5), 273–293.

Mahomoodally, M. F. (2013). Traditional medicines in Africa: An appraisal of ten potent African medicinal plants. *Evidence-Based Complementary and Alternative Medicine, 2013.*

Mahomoodally M. F., Jugreet, S., Sinan, K. I., Zengin, G., Ak, G., Ceylan, R., Jeko, J., & Cziáky, Z. (2021). Pharmacological potential and chemical characterization of *Bridelia ferruginea* Benth-A native tropical African medicinal plant. *Antibiotic, 10*(2), 223.

Mbah, C. C., Akuodor, G. C., Anyalewechi, N. A., Iwuanyanwu, T. C., & Osunkwo, U. A. (2012). In vivo anti-plasmodial activities of aqueous extract of Bridelia ferruginea stem bark against Plasmodium berghei berghei in mice. *Pharmaceutical Biology, 50*(2), 188–194.

Mensah, G. A., Roth, G. A., Sampson, U. K. A., Moran, A. E., Feigin, V. L, & Forouzanfar, M. H. et al. (2015). Mortality from cardiovascular diseases in sub-Saharan Africa, 1990-2013: A systematic analysis of data from the Global Burden of Disease Study 2013. *Cardiovascular Journal of Africa, 26*(2 Suppl 1), S6–S10. DOI: 10.5830/cvja-20115-036.

Mozaffarian, D., Benjamin, E. J., Go, A. S., Arnett, D. K., Blaha, M. J., Cushman, M., . . . & Turner, M. B. (2015). Heart disease and stroke statistics – 2015 update: A report from the American Heart Association. *Circulation, 131*(4), e29–e322.

Murthy, H. N., Dalawai, D., Mamatha, U., Angadi, N. B., Dewir, Y. H., Al-Suhaibani, N. A. (2021). Bioactive constituents and nutritional composition of *Bridelia stipularis L.* Blume fruits. *International Journal of Food Properties,* 24(1): 796–805. DOI: 10.1080/10942912.2021.1924776

Ojo, O. O., & Emoghwa, A. R. (2019). Methanol extracts of *Strophanthus hispidus* exhibit anti-apoptotic effects via alteration of cytochrome *c* and caspase 3 levels in rats with myocardial infarction. *Chemical Papers,* 74, 521–528. Doi.org/10.1007/s11696-019-00894-8

Ojo, O. O., Rotimi, S., Adegbite, O. S., & Ozuem, T. I. (2019). *Bridelia ferruginea* inhibit rat heart and liver Mitochondrial Membrane Permeability Transition pore opening following myocardial infarction. *International Journal for Peptide Research,* 26(1), 1465–1472.

Olajide, O. A., Aderogba, M. A., Okorji, U. P., & Fiebich, B. L. (2012). Bridelia ferruginea produces anti-neuroinflammatory activity through inhibition of nuclear factor-kappa B and p38 MAPK signalling. *Evidence-Based Complementary and Alternative Medicine, 2012.*

Oludele, O., Idris, B., Benard, O., Pius, U., & Olufunso, O. (2018). Mondia whitei, an African spice inhibits mitochondrial permeability transition in Rat Liver. *Preventive Nutrition and Food Science, 23*(3), 206.

Omoboyowa, D. A., Karigidi, K. O., & Aribigbola, T. C. (2020). Bridelia ferruginea Benth leaves attenuates diabetes nephropathy in STZ-induced rats via targeting NGAL/KIM-1/cystatin c gene. *Clinical Phytoscience, 6*(1), 1–10.

Ong, S. B., Kalkhoran, S. B., Cabrera-Fuentes, H. A., & Hausenloy, D. J. (2015). Mitochondrial fusion and fission proteins as novel therapeutic targets for treating cardiovascular disease. *European Journal of Pharmacology, 763*(Pt A), 104–114.

Ramachandra, C. J. A., Hernandez-Resendiz, S., Crespo-Avilan, G. E., Lin, Y. H., Hausenloy, D. J. (2020). Mitochondria in acute myocardial infarction and cardioprotection. *EBioMedicine,* 57, 102884.

Roth, G. A., Johnson, C., Abajobir, A., Abd-Allah, F., Abera, S. F., Abyu, G., . . . & Ukwaja, K. N. (2017). Global, regional, and national burden of cardiovascular diseases for 10 causes, 1990 to 2015. *Journal of the American College of Cardiology, 70*(1), 1–25.

Roth, G. A., Mensah, G. A., Johnson, C. O., Addolorato, G., Ammirati, E., Baddour, L. M., . . . & GBD-NHLBI-JACC Global Burden of Cardiovascular Diseases Writing Group. (2020). Global burden of cardiovascular diseases and risk factors, 1990–2019: Update from the GBD 2019 study. *Journal of the American College of Cardiology*, *76*(25), 2982–3021.

Ruiz-Meana, M., Inserte, J., Fernandez-Sanz, C., Hernando, V., Miro-Casas, E., Barba, I., & Garcia-Dorado, D. (2011). The role of mitochondrial permeability transition in reperfusion-induced cardiomyocyte death depends on the duration of ischemia. *Basic Research in Cardiology*, *106*(6), 1259–1268.

Schupp, J. C., Adams, T. S., Cosme, Jr. C., Raredon, M. S. B. et al. (2021). Integrated single-cell atlas of endothelial cells of the human lung. *Circulation*, *144*(4), 286–302.

Shaito, A., Thuan, D. T. B., Phu, H. T., Nguyen, T. H. D., Hasan, H., Halabi, S., Abdelhady, S., Nasrallah, G. K., Eid, A. H., & Pintus, G. (2020). Herbal medicine for cardiovascular diseases: Efficacy, mechanisms, and safety. *Front. Pharmacol.*, *11*, 422. DOI:10.3389/fphar.2020.00422

Strandberg, T. E., Tilvis, R. S., & Miettinen, T. A. (1989). Variations of hepatic cholesterol precursors during altered flows of endogenous and exogenous squalene in the rat. *Biochimica et FBiophysica Acta (BBA)-Lipids and Lipid Metabolism*, *1001*(2), 150–156.

Tachjian, A., Maria, V., & Jahangir, A. (2010). Use of herbal products and potential interactions in patients with cardiovascular diseases. *Journal of the American College of Cardiology*, *55*(6), 515–525.

Tang, T. T., Li, Y. Y., Li J. J., et al. (2018). Liver-heart crosstalk controls IL-22 activity in cardiac protection after myocardial infarction. *Theranostics*, *8*(16), 4552–4562. DOI:10.7150/thno.24723.

Townsend, N., Wilson, L., Bhatnagar, P., Wickramasinghe, K., Rayner, M., & Nichols, M. (2016). Cardiovascular disease in Europe: Epidemiological update 2016. *European Heart Journal*, *37*(42), 3232–3245.

Townsend, N., Wilson, L., Bhatnagar, P., Wickramasinghe, K., Rayner, M., & Nichols, M. (2016). Cardiovascular disease in Europe: Epidemiological update 2016. *European Heart Journal*, *37*(42), 3232–3245.

Willdenow, C. (1806). Species plantarum. *Editio Quarta*, *4*(2), 978–979.

Yu, J. D., & Miyamoto, S. (2021). Molecular signaling to preserve mitochondrial integrity against ischemic stress in the heart: Rescue or remove mitochondria in danger. *Cells*, *10*(12), 3330.

Zhang, Y., & Fang, X. M. (2021). Hepatocardiac or cardiohepatic interaction: From traditional Chinese medicine to Western medicine. *Evidence-Based Complementary and Alternative Medicine: eCAM*, *2021*, 6655335.

Zhao, D. (2021). Epidemiological features of cardiovascular disease in Asia. *JACC: Asia*, *1*(1), 1–13.

Zhou, X., Li, J., Guo, J., Geng, B., Ji, W., Zhao, Q., Li, J., Liu, X., Liu, J., Guo, Z., Cai, W., Ma, Y., Ren, D., Miao, J., Chen, S., Zhang, Z., Chen, J., Zhong, J., Liu, W., Zou, M., Li, Y., & Cai, J. (2018, April 3). Gut-dependent microbial translocation induces inflammation and cardiovascular events after ST-elevation myocardial infarction. *Microbiome*, *6*(1), 66. DOI:10.1186/s40168-018-0441-4. PMID: 29615110; PMCID: PMC5883284.

Ziegler, M., Wallert, M., Orkowski, S., & Peter, K. (2020). Cardiovascular and metabolic protection by Vitamin E: A matter of treatment strategy? *Antioxidants*, *9*(10), 935.

16 Lingzhi (*Ganoderma lucidum*) and Cardiovascular Disease

Brian Tomlinson, Sze Wa Chan and Paul Chan

CONTENTS

16.1 Introduction 248
16.2 Background...248
16.3 Antioxidant Effects..248
16.4 Anti-Inflammatory Effects 249
16.5 Antihypertensive Effects 249
16.6 Effects on Dyslipidaemia...250
16.7 Hypoglycaemic Activity 250
16.8 Clinical Studies of the Antidiabetic Effects of *G. lucidum*...........................252
16.9 Toxicity and Cautionary Notes 253
16.10 Summary Points 253
References..253

LIST OF ABBREVIATIONS

ACE   Angiotensin converting enzyme
ARB   Angiotensin receptor blocker
CAT   Catalase
DPPH   1,1-diphenyl-2-picrylhydrazyl
FYGL   Fudan-Yueyang-G. lucidum
GPx   Glutathione peroxidase
HbA1c   Glycosylated haemoglobin
HDL-C   High-density lipoprotein cholesterol
HMG-CoA   3-hydroxy-3-methylglutaryl-coenzyme A
hsCRP   High-sensitivity C-reactive protein
IC_{50} 50% of maximal inhibitory concentration
IL   Interleukin
LDL-C   Low-density lipoprotein cholesterol
MDA   Malondialdehyde
OS   Oxidative stress
PTP1B   Protein tyrosine phosphatase 1B
RNS   Reactive nitrogen species
ROS   Reactive oxygen species
SGLT2   sodium-glucose cotransporter 2
SOD   Superoxide dismutase
T2DM   Type 2 diabetes mellitus
TCM   Traditional Chinese medicine
TNFα   Tumour necrosis factor-α

DOI: 10.1201/9781003220329-18

16.1 INTRODUCTION

Ganoderma is a genus of woody mushroom from the family Ganodermataceae that occurs worldwide with many found in tropical regions (Bishop et al. 2015). The different species can be identified by characteristics, such as the shape and colour of the fruiting bodies, the geographical origin and host specificity (Wachtel-Galor et al. 2011). More advanced identification methods include chemical fingerprinting and DNA sequencing (Hennicke et al. 2016). Molecular studies have shown that the *Ganoderma lucidum* commercially cultivated in East Asia is actually a different species from the true *G. lucidum* originally described from Europe (Cao et al. 2012). It was suggested that the East Asian species known as Lingzhi should be named *Ganoderma lingzhi* but most publications still refer to it as *Ganoderma lucidum*.

There are many different commercial products marketed as herbal supplements or nutraceuticals which bear the names Lingzhi, Reishi, or Ganoderma. These contain certain types of extracts obtained from various parts of the mushroom, such as the fruiting bodies, mycelium and spores. Sometimes these are combined with other herbal products (Wachtel-Galor et al. 2011).

16.2 BACKGROUND

Ganoderma lucidum (Curtis) P. Karst is known as Lingzhi in China and Reishi in Japan. It has been used in traditional Chinese medicine (TCM) for over 2000 years (Bishop et al. 2015). It has many different constituents which are biologically active. The major ones include various triterpenes, polysaccharides and proteins (Ahmad et al. 2013). These compounds with pharmacological activity are present in various amounts in different parts of the mushroom.

Triterpenes are derived from squalene and more than 150 triterpenes have been identified from the different parts of *G. lucidum* (Baby et al. 2015). They are extracted with organic solvents and the main types are ganoderic acids and lucidenic acids and less common types include ganodermic acids, ganoderals and ganoderiols (Wachtel-Galor et al. 2011).

Polysaccharides and peptidoglycans are other active components that have been isolated from the spores, mycelia and fruiting bodies of *G. lucidum*. Some of these are thought to have antitumor and immunomodulatory activities (Kao et al. 2013; Xu et al. 2011) and several polysaccharide compounds have gone through clinical trials and have been used to treat various cancers and other diseases in Asia (Wasser 2010).

Several bioactive proteins have also been identified such as a polypeptide known as Lingzhi-8 (LZ-8) which has a structure like an immunoglobulin and is thought to have immunomodulatory activity (Hsu and Cheng 2018).

16.3 ANTIOXIDANT EFFECTS

Free radicals, such as reactive oxygen species (ROS) and reactive nitrogen species (RNS), contain one or more unpaired electrons and are highly reactive and unstable. They are required for certain functions such as the immune system and cell signalling, but when present in excessive amounts they can cause damage such as atherosclerosis, heart disease, diabetes and cancer (Johansen et al. 2005).

Some triterpenoids and polysaccharides from *G. lucidum* show antioxidant activity, in vitro (Ferreira et al. 2015; Krishna et al. 2016). Phenolic compounds from *G. lucidum* showed strong radical scavenging activity for 1,1-diphenyl-2-picrylhydrazyl (DPPH) which correlated with the concentrations of various individual compounds and the total phenolic compounds (Kim et al. 2008). Polysaccharide extracts from *G. lucidum* showed reducing power which correlated with the total amount of phenols and α-glucans, but not with the total amount of polysaccharides and proteins (Kozarski et al. 2012).

In vivo studies showed that *G. lucidum* increased the activity of antioxidant enzymes such as superoxide dismutase (SOD) and catalase (CAT) in rats with streptozotocin-induced diabetes (Vitak et al. 2017). Hot water extract of *G. lucidum* improved oxidative stress (OS) and lipid levels in rats (Rahman et al. 2018). *G. lucidum* extract showed cardioprotective effects attributed to antioxidant properties in an ischemia-reperfusion isolated perfused rat heart model (Lasukova et al. 2015).

Human studies have shown various antioxidant effects with different Lingzhi preparations. Plasma and urine antioxidant capacity increased after a single dose of Lingzhi and after supplementation with 0.72 g per day of Lingzhi for 10 days there were significant increases in fasting plasma lipid standardised alpha-tocopherol concentration and urine antioxidant capacity, but the tendency for increase in fasting plasma ascorbic acid and total alpha-tocopherol concentrations and erythrocyte SOD and glutathione peroxidase (GPx) activities were not significant (Wachtel-Galor et al. 2004a).

A commercially available encapsulated Lingzhi preparation (1.44 g Lingzhi/day; equivalent to 13.2 g fresh mushroom/day) was used in a double-blind, placebo-controlled, cross-over intervention study over 4 weeks and this showed no significant change in a range of antioxidant status biomarkers, and other markers of inflammation, cardiovascular risk, immune status and DNA damage (Wachtel-Galor et al. 2004b).

A placebo-controlled cross-over study in 42 healthy subjects examined the antioxidation and hepatoprotective efficacy of triterpenoids and polysaccharide-enriched *G. lucidum*, which was taken as a 225 mg capsule containing 7% triterpenoid-ganoderic acid (A, B, C, C5, C6, D, E and G), 6% polysaccharide peptides with a few essential amino acids and trace elements, once daily for 6 consecutive months (Chiu et al. 2017). The treatment showed an improvement in total antioxidant capacity, total thiols and glutathione content in plasma, significantly enhanced activities of antioxidant enzymes (SOD, CAT, GPx and glucose-6-phosphate dehydrogenase), and reduced the levels of thiobarbituric acid reactive substances, 8-hydroxy-deoxy-guanosine and hepatic marker enzymes, glutamic-oxaloacetic transaminase and glutamic-pyruvic transaminase. Mild fatty liver detected by abdominal ultrasonic examination was reversed to normal with *G. lucidum* treatment (Chiu et al. 2017).

16.4 ANTI-INFLAMMATORY EFFECTS

Inflammation is important in the development and progression of atherosclerotic plaques (Libby 2021). The inflammatory marker, high-sensitivity C-reactive protein (hsCRP), is often used to determine the inflammatory status.

Anti-inflammatory effects of *G. lucidum* extracts have been shown in several in vitro cellular studies and an in vivo study in rats showed that a water extract of *G. lucidum* had significant anti-inflammatory activity against carrageenan-induced paw oedema (Lin et al. 1993) Methanol and ethyl acetate extracts of *G. lucidum* from South India also showed dose-dependent anti-inflammatory effects in mice (Sheena et al. 2003).

There are few clinical studies of the anti-inflammatory effect of *G. lucidum*. In a clinical trial involving 45 patients with myocardial infarction randomised to polysaccharide peptide of *G. lucidum* (750 mg/day in 3 divided doses for 90 days) there were decreased levels of interleukin (IL)-1 and tumour necrosis factor-α (TNF-α), as well as malondialdehyde (MDA) levels that were not seen with placebo (Sargowo et al. 2019). In another clinical trial in 38 patients with atrial fibrillation, those randomised to *G. lucidum* polysaccharide peptide 3 times a day for 90 days showed significantly reduced IL-1β, IL-6, hsCRP and TNF-α, as well as systolic and diastolic blood pressure, heart rate and LDL-C, compared to placebo-treated patients (Rizal et al. 2020).

16.5 ANTIHYPERTENSIVE EFFECTS

G. lucidum powder was reported to lower blood pressure in spontaneously hypertensive rats many years ago (Kabir et al. 1988). More recent studies have focused on extracts from *G. lucidum* having inhibitory effects on angiotensin converting enzyme (ACE).

ACE inhibitors or angiotensin receptor blockers (ARBs) are considered as first line treatments for hypertension, along with thiazide or thiazide-like diuretics and calcium channel blockers, in recent guidelines for the management of hypertension (Whelton et al. 2018; Williams et al. 2018).

ACE inhibition has been shown in vitro with some triterpenes and proteins from *G. lucidum* (Abdullah et al. 2012; Mohamad Ansor et al. 2013). Three small peptides with ACE-inhibitory activity were isolated from the mycelia of *G. lucidum* (Wu et al. 2019).

In a study using an extract of Reishi, which was auto-digested by the proteases present in the extract, oral administration to spontaneous hypertensive rats resulted in reduction of the systolic blood pressure at 4 and 8 hours (Tran et al. 2014). Four peptides were identified from the extract that showed potent inhibition against ACE.

A study with a water extract of *G. lucidum* administered intragastrically for 7 weeks to adult male rats with inherited stress-induced arterial hypertension found reductions in blood pressure similar to that with the ARB losartan and increased cerebral blood flow which was not seen with losartan (Shevelev et al. 2018).

There have been few clinical trials that examined the effects of Lingzhi in hypertension. An uncontrolled study in Japan showed reductions in blood pressure in subjects with hypertension but not in those with borderline hypertensive or normal blood pressure with a *G. lucidum* extract (240 mg daily) given for 6 months (Kanmatsuse et al. 1985).

More recently, the *G. lucidum* polysaccharides (Ganopoly™) commercial product was used in a double-blind, randomised, placebo-control phase I/II study over 12 weeks in patients with coronary heart disease (Gao et al. 2004a). The average blood pressure was reduced from 142.5/96.4 mmHg to 135.1/92.8 mmHg with the *G. lucidum* product whilst there was no significant change in the control group. There was also a significant reduction in total cholesterol levels and improvement in coronary heart disease symptoms with the active treatment but not with the placebo.

16.6 EFFECTS ON DYSLIPIDAEMIA

Dyslipidaemia includes not only elevated levels of low-density lipoprotein cholesterol (LDL-C) and triglycerides, but also decreased levels of high-density lipoprotein cholesterol (HDL-C). These often occur in combination as an atherogenic dyslipidaemia, which is common in patients with type 2 diabetes mellitus (T2DM) (Tomlinson et al. 2021). Current guidelines for the treatment of lipid disorders recommend starting treatment with the statins or 3-hydroxy-3-methylglutaryl-coenzyme A (HMG-CoA) reductase inhibitors in most cases to reduce the risk of cardiovascular events (Grundy et al. 2019; Mach et al. 2020). The statins were developed from fungal products (Endo 2004), so it may not be surprising that other natural compounds might also inhibit HMG-CoA reductase.

Several triterpenoids from *G. lucidum* can inhibit cholesterol biosynthesis at various steps (Shiao 2003). Some compounds isolated from the fruiting bodies of *G. lucidum* were found to have inhibitory activity against HMG-CoA reductase including ganolucidic acid eta, ganoderenic acid K, ganomycin J and ganomycin B, with ganomycin B (Figure 16.1) being the most potent with an IC_{50} of 14.3 μM (Chen et al. 2017).

Extracts or powder from *G. lucidum* have shown cholesterol-lowering properties in vitro, ex vivo, and in hamsters and minipigs (Berger et al. 2004), but human studies are limited. In one study there was a non-significant trend for increase in HDL-C and reduction in triglycerides in 26 subjects who had borderline elevations of blood pressure and/or cholesterol, after 12 weeks' administration of 1.44 g Lingzhi extract daily (Chu et al. 2012). These effects could be due to an improvement in insulin resistance as this may affect the associated dyslipidaemia (Tomlinson et al. 2021).

16.7 HYPOGLYCAEMIC ACTIVITY

In patients with T2DM, the treatment of hyperglycaemia is important to reduce macrovascular disease and cardiovascular risk, and especially to reduce the risk of microvascular disease (American

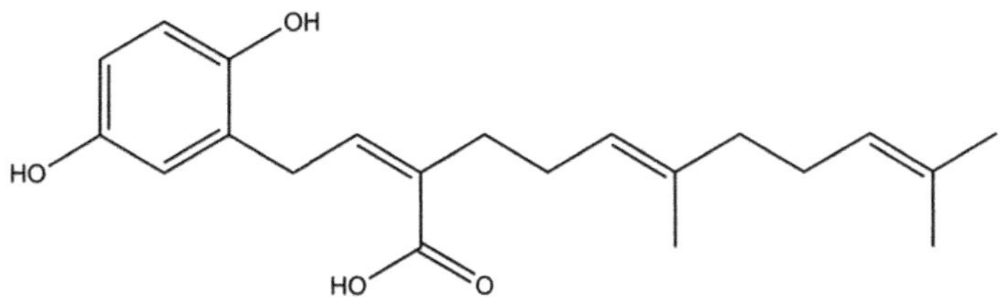

Lingzhi (*Ganoderma lucidum*) and Cardiovascular Disease

FIGURE 16.1   Chemical structure of ganomycin B.

Note: Ganomycin B is a potent inhibitor of HMG-CoA reductase.

Source: Chen et al. (2017).

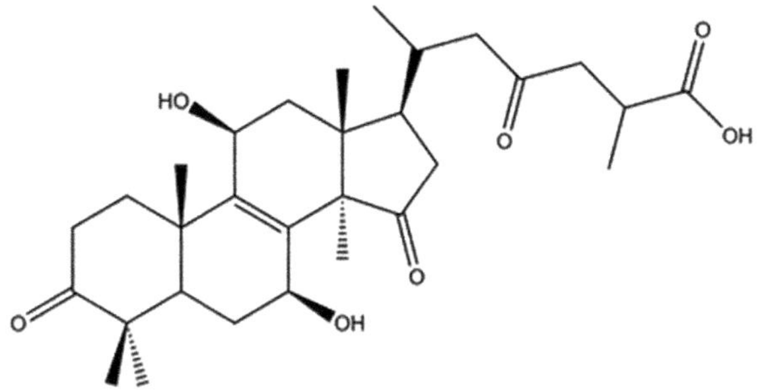

FIGURE 16.2   Chemical structure of Ganoderic acid Df.

Note: Ganoderic acid Df is a potent inhibitor of aldose reductase.

Source: Fatmawati et al. (2010).

Diabetes Association Professional Practice Committee 2021b). Lifestyle intervention is the first-line approach for all patients but pharmacotherapy is often necessary and the guidelines for glycaemic treatment are reviewed annually by the American Diabetes Association (American Diabetes Association Professional Practice Committee 2021a). Some of the current drug treatments have herbal origins such as the biguanides, which were developed from compounds in the plant goat's rue or French lilac (*Galega officinalis*, Linnaeus, Fabaceae) (Witters 2001) and the sodium-glucose cotransporter 2 (SGLT2) inhibitors, which were developed from phlorizin, a natural compound isolated from the bark of apple roots (Hardman et al. 2010).

Various extracts from *G. lucidum* have shown hypoglycaemic activity in in vitro experiments and in animal models of diabetes (Winska et al. 2019). Early studies showed that two peptidoglycans, ganoderans A and B, had hypoglycaemic activity in animal models through various mechanisms (Hikino et al. 1989; Hikino et al. 1985).

An immunomodulatory protein named Ling Zhi-8 (LZ-8), isolated from the mycelial extract of *G. lucidum*, was shown to prevent the development of autoimmune diabetes in a diabetic mouse model (Kino et al. 1989) and it delayed the rejection of transplanted allogeneic pancreatic islets in a rat model (van der Hem et al. 1995).

An inhibitory effect on human aldose reductase activity was shown by a methanol extract from the fruiting bodies of *G. lucidum* and Ganoderic acid Df (Figure 16.2), which is a lanostane-type triterpenoid, and identified as a potent aldose reductase inhibitor (Fatmawati et al. 2009, 2010).

Another triterpenoid isolated from a chloroform extract of *G. lucidum*, Ganoderol B (Figure 16.3), was effective in inhibiting α-glucosidase activity with a stronger inhibitory effect than acarbose, which is a medication used to inhibit α-glucosidase (Fatmawati et al. 2011).

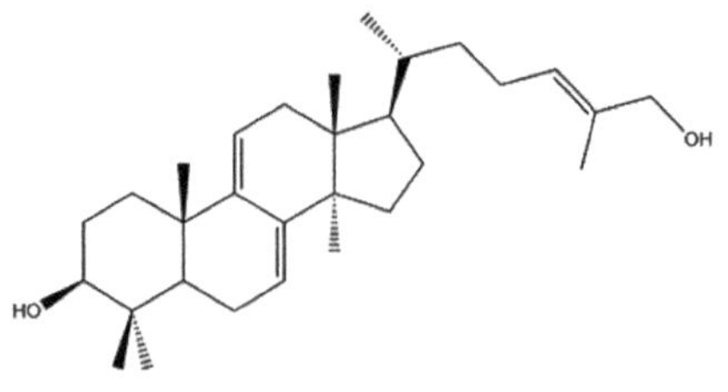

FIGURE 16.3 Chemical structure of Ganoderol B.

Note: Ganoderol B is a potent inhibitor of α-glucosidase.

Source: Fatmawati et al. (2011).

Inhibition of protein tyrosine phosphatase 1B (PTP1B) activity is another potential mechanism for hypoglycaemia activity and a water soluble macromolecular proteoglycan extracted from the fruiting bodies of *G. lucidum* named Fudan-Yueyang-G. lucidum (FYGL), was shown to have this effect (Teng et al. 2011). FYGL showed hypoglycaemic activity in diabetic mice and rat models and improved the associated lipid disorders (Teng et al. 2011; Teng et al. 2012). Further studies in diabetic mice showed the hypoglycaemic effect of FYGL was associated with enhanced insulin secretion, decreased hepatic glucose output and increased adipose and skeletal muscle glucose disposal (Pan et al. 2014; Pan et al. 2013). FYGL was shown to be a hyperbranched heteropolysaccharide bonded with protein via both serine and threonine residues (Pan et al. 2015).

A polysaccharide extract from *G. lucidum* (Gl-PS) has shown hypoglycaemic effects in various animal models which may be related to preventing apoptosis of pancreatic β-cells and enhancing β-cells regeneration (Zhang et al. 2003; Zhang and Lin 2004; Zheng et al. 2012). A β-heteropolysaccharide named F31 isolated from Gl-PS was found to influence glucose metabolism in the liver (Xiao et al. 2018, 2017).

Hypoglycaemic effects have been shown with various types of extract of *G. lucidum* in animal studies without identifying the active constituents (Bach et al. 2018; Sarker 2015; Seto et al. 2009).

16.8 CLINICAL STUDIES OF THE ANTIDIABETIC EFFECTS OF *G. LUCIDUM*

There have been few clinical studies of the hypoglycaemic effects with *G. lucidum* products. Ganopoly™ at a dose of 1800 mg 3 times daily was given for 12 weeks in a placebo-controlled study in 62 patients with T2DM and fasting and postprandial plasma glucose levels and glycosylated haemoglobin (HbA1c) were reduced (Gao et al. 2004b). Another study using a dry extract of *G. lucidum* (3 g) added to the regular oral antidiabetic treatments for 12 weeks showed no effect on HbA1c or fasting glucose but the plasma glucose response during a meal tolerance test improved (Wang et al. 2008).

In a randomised, double-blind, placebo-controlled, cross-over study in 26 subjects with borderline elevations of blood pressure and/or cholesterol and normal plasma glucose levels using 1.44 g daily of a Lingzhi product for 12 weeks, there was no change in plasma glucose but there were reductions in plasma insulin and homeostasis model assessment-insulin resistance with Lingzhi compared to placebo (Chu et al. 2012).

In a study in 84 patients with T2DM and metabolic syndrome, the patients were randomised to administration of a *G. lucidum* preparation containing *G. lucidum* mushroom extract 2240 mg and G. lucidum spores 740 mg daily, alone or in combination with *Cordyceps sinensis* (or *Ophiocordyceps sinensis* (Berk.) G.H. Sung et al.) extract 1000 mg daily, or the placebo excipient for a period of 16 weeks (Klupp et al. 2016). The results from the two intervention groups receiving *G. lucidum*, with or without Cordyceps were combined and there was no significant effect on the

Lingzhi (*Ganoderma lucidum*) and Cardiovascular Disease

primary outcome measures of HbA1c and fasting plasma glucose or any of the secondary outcome measures which included multiple lipid parameters, and blood pressure was also tested.

A systematic review, which included these 4 clinical trials and another one with Ganopoly™ in patients with coronary heart disease mentioned earlier (Gao et al. 2004a), concluded that *G. lucidum* was not an effective treatment for reducing blood glucose, blood pressure or cholesterol (Klupp et al. 2015). It should be noted that the trials mentioned here used different preparations of *G. lucidum* so it may not be appropriate to combine results from the different studies.

16.9 TOXICITY AND CAUTIONARY NOTES

Evidence of safety with *G. lucidum* has come from observational studies and long-term experience. In the *American Herbal Products Association Botanical Safety Handbook* (McGuffin et al. 1997) it is listed in the safest drug class (Class 1 Drug). No herb-drug interactions have been reported. *G. lucidum* may have a mild antithrombotic effect in some doses, which may be due to an antiplatelet effect rather than anticoagulation activity (Kumaran et al. 2011; Shiao 2003). This could increase the effect of other antiplatelet medications, such as aspirin and it is advisable to be cautious in taking any herbal products in combination with warfarin.

A case of hepatotoxicity apparently related to *G. lucidum* mushroom powder was reported, but this may have been due to the excipients in the product (Yuen et al. 2004). Another case of fatal hepatitis in a patient taking Lingzhi powder was reported from Thailand, but whether this was caused by the *G. lucidum* component was not certain (Wanmuang et al. 2007).

The recent clinical trials using *G. lucidum* products have involved laboratory safety parameters and no safety signals have been detected (Klupp et al. 2015, 2016), but these were relatively small studies and larger rigorously controlled clinical trials are needed to confirm the lack of toxicity.

16.10 SUMMARY POINTS

- This chapter focuses on the effects of Lingzhi (*Ganoderma lucidum*) on the major risk factors for cardiovascular disease.
- Various extracts from the fruiting bodies, mycelium and spores of *G. lucidum* have been used in studies in vitro and in vivo.
- Studies in vitro and in animal models have demonstrated antioxidative, anti-inflammatory, antihypertensive, lipid-lowering and hypoglycaemic properties of *G. lucidum* extracts.
- Specific compounds have been shown to inhibit HMG-CoA reductase, aldose reductase and α-glucosidase in vitro.
- Human studies are limited and provide conflicting results, probably because different *G. lucidum* products were used.
- Larger controlled clinical trials with standardised products are needed to demonstrate efficacy and lack of toxicity.

REFERENCES

Abdullah, N., S. M. Ismail, N. Aminudin, A. S. Shuib and B. F. Lau. 2012. Evaluation of Selected Culinary-Medicinal Mushrooms for Antioxidant and ACE Inhibitory Activities. Evid Based Complement Alternat Med 2012: 464238.

Ahmad, M. F., F. A. Ahmad, Z. A. A. Azad, M. I. Alam, J. A. Ansari and B. P. Panda. 2013. Edible Mushrooms as Health Promoting Agent. Adv Sci Focus 1 (3): 189–196.

American Diabetes Association Professional Practice Committee. 2021a. 9. Pharmacologic Approaches to Glycemic Treatment: Standards of Medical Care in Diabetes – 2022. Diabetes Care 45 (Supplement_1): S125–S143.

————. 2021b. 10. Cardiovascular Disease and Risk Management: Standards of Medical Care in Diabetes – 2022. Diabetes Care 45 (Supplement_1): S144–S174.

Baby, S., A. J. Johnson and B. Govindan. 2015. Secondary metabolites from Ganoderma. Phytochemistry 114: 66–101.

Bach, E. E., E. M. B. Hi, A. M. C. Martins, P. A. M. Nascimento and N. S. Y. Wadt. 2018. Hypoglicemic and Hypolipedimic Effects of Ganoderma lucidum in Streptozotocin-Induced Diabetic Rats. Medicines (Basel) 5 (3): 78.

Berger, A., D. Rein, E. Kratky, I. Monnard, H. Hajjaj, I. Meirim, C. Piguet-Welsch, J. Hauser, K. Mace and P. Niederberger. 2004. Cholesterol-lowering properties of Ganoderma lucidum in vitro, ex vivo, and in hamsters and minipigs. Lipids Health Dis 3: 2.

Bishop, K. S., C. H. Kao, Y. Xu, M. P. Glucina, R. R. Paterson and L. R. Ferguson. 2015. From 2000 years of Ganoderma lucidum to recent developments in nutraceuticals. Phytochemistry 114: 56–65.

Cao, Y., S.-H. Wu and Y.-C. Dai. 2012. Species clarification of the prize medicinal Ganoderma mushroom "Lingzhi". Fungal Diversity 56 (1): 49–62.

Chen, B., J. Tian, J. Zhang, K. Wang, L. Liu, B. Yang, L. Bao and H. Liu. 2017. Triterpenes and meroterpenes from Ganoderma lucidum with inhibitory activity against HMGs reductase, aldose reductase and alpha-glucosidase. Fitoterapia 120: 6–16.

Chiu, H. F., H. Y. Fu, Y. Y. Lu, Y. C. Han, Y. C. Shen, K. Venkatakrishnan, O. Golovinskaia and C. K. Wang. 2017. Triterpenoids and polysaccharide peptides-enriched Ganoderma lucidum: A randomized, double-blind placebo-controlled crossover study of its antioxidation and hepatoprotective efficacy in healthy volunteers. Pharm Biol 55 (1): 1041–1046.

Chu, T. T., I. F. Benzie, C. W. Lam, B. S. Fok, K. K. Lee and B. Tomlinson. 2012. Study of potential cardio-protective effects of Ganoderma lucidum (Lingzhi): Results of a controlled human intervention trial. Br J Nutr 107 (7): 1017–1027.

Endo, A. 2004. The origin of the statins. 2004. Atheroscler Suppl 5 (3): 125–130.

Fatmawati, S., K. Kurashiki, S. Takeno, Y.-u. Kim, K. Shimizu, M. Sato, K. Imaizumi, K. Takahashi, S. Kamiya, S. Kaneko and R. Kondo. 2009. The inhibitory effect on aldose reductase by an extract of Ganoderma lucidum. Phytother Res 23 (1): 28–32.

Fatmawati, S., K. Shimizu and R. Kondo. 2010. Ganoderic acid Df, a new triterpenoid with aldose reductase inhibitory activity from the fruiting body of Ganoderma lucidum. Fitoterapia 81 (8): 1033–1036.

Fatmawati, S., K. Shimizu and R. Kondo. 2011. Ganoderol B: A potent alpha-glucosidase inhibitor isolated from the fruiting body of Ganoderma lucidum. Phytomedicine 18 (12): 1053–1055.

Ferreira, I. C. F. R., S. A. Heleno, F. S. Reis, D. Stojkovic, M. J. R. P. Queiroz, M. H. Vasconcelos and M. Sokovic. 2015. Chemical features of Ganoderma polysaccharides with antioxidant, antitumor and anti-microbial activities. Phytochemistry 114: 38–55.

Gao, Y., G. Chen, X. Dai, J. Ye and S. Zhou. 2004a. A Phase I/II Study of Ling Zhi Mushroom *Ganoderma lucidum* (W.Curt.:Fr.) Lloyd (Aphyllophoromycetideae) Extract in Patients with Coronary Heart Disease. Int J Med Mushrooms 6 (4): 8.

Gao, Y., J. Lan, X. Dai, J. Ye and S. Zhou. 2004b. A Phase I/II Study of Ling Zhi Mushroom *Ganoderma lucidum* (W.Curt.:Fr.)Lloyd (*Aphyllophoromycetideae*) Extract in Patients with Type II Diabetes Mellitus. Int J Med Mushrooms 6 (1): 3–9.

Grundy, S. M., N. J. Stone, A. L. Bailey, C. Beam, K. K. Birtcher, R. S. Blumenthal, L. T. Braun, S. de Ferranti, J. Faiella-Tommasino, D. E. Forman, R. Goldberg, P. A. Heidenreich, M. A. Hlatky, D. W. Jones, D. Lloyd-Jones, N. Lopez-Pajares, C. E. Ndumele, C. E. Orringer, C. A. Peralta, J. J. Saseen, S. C. Smith, Jr., L. Sperling, S. S. Virani and J. Yeboah. 2019. 2018 AHA/ACC/AACVPR/AAPA/ABC/ACPM/ADA/AGS/APhA/ASPC/NLA/PCNA Guideline on the Management of Blood Cholesterol: Executive Summary: A Report of the American College of Cardiology/American Heart Association Task Force on Clinical Practice Guidelines. Circulation 139 (25): e1046–e1081.

Hardman, T. C., P. Rutherford, S. W. Dubrey and A. S. Wierzbicki. 2010. Sodium-glucose co-transporter 2 inhibitors: From apple tree to 'Sweet Pee'. Curr Pharm Des 16 (34): 3830–3838.

Hennicke, F., Z. Cheikh-Ali, T. Liebisch, J. G. Maciá-Vicente, H. B. Bode and M. Piepenbring. 2016. Distinguishing commercially grown Ganoderma lucidum from Ganoderma lingzhi from Europe and East Asia on the basis of morphology, molecular phylogeny, and triterpenic acid profiles. Phytochemistry 127: 29–37.

Hikino, H., M. Ishiyama, Y. Suzuki and C. Konno. 1989. Mechanisms of hypoglycemic activity of ganoderan B: A glycan of Ganoderma lucidum fruit bodies. Planta Med 55 (5): 423–8.

Hikino, H., C. Konno, Y. Mirin and T. Hayashi. 1985. Isolation and Hypoglycemic Activity of Ganoderans A and B, Glycans of Ganoderma lucidum Fruit Bodies1. Planta Med 51 (4): 339–340.

Hsu, K. D. and K. C. Cheng. 2018. From nutraceutical to clinical trial: Frontiers in Ganoderma development. Appl Microbiol Biotechnol 102 (21): 9037–9051.

Johansen, J. S., A. K. Harris, D. J. Rychly and A. Ergul. 2005. Oxidative stress and the use of antioxidants in diabetes: Linking basic science to clinical practice. Cardiovasc Diabetol 4: 5.

Kabir, Y., S. Kimura and T. Tamura. 1988. Dietary effect of Ganoderma Lucidum Mushroom on Blood Pressure and Lipid Levels in Spontaneously Hypertensive Rats (SHR). J Nutr Sci Vitaminol (Tokyo) 34 (4): 433–438.

Kanmatsuse, K., N. Kajiwara, K. Hayashi, S. Shimogaichi, I. Fukinbara, H. Ishikawa and T. Tamura. 1985. [Studies on Ganoderma lucidum. I. Efficacy against hypertension and side effects]. Yakugaku Zasshi 105 (10): 942–947.

Kao, C. H. J., A. C. Jesuthasan, K. S. Bishop, M. P. Glucina and L. R. Ferguson. 2013. Anticancer Activities of Ganoderma Lucidum: Active Ingredients and Pathways. Funct Foods Health Dis 3 (2): 48–65.

Kim, M. Y., P. Seguin, J. K. Ahn, J. J. Kim, S. C. Chun, E. H. Kim, S. H. Seo, E. Y. Kang, S. L. Kim, Y. J. Park, H. M. Ro and I. M. Chung. 2008. Phenolic Compound Concentration and Antioxidant Activities of Edible and Medicinal Mushrooms from Korea. Journal of Agricultural and Food Chemistry 56 (16): 7265–7270.

Kino, K., A. Yamashita, K. Yamaoka, J. Watanabe, S. Tanaka, K. Ko, K. Shimizu and H. Tsunoo. 1989. Isolation and Characterization of a New Immunomodulatory Protein, Ling Zhi-8 (LZ-8), from Ganoderma lucidium. J Biol Chem 264 (1): 472–478.

Klupp, N. L., D. Chang, F. Hawke, H. Kiat, H. Cao, S. J. Grant and A. Bensoussan. 2015. Ganoderma Lucidum Mushroom for the Treatment of Cardiovascular Risk Factors. Cochrane Database Syst Rev Issue 2: Art. No.: CD007259.

Klupp, N. L., H. Kiat, A. Bensoussan, G. Z. Steiner and D. H. Chang. 2016. A Double-Blind, Randomised, Placebo-Controlled Trial of Ganoderma Lucidum for the Treatment of Cardiovascular Risk Factors of Metabolic Syndrome. Sci Rep 6: 29540.

Kozarski, M., A. Klaus, M. Nikšić, M. M. Vrvić, N. Todorović, D. Jakovljević and L. J. L. D. Van Griensven. 2012. Antioxidative Activities and Chemical Characterization of Polysaccharide Extracts from the Widely Used Mushrooms Ganoderma Applanatum, Ganoderma Lucidum, Lentinus Edodes and Trametes Versicolor. J Food Compost Anal 26 (1): 144–153.

Krishna, K. V., V. Karuppuraj and K. Perumal. 2016. Antioxidant Activity and Folic Acid Content in Indigenous Isolates of Ganoderma Lucidum. Asian J Pharm Anal 6 (4): 213–215.

Kumaran, S., P. Palani, R. Nishanthi and V. Kaviyarasan. 2011. Studies on Screening, Isolation and Purification of a Fibrinolytic Protease from an Isolate (VK12) of Ganoderma Lucidum and Evaluation of Its Antithrombotic Activity. Med Mycol J 52 (2): 153–162.

Lasukova, T. V., L. N. Maslov, A. G. Arbuzov, V. N. Burkova and L. I. Inisheva. 2015. Cardioprotective Activity of Ganoderma lucidum Extract during Total Ischemia and Reperfusion of Isolated Heart. Bull Exp Biol Med 158 (6): 739–741.

Libby, P. 2021. Inflammation in Atherosclerosis-No Longer a Theory. Clin Chem 67 (1): 131–142.

Lin, J. M., C. C. Lin, H. F. Chiu, J. J. Yang and S. G. Lee. 1993. Evaluation of the Anti-Inflammatory and Liver-Protective Effects of Anoectochilus Formosanus, Ganoderma Lucidum and Gynostemma Pentaphyllum in Rats. Am J Chin Med 21 (1): 59–69.

Mach, F., C. Baigent, A. L. Catapano, K. C. Koskinas, M. Casula, L. Badimon, M. J. Chapman, G. G. De Backer, V. Delgado, B. A. Ference, I. M. Graham, A. Halliday, U. Landmesser, B. Mihaylova, T. R. Pedersen, G. Riccardi, D. J. Richter, M. S. Sabatine, M. R. Taskinen, L. Tokgozoglu, O. Wiklund and E. S. C. S. D. Group. 2020. 2019 ESC/EAS Guidelines for the management of dyslipidaemias: Lipid modification to reduce cardiovascular risk. Eur Heart J 41 (1): 111–188.

McGuffin, M., C. Hobbs, R. Upton and A. Goldberg. 1997. *American Herbal Products Association's botanical safety handbook*. Boca Raton, US: CRC Press.

Mohamad Ansor, N., N. Abdullah and N. Aminudin. 2013. Anti-Angiotensin Converting Enzyme (ACE) Proteins from Mycelia of Ganoderma Lucidum (Curtis) P. Karst. BMC Complement Altern Med 13: 256.

Pan, D., L. Wang, C. Chen, B. Hu and P. Zhou. 2015. Isolation and Characterization of a Hyperbranched Proteoglycan from Ganoderma Lucidum for Anti-Diabetes. Carbohydr Polym 117: 106–114.

Pan, D., L. Wang, B. Hu and P. Zhou. 2014. Structural Characterization and Bioactivity Evaluation of an Acidic Proteoglycan Extract from Ganoderma Lucidum Fruiting Bodies for PTP1B Inhibition and Anti-Diabetes. Biopolymers 101 (6): 613–623.

Pan, D., D. Zhang, J. Wu, C. Chen, Z. Xu, H. Yang and P. Zhou. 2013. Antidiabetic, Antihyperlipidemic and Antioxidant Activities of a Novel Proteoglycan from Ganoderma Lucidum Fruiting Bodies on db/db Mice and the Possible Mechanism. PLoS One 8 (7): e68332.

Rahman, M. A., N. Abdullah and N. Aminudin. 2018. Evaluation of the Antioxidative and Hypo-Cholesterolemic Effects of Lingzhi or Reishi Medicinal Mushroom, Ganoderma Lucidum (Agaricomycetes), in Ameliorating Cardiovascular Disease. International Journal of Medicinal Mushrooms 20 (10): 961–969.

Rizal, A., F. Sandra, M. R. Fadlan and D. Sargowo. 2020. Ganoderma Lucidum Polysaccharide Peptide Reduce Inflammation and Oxidative Stress in Patient with Atrial Fibrillation. Indones Biomed J 12 (4): 384–389.

Sargowo, D., C. R. 'Aissy, U. Kalsum, F. W. Nugroho, P. A. Kamila, D. Irawan, M. Sitio, L. H. Adrian, A. R. Pratama, Y. Arifin, R. Fadlan, D. I. Sari, E. F. Purwanto, F. N. Rahmah, M. P. Sukatman, N. A. Rahmawati and R. Fahmiy. 2019. The role of polysaccharide peptide of Ganoderma lucidum as a potent protective vascular endothelial cell, anti inflammation, and antioxidant in STEMI and NSTEMI patients. AIP Conference Proceedings 2108 (1): 020004.

Sarker, M. M. R. 2015. Antihyperglycemic, Insulin-Sensitivity and Anti-Hyperlipidemic Potential of Ganoderma Lucidum, a Dietary Mushroom, Onalloxan-and Glucocorticoid-Induced Diabetic Long-Evans Rats. Funct Foods Health Dis 5 (12): 450–466.

Seto, S. W., T. Y. Lam, H. L. Tam, A. L. Au, S. W. Chan, J. H. Wu, P. H. Yu, G. P. Leung, S. M. Ngai, J. H. Yeung, P. S. Leung, S. M. Lee and Y. W. Kwan. 2009. Novel Hypoglycemic Effects of Ganoderma Lucidum Water-Extract in Obese/Diabetic (+db/+db) Mice. Phytomedicine 16 (5): 426–436.

Sheena, N., T. A. Ajith and K. K. Janardhanan. 2003. Anti-inflammatory and Anti-Nociceptive Activities of Ganoderma lucidum Occurring in South India. Pharmaceutical Biology 41 (4): 301–304.

Shevelev, O. B., A. A. Seryapina, E. L. Zavjalov, L. A. Gerlinskaya, T. N. Goryachkovskaya, N. M. Slynko, L. V. Kuibida, S. E. Peltek, A. L. Markel and M. P. Moshkin. 2018. Hypotensive and Neurometabolic Effects of Intragastric Reishi (Ganoderma Lucidum) Administration in Hypertensive ISIAH Rat Strain. Phytomedicine 41: 1–6.

Shiao, M. S. 2003. Natural Products of the Medicinal Fungus Ganoderma Lucidum: Occurrence, Biological Activities, and Pharmacological Functions. Chem Rec 3 (3): 172–180.

Teng, B. S., C. D. Wang, H. J. Yang, J. S. Wu, D. Zhang, M. Zheng, Z. H. Fan, D. Pan and P. Zhou. 2011. A protein Tyrosine Phosphatase 1B Activity Inhibitor from the Fruiting Bodies of Ganoderma Lucidum (Fr.) Karst and Its Hypoglycemic Potency on Streptozotocin-Induced Type 2 Diabetic Mice. J Agric Food Chem 59 (12): 6492–500.

Teng, B. S., C. D. Wang, D. Zhang, J. S. Wu, D. Pan, L. F. Pan, H. J. Yang and P. Zhou. 2012. Hypoglycemic Effect and Mechanism of a Proteoglycan from Ganoderma Lucidum on Streptozotocin-Induced Type 2 Diabetic Rats. Eur Rev Med Pharmacol Sci 16 (2): 166–75.

Tomlinson, B., N. G. Patil, M. Fok and C. W. K. Lam. 2021. Managing Dyslipidemia in Patients with Type 2 Diabetes. Expert Opin Pharmacother 22 (16): 2221–2234.

Tran, H. B., A. Yamamoto, S. Matsumoto, H. Ito, K. Igami, T. Miyazaki, R. Kondo and K. Shimizu. 2014. Hypotensive Effects and Angiotensin-Converting Enzyme Inhibitory Peptides of Reishi (Ganoderma lingzhi) Auto-Digested Extract. Molecules 19 (9): 13473–13485.

van der Hem, L. G., J. A. van der Vliet, C. F. Bocken, K. Kino, A. J. Hoitsma and W. J. Tax. 1995. Ling Zhi-8: Studies of a New Immunomodulating Agent. Transplantation 60 (5): 438–443.

Vitak, T. Y., S. P. Wasser, E. Nevo and N. O. Sybirna. 2017. Enzymatic System of Antioxidant Protection of Erythrocytes in Diabetic Rats Treated with Medicinal Mushrooms Agaricus Brasiliensis and Ganoderma Lucidum (Agaricomycetes). Int J Med Mushrooms 19 (8): 697–708.

Wachtel-Galor, S., Y. T. Szeto, B. Tomlinson and I. F. Benzie. 2004a. Ganoderma Lucidum ('Lingzhi'); Acute and Short-Term Biomarker Response to Supplementation. Int J Food Sci Nutr 55 (1): 75–83.

Wachtel-Galor, S., B. Tomlinson and I. F. Benzie. 2004b. Ganoderma Lucidum ("Lingzhi"), a Chinese Medicinal Mushroom: Biomarker Responses in a Controlled Human Supplementation Study. Br J Nutr 91 (2): 263–269.

Wachtel-Galor, S., J. Yuen, J. A. Buswell and I. F. F. Benzie. 2011. "Ganoderma Lucidum (Lingzhi or Reishi): A Medicinal Mushroom" In Herbal Medicine: Biomolecular and Clinical Aspects. 2nd edition, edited by I.F.F. Benzie and S. Wachtel-Galor. Boca Raton (FL): CRC Press/Taylor & Francis.

Wang, C. W., J. S. M. Tschen and W. H. H. Sheu. 2008. Ganoderma Lucidum on Metabolic Control in Type 2 Diabetes Subjects – A Double Blinded Placebo Control Study. Journal of Internal Medicine of Taiwan 19: 54–60.

Wanmuang, H., J. Leopairut, C. Kositchaiwat, W. Wananukul and S. Bunyaratvej. 2007. Fatal Fulminant Hepatitis Associated with Ganoderma Lucidum (Lingzhi) Mushroom Powder. J Med Assoc Thai 90 (1): 179–181.

Wasser, S. P. 2010. Medicinal Mushroom Science: History, Current Status, Future Trends, and Unsolved Problems. Int J Med Mushrooms 12 (1): 1–16.

Whelton, P. K., R. M. Carey, W. S. Aronow, D. E. Casey, Jr., K. J. Collins, C. Dennison Himmelfarb, S. M. DePalma, S. Gidding, K. A. Jamerson, D. W. Jones, E. J. MacLaughlin, P. Muntner, B. Ovbiagele, S. C. Smith, Jr., C. C. Spencer, R. S. Stafford, S. J. Taler, R. J. Thomas, K. A. Williams, Sr., J. D. Williamson and J. T. Wright, Jr. 2018. 2017 ACC/AHA/AAPA/ABC/ACPM/AGS/APhA/ASH/ASPC/NMA/PCNA Guideline for the Prevention, Detection, Evaluation, and Management of High Blood Pressure in Adults: A Report of the American College of Cardiology/American Heart Association Task Force on Clinical Practice Guidelines. Circulation 138 (17): e484–e594.

Williams, B., G. Mancia, W. Spiering, E. Agabiti Rosei, M. Azizi, M. Burnier, D. L. Clement, A. Coca, G. de Simone, A. Dominiczak, T. Kahan, F. Mahfoud, J. Redon, L. Ruilope, A. Zanchetti, M. Kerins, S. E. Kjeldsen, R. Kreutz, S. Laurent, G. Y. H. Lip, R. McManus, K. Narkiewicz, F. Ruschitzka, R. E. Schmieder, E. Shlyakhto, C. Tsioufis, V. Aboyans, I. Desormais and E. S. C. S. D. Group. 2018. 2018 ESC/ESH Guidelines for the Management of Arterial Hypertension. Eur Heart J 39 (33): 3021–3104.

Winska, K., W. Maczka, K. Gabryelska and M. Grabarczyk. 2019. Mushrooms of the Genus Ganoderma Used to Treat Diabetes and Insulin Resistance. Molecules 24 (22).

Witters, L. A. 2001. The Blooming of the French Lilac. J Clin Invest 108 (8): 1105–1107.

Wu, Q., Y. Li, K. Peng, X. L. Wang, Z. Ding, L. Liu, P. Xu and G. Q. Liu. 2019. Isolation and Characterization of Three Antihypertension Peptides from the Mycelia of Ganoderma Lucidum (Agaricomycetes). J Agric Food Chem 67 (29): 8149–8159.

Xiao, C., Q. Wu, Y. Xie, J. Tan, Y. Ding and L. Bai. 2018. Hypoglycemic Mechanisms of Ganoderma Lucidum Polysaccharides F31 in db/db Mice via RNA-seq and iTRAQ. Food Funct 9 (12): 6495–6507.

Xiao, C., Q. Wu, J. Zhang, Y. Xie, W. Cai and J. Tan. 2017. Antidiabetic Activity of Ganoderma Lucidum Polysaccharides F31 Down-Regulated Hepatic Glucose Regulatory Enzymes in Diabetic Mice. J Ethnopharmacol 196: 47–57.

Xu, Z., X. Chen, Z. Zhong, L. Chen and Y. Wang. 2011. Ganoderma Lucidum Polysaccharides: Immunomodulation and Potential Anti-Tumor Activities. Am J Chin Med 39 (1): 15–27.

Yuen, M. F., P. Ip, W. K. Ng and C. L. Lai. 2004. Hepatotoxicity Due to a Formulation of Ganoderma Lucidum (lingzhi). J Hepatol 41 (4): 686–687.

Zhang, H. N., J. H. He, L. Yuan and Z. B. Lin. 2003. In Vitro and in Vivo Protective Effect of Ganoderma Lucidum Polysaccharides on Alloxan-Induced Pancreatic Islets Damage. Life Sci 73 (18): 2307–2319.

Zhang, H. N. and Z. B. Lin. 2004. Hypoglycemic Effect of Ganoderma Lucidum Polysaccharides. Acta Pharmacol Sin 25 (2): 191–195.

Zheng, J., B. Yang, Y. Yu, Q. Chen, T. Huang and D. Li. 2012. Ganoderma Lucidum Polysaccharides Exert Anti-Hyperglycemic Effect on Streptozotocin-Induced Diabetic Rats Through Affecting Beta-Cells. Comb Chem High Throughput Screen 15 (7): 542–550.

17 Mexican Orchid (*Prosthechea karwinskii*) and Use in Cardiovascular Protection
Cellular and Physiological Aspects

Luicita Lagunez Rivera, Gabriela Soledad Barragan Zarate, Rodolfo Solano, Alfonso Alexander Aguilera and Aracely E. Chavez Piña

CONTENTS

17.1 Introduction 260
    17.1.1 The Medicinal Knowledge of *Prosthechea karwinskii* 260
    17.1.2 Cardiovascular Protection of *Prosthechea karwinskii* 263
17.2 Compounds Identified in *P. karwinskii* and Their Protective Effect on Cardiovascular Risk 263
17.3 Decreased Weight and Pericardial Fat by *P. karwinskii* and Its Effect on Cardiovascular Risk 263
17.4 Hypoglycemic Effect of *P. karwinskii* and Its Effect on Cardiovascular Risk 272
17.5 Anti-Inflammatory Effect of *P. karwinskii* and Its Effect on Cardiovascular Risk 273
17.6 Increase in Adiponectin Levels by *P. karwinskii* Extract and Its Effect on Cardiovascular Risk 274
17.7 Capacity of *P. karwinskii* to Inhibit ROS and Its Effect on Cardiovascular Risk 275
17.8 Physiological Aspects Protected with *Prosthechea karwinskii* in Cardiovascular Risk 276
17.9 Toxicity and Cautionary Notes 276
17.10 Summary Points 276
References 276

LIST OF ABBREVIATIONS

CVD   Cardiovascular diseases
eNOS   Endothelial nitric oxide synthase
HDL   High-density lipoproteins
HS-CRP   High-sensitivity C-reactive protein
IR   Insulin resistance
MS   Metabolic syndrome
NO   Nitric oxide
$ONOO^-$ Peroxynitrite

DOI: 10.1201/9781003220329-19

ROS   Reactive oxygen species
TNF-α   Tumor necrosis factor alpha

17.1 INTRODUCTION

17.1.1 THE MEDICINAL KNOWLEDGE OF *PROSTHECHEA KARWINSKII*

Prosthechea karwinskii (Mart.) J.M.H. Shaw.
Cozticoatzontecoxochitl (Náhuatl, snake-shape yellow flower); monja amarilla (Spanish, yellow nun), ita ndeka amarilla (Mixtec, yellow flower growing on oak), Lirio amarillo (Spanish, yellow lily).

Prosthechea karwinskii is an epiphytic orchid, growing in oak forests, at 1850–2500 m elevation in western and southern Mexico (Solano et al. 2020). This species has yellow flowers producing a pleasant citrus fragrance (Figure 17.1). It has been culturally important and is one of the distinctive orchids in Mexican flora. In pre-Hispanic times the species was a source of mucilage used in

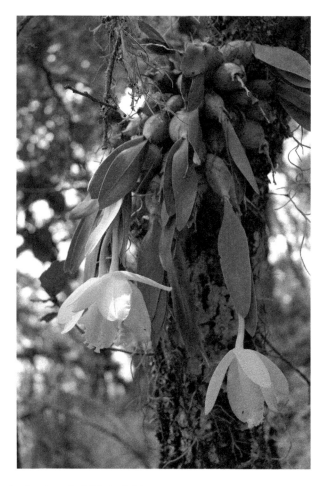

FIGURE 17.1 *Prosthechea karwinskii* in its habitat.
Source: Photo by R. Solano.

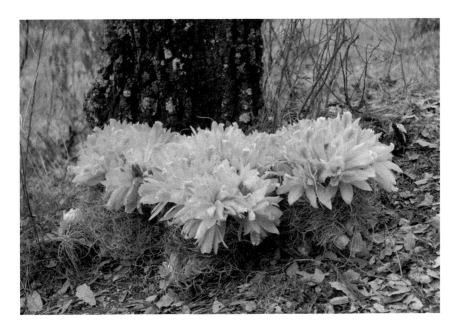

FIGURE 17.2 *Prosthechea karwinskii* are extracted from their habitat to be sold as ephemeral decorations in traditional markets, Oaxaca, Mexico.

Source: Photo by R. Solano.

plumeria (feather) art (Hágsater et al. 2005). During the Colonial period, this mucilage was used to make religious images used in Catholic processions because of their light weight.

During its blooming in spring, specimens of *P. karwinskii* are extracted from its habitat to be sold as ephemeral decorations in traditional markets in several Mexican cities; the species is one of the most extracted orchids in Mexico for local trade (Cruz-Garcia et al. 2015) (Figure 17.2). But there is also extraction that does not generate economic benefits, when specimens are extracted to be used as ornaments in Catholic temples during Easter (Solano et al. 2010) (Figure 17.3). In Mexico *P. karwinskii* is considered as a species at risk (SEMARNAT 2019) due to the extraction of specimens for trade and religious use, the transformation of its habitat, and the environmental effects caused by climate change (Solano and Huerta-Espinosa 2019; Solano et al. 2020).

This plant is part of a biocultural heritage in ethnicities from Oaxaca, Mexico. Like other orchids, *P. karwinskii* is considered as a fine flower, different from other plants because of its shape, size, color, and scent. For Mixtec people in Oaxaca, epiphytic orchids are named "ita ndeka," which means "flor que crece sobre encino" (flower growing on oak) in Spanish, because the species grows on these trees. To distinguish it from other epiphytic orchids, the flower color is added to the name, so for Mixtec the species is known as "ita ndeka amarilla" (yellow oak flower).

According to Cruz-Garcia et al. (2014) Mixtec use pseudobulbs, leaves, and flowers of *P. karwinskii* in the traditional medicine (Table 17.1). From pseudobulbs an infusion is prepared to treat cough and diabetes, consumed as drinking water; the pseudobulbs are also prepared as poultice to treat wounds and burns. The leaves are chewed, and the sap swallowed as treatment for diabetes. The flowers are used in an infusion to treat cough, to prevent spontaneous abortion, and to assist childbirth; sometimes "gordolobo" (cudweed, *Gnaphalium* sp.) branches are added to the infusion. Sometimes flower infusion seems to imply a magical or superstitious belief when a gold coin,

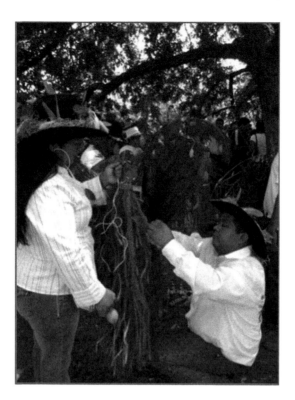

FIGURE 17.3 Hat adorned with *Prosthechea karwinskii* and *Disocactus ackermanii* flowers during Easter commemoration in Zaachila, Oaxaca, Mexico.

Source: Photo by G. Cruz-Lustre.

TABLE 17.1
Summary of Medicinal Practices Documented for *Prosthechea karwinskii* in Tlaxiaco, Oaxaca, Mexico.

Health Problem	Part of the Plant Used	Mode of Preparation	Doses
Cough	Pseudobulbs	Infusion	Three days
			Taken at the night
	Flowers	Infusion	Three days
		Two cudweed branches are added	Taken as drinking water
Burns and wounds	Pseudobulbs	Poultice	Until the burn or wound heals
Diabetes	Pseudobulbs	Infusion	Taken as drinking water
			Until obtaining stability in glucose levels
	Leaves	Chewed	Daily
			Until obtaining stability in glucose levels
To prevent spontaneous abortion, childbirth	Flowers	Infusion	During a month
		A gold coin or a jewel is added	Taken as drinking water
	Flowers	Infusion	Drinking for several days.
		A gold coin, a jewel, or a potter wasp is added	

Source: Based on Cruz-Garcia et al. (2014, Rev. Bras. Pharmacog.).

Mexican Orchid (*Prosthechea karwinskii*)

a jewel, or a potter wasp (*Eumenes* sp.) is added to it. *Prosthechea karwinskii* has potential for pharmacological research, thus it is necessary to evaluate its biological activity and identify the compounds responsible for it.

17.1.2 CARDIOVASCULAR PROTECTION OF *PROSTHECHEA KARWINSKII*

Cardiovascular diseases (CVD) are one of the leading causes of death worldwide (WHO 2018). Natural products such as phenolics have cardioprotective potential and are present in the orchid *P. karwinskii*. The evaluation in an animal model (Wistar rats) of the foliar extract of this plant affects parameters associated with CVD and metabolic syndrome (MS). Wistar rats with MS increased insulin resistance (IR), tumor necrosis factor-alpha (TNF-α), high-sensitivity C-reactive protein (HS-CRP) levels, and pericardial fat (all CVD factors), as well as a decrease in adiponectin levels, compared to healthy rats. The extract administered to rats with MS causes these parameters to change to the normal levels present in healthy rats. Since MS promotes the development of CVD (Zheng et al. 2020) and *P. karwinskii* extract can decrease cardiovascular risk in rats with MS, this means that *P. karwinskii* could be a natural product with potential in the treatment of CVD.

17.2 COMPOUNDS IDENTIFIED IN *P. KARWINSKII* AND THEIR PROTECTIVE EFFECT ON CARDIOVASCULAR RISK

Table 17.2 shows the compounds present in the leaves, flowers, and pseudobulbs of *P. karwinskii*. The compounds present in *P. karwinskii* extract with a history of protection against cardiovascular risk are chlorogenic acid, which has an antihypertensive effect by improving the bioavailability of nitric oxide (NO), improving endothelial function in the arterial vasculature (Zhao et al. 2012), and inhibiting platelet aggregation and thrombus formation (Fuentes et al. 2014); embelin, a compound which reduces isoproterenol-induced myocardial damage in rats by restoring myocardial antioxidant defense (Sahu et al. 2014); and rutin, which reverses vascular calcification (Su et al. 2022).

17.3 DECREASED WEIGHT AND PERICARDIAL FAT BY *P. KARWINSKII* AND ITS EFFECT ON CARDIOVASCULAR RISK

The administration of the extract to the diet in rats with MS decreased the weight of the rats, as well as the accumulation of pericardial fat (Figure 17.4). This effect has an impact on cardiovascular risk.

Weight reduction is essential as decreasing obesity may help reduce the risk of CVD by inhibiting inflammatory mechanisms (Hamjane et al. 2020). In obese patients, myocardiocytes are progressively replaced by adipocytes and irregular bands of fat tissue that determine an adverse global structural change of the heart with cardiac hypertrophy and contractile dysfunction (Formica et al. 2020).

Pericardial fat is also associated with CVD (Shah et al. 2017) and the development of coronary artery disease (Kahl et al. 2017). Increased levels of pericardial fat are associated with a high prevalence of cardiometabolic risk factors, including dysglycemia, dyslipidemia, hypertension, adiposity-associated inflammation (Shah et al. 2017), an increase in body mass index, abdominal circumference, triglyceride, and HS-CRP levels, as well as a decrease in high-density lipoprotein (HDL) levels (Joo 2017). Pericardial fat volume is also associated with heart problems such as increased left ventricular mass, left atrial enlargement, impaired left ventricular diastolic function, coronary artery disease, atherosclerosis, and adverse cardiovascular events (Drossos et al. 2014; Sharma et al. 2022).

TABLE 17.2

Compounds in the Different Parts of *Prosthechea karwinskii*

Compound	RT (min)	m/z (M-H)⁻	Compound (Chemical Formula)	Chemical Structure	Part of the Plant
1	0.65	179.0555	D-Tagatose[d] ($C_6H_{12}O_6$)		Flowers
2	0.7	191.0557	Quinic Acid[c] ($C_7H_{12}O_6$)		Leaves, pseudobulbs and flowers
3	0.8	133.0140	Malic acid[c] ($C_4H_6O_5$)		Leaves, pseudobulbs and flowers
4	1.2	117.0191	Succinic acid[c] ($C_4H_6O_4$)		Leaves, pseudobulbs and flowers
5	2.3	164.0712	L-(–)-Phenylalanine[d] ($C_9H_{11}NO_2$)		Leaves and flowers
6	2.7	282.0833	Guanosine[d] ($C_{10}H_{13}N_5O_5$)		Leaves and flowers

7	3.1	331.1025	1,3,4,6-tetra-O-acetyl-2-deoxyhexopyranose[e] ($C_{14}H_{20}O_9$)		Flowers
8	3.7	299.0762	1-O-salicyl-D-glucose[e] ($C_{13}H_{16}O_8$)		Flowers
9	6.0	353.0867	Neochlorogenic acid[b] ($C_{16}H_{18}O_9$)		Leaves and pseudobulbs
10	6.1	145.0502	3-Methylglutaric acid[d] ($C_6H_{10}O_4$)		Pseudobulbs

(*Continued*)

TABLE 17.2 *(Continued)*

Compounds in the Different Parts of *Prosthechea karwinskii*

Compound	RT (min)	m/z (M-H)⁻	Compound (Chemical Formula)	Chemical Structure	Part of the Plant
11	6.3	353.0866	Chlorogenic acid[b] ($C_{16}H_{18}O_9$)		Leaves and pseudobulbs
12	6.0	329.0866	1-O-vanilloyl-beta-D-glucose[e] ($C_{14}H_{18}O_9$)		Flowers
13	6.2	451.2170	Calaliukiuenoside[e] ($C_{20}H_{36}O_{11}$)		Flowers

| 14 | 6.4 | 403.1595 | 2-Methyl-2-propanyl 2,3,4,6-tetra-O-acetyl-D-glucopiranoside[e] ($C_{18}H_{28}O_{10}$) | | Flowers |
| 15 | 6.5 | 609.1438 | Rutin[a,d] ($C_{27}H_{30}O_{16}$) | | Leaves and pseudobulbs |

(*Continued*)

TABLE 17.2 *(Continued)*

Compounds in the Different Parts of *Prosthechea karwinskii*

Compound	RT (min)	m/z (M-H)⁻	Compound (Chemical Formula)	Chemical Structure	Part of the Plant
16	6.6	593.1489	Kaempferol-3-O-rutinoside[d] ($C_{27}H_{30}O_{15}$)		Leaves
17	6.6	217.1074	2-Hydroxysebacic acid[d] ($C_{10}H_{18}O_5$)		Pseudobulbs
18	6.6	425.1800	(+)-abscisic acid β-D-glucopyranosyl ester[e] ($C_{21}H_{30}O_9$)		Flowers

19	6.7	Myricitrin-5-methyl ether[e] ($C_{22}H_{22}O_{12}$)	Flowers
20	6.8	Azelaic acid[e] ($C_9H_{16}O_4$)	Leaves, pseudobulbs and flowers
21	7.0	Phloridzin[d] ($C_{21}H_{24}O_{10}$)	Pseudobulbs
22	7.2	Sebacic acid[e] ($C_{10}H_{18}O_4$)	Leaves and pseudobulbs

(Continued)

TABLE 17.2 *(Continued)*

Compounds in the Different Parts of *Prosthechea karwinskii*

Compound	RT (min)	m/z (M-H)⁻	Compound (Chemical Formula)	Chemical Structure	Part of the Plant
23	7.2	263.1278	Abscisic acid[d] ($C_{15}H_{20}O_4$)		Flowers
24	8.0	242.1756	N-undecanoylglycine[e] ($C_{13}H_{25}NO_3$)		Leaves and pseudobulbs
25	8.2	329.2321	Pinellic acid[e] ($C_{18}H_{34}O_5$)		Leaves, pseudobulbs and flowers
26	8.8	359.2063	(1R,3S,4R)-1-[(3R-4S-6R)-3,4,5,6-tetrahydroxy-6-methoxy-hexoxy] hexane-1,2,3,4,6-pentol[c] ($C_{13}H_{28}O_{11}$)		Flowers

| 27 | 9.2 | 329.1379 | Gibberellin A7[c] (C$_{19}$H$_{22}$O$_5$) | | Pseudobulbs |
| 28 | 11.5 | 293.2112 | Embelin[e] (C$_{17}$H$_{26}$O$_4$) | | Leaves |

Source: Superscripts correspond to the reference used for identifying the compound: [a]De Souza et al. (2016), [b]Liu et al. (2016), [c]MassBank library, [d]Bruker's MetaboBase library, [e]Compound-Crawler. RT: Retention time.

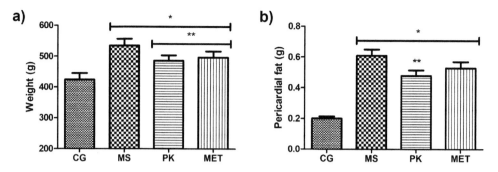

FIGURE 17.4 Weight gain and pericardial fat at the end of the experimental diet with *Prosthechea karwinskii* extract.

Note: Values expressed as mean ± standard deviation (n = 5). * Indicates a significant difference ($p < 0.05$) with respect to CG. **Indicates a significant difference ($p < 0.05$) with respect to MS. CG = control group, MS = group with metabolic syndrome, PK = group with metabolic syndrome and extract at a dose of 300 mg/kg p.o., MET = group with metabolic syndrome and metformin at a dose of 200 mg/kg p.o.

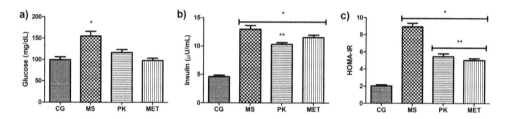

FIGURE 17.5 Effect of *Prosthechea karwinskii* extract on glucose levels, insulin, and HOMA-IR index.

Note: Values expressed as mean ± standard deviation (n = 5). * Indicates a significant difference ($p < 0.05$) with respect to CG. **Indicates a significant difference ($p < 0.05$) with respect to MS. CG = control group, MS = group with metabolic syndrome, PK = group with metabolic syndrome and extract at a dose of 300 mg/kg p.o., MET = group with metabolic syndrome and metformin at a dose of 200 mg/kg p.o., HOMA-IR = Homeostatic Model Assessment of Insulin Resistance.

17.4 HYPOGLYCEMIC EFFECT OF *P. KARWINSKII* AND ITS EFFECT ON CARDIOVASCULAR RISK

The leaves and pseudobulbs of the orchid are used in traditional medicine to treat diabetes (Cruz-Garcia et al. 2014). As seen in Figure 17.5, *P. karwinskii* extract can decrease glucose, insulin, and IR levels in rats with MS; this decreases cardiovascular risk.

High insulin levels as well as IR induce the formation of atheroma plaques and increase peripheral vascular resistance, leading to cardiovascular complications (Formica et al. 2020). Insulin plays an important role in metabolic and cardiovascular homeostasis, as it stimulates NO production in vascular endothelial cells, inducing vasodilatation with increased blood flow, reduced NO production is a hallmark condition of IR (Formica et al. 2020; Andreadi et al. 2021). NO has an important role in reducing platelet aggregation and local inflammation, thus preventing atherosclerotic disease (Wu and Meininger 2009; Formica et al. 2020).

Insulin resistance is a cardiovascular risk factor in subjects with and without diabetes, independent of other cardiovascular risk factors. IR is associated with a latent vascular injury even before the clinical onset of diabetes, and lowering IR has beneficial effects on cardiovascular health in healthy subjects and diabetic patients (Adeva-Andany et al. 2019).

Diabetes is associated with pathological changes in the cardiovascular system, including microvascular and macrovascular abnormalities. Microvascular complications involve capillary damage that reduces glucose and insulin delivery to skeletal muscle, making glucose uptake difficult. Macrovascular damage affects larger blood vessels and is manifested through impaired endothelial function, increased arterial stiffness, elevated resting blood pressure, abnormal blood lipid profiles, reduced oxygen supply to tissues, and often results in myocardial ischemia (Brown et al. 2020).

Diabetes is associated with an increased risk of heart failure, commonly referred to as diabetic cardiomyopathy, which is characterized by increased cardiac fibrosis, pathological hypertrophy, increased oxidative and endoplasmic reticulum stress, and diastolic dysfunction. Diabetic lesions in the myocardium contribute to the development of the impaired cardiac function, and a progression of the disease called diabetic cardiomyopathy (Sharma et al. 2022).

17.5 ANTI-INFLAMMATORY EFFECT OF *P. KARWINSKII* AND ITS EFFECT ON CARDIOVASCULAR RISK

Prosthechea karwinskii extract was able to decrease the pro-inflammatory state of metabolic syndrome rats with decreased levels of TNF-α (Figure 17.6) and HS-CRP (Figure 17.7). This decrease in the pro-inflammatory state decreases the cardiovascular risk presented.

Inflammatory mediators accelerate the progression of CVD, as chronic inflammation contributes to atherogenesis. Systemic inflammation has also been associated with heart failure, atrial fibrillation, and acute myocardial infarction (Silva Dias et al. 2022).

Elevated levels of TNF-α are associated with an increased risk of cardiovascular diseases such as atherothrombotic disease (coronary artery disease and ischemic stroke) and venous thromboembolism. Inhibition of TNF-α in patients with rheumatoid arthritis decreases carotid intima-medial thickness and aortic stiffness, also reduces the risk of cardiovascular events such as myocardial infarction and stroke (Yuan et al. 2020). Elevated TNF-α levels are associated with abdominal obesity and increased risk of myocardial injury in humans (Hamjane et al. 2020).

Following the increase in dysfunctional adipose tissue, several inflammatory mediators increase, including HS-CRP, which exerts prothrombotic and antifibrinolytic effects on endothelial cells and contributes to plaque formation through the generation of foam cells in blood vessels (Formica

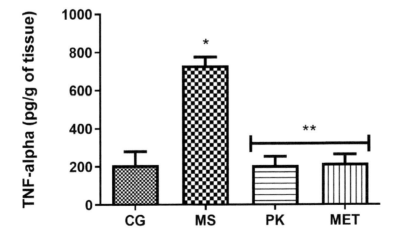

FIGURE 17.6 Effect of *Prosthechea karwinskii* leaves extract on TNF-α levels.

Note: Values expressed as mean ± standard deviation (n = 5). * Indicates a significant difference ($p < 0.05$) with respect to CG. **Indicates a significant difference ($p < 0.05$) with respect to MS. CG = control group, MS = metabolic syndrome group, PK = metabolic syndrome group treated with 300 mg/kg extract p.o., MET = metabolic syndrome group treated with 200 mg/kg metformin p.o.

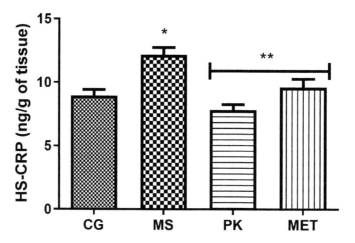

FIGURE 17.7 Effect of *Prosthechea karwinskii* leaves extract on HS-CRP levels.

Note: Values expressed as mean ± standard deviation (n = 5). * Indicates a significant difference ($p < 0.05$) with respect to CG. **Indicates a significant difference ($p < 0.05$) with respect to MS. CG = control group, MS = metabolic syndrome group, PK = metabolic syndrome group treated with 300 mg/kg extract p.o., MET = metabolic syndrome group treated with 200 mg/kg metformin p.o.

et al. 2020). HS-CRP is a marker of inflammation that is recommended to be measured as part of coronary risk assessment (Ajmal et al. 2014). Increased HS-CRP levels are related to several aspects of MS and CVD (Mirhafez et al. 2016; Yoon et al. 2018); this parameter is a predictor of risk for hypertension and cardiovascular events (Ridker et al. 2008).

17.6 INCREASE IN ADIPONECTIN LEVELS BY *P. KARWINSKII* EXTRACT AND ITS EFFECT ON CARDIOVASCULAR RISK

The administration of *P. karwinskii* extract increased adiponectin levels to levels similar to those of the control group, as shown in Figure 17.8. This increase in adiponectin levels by the extract has a cardioprotective effect.

Adiponectin is a protein found not only in adipose tissues but also in hepatocytes, skeletal muscle, bone cells, and cardiomyocytes (Silva Dias et al. 2022). Cardiomyocyte-derived adiponectin is biologically active and protects cardiomyocytes from ischemia-reperfusion injury and directly impacts cardiac metabolism; it can also prevent cardiomyocyte hypertrophy, cardiac fibrosis, oxidative stress, and inflammation, all of which are commonly associated with cardiomyopathy and diastolic dysfunction. There is also an association between low adiponectin levels and the progression of left ventricular hypertrophy (Sharma et al. 2022).

Adiponectin exerts beneficial effects on the vascular endothelium, where it increases endothelial nitric oxide synthase (eNOS) activity and NO production. It also inhibits the expression of reactive oxygen species (ROS) and TNF-α, leading to a reduction in the expression of adhesion molecules, contributing to the control of inflammation and endothelial dysfunction. Adiponectin deficiency promotes cardiac hypertrophy, fibrosis, and remodeling, which are key factors of diastolic dysfunction by promoting left ventricular wall stiffness (Sharma et al. 2022).

Adiponectin is secreted by adipocytes and acts in anti-atherogenesis and vasodilation (Srikanthan et al. 2016). Depletion of this hormone contributes to the pathogenesis of CVD (Calle et al. 2012; Ghadge et al. 2018); low levels of adiponectin are predictors of myocardial infarction (Nakamura et al. 2004; Pischon et al. 2004; Ghadge et al. 2018). On the other hand, adiponectin is inversely correlated with hypertension (Hamjane et al. 2020).

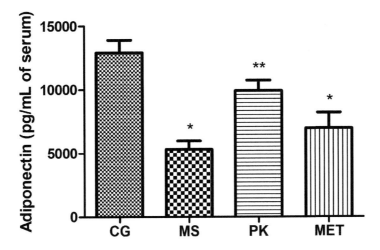

FIGURE 17.8 Effect of *Prosthechea karwinskii* leaves extract on adiponectin levels.

Note: Values are expressed as mean ± standard deviation (n = 5). * Indicates a significant difference ($p < 0.05$) with respect to CG. ** Indicates a significant difference ($p < 0.05$) with respect to MS. CG = control group, MS = metabolic syndrome group, PK = metabolic syndrome group treated with 300 mg/kg extract p.o., MET = metabolic syndrome group treated with 200 mg/kg metformin p.o.

TABLE 17.3
Inhibition of ROS by *Prosthechea karwinskii* Leaves Extract at Different Concentrations

Extract Concentration (µg/mL)	ROS Inhibition (%)
10	23.15 ± 6.02*
100	40.81 ± 8.23**
250	55.40 ± 7.49***
500	68.26 ± 7.48***
1000	68.24 ± 2.89***

Note: Values are expressed as mean ± standard deviation (n = 5). Different superscripts indicate significant differences ($p < 0.05$). ROS = Reactive oxygen species.

17.7 CAPACITY OF *P. KARWINSKII* TO INHIBIT ROS AND ITS EFFECT ON CARDIOVASCULAR RISK

Prosthechea karwinskii leaves extract can inhibit ROS in peripheral blood mononuclear cells as seen in Table 17.3. Inhibition of ROS decreases cardiovascular risk.

Reactive oxygen species are important messengers in the heart, involved in multiple physiological processes, such as differentiation, proliferation, and excitation-contraction coupling. However, when ROS production exceeds the buffering capacity of the heart's antioxidant defense systems, oxidative stress arises, resulting in cardiac dysfunction, ischemia-reperfusion injury, hypertrophy, cell death, and heart failure. In addition, O^{2-} is one of the ROS that can react with NO, leading to the generation of peroxynitrite ($ONOO^-$) and endothelial dysfunction. In the heart, all these events could trigger cardiomyocyte dysfunction and death through apoptosis and cause contractile dysfunction, cardiac remodeling, fibrosis, hypertrophy, and heart failure. Cardiomyocyte apoptosis plays an important role in the development of cardiovascular diseases (D'Oria et al. 2020).

Excessive ROS generation and oxidative stress are directly associated with cardiovascular diseases, as cardiac tissue is more susceptible to oxidative stress than other tissues, due to lower antioxidant enzyme activity in cardiac tissues (Sahu et al. 2014).

17.8 PHYSIOLOGICAL ASPECTS PROTECTED WITH *PROSTHECHEA KARWINSKII* IN CARDIOVASCULAR RISK

Obesity favors the development of cardiovascular disease through ectopic lipid deposition, hyperglycemia, and the development of a procoagulant state (Meghatria et al. 2021). Obesity is further considered a state of chronic inflammation (Ballak et al. 2015; El-shiekh et al. 2019), where adipose tissue plays an essential role in the regulation of glucose and lipid metabolism through the secretion of inflammation-related cytokines such as adiponectin and TNF-α (Ghadge et al. 2018). Changes in heart structure may precede for several years the manifestation of dilated cardiomyopathy and heart failure. In this regard, adipose tissue can be considered a very active player in the innate immune response, in which adipocytes and macrophages are intertwined in a paracrine loop and contribute to chronic low-grade inflammation that represents a favorable niche for widespread cardiovascular damage (Formica et al. 2020).

Prosthechea karwinskii orchid decreases cardiovascular risk, as it has been shown to have the ability to reduce obesity by decreasing body weight, as well as accumulated pericardial fat; it also reduced IR, inflammatory status by decreasing TNF-α and HS-CRP, decreased ROS, and increased adiponectin levels in rats with metabolic syndrome. All these are risk factors that generate an environment conducive to the development of cardiovascular diseases, so the orchid could reduce the onset and progression of these diseases.

17.9 TOXICITY AND CAUTIONARY NOTES

Although no toxicological studies have been conducted on *Prosthechea karwinskii* orchid to date, studies have been conducted in animal models of inflammation, gastric damage, and metabolic syndrome in Wistar rats. In these evaluations, doses ranging from 100 mg/kg to 1000 mg/kg have been administered and no indicators of toxicity were observed in the animals. In the metabolic syndrome model, the extract was administered at doses of 100, 200, and 300 mg/kg for 4 weeks, and nothing was observed to indicate any type of damage in the behavior of the rats, nor in the measured parameters or organs.

17.10 SUMMARY POINTS

- This chapter focuses on the potential of the *Prosthechea karwinskii* orchid to treat cardiovascular diseases.
- The *Prosthechea karwinskii* orchid is endemic to southern Mexico.
- This plant is used in traditional medicine to treat problems such as diabetes, coughs, wounds, burns, to prevent miscarriage, and is used in labor.
- The orchid can decrease cardiovascular risk by decreasing obesity, insulin resistance, inflammation, reactive oxygen species, and increasing adiponectin levels.
- Compounds present in the orchid also have the potential to treat cardiovascular problems.

REFERENCES

Adeva-Andany, María M., Julia Martínez-Rodríguez, Manuel González-Lucán, Carlos Fernández-Fernández, and Elvira Castro-Quintela. 2019. "Insulin Resistance Is a Cardiovascular Risk Factor in Humans." *Diabetes and Metabolic Syndrome: Clinical Research and Reviews* 13 (2): 1449–1455. doi:10.1016/j.dsx.2019.02.023.

Ajmal, Masihur Rehman, Monika Yaccha, Mohammed Azharuddin Malik, M. U. Rabbani, Ibne Ahmad, Najmul Isalm, and Nasar Abdali. 2014. "Prevalence of Nonalcoholic Fatty Liver Disease (NAFLD) in Patients of Cardiovascular Diseases and Its Association with Hs-CRP and TNF-α." *Indian Heart Journal* 66 (6). Elsevier Ltd and IIR: 574–579. doi:10.1016/j.ihj.2014.08.006.

Andreadi, Aikaterini, Alfonso Bellia, Nicola Di Daniele, Marco Meloni, Renato Lauro, David Della-Morte, and Davide Lauro. 2022. "The Molecular Link between Oxidative Stress, Insulin Resistance, and Type 2 Diabetes: A Target for New Therapies against Cardiovascular Diseases." *Current Opinion in Pharmacology* 62 (Dm). Elsevier Ltd: 85–96. doi:10.1016/j.coph.2021.11.010.

Ballak, Dov B., Rinke Stienstra, Cees J. Tack, Charles A. Dinarello, and Janna A. van Diepen. 2015. "IL-1 Family Members in the Pathogenesis and Treatment of Metabolic Disease: Focus on Adipose Tissue Inflammation and Insulin Resistance." *Cytokine* 75 (2). Elsevier Ltd: 280–290. doi:10.1016/j.cyto.2015.05.005.

Brown, Elise C., Barry A. Franklin, Judith G. Regensteiner, and Kerry J. Stewart. 2020. "Effects of Single Bout Resistance Exercise on Glucose Levels, Insulin Action, and Cardiovascular Risk in Type 2 Diabetes: A Narrative Review." *Journal of Diabetes and Its Complications* 34 (8). Elsevier Inc.: 107610. doi:10.1016/j.jdiacomp.2020.107610.

Calle, M. C., and M. L. Fernandez. 2012. "Inflammation and Type 2 Diabetes." *Diabetes and Metabolism* 38 (3). Elsevier Masson SAS: 183–191. doi:10.1016/j.diabet.2011.11.006.

Cruz-Garcia, Gabriela, Rodolfo Solano, and Luicita Lagunez-Rivera. 2014. "Documentation of the Medicinal Knowledge of *Prosthechea Karwinskii* in a Mixtec Community in Mexico Gabriela Cruz Garcia." *Revista Brasileira de* Farmacognosia 24: 153–58. doi:http://dx.doi.org/10.1016/j.bjp.2014.03.002.

Cruz-Garcia, Gabriela, Luicita Lagunez-Rivera, Manuel Gerardo Chavez-Angeles, and Rodolfo Solano. 2015. "The wild orchid trade in a Mexican local market: Diversity and economics." Economic Botany 69: 291–305. doi:10.1007/s12231-015-9321-z.

D'Oria, Rossella, Rossella Schipani, Anna Leonardini, Annalisa Natalicchio, Sebastio Perrini, Angelo Cignarelli, Luigi Laviola, and Francesco Giorgino. 2020. "The Role of Oxidative Stress in Cardiac Disease: From Physiological Response to Injury Factor." *Oxidative Medicine and Cellular Longevity* 2020. doi:10.1155/2020/5732956.

Drossos, George, Charilaos Panagiotis Koutsogiannidis, Olga Ananiadou, George Kapsas, Fotini Ampatzidou, Athanasios Madesis, Kalliopi Bismpa, Panagiotis Palladas, and Labros Karagounis. 2014. "Pericardial Fat Is Strongly Associated with Atrial Fibrillation after Coronary Artery Bypass Graft Surgery." *European Journal of Cardio-Thoracic Surgery* 46 (6): 1014–1020. doi:10.1093/ejcts/ezu043.

El-shiekh, Riham A., Dalia A. Al-Mahdy, Samar M. Mouneir, Mohamed S. Hifnawy, and Essam A. Abdel-Sattar. 2019. "Anti-Obesity Effect of Argel (Solenostemma Argel) on Obese Rats Fed a High Fat Diet." *Journal of Ethnopharmacology* 238. Elsevier B.V.: 111893. doi:10.1016/j.jep.2019.111893.

Formica, V., C. Morelli, S. Riondino, N. Renzi, D. Nitti, N. Di Daniele, M. Roselli, and M. Tesauro. 2020. "Obesity and Common Pathways of Cancer and Cardiovascular Disease." *Endocrine and Metabolic Science* 1 (3–4). Elsevier Ltd: 100065. doi:10.1016/j.endmts.2020.100065.

Fuentes, Eduardo, Julio Caballero, Marcelo Alarcón, Armando Rojas, and Iván Palomo. 2014. "Chlorogenic Acid Inhibits Human Platelet Activation and Thrombus Formation." *PLoS ONE* 9 (3): 1–14. doi:10.1371/journal.pone.0090699.

Ghadge, Abhijit A., Amrita A. Khaire, and Aniket A. Kuvalekar. 2018. "Adiponectin: A Potential Therapeutic Target for Metabolic Syndrome." *Cytokine and Growth Factor Reviews* 39. Elsevier Ltd: 151–158. doi:10.1016/j.cytogfr.2018.01.004.

Hágsater, E., M. Á. Soto-Arenas, G. A. Salazar-Chávez, R. Jiménez-Machorro, M. A. López-Rosas, and R. L. Dressler. 2005. "Las orquídeas de México." *Instituto Chinoín México*, D.F. 304 pp

Hamjane, Nadia, Fatiha Benyahya, Naima Ghailani Nourouti, Mohcine Bennani Mechita, and Amina Barakat. 2020. "Cardiovascular Diseases and Metabolic Abnormalities Associated with Obesity: What Is the Role of Inflammatory Responses? A Systematic Review." *Microvascular Research* 131 (May). Elsevier: 104023. doi:10.1016/j.mvr.2020.104023.

Joo, N. S. 2017. "Cutoff Value of Pericardial Adipose Tissues in Association with Metabolic Syndrome in Aging Koreans." *Maturitas* 100, 184. doi:10.1016/j.maturitas.2017.03.220.

Kahl, K. G., J. Herrmann, B. Stubbs, T. H. C. Krüger, J. Cordes, M. Deuschle, U. Schweiger, et al. 2017. "Pericardial Adipose Tissue and the Metabolic Syndrome Is Increased in Patients with Chronic Major Depressive Disorder Compared to Acute Depression and Controls." *Progress in Neuro-Psychopharmacology and Biological Psychiatry* 72. Elsevier B.V.: 30–35. doi:10.1016/j.pnpbp.2016.08.005.

Liu, Qingfeng, Jiao, Zheng, Liu, Yi, Li, Zhong, Shi, Xiaojin, Wang, Wenjian, Wang, Bin, Zhong, Mingkang. 2016. "Chemical profiling of San-Huang decoction by UPLC – ESI-Q-TOF-MS." *J. Pharm. Biomed. Anal.* 131, 20–32. doi:10.1016/j.jpba.2016.07.036

Meghatria, Farida, and Omar Belhamiti. 2021. "Predictive Model for the Risk of Cardiovascular Disease and Type 2 Diabetes in Obese People." *Chaos, Solitons and Fractals* 146. Elsevier Ltd: 110834. doi:10.1016/j.chaos.2021.110834.

Mirhafez, S. R., M. Ebrahimi, M. Saberi Karimian, A. Avan, M. Tayefi, A. Heidari-Bakavoli, M. R. Parizadeh, et al. 2016. "Serum High-Sensitivity C-Reactive Protein as a Biomarker in Patients with Metabolic Syndrome: Evidence-Based Study with 7284 Subjects." *European Journal of Clinical Nutrition* 70 (11): 1298–1304. doi:10.1038/ejcn.2016.111.

Nakamura, Y., K. Shimada, D. Fukuda, Y. Shimada, S. Ehara, M. Hirose, T. Kataoka, K. Kamimori, S. Shimodozono, Y. Kobayashi, M. Yoshiyama, K. Takeuchi, and J. Yoshikawa. 2004. "Implications of Plasma Concentrations of Adiponectin in Patients with Coronary Artery Disease." *Heart* 90(5): 528–533. https://doi.org/10.1136/hrt.2003.011114

Pischon, T., C. J. Girman, G. S. Hotamisligil, N. Rifai, F. B. Hu, and E. B. Rimm. 2004. "Plasma Adiponectin Levels and Risk of Myocardial Infarction in Men." *J Am Med Assoc*. 291(14), 1730–1737. https://doi.org/10.1001/jama.291.14.1730

Ridker, Paul M., Nina P. Paynter, Nader Rifai, J. Michael Gaziano, and Nancy R. Cook. 2008. "C-Reactive Protein and Parental History Improve Global Cardiovascular Risk Prediction: The Reynolds Risk Score for Men." *Circulation* 118 (22): 2243–2251. doi:10.1161/CIRCULATIONAHA.108.814251.

Sahu, Bidya Dhar, Harika Anubolu, Meghana Koneru, Jerald Mahesh Kumar, Madhusudana Kuncha, Shyam Sunder Rachamalla, and Ramakrishna Sistla. 2014. "Cardioprotective Effect of Embelin on Isoproterenol-Induced Myocardial Injury in Rats: Possible Involvement of Mitochondrial Dysfunction and Apoptosis." *Life Sciences* 107 (1–2). Elsevier Inc.: 59–67. doi:10.1016/j.lfs.2014.04.035.

SEMARNAT. 2019. Norma Oficial Mexicana NOM-059-SEMARNAT-2010, Protección ambiental – Especies nativas de México de flora y fauna silvestres – Categorías de riesgo y especificaciones para su inclusión, exclusión o cambio – Lista de especies en riesgo. Modificación del Anexo Normativo III, publicado en el Diario Oficial de la Federación el 14 November 2019. (www.dof.gob.mx/nota_detalle.php?codigo=5578808&fecha=14/11/2019)

Shah, Ravi V., Amanda Anderson, Jingzhong Ding, Matthew Budoff, Oliver Rider, Steffen E. Petersen, Majken Karoline Jensen, et al. 2017. "Pericardial, But Not Hepatic, Fat by CT Is Associated With CV Outcomes and Structure: The Multi-Ethnic Study of Atherosclerosis." *JACC: Cardiovascular Imaging* 10 (9): 1016–1027. doi:10.1016/j.jcmg.2016.10.024.

Sharma, Abhipree, Michael Mah, Rebecca H. Ritchie, and Miles J. De Blasio. 2022. "The Adiponectin Signalling Pathway – A Therapeutic Target for the Cardiac Complications of Type 2 Diabetes?" *Pharmacology and Therapeutics* 232. Elsevier Inc.: 108008. doi:10.1016/j.pharmthera.2021.108008.

Silva Dias, I. C., S. M. de Campos-Carli, E. L. Marciano Vieira, A. P. Lucas Mota, P. Santos Azevedo, V. T. da Silveira Anício, F. Carneiro Guimarães, L. Machado Mantovani, B. Fiusa Cruz, A. Lucio Teixeira, and J. Vinicius Salgado. 2022. "Adiponectin and Stnfr2 Peripheral Levels are Associated with Cardiovascular Risk in Patients with Schizophrenia." *Journal of Psychiatric Research* 149: 331–338. doi:10.1016/j.jpsychires.2021.11.020.

Solano Rodolfo, Gabriela Cruz-Lustre, Aaron Martinez-Feria, and Luicita Lagunez-Rivera. 2010. "Plantas utilizadas en la celebración de la Semana Santa en Zaachila, Oaxaca, México." Polibotanica 29: 263–279.

Solano Rodolfo, and Hector Huerta-Espinosa. 2019. Propuesta de inclusión en la Norma Oficial Mexicana 059-SEMARNAT-2010: *Prosthechea karwinskii* en la categoría de Sujeta a Protección Especial (Pr). http://187.191.71.192/expediente/17979/mir/47782/anexo/5317332

Solano Rodolfo, Luicita Laguez-Rivera, and Gabriela Cruz-Garcia. 2020. "*Prosthechea karwinskii*. Una orquidea emblemática de Mexico." Boletin AMO Septiembre-Octubre 2020: 8–18.

Souza, Mayane P. de, Giovana A. Bataglion, Felipe M. A. da Silva, Richardson A. de Almeida, Weider H. P. Paz, Thaís A. Nobre, Jane V. N. Marinho, et al. 2016. "Phenolic and Aroma Compositions of Pitomba Fruit (Talisia Esculenta Radlk.) Assessed by LC-MS/MS and HS-SPME/GC-MS." *Food Research International* 83: 87–94. doi:10.1016/j.foodres.2016.01.031.

Srikanthan, K., A. Feyh, H. Visweshwar, J. I. Shapiro, and K. Sodhi. 2016. "Systematic Review of Metabolic Syndrome Biomarkers: A Panel for Early Detection, Management, and Risk Stratification in the West Virginian Population." *International Journal of Medical Sciences* 13: 25–38. https://doi.org/10.7150/ijms.13800.

Su, Ruijun, Xiaoting Jin, Wenjing Zhao, Xiaoying Wu, Feihong Zhai, and Zhuoyu Li. 2022. "Rutin Ameliorates the Promotion Effect of Fine Particulate Matter on Vascular Calcification in Calcifying Vascular Cells and ApoE-/- Mice." *Ecotoxicology and Environmental Safety* 234 (March). Elsevier Inc.: 113410. doi:10.1016/j.ecoenv.2022.113410.

WHO. 2018. (World Health Organization) www.who.int/news-room/fact-sheets/detail/diabetes

Wu, Guoyao, and Cynthia J. Meininger. 2009. "Nitric Oxide and Vascular Insulin Resistance." *BioFactors* 35 (1): 21–27. doi:10.1002/biof.3.

Yoon, K., S. Ryu, J. Lee, J. D. Park. 2018. "Higher and Increased Concentration of hs-CRP Within Normal Range Can Predict the Incidence of Metabolic Syndrome in Healthy Men." *Diabetes and Metabolic Syndrome: Clinical Research and Reviews* 12 (6): 977–983. https://doi.org/10.1016/j.dsx.2018.06.008.

Yuan, Shuai, Paul Carter, Maria Bruzelius, Mathew Vithayathil, Siddhartha Kar, Amy M. Mason, Ang Lin, Stephen Burgess, and Susanna C. Larsson. 2020. "Effects of Tumour Necrosis Factor on Cardiovascular Disease and Cancer: A Two-Sample Mendelian Randomization Study." *EBioMedicine* 59. Elsevier B.V. doi:10.1016/j.ebiom.2020.102956.

Zhao, Youyou, Wang, Junkuan, Ballevre, Olivier, Luo, Hongliang, and Zhang, Weiguo. 2012. "Antihypertensive Effects and Mechanisms of Chlorogenic Acids." *Hypertens. Res.* 35, 370–374. https://doi.org/10.1038/hr.2011.195

Zheng, Junping, Jing Zhang, Yanlei Guo, Huabing Yang, Aizhen Lin, Baifei Hu, Qinghua Gao, Yunzhong Chen, and Hongtao Liu. 2020. "Improvement on Metabolic Syndrome in High Fat Diet-Induced Obese Mice through Modulation of Gut Microbiota by Sangguayin Decoction." *Journal of Ethnopharmacology* 246 (August 2019). Elsevier Ireland Ltd: 112225. doi:10.1016/j.jep.2019.112225.

18 Mushrooms and Cardiovascular Protection
Molecular, Cellular, and Physiological Aspects

Rachel B. Wilson and Nica M. Borradaile

CONTENTS

18.1 Introduction 282
18.2 Background..282
18.3 Whole Mushrooms and Mushroom Extracts...283
    18.3.1 Preclinical evidence..283
        18.3.1.1 Effects on Plasma Lipids and Blood Glucose....................283
        18.3.1.2 Effects on Liver Lipid Metabolism....................................283
            18.3.1.2.1 Liver Lipid Accumulation 283
            18.3.1.2.2 Hepatic Molecular Mechanisms for Hepatic and Plasma Lipid-Lowering.................................285
        18.3.1.3 Effects on Liver Glucose Metabolism 285
        18.3.1.4 Effects on Atherosclerosis 285
    18.3.2 Clinical Evidence..286
18.4 Mushroom Dietary Fiber and Polysaccharides...286
    18.4.1 Preclinical Evidence 286
        18.4.1.1 Effects on Plasma Lipids and Blood Glucose....................286
        18.4.1.2 Effects on Liver Lipid Metabolism....................................287
            18.4.1.2.1 Liver Lipid Accumulation 287
            18.4.1.2.2 Hepatic Molecular Mechanisms for Liver and Plasma Lipid-Lowering Effects....................288
        18.4.1.3 Effects on Liver Glucose Metabolism 288
        18.4.1.4 Effects on Atherosclerosis 288
    18.4.2 Clinical Evidence..289
18.5 Ergothioneine..289
    18.5.1 Preclinical Evidence 289
        18.5.1.1 Effects on Plasma Lipids and Blood Glucose....................289
        18.5.1.2 Effects on Liver Metabolism 289
        18.5.1.3 Effects on Atherosclerosis 290
    18.5.2 Clinical Evidence..290
18.6 Toxicity and Cautionary Notes 290
    18.6.1 Safety and Toxicity Concerns...290
    18.6.2 Need for High-Quality Clinical Studies.......................................290
18.7 Summary Points 290
18.8 Acknowledgements 291
References...291

DOI: 10.1201/9781003220329-20

LIST OF ABBREVIATIONS

ABCA1	ATP binding cassette subfamily A member 1
ACAT2	acetyl-coA acetyltransferase 2
ACC	acetyl-coA carboxylase
ACOX1	acyl-coA oxidase 1
AKT	protein kinase B
BSEP	bile salt export pump
ChREBP	carbohydrate response element binding protein
CPT1A	carnitine palmitoyltransferase 1A
CYP7A1	cytochrome P450 family 7 subfamily A member 1
DGAT1	diacylglycerol O-acyltransferase 1
EGT	ergothioneine
FASN	fatty acid synthase
HDL	high-density lipoprotein
HMGCR	3-hydroxy-3-methyl-glutaryl-coenzyme A reductase
LDL	low-density lipoprotein
LDLR	low-density lipoprotein receptor
LXRα	liver X receptor alpha
NAFLD	non-alcoholic fatty liver disease
PI3K	phosphoinositide 3-kinase
PPARα	peroxisome proliferator-activated receptor alpha
SREBP1/2	sterol regulatory element-binding protein 1/2
VLDL	very low-density lipoprotein

18.1 INTRODUCTION

Mushroom consumption is significantly associated with reduced risk of all-cause mortality (Ba et al. 2021b; Ba et al. 2021a). Given that cardiovascular disease is the leading cause of death worldwide, there is strong rationale to examine the potential impact of mushroom consumption on cardiovascular risk. In this chapter, we focus on the effects of edible mushrooms on cardiovascular protection, with emphasis on their modulation of liver lipid and glucose metabolism in relation to cardiovascular health. We review the effects of whole mushroom preparations, mushroom extracts, and mushroom-specific compounds (polysaccharides and ergothioneine) on liver metabolism and cardiovascular protection. The chapter is structured to summarize the effects of mushrooms from molecular to physiological levels, and from preclinical to clinical studies, focusing on publications from the last 12 years (2010–present).

18.2 BACKGROUND

Mushrooms have long been recognized for their nutritional, medicinal, and culinary value. The earliest evidence of mushroom consumption dates to the Upper Paleolithic period (~18,700 years ago) (Power et al. 2015). The first potential indication of humans using mushrooms as medicine dates to the Neolithic period, more than 5000 years ago. In 1991, a natural mummy, referred to colloquially as the 'Ice Man', was discovered in a glacier in Northern Italy. It was found with a bracket fungus called birch polyphore, or *Fomitopsis betulina*, now known to contain oils that have antibiotic and antiparasitic properties. Further analysis revealed the Ice Man had had intestinal parasites, raising the possibility that he may have been using the fungus to treat his parasitic infection (Capasso 1998). Ancient civilizations of China, Rome, Egypt, and Central America recognized the nutritional and medicinal value of mushrooms, and used them as food and medicine. In fact, in ancient Egypt, mushrooms were reserved for royalty only (Niksic et al. 2016). While many countries have

Mushrooms and Cardiovascular Protection

cultivated mushrooms throughout history, China has the longest history of mushroom cultivation and is currently the largest mushroom producer in the world. The first known intentional cultivation of mushrooms occurred in China around 600 AD, with the cultivation of *Auricularia* (Brenneman and Guttman 1994). Additionally, mushrooms have long been part of Chinese herbal medicine, with their medicinal use documented in the *Compendium of Materia Medica* written during the Ming dynasty in the 16th century (Niksic et al. 2016). Today, mushrooms are increasingly recognized by the scientific community for their potential benefits to human health and for treatment of several chronic diseases, including cardiovascular disease (Roncero-Ramos and Delgado-Andrade 2017).

18.3 WHOLE MUSHROOMS AND MUSHROOM EXTRACTS

18.3.1 PRECLINICAL EVIDENCE

18.3.1.1 Effects on Plasma Lipids and Blood Glucose

Considerable evidence from animal models suggests benefits of whole mushroom preparations and mushroom extracts for cardiovascular risk factors, such as hyperlipidemia and hyperglycemia (Figure 18.1). Mushrooms of genus *Agaricus* provide benefit in rat models of diabetes mellitus and hypercholesterolemia. In a rat model of type 1 diabetes, *A. bisporus* (white button mushroom) (Jeong et al. 2010) and *A. sylvaticus* (scaly wood mushroom) (Mascaro et al. 2014) reduced blood glucose and improved plasma lipid profiles. Similarly, in rodent models of hypercholesterolemia, *A. blazei* (sun mushroom) reduced plasma total cholesterol and LDL-cholesterol (LDL-c) (De Miranda et al. 2014; De Miranda et al. 2017), while *A. bisporus* also increased cardioprotective HDL-cholesterol (HDL-c) (Jeong et al. 2010). Some studies suggest mushrooms of genus *Pleurotus* also provide benefit in hyperglycemia and hyperlipidemia. In rodent models of hypercholesterolemia or diabetes, *P. ostreatus* (oyster mushroom) reduced blood glucose and plasma total cholesterol, triglyceride (Sato et al. 2011), LDL-c, and VLDL-cholesterol (VLDL-c), and in some work, increased HDL-c (Ravi et al. 2012; Anandhi et al. 2013). Other studies revealed similar effects on plasma lipids and blood glucose in response to *P. eryngii* var. *ferulae* (a variety of king trumpet mushroom associated with *Ferula communis*, the giant fennel) (Alam et al. 2011b), *P. pulmonarius* (Indian oyster mushroom) (Balaji et al. 2020), and *P. citrinopileatus* (golden oyster mushroom) (Sheng et al. 2019). In high-fat diet-fed rodents, *Lentinula edodes* (shiitake mushroom) reduced plasma total cholesterol and triglyceride (Kim et al. 2019; Drori et al. 2017; Spim et al. 2017; Yang et al. 2013), and in certain studies, reduced plasma LDL-c (Kim et al. 2019; Drori et al. 2017; Yang et al. 2013) and blood glucose (Spim et al. 2017; Drori et al. 2017). Several other studies showed benefits of various mushrooms for lipid profiles and/or glucose homeostasis in rodent models of hyperlipidemia and/or diabetes, including *Flammulina velutipes* (enoki mushroom) (Yeh et al. 2014), *Grifola frondosa* (maitake mushroom) (Aoki et al. 2018), *Panellus serotinus* (late oyster mushroom) (Inoue et al. 2013), *Hericium erinaceus* (lion's mane mushroom) (Hiwatashi et al. 2010), *Inonotus obliquus* (chaga mushroom) (Lu et al. 2010; Zhang et al. 2021), and a recently identified edible mushroom *Ceraceomyces tessulatus* (Basidiomycetes-X) (Khatun et al. 2020).

18.3.1.2 Effects on Liver Lipid Metabolism

18.3.1.2.1 Liver Lipid Accumulation

Many mushroom species described in the previous section elicit effects on liver lipid metabolism (Figure 18.2), which may contribute to their plasma lipid-lowering properties in animal models. There is extensive evidence suggesting that mushrooms can reduce liver lipid accumulation, which, depending on the metabolic fate of these lipids, could beneficially impact hyperlipidemia. Additionally, non-alcoholic fatty liver disease (NAFLD), which is defined by hepatocyte lipid accumulation, is independently associated with subclinical atherosclerosis, a concept we have previously reviewed (Peters et al. 2018). Therefore, reducing hepatic lipid accumulation may be beneficial in

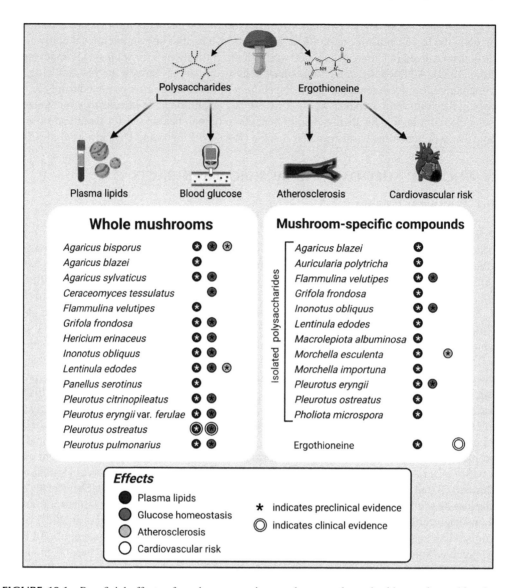

FIGURE 18.1 Beneficial effects of mushroom species, mushroom polysaccharides, and ergothioneine on cardiovascular risk factors and cardiovascular disease.

Note: Effects supported by preclinical or clinical evidence are indicated by symbols in the legend. Evidence which suggested no benefit on a given parameter is not included in this figure.

reducing cardiovascular risk. *A. bisporus* reduced liver triglyceride and cholesterol accumulation in hypercholesterolemic rats (Jeong et al. 2010) and lipid droplet accumulation in Huh7 hepatoma cells exposed to lipid excess (Rojas et al. 2018). Some evidence suggests that mushrooms of the *Pleurotus* genus, specifically *P. ostreatus* and *P. eryngii* var. *ferulae*, can reduce liver lipid accumulation in rodent models (Sato et al. 2011; Alam et al. 2011a; Alam et al. 2011b). In mice fed high-fat and/or high-cholesterol diets, *L. edodes* reduced liver lipid accumulation (Gil-Ramírez et al. 2016; Drori et al. 2017; Yang et al. 2013). Several other mushroom species also reduced hepatic lipids, including *G. frondosa* (Sato et al. 2011; Aoki et al. 2018), *F. velutipes* (Yeh et al. 2014), *P. serotinus* (Inoue et al. 2013), *H. erinaceus* (Hiwatashi et al. 2010), and *Sparassis crispa* (cauliflower mushroom) (Takeyama et al. 2018).

18.3.1.2.2 Hepatic Molecular Mechanisms for Hepatic and Plasma Lipid-Lowering

A significant body of work suggests that extracts from several mushroom species inhibit 3-hydroxy-3-methyl-glutaryl-coenzyme A reductase (HMGCR) (Figure 18.2), which is the mechanism underlying the LDL-c-lowering effect of the statin class of antihyperlipidemic drugs. An interesting study conducted by Gil-Ramírez et al. (2013a) involved screening water extracts from 26 mushroom species for potency of HMGCR inhibition. An extract from *L. edodes* was identified as the most potent inhibitor of HMGCR, with an inhibitory activity of 76%, comparable to pravastatin's inhibitory activity of 83% (Gil-Ramírez et al. 2013a). The HMGCR inhibitory activity of *L. edodes* was subsequently confirmed by other groups (Morales et al. 2018; Rahman et al. 2018). In addition, extracts from *P. ostreatus* and *P. pulmonarius* were among the top five most potent inhibitors of HMGCR (Gil-Ramírez et al. 2013a). Other mushrooms with documented HMGCR inhibitory activity include *A. bisporus* (Gil-Ramírez et al. 2013b) and *H. erinaceus* (Rahman et al. 2014). This mechanism may contribute to the cholesterol-lowering effects of these mushrooms, described in the previous section. Furthermore, preliminary evidence in rodent models suggests that the mushrooms *A. blazei* (De Miranda et al. 2017), *P. ostreatus* (Sato et al. 2011), and *Hypsizygus marmoreus* (beech mushroom) (Sato et al. 2011) may upregulate hepatic *Ldlr* mRNA expression, which could result in increased hepatic clearance of LDL from the circulation, thereby decreasing cardiovascular risk. Gil-Ramírez et al. (2016) developed an *in vitro* model of intestine-liver communication via the portal vein using Caco-2 colorectal adenocarcinoma and HepG2 hepatoma cell lines. Conditioned media collected from the basolateral surface of *L. edodes*-treated Caco-2 cells modulated the expression of genes involved in cholesterol synthesis and secretion in HepG2 cells (Gil-Ramírez et al. 2016); this suggests a mechanism whereby *L. edodes* can regulate enterocyte basolateral secretions to subsequently alter hepatocyte lipid metabolism. However, whether this axis functionally alters hepatocyte lipid metabolism and lipoprotein secretion remains to be demonstrated. Finally, some work has suggested that certain mushrooms may modulate hepatic *de novo* lipogenesis and fatty acid oxidation. In rodent models, *S. crispa* (Takeyama et al. 2018) and *P. serotinus* (Inoue et al. 2013) reduced hepatic fatty acid synthase (FASN) activity and, in the case of *S. crispa*, activities of other enzymes that contribute to *de novo* lipogenesis (Takeyama et al. 2018). *P. ostreatus* has also been shown to robustly upregulate expression of *Cpt1a* mRNA in mouse liver by cDNA microarray analyses, but this is not yet validated by quantitative methods (Sato et al. 2011). The latter mechanisms may contribute to the liver triglyceride-lowering effects of these mushrooms, described in the previous section.

18.3.1.3 Effects on Liver Glucose Metabolism

While many studies have described glucose-lowering effects of edible mushrooms in animal models, few have investigated potential hepatic mechanisms through which this may occur. It stands to reason that, by lowering liver lipids, mushrooms could improve hepatic insulin sensitivity and thereby reduce hepatic glucose production to improve glucose homeostasis, but this has yet to be demonstrated. A study conducted by Zhang et al. (2021) in a mouse model of type 2 diabetes showed that *I. obliquus* extract increased hepatic glycogen levels and hepatic markers of PI3K/AKT signaling (Figure 18.2), which suggests improved hepatic glucose storage and insulin sensitivity (Zhang et al. 2021). The potential molecular mechanisms underlying hepatic glucose regulation by edible mushroom species is an area that warrants further investigation.

18.3.1.4 Effects on Atherosclerosis

Although there is extensive preclinical evidence suggesting benefits of mushrooms for cardiovascular risk factors (e.g. hyperlipidemia, hyperglycemia), evidence of their benefit in preventing atherosclerotic lesion development or progression in animal models is more limited (Figure 18.1). A study conducted by Kim et al. (2019) in high-fat diet-fed LDL receptor-deficient mice showed robust reduction of aortic atherosclerotic lesion area and aortic tricuspid valve plaque area in response to *L. edodes* dietary supplementation (Kim et al. 2019), which is consistent with earlier preliminary evidence (Yang et al. 2013). These authors also reported a significant decrease in aortic tricuspid valve plaque area in response to supplementation with portobello mushroom, the mature form of *A. bisporus* (Kim et al. 2019). The effects and potential mechanisms whereby mushrooms impact atherosclerosis is another area warranting further study.

18.3.2 Clinical Evidence

In contrast to preclinical data, clinical evidence for benefits of mushrooms on hyperlipidemia, hyperglycemia, and cardiovascular risk is quite limited (Figure 18.1). Although preliminary, the majority of work in this area involves *P. ostreatus*. A handful of small studies showed lipid- (Sayeed et al. 2014; Choudhury, Hossain et al. 2013; Schneider et al. 2011) and glucose-lowering (Sayeed et al. 2014; Choudhury, Rahman et al. 2013; Jayasuriya et al. 2015) effects of *P. ostreatus* in humans. Accordingly, a systematic review by Dicks and Ellinger (2020) suggested possible cardiometabolic benefits of *P. ostreatus* intake, but that evidence for this is minimal (Dicks and Ellinger 2020). Calvo et al. (2016) performed a retrospective analysis on 37 subjects with metabolic syndrome who consumed 100 g of *A. bisporus* daily for 16 weeks and found significant reductions in serum levels of certain advanced glycation end products, which may have implications for vascular complications of diabetes (Calvo et al. 2016). However, large-scale studies suggest that the effects of mushroom consumption on cardiovascular risk are unclear. Lee et al. (2019) followed two prospective subject cohorts, comprising over 100,000 individuals, and found no association between mushroom consumption and biomarkers or risk of cardiovascular disease (Lee et al. 2019). Furthermore, a systematic review performed by Krittanawong et al. (2021) reported that edible mushroom consumption may improve blood lipid profiles, but does not conclusively affect cardiovascular risk (Krittanawong et al. 2021). In summary, further prospective clinical studies should be performed to determine potential effects of mushroom consumption on human cardiovascular risk.

18.4 MUSHROOM DIETARY FIBER AND POLYSACCHARIDES

18.4.1 Preclinical Evidence

18.4.1.1 Effects on Plasma Lipids and Blood Glucose

Several studies indicate that polysaccharides isolated from certain mushrooms of the *Pleurotus* genus may provide benefit in hyperlipidemia and hyperglycemia (Figure 18.1). Various polysaccharide fractions derived from *P. eryngii* (king trumpet mushroom) reduced plasma total cholesterol, LDL-c (Nakahara et al. 2020; Zhang et al. 2017; Chen et al. 2016; Xu et al. 2017), and triglyceride (Zhang et al. 2017; Chen et al. 2016; Xu et al. 2017), increased plasma HDL-c (Chen et al. 2016; Xu et al. 2017), and improved glucose homeostasis (Nakahara et al. 2020; Chen et al. 2016) in rodent models of diet-induced obesity, hyperlipidemia, or type 2 diabetes. Additionally, a β-glucan-enriched extract from *P. ostreatus* reduced plasma total cholesterol and LDL-c in hypercholesterolemic mice (Caz et al. 2016). Some studies suggest lipid-lowering effects of polysaccharides from *Morchella* (morel) mushrooms. A comprehensive study conducted by Wang et al. (2021) investigated the effects of a novel polysaccharide MCP isolated from *M. esculenta* in high-fat diet-fed LDL receptor-deficient mice, and showed robust decreases in plasma total cholesterol, LDL-c, and triglyceride (Wang et al. 2021). Furthermore, *M. importuna* polysaccharides reduced plasma triglyceride in mice with carbon tetrachloride-induced hepatotoxicity (Xu et al. 2021). In hyperlipidemic mice, administration of water-soluble polysaccharides extracted from *L. edodes* reduced plasma total cholesterol, LDL-c (Caz et al. 2016; Zhu et al. 2013), and triglyceride (Zhu et al. 2013), and increased plasma HDL-c (Zhu et al. 2013). Similar effects were also reported for a β-glucan-enriched *L. edodes* extract (Morales et al. 2019). Insoluble dietary fiber and the polysaccharide chitosan isolated from *F. velutipes* reduced plasma total cholesterol, triglyceride (Yang et al. 2021; Miyazawa et al. 2018), and LDL-c, increased HDL-c (Miyazawa et al. 2018), and

Mushrooms and Cardiovascular Protection

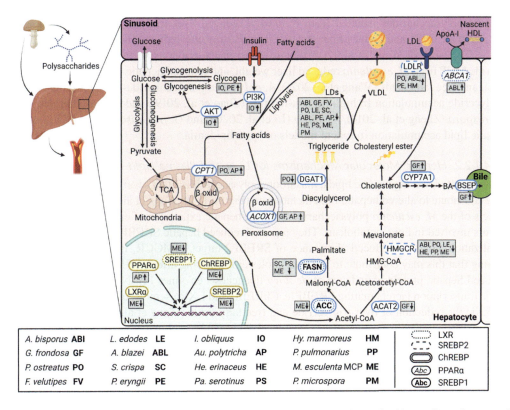

FIGURE 18.2 Molecular effects of mushroom species and mushroom polysaccharides on liver glucose and lipid metabolism in relation to cardiovascular disease.

Note: Effects of mushroom polysaccharides have been combined with effects of the corresponding whole mushroom preparation for clarity. Molecular targets altered by mushroom species and mushroom polysaccharides are indicated by the text with blue (non-transcription factor) and yellow (transcription factor) fill and borders. Targets of various transcription factors are indicated by different borders or text, as shown in the legend. Codes assigned to mushrooms in the legend are used to indicate the specific molecular alterations associated with a given mushroom (two- or three-letter codes in gray boxes beside each molecular target), and the arrow indicates the direction of the effect. LDs, lipid droplets.

improved oral glucose tolerance (Yang et al. 2021) in mice. Polysaccharide-peptides (Zhao et al. 2019) and soluble polysaccharides (Zhao et al. 2015) isolated from *Auricularia polytricha* (cloud ear fungus) reduced plasma total cholesterol, LDL-c, and triglyceride (Zhao et al. 2019, 2015), and increased HDL-c (Zhao et al. 2019) in rodent models of hyperlipidemia. Lipid-lowering effects of polysaccharides from *Pholiota microspora* (nameko mushroom) (Li et al. 2010; Zheng et al. 2014), *A. blazei* (Li et al. 2020), *G. frondosa* (Li et al. 2019), *I. obliquus* (Wang et al. 2017), and *Macrolepiota albuminosa* (termite mushroom) (Zhao et al. 2016) have been demonstrated in various rodent models of hyperlipidemia and type 2 diabetes. *I. obliquus* polysaccharides also reduced fasting blood glucose and plasma insulin, and improved oral glucose tolerance in a mouse model of type 2 diabetes (Wang et al. 2017).

18.4.1.2 Effects on Liver Lipid Metabolism

18.4.1.2.1 Liver Lipid Accumulation

As with whole mushroom preparations and mushroom extracts, polysaccharides isolated from various mushrooms affect liver lipid accumulation (Figure 18.2). In mouse models of hyperlipidemia, specific polysaccharides isolated from *P. eryngii* reduced liver triglyceride and total cholesterol (Zhang et al. 2017), and dietary fiber isolated from *P. ostreatus* reduced liver triglyceride (Caz et al. 2015). The work of Wang et al. (2021), highlighted in the previous section, showed that polysaccharide MCP from *M. esculenta* reduced liver weight, and reduced hepatic triglyceride, total cholesterol, and free fatty acids (Wang et al. 2021). *A. polytricha* polysaccharide-peptides reduced hepatic triglyceride accumulation in high-fat diet-fed rats (Zhao et al. 2019), and polysaccharides from *P. microspora* (Zheng et al. 2014), *A. blazei* (Li et al. 2020), and *G. frondosa* (Li et al. 2019) reduced hepatic lipid accumulation in rodent models of hyperlipidemia.

18.4.1.2.2 Hepatic Molecular Mechanisms for Liver and Plasma Lipid-Lowering Effects

In addition to lowering hepatic lipids, mushroom polysaccharides elicit several molecular changes that may contribute to altered hepatic lipid metabolism (Figure 18.2). Wang et al. (2021) characterized the effects of the *M. esculenta* polysaccharide MCP on hepatic expression of enzymes and transcription factors involved in lipid metabolism. They reported reduced hepatic SREBP2 processing and nuclear localization alongside reduced abundance of SREBP2 target, HMGCR, in response to MCP, suggesting that this may contribute to the liver cholesterol-lowering effects of MCP. Furthermore, MCP reduced hepatic protein abundance of *de novo* lipogenesis enzymes FASN and ACC1, and of lipogenic transcription factors mature SREBP1c, ChREBP, and LXRα – molecular alterations which may underlie the reduction of liver triglyceride and free fatty acids (Wang et al. 2021). Other mushroom polysaccharides also alter molecular targets involved in cholesterol metabolism and handling. Water-soluble polysaccharides isolated from *L. edodes* inhibited HMGCR activity by 76% (Gil-Ramírez et al. 2016), and *P. eryngii* polysaccharides induced hepatic *Ldlr* mRNA expression in high-fat diet-fed mice (Nakahara et al. 2020); both mechanisms have implications for LDL-c-lowering in cardiovascular disease. Furthermore, in high-fat diet-fed rats, polysaccharides from *G. frondosa* upregulated *Cyp7a1* and *Bsep* mRNAs and downregulated *Acat2* mRNA, which may explain the effects of these polysaccharides in reducing hepatic and plasma total cholesterol (Li et al. 2019). Finally, *A. blazei* polysaccharides induced ABCA1 expression in livers of high-fat diet-fed rats, which likely contributed to the observed increase in plasma HDL-c (Li et al. 2020). Additional molecular mechanisms through which mushroom polysaccharides may reduce liver triglyceride have also been identified. *A. polytricha* polysaccharide-peptides (Zhao et al. 2019) and *G. frondosa* polysaccharides (Li et al. 2019) increased mRNA expression of genes involved in β-oxidation, including ACOX1 (Zhao et al. 2019; Li et al. 2019), CPT1, and PPARα (Zhao et al. 2019) in HepG2 hepatoma cells exposed to high fatty acids and ethanol (Zhao et al. 2019) or high-fat diet-fed rat liver (Li et al. 2019). Unrelated to β-oxidation, dietary fiber from *P. ostreatus* reduced hepatic *Dgat1* mRNA in hypercholesterolemic mice, which may have contributed to its liver triglyceride-lowering effect (Caz et al. 2015).

18.4.1.3 Effects on Liver Glucose Metabolism

While some preclinical evidence exists for benefits of mushroom polysaccharides on glucose homeostasis, few studies have characterized their effects on hepatic glucose metabolism. In addition to improving plasma lipid profiles and glucose homeostasis in mouse models of type 2 diabetes, *P. eryngii* (Chen et al. 2016) and *I. oliquus* (Wang et al. 2017) polysaccharides increased liver glycogen (Figure 18.2), which suggests enhanced hepatic glucose storage and thus improved hepatic insulin sensitivity. Preliminary evidence suggests that *I. obliquus* polysaccharides enhance hepatic PI3K/AKT signaling (Wang et al. 2017) (Figure 18.2), in further support of improved hepatic insulin sensitivity. Additionally, mushroom polysaccharides have been reported to increase hepatic expression or phosphorylation of metabolic regulator AMPK (Zhao et al. 2019; Li et al. 2019; Wang et al. 2021), which has implications for hepatic glucose and lipid metabolism.

18.4.1.4 Effects on Atherosclerosis

Preclinical studies on the effects of mushroom polysaccharides on atherosclerosis are limited. However, Wang et al. (2021) provided extensive evidence for the benefits of the *M. esculenta*

Mushrooms and Cardiovascular Protection

polysaccharide MCP in atherosclerosis (Figure 18.1). In high-fat diet-fed LDL receptor-deficient mice, MCP reduced atherosclerotic lesion area in whole aorta and aortic root cross-sections. MCP also reduced macrophage accumulation and increased vascular smooth muscle cell content in the arterial wall of the aortic root, the latter suggestive of increased plaque stability (Wang et al. 2021). Further work is required to elucidate the effects of polysaccharides from other mushroom species on atherosclerosis in animal models.

18.4.2 Clinical Evidence

Only one small study exists on the effects of edible mushroom polysaccharides on cardiovascular risk. Morales et al. (2021) conducted a randomized, controlled, double-blind clinical trial in 52 subjects with untreated mild hypercholesterolemia to study the effects of a β-glucan-enriched extract from *L. edodes* on cardiovascular risk factors. The authors reported no effect of the extract on plasma total cholesterol, HDL-c, LDL-c, and triglyceride after eight weeks of intervention (Morales et al. 2021). Given the preclinical evidence for lipid-lowering effects of mushroom polysaccharides, further clinical studies are required to determine whether these effects, and benefits for cardiovascular risk, translate to humans.

18.5 ERGOTHIONEINE

Ergothioneine (EGT) is a modified amino acid synthesized in certain bacteria and fungi and is thought to accumulate in higher order plant and animal food sources by uptake from the environment. While EGT is present to some degree in various plant and animal dietary sources, the highest concentrations of EGT have been detected in certain mushrooms. EGT is well known for its antioxidant effects, and therefore may have important implications for cardiovascular disease. We previously reviewed the effects of EGT on the vasculature as it relates to atherosclerosis (Lam-Sidun et al. 2021). As with earlier sections, we will focus on preclinical and clinical evidence for the effects of EGT on plasma lipids and blood glucose, liver metabolism, and atherosclerosis.

18.5.1 Preclinical Evidence

18.5.1.1 Effects on Plasma Lipids and Blood Glucose

Much research related to EGT is focused on its role as an antioxidant and as a cytoprotectant; thus, evidence of its effects on plasma lipid profiles and glucose homeostasis is relatively limited (Figure 18.1). However, two recent studies by Dare et al. suggested benefits of EGT in hypertriglyceridemia in a rodent model of type 2 diabetes. Using a rat model of type 2 diabetes, the authors showed a significant reduction in plasma triglyceride in response to EGT administration, but no effect on glucose homeostasis (Dare et al. 2021b, 2021a) or liver triglyceride (Dare et al. 2021b). EGT did, however, significantly reduce markers of oxidative stress in liver and kidney, and improved serum indicators of liver and kidney function (Dare et al. 2021b, 2021a), consistent with its well-documented antioxidant and cytoprotectant effects.

18.5.1.2 Effects on Liver Metabolism

EGT is known to accumulate in liver (Tang et al. 2018), and its hepatic accumulation correlates significantly with hepatic cholesterol content in guinea pigs fed high-cholesterol diet (Cheah et al. 2016), suggesting that its accumulation in the liver may defend against metabolic stress. Antioxidants have been shown to reduce hepatic lipid accumulation (Imai et al. 2018) and improve hepatic insulin resistance (Pereira et al. 2014). Therefore, it stands to reason that EGT, through its function as an antioxidant, could also reduce liver lipid accumulation and improve liver insulin sensitivity, which may improve plasma lipid profiles and glucose homeostasis in the setting of cardiovascular disease. However, further research is needed to support this hypothesis.

18.5.1.3 Effects on Atherosclerosis

No preclinical studies have directly investigated the effects of EGT on atherosclerotic lesion formation. As cited in a previous section, work by Kim et al. (2019), which compared the effects of supplementation with portobello mushroom or shiitake mushroom on atherosclerosis in LDL receptor-deficient mice, provides some preliminary evidence for potential benefits of EGT in atherosclerosis. Shiitake mushroom elicited a stronger improvement on measures of atherosclerosis compared to portobello mushroom, which is particularly interesting because the EGT content of shiitake mushrooms is four-fold that of portobello mushrooms (Kim et al. 2019). While this differential effect could result from other differences in nutritional composition between the two species, the work provides rationale to investigate the effects of EGT on atherosclerosis in animal models.

18.5.2 CLINICAL EVIDENCE

Very little evidence exists to support potential benefits of EGT for cardiovascular disease in humans. However, work by Smith et al. (2020) used a metabolomics approach to identify plasma metabolites associated with cardiovascular risk, and indicated that EGT was independently associated with lower risk of coronary artery disease, cardiovascular mortality, and overall mortality (Smith et al. 2020) (Figure 18.1). While this association does not imply causality, it provides strong rationale to conduct both preclinical and clinical studies investigating the effects of EGT supplementation on cardiovascular disease.

18.6 TOXICITY AND CAUTIONARY NOTES

18.6.1 SAFETY AND TOXICITY CONCERNS

Of the preclinical studies suggesting potential benefits of mushrooms on cardiovascular risk factors, few animal studies have shown negative effects of mushrooms on cardiometabolic disease. One study showed that dietary supplementation with *A. blazei* increased atherosclerotic lesion area and inflammation in ApoE-deficient mice (Gonçalves et al. 2012). This finding is not consistent with studies described earlier for *A. blazei*, which suggested a reduction in cardiovascular risk (De Miranda et al. 2014; De Miranda et al. 2017). This discrepancy may be related to the dose used, as the former study used a five-fold greater dose of *A. blazei* than the latter studies. Furthermore, a high dose of *L. edodes* lowered plasma triglyceride (Handayani et al. 2011), but increased liver triglyceride, in high-fat diet-fed rats (Handayani et al. 2014), suggesting concomitant benefits for cardiovascular disease and risks for NAFLD.

18.6.2 NEED FOR HIGH-QUALITY CLINICAL STUDIES

Overall, there is insufficient clinical evidence of beneficial effects of mushrooms on cardiovascular risk factors and outcomes. Therefore, while the preclinical evidence summarized in this chapter is quite promising, high-quality clinical studies should be conducted to evaluate whether these effects translate to humans.

18.7 SUMMARY POINTS

- Mushrooms have long been recognized for their nutritional, medicinal, and culinary properties.
- Strong preclinical evidence exists for benefits of mushrooms on plasma lipids and glucose homeostasis.
- Many mushrooms also beneficially alter liver lipid and glucose metabolism in preclinical models.

Mushrooms and Cardiovascular Protection

- Few studies have examined the effects of mushrooms on atherosclerosis in preclinical models.
- Clinical evidence for benefits of mushrooms for cardiovascular risk factors and outcomes is lacking.

18.8 ACKNOWLEDGEMENTS

NMB holds funding from the Natural Sciences and Engineering Research Council of Canada (RGPIN-2017–04646). RBW is supported by an NSERC doctoral scholarship. Figures were created in BioRender.com.

REFERENCES

Alam, N., Yoon, K.N., and Lee, T.S. 2011a. Antihyperlipidemic Activities of Pleurotus Ferulae on Biochemical and Histological Function in Hypercholesterolemic Rats. *Journal of Research in Medical Sciences* 16: 776–786.

Alam, N., Yoon, K.N., Lee, T.S., and Lee, U.Y. 2011b. Hypolipidemic Activities of Dietary Pleurotus Ostreatus in Hypercholesterolemic Rats. *Mycobiology* 39: 45–51.

Anandhi, R., Annadurai, T., Anitha, T.S., Muralidharan, A.R., Najmunnisha, K., Nachiappan, V., Thomas, P.A. et al. 2013. Antihypercholesterolemic and Antioxidative Effects of an Extract of the Oyster Mushroom, Pleurotus Ostreatus, and Its Major Constituent, Chrysin, in Triton WR-1339-Induced Hypercholesterolemic Rats. *J Physiol Biochem* 69: 313–323.

Aoki, H., Hanayama, H., Mori, K., and Sato, R. 2018. Grifola Frondosa (Maitake) Extract Activates PPARδ and Improves Glucose Intolerance in High-Fat Diet-Induced Obese Mice. *Bioscience, Biotechnology, and Biochemistry* 82: 1550–1559.

Ba, D.M., Gao, X., Al-Shaar, L., Muscat, J., Chinchilli, V.M., Ssentongo, P., Zhang, X., Liu, G., Beelman, R.B., and Richie Jr., J.P. 2021a. Prospective Study of Dietary Mushroom Intake and Risk of Mortality: Results from Continuous National Health and Nutrition Examination Survey (NHANES) 2003–2014 and a Meta-Analysis. *Nutrition Journal* 20:80.

Ba, D.M., Gao, X., Muscat, J., Al-Shaar, L., Chinchilli, V., Zhang, X., Ssentongo, P., Beelman, R.B., and Richie Jr., J.P. 2021b. Association of Mushroom Consumption with All-Cause and Cause-Specific Mortality among American Adults: Prospective Cohort Study Findings from NHANES III. *Nutrition Journal* 20:38.

Balaji, P., Madhanraj, R., Rameshkumar, K., Veeramanikandan, V., Eyini, M., Arun, A., Thulasinathan, B. et al. 2020. Evaluation of Antidiabetic Activity of Pleurotus Pulmonarius against Streptozotocin-Nicotinamide Induced Diabetic Wistar Albino Rats. *Saudi Journal of Biological Sciences* 27:913–924.

Brenneman, J.A. and M.C. Guttman. 1994. The Edibility & Cultivation of the Oyster Mushroom. *American Biology Teacher* 56:291–293.

Calvo, M.S., Mehrotra, A., Beelman, R.B., Nadkarni, G., Wang, L., Cai, W., Goh, B.C., Kalaras, M.D., and Uribarri J. 2016. A Retrospective Study in Adults with Metabolic Syndrome: Diabetic Risk Factor Response to Daily Consumption of Agaricus Bisporus (White Button Mushrooms). *Plant Foods Hum Nutr.* 71:245–251.

Capasso, L. 1998. 5300 Years Ago, the Ice Man Used Natural Laxatives and Antibiotics. *The Lancet* 352:1864.

Caz, V., Gil-Ramírez, A., Largo, C., Tabernero, M., Santamaría, M., Martín-Hernández, R., Marín, F.R., Reglero, G., and Soler-Rivas, C. 2015. Modulation of Cholesterol-Related Gene Expression by Dietary Fiber Fractions from Edible Mushrooms. *Journal of Agricultural and Food Chemistry* 63:7371–7380.

Caz, V., Gil-Ramírez, A., Santamaría, M., Tabernero, M., Soler-Rivas, C., Martín-Hernández, R., Marín, F.R., Reglero, G., and Largo, C. 2016. Plasma Cholesterol-Lowering Activity of Lard Functionalized with Mushroom Extracts Is Independent of Niemann–Pick C1-Like 1 Protein and ABC Sterol Transporter Gene Expression in Hypercholesterolemic Mice. *Journal of Agricultural and Food Chemistry* 64:1686–1694.

Cheah, I.K., Tang, R., Ye, P., Yew, T.S.Z., Lim, K.H.C., and Halliwell, B. 2016. Liver Ergothioneine Accumulation in a Guinea Pig Model of Non-Alcoholic Fatty Liver Disease: A Possible Mechanism of Defence? *Free Radical Research* 50:14–25.

Chen, L., Zhang, Y., Sha, O., Xu, W., and Wang, S. 2016. Hypolipidaemic and Hypoglycaemic Activities of Polysaccharide from Pleurotus Eryngii in Kunming Mice. *International Journal of Biological Macromolecules* 93:1206–1209.

Choudhury, B.K., Hossain, S., Hossain, M., Kakon, A.J., Choudhury, M.A.K., Ahmed, N.U., and Rahman, T. 2013. Pleurotus Ostreatus Improves Lipid Profile of Obese Hypertensive Nondiabetic Males. *Bangladesh Journal of Mushroom* 7:37–44.

Choudhury, M.B.K., Rahman, T., Kakon, A.J., Hoque, N., Akhtaruzzaman, M., Begum, M.M., Choudhuri, M.S.K., and Hossain, M.S. 2013. "Effects of Pleurotus Ostreatus on Blood Pressure and Glycemic Status of Hypertensive Diabetic Male Volunteers." *Bangladesh Journal of Medical Biochemistry* 6:5–10.

Dare, A., Channa, M.L., and Nadar, A. 2021a. L-Ergothioneine and Its Combination with Metformin Attenuates Renal Dysfunction in Type-2 Diabetic Rat Model by Activating Nrf2 Antioxidant Pathway. *Biomedicine & Pharmacotherapy* 141:111921.

Dare, A., Channa, M.L., and Nadar, A. 2021b. L-Ergothioneine and Metformin Alleviates Liver Injury in Experimental Type-2 Diabetic Rats via Reduction of Oxidative Stress, Inflammation, and Hypertriglyceridemia. *Canadian Journal of Physiology and Pharmacology* 99:1137–1147.

Dicks, L. and Ellinger, S. 2020. Effect of the Intake of Oyster Mushrooms (Pleurotus Ostreatus) on Cardiometabolic Parameters – A Systematic Review of Clinical Trials. *Nutrients* 12:1134.

Drori, A., Rotnemer-Golinkin, D., Avni, S., Drori, A., Danay, O., Levanon, D., Tam, J., Zolotarev, L., and Ilan, Y. 2017. Attenuating the Rate of Total Body Fat Accumulation and Alleviating Liver Damage by Oral Administration of Vitamin D-Enriched Edible Mushrooms in a Diet-Induced Obesity Murine Model Is Mediated by an Anti-Inflammatory Paradigm Shift. *BMC Gastroenterology* 17:130.

Gil-Ramírez, A., Caz, V., Smiderle, F.R., Martin-Hernandez, R., Largo, C., Tabernero, M., Marín, F.R., Iacomini, M., Reglero, G., and Soler-Rivas, C. 2016. Water-Soluble Compounds from Lentinula Edodes Influencing the HMG-CoA Reductase Activity and the Expression of Genes Involved in the Cholesterol Metabolism. *Journal of Agricultural and Food Chemistry* 64:1910–1920.

Gil-Ramírez, A., Clavijo, C., Palanisamy, M., Ruiz-Rodríguez, A., Navarro-Rubio, M., Pérez, M., Marín, F.R., Reglero, G., and Soler-Rivas, C. 2013a. Screening of Edible Mushrooms and Extraction by Pressurized Water (PWE) of 3-Hydroxy-3-Methyl-Glutaryl CoA Reductase Inhibitors." *Journal of Functional Foods* 5:244–250.

Gil-Ramírez, A., Clavijo, C., Palanisamy, M., Ruiz-Rodríguez, A., Navarro-Rubio, M., Pérez, M., Marín, F.R., Reglero, G., and Soler-Rivas, C. 2013b. Study on the 3-Hydroxy-3-Methyl-Glutaryl CoA Reductase Inhibitory Properties of Agaricus Bisporus and Extraction of Bioactive Fractions Using Pressurised Solvent Technologies. *Journal of the Science of Food and Agriculture* 93:2789–2796.

Gonçalves, J.L., Roma, E.H., Gomes-Santos, A.C., Aguilar, E.C., Cisalpino, D., Fernandes, L.R. et al. 2012. Pro-Inflammatory Effects of the Mushroom Agaricus Blazei and Its Consequences on Atherosclerosis Development. *European Journal of Nutrition* 51:927–937.

Handayani, D., Chen, J., Meyer, B.J., and Huang, X.F. 2011. Dietary Shiitake Mushroom (Lentinus Edodes) Prevents Fat Deposition and Lowers Triglyceride in Rats Fed a High-Fat Diet. *Journal of Obesity* 2011:258051.

Handayani, D., Meyer, B.J., Chen, J., Brown, S.H.J., Mitchell, T.W., and Huang, X.F. 2014. A High-Dose Shiitake Mushroom Increases Hepatic Accumulation of Triacylglycerol in Rats Fed a High-Fat Diet: Underlying Mechanism. *Nutrients* 6:650–662.

Hiwatashi, K., Kosaka, Y., Suzuki, N., Hata, K., Mukaiyama, T., Sakamoto, K., Shirakawa, H., and Komai, M. 2010. Yamabushitake Mushroom (Hericium Erinaceus) Improved Lipid Metabolism in Mice Fed a High-Fat Diet. *Bioscience, Biotechnology, and Biochemistry* 74:1447–1451.

Imai, Y., Fink, B.D., Promes, J.A., Kulkarni, C.A., Kerns, R.J., and Sivitz, W.I. 2018. Effect of a Mitochondrial-Targeted Coenzyme Q Analog on Pancreatic β-Cell Function and Energetics in High Fat Fed Obese Mice. *Pharmacology Research & Perspectives* e00393.

Inoue, N., Inafuku, M., Shirouchi, B., Nagao, K., and Yanagita, T. 2013. Effect of Mukitake Mushroom (Panellus Serotinus) on the Pathogenesis of Lipid Abnormalities in Obese, Diabetic ob/ob Mice. *Lipids in Health and Disease* 12:18.

Jayasuriya, W.J.A.B.N., Wanigatunge, C.A., Fernando, G.H., Abeytunga, D.T.U., and Suresh, T.S. 2015. Hypoglycaemic Activity of Culinary Pleurotus Ostreatus and P. Cystidiosus Mushrooms in Healthy Volunteers and Type 2 Diabetic Patients on Diet Control and the Possible Mechanisms of Action. *Phytotherapy Research* 29:303–309.

Jeong, S.C., Jeong, Y.T., Yang, B.K., Islam, R., Koyyalamudi, S.R., Pang, G., Cho, K.Y., and Song, C.H. 2010. White Button Mushroom (Agaricus Bisporus) Lowers Blood Glucose and Cholesterol Levels in Diabetic and Hypercholesterolemic Rats. *Nutrition Research* 30:49–56.

Khatun, M.A., Sato, S., and Konishi, T. 2020. Obesity Preventive Function of Novel Edible Mushroom, Basidiomycetes-X (Echigoshirayukidake): Manipulations of Insulin Resistance and Lipid Metabolism. *Journal of Traditional and Complementary Medicine* 10:245–251.

Mushrooms and Cardiovascular Protection

Kim, S.H., Thomas, M.J., Wu, D., Carman, C.V., Ordovás, J.M., and Meydani, M. 2019. Edible Mushrooms Reduce Atherosclerosis in Ldlr-/- Mice Fed a High-Fat Diet. *The Journal of Nutrition* 149:1377–1384.

Krittanawong, C., Isath, A., Hahn, J., Wang, Z., Fogg, S.E., Bandyopadhyay, D., Jneid, H., Virani, S.S., and Tang, W.H.W. 2021. Mushroom Consumption and Cardiovascular Health: A Systematic Review. *The American Journal of Medicine* 134:637–642.

Lam-Sidun, D., Peters, K.M., and Borradaile, N.M. 2021. Mushroom-Derived Medicine? Preclinical Studies Suggest Potential Benefits of Ergothioneine for Cardiometabolic Health. *International Journal of Molecular Sciences* 22:3246.

Lee, D.H., Yang, M., Giovannucci, E.L., Sun, Q., and Chavarro, J.E. 2019. Mushroom Consumption, Biomarkers, and Risk of Cardiovascular Disease and Type 2 Diabetes: A Prospective Cohort Study of US Women and Men. *The American Journal of Clinical Nutrition* 110:666–674.

Li, H., Zhang, M., and Ma, G. 2010. Hypolipidemic Effect of the Polysaccharide from Pholiota Nameko. *Nutrition* 26:556–562.

Li, L., Guo, W., Zhang, W., Xu, J., Qian, M., Bai, W., Zhang, Y., Rao, P., Ni, L., and Lv, X. 2019. Grifola Frondosa Polysaccharides Ameliorate Lipid Metabolic Disorders and Gut Microbiota Dysbiosis in High-Fat Diet Fed Rats. *Food & Function* 10:2560–2572.

Li, Y., Sheng, Y., Lu, X., Guo, X., Xu, G., Han, X., An, L., and Du, P. 2020. Isolation and Purification of Acidic Polysaccharides from Agaricus Blazei Murill and Evaluation of Their Lipid-Lowering Mechanism. *International Journal of Biological Macromolecules* 157:276–287.

Lu, X., Chen, H., Dong, P., Fu, L., and Zhang, X. 2010. Phytochemical Characteristics and Hypoglycaemic Activity of Fraction from Mushroom Inonotus Obliquus. *Journal of the Science of Food and Agriculture* 90:276–280.

Mascaro, M.B., França, C.M., Esquerdo, K.F., Lara, M.A.N., Wadt, N.S.Y., and Bach, E.E. 2014. Effects of Dietary Supplementation with Agaricus Sylvaticus Schaeffer on Glycemia and Cholesterol after Streptozotocin-Induced Diabetes in Rats. *Evidence-Based Complementary and Alternative Medicine* 2014:107629.

de Miranda, A.M., Rossoni Júnior, J.V., e Silva, L.S., dos Santos, R.C., Silva, M.E., and Pedrosa, M.L. 2017. Agaricus Brasiliensis (Sun Mushroom) Affects the Expression of Genes Related to Cholesterol Homeostasis. *European Journal of Nutrition* 56:1707–1717.

de Miranda, A.M., Ribeiro, G.M., Cunha, A.C., Silva, L.S., dos Santos, R.C., Pedrosa, M.L., and Silva, M.E. 2014. Hypolipidemic Effect of the Edible Mushroom Agaricus Blazei in Rats Subjected to a Hypercholesterolemic Diet. *Journal of Physiology and Biochemistry* 70: 215–224.

Miyazawa, N., Yoshimoto, H., Kurihara, S., Hamaya, T., and Eguchi, F. 2018. Improvement of Diet-Induced Obesity by Ingestion of Mushroom Chitosan Prepared from Flammulina Velutipes. *Journal of Oleo Science* 67:245–254.

Morales, D., Piris, A.J., Ruiz-Rodriguez, A., Prodanov, M., and Soler-Rivas, C. 2018. Extraction of Bioactive Compounds against Cardiovascular Diseases from Lentinula Edodes Using a Sequential Extraction Method. *Biotechnology Progress* 34:746–755.

Morales, D., Shetty, S.A., López-Plaza, B., Gómez-Candela, C., Smidt, H., Marín, F.R., and Soler-Rivas, C. 2021. Modulation of Human Intestinal Microbiota in a Clinical Trial by Consumption of a β-d-Glucan-Enriched Extract Obtained from Lentinula Edodes. *European Journal of Nutrition* 60:3249–3265.

Morales, D., Tejedor-Calvo, E., Jurado-Chivato, N., Polo, G., Tabernero, M., Ruiz-Rodríguez, A., Largo, C., and Soler-Rivas, C. 2019. In Vitro and in Vivo Testing of the Hypocholesterolcmic Activity of Ergosterol- and β-Glucan-Enriched Extracts Obtained from Shiitake Mushrooms (Lentinula Edodes). *Food & Function* 10:7325–7332.

Nakahara, D., Nan, C., Mori, K., Hanayama, M., Kikuchi, H., Hirai, S., and Egashira, Y. 2020. Effect of Mushroom Polysaccharides from Pleurotus Eryngii on Obesity and Gut Microbiota in Mice Fed a High-Fat Diet. *European Journal of Nutrition* 59:3231–3244.

Niksic, M., Klaus, A., and Argyropoulos, D. 2016. Safety of Foods Based on Mushrooms. In *Regulating Safety of Traditional and Ethnic Foods*, ed. V Prakash, O Martín-Belloso, L Keener, S Astley, S Braun, H McMahon, and H Lilieveld, 421–439. Academic Press.

Pereira, S., Park, E., Mori, Y., Haber, C.A., Han, P., Uchida, T., Stavar, L., et al. 2014. FFA-Induced Hepatic Insulin Resistance in Vivo Is Mediated by PKCδ, NADPH Oxidase, and Oxidative Stress. *American Journal of Physiology – Endocrinology and Metabolism* 307:E34–E46.

Peters, K.M., Wilson, R.B., and Borradaile, N.M. 2018. Non-Parenchymal Hepatic Cell Lipotoxicity and the Coordinated Progression of Non-Alcoholic Fatty Liver Disease and Atherosclerosis. *Current Opinion in Lipidology* 29:417–422.

Power, R.C., Salazar-García, D.C., Straus, L.G., Morales, M.R.G., and Henry, A.G. 2015. Microremains from El Mirón Cave Human Dental Calculus Suggest a Mixed Plant-Animal Subsistence Economy during the Magdalenian in Northern Iberia. *Journal of Archaeological Science* 60:39–46.

Rahman, M.A., Abdullah, N., and Aminudin, N. 2014. Inhibitory Effect on In Vitro LDL Oxidation and HMG Co-A Reductase Activity of the Liquid-Liquid Partitioned Fractions of Hericium Erinaceus (Bull.) Persoon (Lion's Mane Mushroom). *BioMed Research International* 2014:828149.

Rahman, M.A., Abdullah, N., and Aminudin, N. 2018. Lentinula Edodes (Shiitake Mushroom): An Assessment of in Vitro Anti-Atherosclerotic Bio-Functionality. *Saudi Journal of Biological Sciences* 25:1515–1523.

Ravi, B., Renitta, R.E., Prabha, M.L., Issac, R., and Naidu, S. 2012. Evaluation of Antidiabetic Potential of Oyster Mushroom (Pleurotus Ostreatus) in Alloxan-Induced Diabetic Mice. *Immunopharmacology and Immunotoxicology* 35:101–9.

Rojas, Á., Gallego, P., Gil-Gómez, A., Muñoz-Hernández, R., Rojas, L., Maldonado, R., Gallego-Durán, R., et al. 2018. Natural Extracts Abolished Lipid Accumulation in Cells Harbouring Non-Favourable PNPLA3 Genotype. *Annals of Hepatology* 17:242–249.

Roncero-Ramos, I., and Delgado-Andrade, C. 2017. The Beneficial Role of Edible Mushrooms in Human Health. *Current Opinion in Food Science* 14:122–128.

Spim, S.R.V., de Oliveira, B.G.C.C., Leite, F.G., Gerenutti, M., and Grotto, D. 2017. Effects of Lentinula Edodes Consumption on Biochemical, Hematologic and Oxidative Stress Parameters in Rats Receiving High-Fat Diet. *European Journal of Nutrition* 56:2255–2264.

Sato, M., Tokuji, Y., Yoneyama, S., Fujii-Akiyama, K., Kinoshita, M., and Ohnishi, M. 2011. Profiling of Hepatic Gene Expression of Mice Fed with Edible Japanese Mushrooms by DNA Microarray Analysis: Comparison among Pleurotus Ostreatus, Grifola Frondosa, and Hypsizigus Marmoreus. *Journal of Agricultural and Food Chemistry* 59:10723–10731.

Sayeed, M.A., Banu, A., Khatun, K., Khanam, P.A., Begum, T., Mahtab, H., and Haq, J.A. 2014. Effect of Edible Mushroom (Pleurotus Ostreatus) on Type-2 Diabetics. *Ibrahim Medical College Journal* 8:6–11.

Schneider, I., Kressel, G., Meyer, A., Krings, U., Berger, R.G., and Hahn, A. 2011. Lipid Lowering Effects of Oyster Mushroom (Pleurotus Ostreatus) in Humans. *Journal of Functional Foods* 3:17–24.

Sheng, Y., Zhao, C., Zheng, S., Mei, X., Huang, K., Wang, G., and He, X. 2019. Anti-Obesity and Hypolipidemic Effect of Water Extract from Pleurotus Citrinopileatus in C57BL/6J Mice. *Food Science and Nutrition* 7:1295–1301.

Smith, E., Ottosson, F., Hellstrand, S., Ericson, U., Orho-Melander, M., Fernandez, C., and Melander, O. 2020. Ergothioneine Is Associated with Reduced Mortality and Decreased Risk of Cardiovascular Disease. *Heart* 106:691–697.

Takeyama, A., Nagata, Y., Shirouchi, B., Nonaka, C., Aoki, H., Haraguchi, T., Sato, M., Tamaya, K., Yamamoto, H., and Tanaka, K. 2018. Dietary Sparassis Crispa Reduces Body Fat Mass and Hepatic Lipid Levels by Enhancing Energy Expenditure and Suppressing Lipogenesis in Rats. *J. Oleo Sci* 67:1137–1147.

Tang, R.M.Y., Cheah, I.K., Yew, T.S.K., and Halliwell, B. 2018. Distribution and Accumulation of Dietary Ergothioneine and Its Metabolites in Mouse Tissues. *Scientific Reports* 8:1601.

Wang, D., Yin, Z., Ma, L., Han, L., Chen, Y., Pan, W., Gong, K., et al. 2021. Polysaccharide MCP Extracted from Morchella Esculenta Reduces Atherosclerosis in LDLR-Deficient Mice. *Food & Function* 12:4842–4854.

Wang, J., Wang, C., Li, S., Li, W., Yuan, G., Pan, Y., and Chen, H. 2017. Anti-Diabetic Effects of Inonotus Obliquus Polysaccharides in Streptozotocin-Induced Type 2 Diabetic Mice and Potential Mechanism via PI3K-Akt Signal Pathway. *Biomedicine and Pharmacotherapy* 95:1669–1677.

Xu, N., Ren, Z., Zhang, J., Song, X., Gao, Z., Jing, H., Li, S., Wang, S., and Jia, L. 2017. Antioxidant and Anti-Hyperlipidemic Effects of Mycelia Zinc Polysaccharides by Pleurotus Eryngii Var. Tuoliensis. *International Journal of Biological Macromolecules* 95:204–214.

Xu, Y., Xie, L., Tang, J., He, X., Zhang, Z., Chen, Y., Zhou, J., Gan, B., and Peng, W. 2021. Morchella Importuna Polysaccharides Alleviate Carbon Tetrachloride-Induced Hepatic Oxidative Injury in Mice. *Frontiers in Physiology* 12:669331.

Yang, H., Hwang, I., Kim, S., Hong, E., and Jeung, E. 2013. Lentinus Edodes Promotes Fat Removal in Hypercholesterolemic Mice. *Experimental and Therapeutic Medicine* 6:1409–1413.

Yang, X., Dai, J., Zhong, Y., Wei, X., Wu, M., Zhang, Y., Huang, A., et al. 2021. Characterization of Insoluble Dietary Fiber from Three Food Sources and Their Potential Hypoglycemic and Hypolipidemic Effects. *Food & Function* 12:6576–6587.

Yeh, M., Ko, W., and Lin, L. 2014. Hypolipidemic and Antioxidant Activity of Enoki Mushrooms (Flammulina Velutipes). *BioMed Research International* 2014:352385.

Zhang, C., Li, J., Wang, J., Song, X., Zhang, J., Wu, S., Hu, C., Gong, Z., and Jia, L. 2017. Antihyperlipidaemic and Hepatoprotective Activities of Acidic and Enzymatic Hydrolysis Exopolysaccharides from Pleurotus Eryngii SI-04. *BMC Complementary and Alternative Medicine* 17:403.

Zhang, Z., Liang, X., Tong, L., Lv, Y., Yi, H., Gong, P., Tian, X., Cui, Q., Liu, T., and Zhang, L. 2021. Effect of Inonotus Obliquus (Fr.) Pilat Extract on the Regulation of Glycolipid Metabolism via PI3K/Akt and AMPK/ACC Pathways in Mice. *Journal of Ethnopharmacology* 273:113963.

Zhao, H., Li, S., Zhang, J., Che, G, Zhou, M., Liu, M, Zhang, C., et al. 2016. The Antihyperlipidemic Activities of Enzymatic and Acidic Intracellular Polysaccharides by Termitomyces Albuminosus. *Carbohydrate Polymers* 151:1227–1234.

Zhao, S., Rong, C., Liu, Y., Xu, F., Wang, S., Duan, C., Chen, J., and Wu, X. 2015. Extraction of a Soluble Polysaccharide from Auricularia Polytricha and Evaluation of Its Anti-Hypercholesterolemic Effect in Rats. *Carbohydrate Polymers* 122:39–45.

Zhao, S., Zhang, S., Zhang, W., Gao, Y., Rong, C., Wang, H., Liu, Y., Wong, J.H., and Ng, T. 2019. First Demonstration of Protective Effects of Purified Mushroom Polysaccharide-Peptides against Fatty Liver Injury and the Mechanisms Involved. *Scientific Reports* 9:13725.

Zheng, L., Zhai, G., Zhang, J., Wang, L., Ma, Z., Jia, M., and Jia, L. 2014. Antihyperlipidemic and Hepatoprotective Activities of Mycelia Zinc Polysaccharide from Pholiota Nameko SW-02. *International Journal of Biological Macromolecules* 70:523–529.

Zhu, M., Nie, P., Liang, Y., and Wang, B. 2013. Optimizing Conditions of Polysaccharide Extraction from Shiitake Mushroom Using Response Surface Methodology and Its Regulating Lipid Metabolism. *Carbohydrate Polymers* 95:644–648.

19 Pomegranate *(Punica granatum)* and Cardiovascular Protection
Molecular, Cellular, and Metabolic Aspects

María del Rocío Thompson Bonilla and
María Eugenia Jaramillo Flores

CONTENTS

19.1 Introduction 298
19.2 Effects of Pomegranate and Its Bioactive Compounds on the Modulation of the Lipid Profile 299
19.3 Hyperlipidemia Reduction by the Consumption of Pomegranate and Its Bioactive Compounds 299
19.4 Pomegranate Improves Dyslipidemia 300
19.5 Effect of Pomegranate Consumption and Its Bioactive Compounds on Hypertension 300
19.6 The Consumption of Pomegranate and Its Bioactive Compounds Ameliorate Diabetes 302
19.7 The Consumption of Pomegranate and Its Bioactive Compounds Ameliorate the Comorbidities of Obesity 303
19.8 Reduction of Inflammation and Inhibition of Atherosclerosis 305
19.9 Other Foods, Herbs, Spices, and Botanicals Used in Cardiovascular Health and Disease 307
19.10 Toxicity and Cautionary Notes 308
19.11 Conclusions 308
19.12 Summary Points 308
References 309

LIST OF ABBREVIATIONS

AMPK	Activated protein kinase
EA	Ellagic acid
eNOS	Endothelial nitric oxide synthetase
ICAM-1	Intracellular Adhesion Molecule 1
INF-γ	Interferon-γ
iNOS	Inducible nitric oxide synthase
JP	Pomegranate juice
LDL	Low-Density Lipoproteins
LSH	hormone sensitive lipase
MAPK	Mitogen-activated protein kinase
MCP-1	Monocyte Chemotray Protein 1

DOI: 10.1201/9781003220329-21

NF-κB	Nuclear factor kappa B
PAI-1	Plasminogen activator inhibitor
PAMP	Molecular patterns associated with pathogens
PDGFR α/β	Platelet-derived growth factor α
ROS	Reactive Oxygen Species
sE-S	Selectin soluble
SOD	Superoxide dismutase
SREBP1	Sterol Regulatory Element Binding Protein 1
TNF-α	Tumor necrosis factor α
VCAM	Vascular Cell Adhesion Protein 1
VEGF	Vascular Endothelial Growth Factor
VLDL	Very Low-Density Lipoprotein
VWF	Von Willebrand Factor

19.1 INTRODUCTION

Cardiovascular diseases are the main cause of death around the world, estimated around 17.9 million deaths each year (WHO 2022). CVDs are a group of disorders of the heart and blood vessels and include cerebrovascular and coronary heart disease (CHO); this last is the major source of fatality, followed by stroke, which is the second prime cause of death. CVDs comprise a group of comorbidities related to the heart and blood vessels, among others peripheral arterial disease, stroke, atherosclerosis, hypertension, CHO, cerebrovascular disease, and rheumatic cardiac disease.

Deaths due to cardiovascular diseases include risk factors, many of which can be controlled, such as hypertension, obesity, tobacco and alcohol consumption, diabetes, unhealthy dietary habits, lack of physical activity, hyperlipidemia, salt intake (Behl et al. 2020; Liu et al. 2019).

According to various epidemiological, preclinical, and clinical studies, it has been found that adequate consumption of plant-based foods significantly reduces the risk of suffering from chronic diseases. Within this context, the pomegranate has been studied for being an excellent source of dietary fiber and health benefiting nutrients, including vitamins (i.e., vitamin C, A, folic acid) and minerals (such as potassium). It is also a rich source of bioactive polyphenols compounds (ellagitannins, gallotannins, and flavonoids), some alkaloids, triterpenes, sterols, unsaturated fatty acids like the omega 5 punicic acid that constitutes around 70% of pomegranate seed oil. It is widely documented that these compounds exert numerous beneficial health activities and are the basis for considering pomegranate as a possible functional food (Table 19.1). The peel represents approximately 50% of the total weight of the pomegranate fruit and contains a higher content of polyphenols than the edible arils. Ellagitannins (punicalin and two isomers of punicalagin),

TABLE 19.1
Main Bioactive Components of *Punica granatum*

	Functional Biomolecules
Juice	Anthocyanins, ellagic acid, gallic acid, caffeic acid, catechins, quercetin, rutin
Pericarp (Peel, Bark)	Punicalagin, punicalin, peduncalagin, ellagic acid, gallic acid, luteolin, fatty acids, catechin, quercetin, rutin kaempferol, flavonols, flavones, flavanones, and anthocyanidins
Leaves	Tannins (punicalin and punicafolin) and flavone glycosides such as luteolin and apigenin.
Flowers	Gallic acid, ursolic acid, triterpenoids such as maslinic and asiatic acid
Roots and Bark	Ellagitannins (punicalin and punicalagin) and numerous piperidine alkaloids

Source: Adapted from Jurenka (2008)

Note: This table shows the main components with biological activity of pomegranate on cardiovascular diseases.

Pomegranate (*Punica granatum*) and Cardiovascular Protection

gallotannins, proanthocyanidins, and ellagic acid derivatives are the primary peel polyphenols. Anthocyanins are the minor phenolics present and are responsible for the characteristic pomegranate color (Gimenez Bastida et al. 2021).

The high antioxidant capacity of pomegranate juice is due to the high content of phenolic compounds present in both the arils and the peel, including punicalagin. This is why one of the main mechanisms by which it exerts its beneficial effects is the reduction of oxidative stress in addition to inhibiting lipid peroxidation. The reduction of oxidative stress is carried out either by direct neutralization of ROS, improving the activity and/or expression of antioxidant enzymes, by metal chelation, and/or by activating or inhibiting transcription factors such as SREBP, nuclear factor kappa B (NF-κB), and peroxisome proliferator-activated receptor gamma (PPARγ).

19.2 EFFECTS OF POMEGRANATE AND ITS BIOACTIVE COMPOUNDS ON THE MODULATION OF THE LIPID PROFILE

Cholesterol is an essential molecule that is part of the group of lipids or fats of the cell's membranes and necessary for the formation of hormones, metabolism of vitamin D, and the absorption of calcium and bile acids. The high levels of low-density lipoproteins cholesterol (LDL-C), the low levels in high-density lipoprotein cholesterol (HDL-C), and altered serum LDL-C/HDL-C ratio are highly associated with CVDs. The high LDL-C concentrations lead to the accumulation of fatty substances in the wall of the arteries (atherosclerosis) and cause various other complications and the elevated serum LDL-C/HDL-C ratio was found to be independently associated with sudden cardiac death (Behl et al. 2020).

High consumption of saturated fat, high cholesterol diets, low intake of fruits, vegetables, and whole grain fibers can lead to hypercholesterolemia and atherosclerosis, especially in genetically predisposed individuals.

Pomegranate peel significantly decreased levels of serum TC, LDL-C, and TG and increased HDL-C. There is a large body of evidence indicating decrease in Systolic Blood Pressure (SBP) levels and hs-CRP whereas Diastolic Blood Pressure (DBP) levels and BMI remained unchanged (Haghighian et al. 2016).

19.3 HYPERLIPIDEMIA REDUCTION BY THE CONSUMPTION OF POMEGRANATE AND ITS BIOACTIVE COMPOUNDS

Hyperlipidemia, characterized by high lipid content in the bloodstream, leads to tissue injury in various pathophysiological conditions, like diabetes, obesity, and CVDs. This tissue damage leads to endothelial dysfunction, whereas the endothelium of the blood vessels is constantly and directly exposed to the deleterious consequences of hyperlipidemia and recognized as one of the most important factors leading up to atherosclerosis. The role of NO not only as a vasodilator, but also as an inhibitor of neutrophil adhesion and platelet aggregation, is essential for the maintenance of endothelial function. Endothelial dysfunction is caused by reduced NO bioavailability and/or eNOS expression, and in the pathogenesis of endothelial dysfunction, both vascular inflammation and oxidative stress are interrelated factors. Interventions to improve mitochondrial function have been shown to correct endothelial abnormalities, although the mechanisms by which hyperlipidemia and mitochondrial dysfunction generate endothelial dysfunction are not precisely understood.

Various studies have shown that hyperlipidemia generated by the accumulation of triacylglycerols and cholesterol in serum, endothelial dysfunction, and mitochondrial dysfunction of the thoracic aorta are reduced by the administration of punicalagin, one of the active components of pomegranate, even though some studies with pomegranate juice coincide with the effects on the lipid profile, except for triglycerides. Punicalagin activates the FOXO1 signaling pathway, increases protein, and enhances translocation to the nucleus, inducing mitochondrial biogenesis, preventing mitochondria loss, and preventing vascular dysfunction (Liu et al. 2019).

19.4 POMEGRANATE IMPROVES DYSLIPIDEMIA

Dyslipidemia is one of the most important risk factors for cardiovascular disease and is characterized by elevated levels of total cholesterol (TC), triglycerides (TG), low-density lipoprotein cholesterol (LDL-C), and decreased levels of high-density lipoprotein cholesterol (HDL-C). Pomegranate and its polyphenols may have hypolipidemic effects. Lowering blood lipids with nutritional interventions is an important strategy that plays a key role in reducing cardiovascular diseases. A 10% reduction of total serum cholesterol reduces cardiovascular diseases (CVD) incidence by about 30%. Both preclinical and clinical trial showed reduction in serum TC, LDL-C, and TG levels and increase in serum HDL-C using pomegranate peel extract.

The consumption of pomegranate juice shows reduction of hs-CRP and inflammatory biomarkers. Punicalagin, punicalin, strictinin A, and granatin B have anti-inflammatory properties and could significantly reduce production of nitric oxide and prostaglandin E2 (PGE2) by inhibiting the expression of pro\-inflammatory proteins. Expression studies have shown reduced expression of TNF-α, IL-1β, IL-6, and IL-10, with a greater reduction in expression with pomegranate peel than juice (Haghighian et al. 2016).

The supplementation of dyslipidemic patients with two 500 mg pomegranate peel extract per day for 8 weeks remarkably decreased high sensitive C reactive protein (hs-CRP) levels. The peel active component presents inhibitory effects against inflammation compared to indomethacin after 6 h of treatment. Additionally, a pomegranate peel aqueous extract at a 50 ng/ml concentration inhibited neutrophil myeloperoxidase activity and the enzymatic production of hydrochloric acid from hydrogen peroxide. Through the suppression of various inflammatory pathways, the anti-inflammatory properties of pomegranate and its components have been revealed, inhibiting the production of proinflammatory cytokines such as IL-1, IL-2, and INF-γ. However, there are contradictory results due, among others, to changes in the profiles of the bioactive compounds present, as well as the concentrations, type, and duration of the test, and the pathology under study (obesity, diabetes, hypertension, etc.). More clinical trials are needed to explain this conflict of results in vitro and in vivo studies (Haghighian et al. 2016).

FOXO1 (class O of forkhead box) is a transcription factor that suppresses endothelial growth and proliferation, which under conditions of hyperglycemia and insulin resistance modulates myocardial function, preventing mitochondrial dysfunction via activation of FoxOl/PGC-1a (peroxisome proliferator receptor and coactivator 1a). Furthermore, in vascular endothelial cells, FoxOl promotes inducible NOS-dependent peroxynitrite generation of NO, which in turn leads to LDL oxidation and eNOS dysfunction. FoxOl downregulates eNOS, such that eNOS expression depends on FoxOl expression levels. However, it is unknown whether FoxOl is involved in hyperlipidemia-induced vascular damage. It has also been shown that punicalagin ameliorated cardiac mitochondrial impairment in obese rats via AMPK activation. Furthermore, it is known that ROS leads to the generation of intracellular signals that stimulate inflammation, including p38 MAPK. Regarding p38 MAPK, PU reduces its phosphorylation as well as the activation of NF-κB nuclear translocation by suppressing iKBa phosphorylation.

One study showed that a concentrate of pomegranate juice, increased eNOS expression in EC cultures and in atherosclerosis-prone areas of hyperlipidemic mice, indicating that oral administration of pomegranate juice at various stages of disease significantly reduces the progression of atherosclerosis (Liu et al. 2019).

19.5 EFFECT OF POMEGRANATE CONSUMPTION AND ITS BIOACTIVE COMPOUNDS ON HYPERTENSION

Elevated blood pressure (BP), commonly known as hypertension, is also a significant contributing factor of CVDs such as stroke, heart attack, and sudden cardiac failure. It has been reported that about 40% patients with essential hypertension also possess hypercholesterolemia. A strong correlation between hypertension and dyslipidemia has been established. Hypertension it is usually present with type 2 DM, such that the occurrence of hypertension in diabetic patients is approximately double as compared to those without diabetes.

Hypertension is defined as the level of blood pressure above normal pressure levels ranging from 100–120 mmHg in systolic pressure and 84–90 mmHg in diastolic pressure in (Valido Díaz et al. 2018) which therapeutic intervention has clinical benefits. It is the most common chronic cardiovascular disease and is associated with several pathological states, being an important cause of morbidity and mortality throughout the world. Hypertension is associated with vascular inflammation, increased levels of vascular cytokines, and immune cell infiltration of the vasculature, kidneys, and heart. Vascular inflammation is associated with the I-kappa B/nuclear factor kappa B inflammation pathway, which mediates most inflammatory responses such as atherosclerosis characterized by chronic inflammation of the vascular wall, via angiotensin and endothelin-1 (Virdis and Schiffrin 2003). Various pathophysiological factors are considered in the genesis of hypertension due to obesity and insulin resistance, which contribute to hypertension through different mechanisms: 1) insulin resistance; 2) altered lipid metabolism; 3) endothelial dysfunction; 4) decreased levels of adiponectin; 5) hyperactivity of the sympathetic nervous system (SNS); 6) the renin-angiotensin-aldosterone system (RAAS); 7) Renin-Angiotensin System (López De Fez et al. 2004).

Arterial hypertension generates a vicious circle (Figure 19.1) that activates various mechanisms producing greater hypertension, so that when a constant increase in blood pressure occurs, it produces a deregulation in the interaction of the mechanisms (renin-angiotensin-aldosterone system (RAAS), sympathetic nervous system (SNS), nitric oxide, and ACE) that maintain pressure and flow homeostasis (Gamboa 2006). In a state of obesity and hypertension, the renin-angiotensin-aldosterone system is affected by increasing aldosterone levels and producing angiotensin II, causing vasoconstriction, thrombosis by increasing PA-1 levels, platelet aggregation, production of superoxides and growth of the myocyte. Obesity causes oxidative stress and endothelial damage. Clinical studies have shown that in humans with hypertension, the production of reactive oxygen species increases and the activity of antioxidant enzymes (superoxide dismutase (SOD), glutathione peroxidase (GPx), and catalase) decreases; on the other hand, endothelial damage produces and releases vasoconstrictor substances such as endothelins and thromboxane and decreases the production and release of nitric oxide, causing vasoconstriction, platelet aggregation, inflammation, thrombosis (increase in PAI-1 levels) (Gamboa 2006; López De Fez et al. 2004).

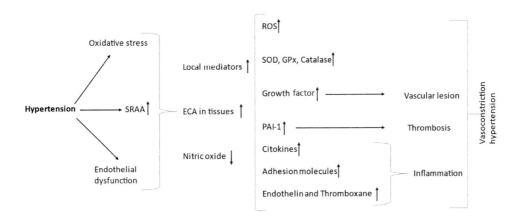

FIGURE 19.1 Vicious circle of hypertension.

Note: This figure shows the different causes and effects that generate hypertension and vasoconstriction, and the feedback of those causes and effects.

The most common form of hypertension, accounting for 90–95% of all cases, is primary (also known as "essential") hypertension, resulting from a complex interaction of genes and environmental factors. Chronic hypertension in combination with atherosclerosis is the leading risk factor for stroke, coronary heart disease, congestive heart failure, and end-stage renal disease. Obesity can increase the risk of hypertension compared to normal weight, and more than 85% of hypertension cases can be attributed to a body mass index greater than 25 (Bomfim et al. 2019; Carlberg et al. 2016).

In relation to blood pressure, in a preclinical study in obese rats, it was shown that treatments with peel, juice, and ellagic acid decrease systolic pressure to values of 120 mm Hg, 112.6 mm Hg, and 110.6 mm Hg, which corresponds to a 15%, 21%, and 22% decrease respectively. The treatments also reduced diastolic pressure to values of 99.6 mm Hg, 89 mm Hg, and 91 mm Hg which is equivalent to a reduction of 15%, 24%, and 22% respectively, compared to the group with hyperlipidic diet. The results suggest that pomegranate juice, peel, and ellagic acid reduce the risk of hypertension and therefore cardiovascular diseases in obesity, since its effect lowers blood pressure to normal pressure levels, which is probably due to the polyphenols (anthocyanins, punicalagin, and ellagic acid) present in pomegranate juice and pomegranate peel, according to various studies of pomegranate's beneficial effects on vascular diseases (Danesi and Ferguson 2017).

A clinical study evaluated the effects of 250 mg of ethanolic extract of pomegranate peel on blood pressure in diabetic patients for 8 weeks, showing a decrease in systolic blood pressure from 136.31 mm Hg to 130.26 mm Hg, as well as in diastolic pressure in diabetic patients from 82.89 mmHg to 80.79 mmHg (Grabež et al. 2020). In contrast, another double-blind, placebo-controlled clinical trial, which included 55 participants (men and women, without symptomatic disease), were treated with 210 mg of pomegranate extract for 8 weeks, lowering diastolic blood pressure, but with no change of systolic pressure (Stockton et al. 2017). It has been found that pomegranate peel (dry powdered peel) has a greater effect in lowering blood pressure than an ethanolic extract thereof, possibly due to the synergy of the phenolic compounds present (punicalagin and ellagic acid in higher concentration).

Ellagic acid, a flavonoid present in both pomegranate juice and peel, appears to be largely the compound responsible for the blood pressure-lowering effect in obese rats, thus promoting the reduction of risk of cardiovascular diseases.

A clinical study evaluated the effects of 250 mg of pomegranate ethanolic extract in rats with hypertension induced with 60 mg of Nω-Nitro-L-arginine methyl ester hydrochloride (L-NAME), and the effect of ellagic acid on the vascular damage caused by hypertension. Rats were co-administered with 10 and 30 mg/kg/day of ellagic acid for 6 weeks, where they found that 10 mg/kg of ellagic acid reduced systolic blood pressure by 16.8% while 30 mg/kg of ellagic acid reduced systolic blood pressure by 21.6%. The reduction in systolic pressure was 21.6%, so that ellagic acid decreases hypertension, possibly improving the availability of nitric oxide (Jordão et al. 2017).

It was shown that some polyphenols such as punicalagin activates the endothelial nitric oxide (NO) synthase and acts as a vasodilator. It could be a mechanism of observed hypotensive effect of pomegranate peel extract.

It has also been found that impaired mitochondrial oxidative phosphorylation and myocardial mitochondrial biogenesis lead to diastolic dysfunction, and this mitochondrial dysfunction brings with it lipid accumulation, ultimately leading to a further aggravation of mitochondrial dysfunction.

19.6 THE CONSUMPTION OF POMEGRANATE AND ITS BIOACTIVE COMPOUNDS AMELIORATE DIABETES

Diabetes is a metabolic disorder which is characterized by the presence of high concentration of blood glucose levels in the blood. It is also a prominent risk factor in the development and progression of CVDs. CHO is the causal agent of fatality in type 2 DM patients, which also enhances the risk for acute myocardial infraction (MI). High blood glucose levels may lead to artery wall destruction, forming atheroma (deposition of fats) in the arteries. The deposition of fatty substances, occurring in the coronary arteries, may lead to CHO and cardiac failure.

TABLE 19.2

Outcome of Clinical Studies Involving Intake of Pomegranate Juice or Peel Hydro Alcoholic Extract

Type of Study/Number of Probands	Clinical Outcome	References
In hypertensive patients ($N = 10$), consumption of pomegranate juice, every day for 2 weeks	They observed a 36% reduction in ACE activity and 5% of systolic blood pressure	Aviram and Dornfeld (2001)
In a study with 19 patients with carotid stenosis, for a long duration intake of pomegranate juice for 3 years	They observed a 12% reduction in systolic blood pressure and decrease in common carotid intima-media thickness up to 30%	Aviram et al. (2004)
A 4-week consumption of pomegranate juice by healthy women ($N = 51$)	A mild, but significant reduction in blood pressure (without significantly changing serum ACE activity)	Lynn et al. (2012)
In a study of hypertensive men ($N = 13$), who ingested pomegranate juice	Parameters as serum concentrations of CRP, E-selectin, VCAM-1, ICAM-1, and IL-6, remain unchanged, only they observed decrease in blood pressure	Asgary et al. (2013)
In a study with hypertensive patients ($N = 21$), with consumption of pomegranate juice	They found a significant reduction in systolic and diastolic blood pressure	Asgary et al. (2014)
In 38 obese women with dyslipidemia, whose intake of pomegranate peel hydro alcoholic extract were evaluated.	They observed a significant reduction in systolic blood pressure	Haghighian et al. (2016)

Note: This table shows the effect of pomegranate extracts or compounds and doses used, on biomarkers of cardiovascular diseases in humans.

Moreover, impaired fasting plasma glucose (FPG) and impaired glucose tolerance are significantly associated with various cardiovascular diseases. Epidemiological data also suggests that hyperglycemia, insulin resistance, and hyperinsulinemia exhibit direct effects on the progression of endothelial dysfunction and atherosclerosis.

The prevalence of the diabetic heart is the main cause of sickness and death in the diabetic and obese population. Conditions of low glycemic control and an increase in ROS, which stimulate cell damage and activate the mitochondrial pathway, result in increased apoptosis of cardiomyocytes in diabetic patients.

A study showed that the heart of diabetic rats presented a disorganized matrix of myocardial structure, myofibrillar disruption, degeneration of myocytes and pyknotic nuclei. Those animals that were treated with punicalagin presented uniform size and regular arrangement of cardiac muscle fibers, with centrally located round or oval nuclei. Punicalagin treatment of diabetic rats has cardioprotective effects in STZ-induced diabetes, reducing the risk of diabetes-induced cardiac apoptosis. Oxidative stress is one of the main causes of hyperglycemia-induced cardiac injury, so antioxidant compounds can be used to block pathological changes and protect cardiac function. Additionally, pomegranate juice can lead to a reduction in inflammation associated with diabetes by the decrease in levels of E-selectin and NF-κB and increase in levels of SIRT-1 (Sohrab et al. 2018).

19.7 THE CONSUMPTION OF POMEGRANATE AND ITS BIOACTIVE COMPOUNDS AMELIORATE THE COMORBIDITIES OF OBESITY

Obesity is a global health problem characterized by the excessive accumulation of energy in the form of fat in adipose tissue (González-Muniesa et al. 2017), which is the result of the combination of genetic factors, inadequate nutrition, and lack of regular physical activity (Manzur et al. 2010). The energy imbalance arises from the intake of a high-fat diet and/or increases in the consumption of processed carbohydrates with a high glycemic load, and it is the main cause of visceral or central obesity (San-Cristobal et al. 2020; Ludwig and Ebbeling, 2018), producing hormonal changes that promote energy storage in adipose tissue, exacerbating hunger, and reducing energy expenditure (Ludwig and Ebbeling 2018). The energy reserves found in adipose tissue promote hypertrophy and hyperplasia (increase in size and number) in adipocytes, as well as metabolic dysfunction, hypoxia, an increase in proinflammatory cytokines, and the release of fatty acids in the adipose tissue, promoting macrophage infiltration thus leading to a state of chronic low-grade inflammation, insulin resistance, and endothelial dysfunction (Manzur et al. 2010; Reyes 2012).

Obesity is related to various pathophysiologies and alterations in glycolipid metabolism, as well as proinflammatory and prothrombotic states. The link between all of them is attributed to insulin resistance, favored by the increase in free fatty acids, related to overweight and obesity (Redinger 2007).

The first indication for increased cytokine release in obesity was the identification of increased expression of TNF-α, a proinflammatory cytokine that is expressed and produced primarily in adipose tissue, macrophages, and/or peripheral tissues, and induces cell-specific inflammation of tissue through the generation of reactive oxygen species (ROS) and the activation of several transcription-mediated molecular and metabolic pathways. The elevated level of TNF-α induces insulin resistance in adipocytes and peripheral tissues by altering insulin signaling through serine phosphorylation that leads to the development of type 2 diabetes, its levels correlating with the degree of adiposity and the insulin resistance (Akash et al. 2018; Tzanavari et al. 2010).

Another cytokine implicated in obesity is interleukin-6, a multifunctional cytokine that performs immune and hematopoietic activities (Simpson et al. 1997). In obese patients, elevated levels of IL-6 are regulated by different physiological or pathological factors such as hormones, cytokines, diet, physical activity, stress, and hypoxia (Eder et al. 2009). Its gene expression is strictly controlled by transcriptional and post-transcriptional mechanisms, continuously deregulated synthesis of IL-6, and has a pathological effect on chronic inflammation and autoimmunity (Tanaka et al. 2014). Adipose-derived IL-6 may have an effect on metabolism through several mechanisms, including adipose-specific gene expression, triglyceride release, lipoprotein lipase downregulation, and insulin sensitivity (Eder et al. 2009).

Plasminogen activator inhibitor 1 (PAI-1) is the main regulatory protein of the fibrinolytic system in vivo (Van Meijer and Pannekoek 1995). Clinical studies have shown a strong association between PAI-1 and the metabolic components of insulin resistance, suggesting that insulin resistance may regulate circulating PAI-1 (Bastard and Piéroni 1999). PAI-1 is also considered an acute phase reactant, which is highly influenced by inflammatory cytokines: IL-6, IL-1, TNF-α; growth factors: tissue growth factor-β (TGF-β); and hormones: insulin, glucocorticoids, and adrenaline (Cesari et al. 2010). The levels and activity of PAI-1 are increased in obesity and metabolic syndrome, whose previous studies have implicated it in the expansion of adipose tissue. A high-fat diet is a link between obesity, insulin resistance, and cardiovascular disease, where PAI-1 is a key component of fibrinolysis and increased cardiovascular risk in obese people due to dyslipidemia, hypertension, and insulin intolerance (Wang et al. 2018).

Monocyte chemoattractant protein 1 (MCP-1) is a member of the CC chemokine subfamily, which controls the migration of neutrophils, lymphocytes, and antigen-presenting cells (dendritic cells, monocytes, and macrophages) (Yadav et al. 2010). The expression of this proinflammatory chemokine is increased in the adipose tissue of obese people and in atherosclerotic lesions in patients with atherosclerosis. Inhibition of its expression or that of its receptor (CC chemokine receptor 2 (CCR2)) reduces the degree of atheroma formation and inflammation (Kanda et al. 2006).

In pathological conditions such as obesity, the anti-inflammatory response may be insufficient to counteract inflammatory activity or, on the contrary, act and inhibit the immune system (De Pablo Sánchez et al. 2005).

Interleukin-10 (IL-10) is a Th2-type cytokine that inhibits the synthesis and activity of proinflammatory cytokines and counteracts inflammation mediated by Toll-like receptors (Dagdeviren et al. 2016). IL-10 is also a protective factor against high-fat diet-induced insulin resistance in the liver (Febbraio 2014).

Fatty acid synthase (FAS) has been recognized as a potential therapeutic target for obesity. The inhibitory effect of pomegranate husk extract, punicalagin, and ellagic acid on FAS was with half-inhibitory concentration values (IC50) of 4.1 µg/ml (pomegranate husk extract), 4.2 µg/ml (4.50 µM, punicalagin), and 1.31 µg/ml (4.34 µM, ellagic acid), respectively. Many of them exhibited time-dependent inactivation of FAS. Punicalagin and ellagic acid inhibited FAS with different mechanisms compared to previously reported inhibitors, through inactivating acetyl/malonyl transferase and α-ketoacyl synthase domains, respectively. FAS plays a key role in the biosynthesis pathway of fatty acid; these findings suggest that pomegranate husk extract, punicalagin, and ellagic acid have potential in the prevention and treatment of obesity. It was reported that the body weight and food intake of obese mice obviously reduced after they were treated with FAS inhibitors. The actions were due to inhibition of the expression of signal neuropeptide Y in hypothalamus, which is mediated by Mal-CoA, one of the substrates of FAS (Wu 2013).

Although there are various studies on the bioavailability of flavonoids, ellagitannins, punicalagin, ellagic acid, and phenolic compounds in general (Figure 19.2), they are still insufficient, and although progress has been made in this regard, little is known about the precise mechanisms of their absorption and transformation. But nevertheless, it was reported that daily intake of pomegranate juice containing 6% punicalagin ranged from 0.6 to 1.2 g, and the plasma concentration of punicalagin was detected at around 30 µg/ml (Wu 2013).

19.8 REDUCTION OF INFLAMMATION AND INHIBITION OF ATHEROSCLEROSIS

Atherosclerosis, a chronic inflammatory disorder, plays a significant role in the progression of CVDs. Accumulation of apolipoprotein B, including lipoprotein and LDL, promotes dysfunction of endothelial cells. This dysfunction of the endothelial cells causes infiltration of LDL. Additionally,

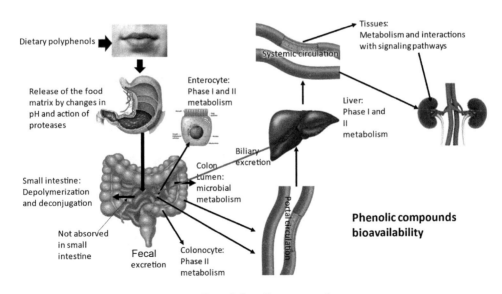

FIGURE 19.2 Absorption and bioavailability of phenolic compounds.

Note: The figure shows the absorption/digestion/transformation process of phenolic compounds and their polymers during their passage through the gastrointestinal tract.

there is an increment in both the release of chemokines from endothelial cells and expression of adhesion protein on their surface, which further triggers the recruitment of monocytes. On the surface, monocytes convert into macrophages and undergo lipoprotein uptake to modify into foam cells. The formation of foam cells are the signatures of early atherosclerosis in arterial intima. With the passage of time, necrosis and apoptosis of these cells is observed, resulting in the progression of a lipid-rich necrotic core, subsequently leading to a chronic inflammatory response. Extracellular matrix (ECM), formed by smooth muscle cells, covers this lipid-rich necrotic core with a fibrous cap that transfers and proliferates to the intima from the media. Inflammatory mediators and increased expressions facilitate the activity of fibrous cap, which enhances the destruction of the ECM and also provides stability to the lesions, as a result of plaque rupture.

However, different stages involved in the pathogenesis serve as favorable targets for different therapeutic approaches in the treatment of atherosclerosis. The management of lipid homeostasis is a major success accomplished by therapeutic agents.

The prevalence of the diabetic heart has markedly increased in the past few years and is now considered the main cause of sickness and death among the diabetic and obese population. Diabetic cardiomyopathy is associated with increased oxidative stress that stimulates cellular injury and contributes to the development and progression of complications associated with diabetes. Apoptosis is a key process in diabetic cardiac diseases derived from poor glycemic control. A number of studies have documented an increased occurrence of apoptosis in the cardiomyocytes of diabetic patients and experimentally induced diabetic animals. It is mediated, at least in part, by the activation of the mitochondrial pathway, which is often triggered by reactive oxygen species (ROS).

Maintaining normal serum lipid levels through nutrition programs is an effective approach to decrease the major risk of cardiovascular disease and related disease complications. Punicalagin treatment reduces levels of total cholesterol, LDL-cholesterol, VLDL-cholesterol, and triglyceride levels in the serum while the pomegranate extract improves abnormal cardiac lipid metabolism by activating peroxisome proliferator-activated receptor-alpha (PPAR-α) (cardiac transcription factor involved in myocardial energy production via fatty acid uptake and oxidation). Pomegranate reduced cholesterol absorption, increased cholesterol excretion in feces, exerted positive effects on cholesterol metabolizing enzymes, markedly decreased total and LDL-cholesterol and improved the total/HDL and LDL/HDL-cholesterol ratios. Furthermore, in macrophages punicalagin modulates the expression of PPARγ reducing oxidative stress in vitro (El-Missiry et al. 2015).

Regarding the levels of E-selectin modulated by juice pomegranate treatments, contradictory results have been obtained, since while some studies have found a significant decrease in the level of E-selectin, other studies found a significant elevation in the levels of E-selectin. More evidence is required to know the causes of the differences in the results of E-selectin, given the importance of the downstream genes FOXO1 than promote endothelial cell migration, also like VCAM-1Y (Kelishadi et al. 2011, Asgary et al. 2014, Sohrab et al. 2018).

Cyanidin glucoside is a type of anthocyanin found in pomegranate juice, which leads to a decrease in the levels of nuclear factor-κB (NF-κB) and SIRT1 (Sohrab et al. 2018). Using peel extract of pomegranate and punicalagin on human monocytic cell line THP-1, it was shown to decrease the release of ICAM-1, but in contrast, no effect was observed on release of VCAM-1 by the THP-1 cell line (Sohrab et al. 2018).

Different studies, both in animal and cell models, have shown that preventive and/or therapeutic effect of pomegranate against cardiovascular disease. Administration of pomegranate juice (100 or 300 mg/kg) for 4 weeks led to a reduction in the serum angiotensin-converting enzyme activity and as a consequence decreased the mean arterial blood pressure in diabetic hypertensive rats. The evidence indicates that anti-atherogenic properties of pomegranate juice can prevent foam cell progression and cellular cholesterol accumulation in macrophages by suppressing cholesterol biosynthesis and oxidized low-density lipoprotein degradation. Like a source of anti-oxidants, pomegranate pretreatment reduced the cardiac damage inhibiting lipoperoxidation and inflammatory processes in daunorubicin-induced cardiotoxicity in rats. The cardiac biomarkers

Pomegranate (*Punica granatum*) and Cardiovascular Protection

troponin I, malondialdehyde, and IL-17 were decreased using pomegranate in rats (Fuhrman et al. 2005; Mohan et al. 2010, Asgary 2021).

19.9 OTHER FOODS, HERBS, SPICES, AND BOTANICALS USED IN CARDIOVASCULAR HEALTH AND DISEASE

Epicatechin is found in a wide variety of foods such as tea (51%), apples (28%), and cocoa (7%), with antioxidant, anti-inflammatory and antihypertensive properties. The intake (15.2 ± 7.7 mg/d), is inversely related to CHD mortality in elderly men and to CVD mortality in prevalent cases of CVD. However, more studies are needed before conclusions can be drawn. Epicatechin's vascular responses and cardioprotective effects are mediated through opioid receptors, nitric oxide, potassium channel and calcium channel activation and highlight the importance of the endothelium/nitric oxide in epicatechin-mediated vasorelaxation (Dower et al. 2016; MacRae et al. 2019).

Curcumin and its antioxidant, anti-inflammatory, and anti-apoptotic properties have been reported to be effective in improving cardiac hypertrophy, heart failure, diabetic cardiovascular complications, and cardiotoxicity (Wongcharoen et al. 2009).

Ginger can prevent blood clotting. A single dose of 10 grams prevented clotting in patients with heart disease, and enhanced the effects of the blood pressure medication nifedipine; however, while this effect could have health benefits, it could also prove problematic, such that it is recommended that patients using anticoagulants or nifedipine stay cautious about their ginger use (Dülger 2012; Ruivo 2016).

Cinnamon consists of a variety of resinous compounds, including cinnamaldehyde, cinnamate, cinnamic acid, and numerous essential oils. Cinnamon inhibits the release of inflammatory fatty acids such as arachidonic acid from the blood's platelet membranes. It also works to reduce the

TABLE 19.3
Cardioprotective Abilities of Fruits

Fruit Pomegranate	Subject	Study Type	Dose	Main Effects	References
PE	SR-B1/apoE double KO mice	In vivo	307.5 µl/L in water	Oxidative stress and inflammation in the vessel wall↓, aortic sinus and coronary artery atherosclerosis↓, was observed	Al-Jarallah (2013)
PE with 40% punicalagin	SHR	In vivo	150 mg/Kg/day	They observed mitochondrial, superoxide anion levels↓, mitochondrial function↑, BP↓, cardiac hypertrophy↓, oxidative stress↓, antioxidant defense, system↑, paraventricular nucleus inflammation↓.	Sun (2016)
PE with 40% punicalagin	Heart of a high-fat diet-induced obesity rat model	In vivo	150 mg/Kg/day	cardiac, metabolic disorders↓, mitochondrial biogenesis↑, oxidative stress↓, phase II enzymes↑.	Cao (2015)
Pomegranate seed extract	CHI rat model	In vivo	100, 200, 400, 800 mg/Kg/day	motor and cognitive coordination↑	Hajipour (2014)

Note: This table shows the effect of pomegranate extracts or compounds and doses used, on biomarkers of cardiovascular diseases in animal models.

formation of thromboxane A2, which is an inflammatory molecule found in the blood stream. It was able to interfere with monocyte differentiation and macrophage scavenger activity, indicating its potential in preventing the development of atherosclerotic lesions (Hariri and Reza 2016).

Garlic (organic sulfides), onion (quercetin and alkenyl cysteine sulfoxides), black peppers (piperine), chili peppers (capsaicin), and green tea have beneficial effects on the prevention of various aspects of cardiovascular disease, including hypertension and dyslipidemia. The treatment of hypercholesterolemia using garlic is through the inhibition of cholesterol biosynthesis in the liver, and the inhibition of the oxidation of low-density lipoproteins (Steiner and Li 2001; Qidwai et al. 2013).

19.10 TOXICITY AND CAUTIONARY NOTES

Pomegranate juice and punicalagin, its major component, inhibited 1-naphthol sulfoconjugation in Caco-2 cells in a dose-time dependent manner. No inhibition of 1-naphthol glucuronidation was observed in Caco-2 cells. On the other hand, both pomegranate juice and punicalagin inhibit phenol sulfotransferase activity in Caco-2 cells. Pomegranate juice, however, shows no effect on the expression of the SULT1A sulfotransferase gene family (SULT1A1 and SULT1A3) in Caco-2 cells. This indicates that the reduction in 1-naphthylsulfate accumulation is due to the inhibition of sulfotransferase activity by punicalagin. Therefore, some constituents of pomegranate juice, most likely punicalagin, impair enteric sulfoconjugation functions and this could have effects on the bioavailability of drugs and other compounds present in food and in the environment.

Ellagic acid, although its safety has not been proven, is sold in supplement form. It can affect certain enzymes in the liver, which could alter the levels of some drugs in the body. For this reason, people who take medications or other dietary supplements should talk to their doctors or pharmacists about all of their medications and supplements before taking ellagic acid.

Ellagic acid can increase the hepatotoxic activities of paracetamol, while on the other hand, excretion of ellagic acid can be decreased when combined with different types of third-generation antibiotics, benzopyrans, and a number of drugs such as acetylsalicylic acid.

Due to this, it is necessary to carry out preclinical and clinical studies in relation to the chronic toxicity of ellagic acid, as well as the interactions with drugs of massive use such as those used for diabetics, hypertensive patients, etc.

19.11 CONCLUSIONS

The results of various studies carried out in vitro and in vivo suggest that pomegranate has cardioprotective effects, include diminishing of oxidative stress; positive influencing on macrophage, endothelial cell, and platelet function; lowering lipid oxidation; reducing blood glucose levels; vasodilatory effects; as well as decreasing blood pressure via an inhibition of ACE activity, when consumed properly, but it has also been seen that excessive consumption of this functional food can produce diarrhea. In general, studies suggest that it has a lot of potential as a functional food, and perhaps that explains why it has been consumed since ancient times and why society has attributed aphrodisiac properties to it.

They are undoubtedly compounds with great potential to improve cardiovascular health; however, there is still little information on the mechanisms of action of each of the compounds that can work as therapeutics or as adjuvants, as well as the appropriate doses, since the information existing shows a great diversity of doses tested.

19.12 SUMMARY POINTS

- This chapter focuses on the study of the effects of pomeranate, its components (juice, peel, arils), and the compounds it contains on cardiovascular health.
- Pomegranate contains compounds with antihypertensive and anti-inflammatory activity.

Pomegranate (*Punica granatum*) and Cardiovascular Protection

- The compounds contained in pomegranate reduce oxidative stress.
- Punicalagin induces mitochondrial biogenesis.
- The compounds contained in the pomegranate modify the lipid metabolism.
- The compounds contained in pomegranate prevent atherosclerosis.

REFERENCES

Akash, M. S. H., Rehman, K., & Liaqat, A. 2018. Tumor necrosis factor-alpha: Role in development of insulin resistance and pathogenesis of type 2 diabetes mellitus. *Journal of Cellular Biochemistry, 119*(1), 105–110. https://doi.org/10.1002/jcb.26174

Al-Jarallah, A., Igdoura, F., Zhang, Y., Tenedero, C. B., White, E. J., MacDonald, M. E., Igdoura, S. A., & Trigatti, B. L. 2013. The effect of pomegranate extract on coronary artery atherosclerosis in SR-BI/APOE double knockout mice. *Atherosclerosis, 228*, 80–89.

Asgary, S., Karimi, R., Joshi, T., Kilpatrick, K. L., Moradi, S., Samini, Z., Mohammadi, E., Farzai, M. H., & Bishayee, A. 2021. Effect of pomegranate juice on vascular adhesion factors: A systematic review and meta-analysis. *Phytomedicine, 80*, 153359. https://doi.org/10.1016/j.phymed.2020.153359

Asgary, S., Keshvari, M., Sahebkar, A., Hashemi, M., & Rafieian-Kopaei, M. 2013. Clinical investigation of the acute effects of pomegranate juice on blood pressure and endothelial function in hypertensive individuals. *ARYA Atherosclerosis, 9*, 326–331.

Asgary, S., Sahebkar, A., Afshani, M. R., Keshvari, M., Haghjooyjavanmard, S., & Rafieian-Kopaei, M. 2014. Clinical evaluation of blood pressure lowering, endothelial function improving, hypolipidemic and anti-inflammatory effects of pomegranate juice in hypertensive subjects. *Phytotherapy Research 28*(2), 193–199. doi: 10.1002/ptr.4977

Aviram, M., & Dornfeld, L. 2001. Pomegranate juice consumption inhibits serum angiotensin converting enzyme activity and reduces systolic blood pressure. *Atherosclerosis, 158*, 195–198. doi: 10.1016/S0021–9150(01)00412–9

Aviram, M., Rosenblat, M., Gaitini, D., Nitecki, S., Hoffman, A., Dornfeld, L., et al. 2004. Pomegranate juice consumption for 3 years by patients with carotid artery stenosis reduces common carotid intima-media thickness, blood pressure and LDL oxidation. *Clinical Nutrition, 23*, 423–433. doi: 10.1016/j.clnu.2003.10.002

Bastard, J. P., & Piéroni, L. 1999. Plasma plasminogen activator inhibitor 1, insulin resistance and android obesity. *Biomedicine and Pharmacotherapy, 53*(10), 455–461. https://doi.org/10.1016/S0753-3322(00)88103-2

Behl, T., Bungau, S., Kumar, K., Zengin C. G., & Khan, F. 2020. Pleotropic effects of polyphenols in cardiovascular system. *Biomedicine and Pharmacotherapy, 130*, 110714.

Bomfim, G. F., Bruno Assis Cau, S., Santos Bruno, A., Garcia Fedoce, A., & Carneiro, F. S. 2019. Hypertension: A new treatment for an old disease? Targeting the immune system. *British Journal of Pharmacology*. https://doi.org/10.1111/bph.14436

Cao, K., Xu, J., Pu, W. J., Dong, Z. Z., Sun, L., Zang, W. J., Gao, F., Zhang, Y., Feng, Z. H., & Liu, J. K. 2015. Punicalagin, an active component in pomegranate, ameliorates cardiac mitochondrial impairment in obese rats via AMPK activation. *Scientific Reports, 5*, 14014.

Carlberg, C., Ulven, S. M., & Molnár, F. 2016. Hypertension, atherosclerosis and dyslipidemias in Nutrigenomics, ed. C. Carlberg, S. M. Ulven, & F. Molnár, 195–208, Springer. doi: 10.1007/978-3-319-30415-1_11

Cesari, M., Pahor, M., & Incalzi, R. A. 2010. Plasminogen activator inhibitor-1 (PAI-1): A key factor linking fibrinolysis and age-related subclinical and clinical conditions. *Cardiovascular Therapeutics, 28*(5), 72–91. https://doi.org/10.1111/j.1755-5922.2010.00171.x

Dagdeviren, S., Jung, D. Y., Lee, E., Friedline, R. H., Noh, H. L., Kim, J. H., . . . Kim, J. K. 2016. Altered interleukin-10 signaling in skeletal muscle regulates obesity-mediated inflammation and insulin resistance. *Molecular and Cellular Biology, 36*(23), 2956–2966. https://doi.org/10.1128/mcb.00181-16

Danesi, F., & Ferguson, L. R. 2017. Could pomegranate juice help in the control of inflammatory diseases? *Nutrients, 9*(9). https://doi.org/10.3390/nu9090958

De Pablo Sánchez, R., Monserrat Sanz, J., Prieto Martín, A., Reyes Martín, E., Alvarez De Mon Soto, M., & Sanchez Garcia, M. 2005. Balance entre citocinas pro y antiinflamatorias en estados sépticos. *Medicina Intensiva, 29*(3), 151–158. https://doi.org/10.1016/s0210-5691(05)74222-4

Dower, J. I., Geleijnse, J. M., Hollman, P. C., Soedamah-Muthu, S. S., & Kromhout, D. 2016. Dietary epicatechin intake and 25-y risk of cardiovascular mortality: The Zutphen Elderly Study. *American Journal of Clinical Nutrition, 104*(1), 58–64. doi: 10.3945/ajcn.115.128819

Dülger, G. 2012. Herbal drugs and drug interactions. *Marmara Pharmaceutical Journal, 16*, 9–22. doi: 10.12991/201216415

Eder, K., Baffy, N., Falus, A., & Fulop, A. K. 2009. The major inflammatory mediator interleukin-6 and obesity. *Inflammation Research*, *58*(11), 727–736. https://doi.org/10.1007/s00011-009-0060-4

El-Missiry, M. A., Amer, M. A., Hemieda, F. A. E., Othman, A. I., Sakr, D. A., & Abdulhadi, H. L. 2015. Cardioameliorative effect of punicalagin against streptozotocin-induced apoptosis, redox imbalance, metabolic changes and inflammation. *Egyptian Journal of Basic and Applied Sciences*, *2*, 247–260. https://doi.org/10.1016/j.ejbas.2015.09.004

Febbraio, M. A. 2014. Role of interleukins in obesity: Implications for metabolic disease. *Trends in Endocrinology and Metabolism*, *25*(6), 312–319. https://doi.org/10.1016/j.tem.2014.02.004

Fuhrman, B., Volkova, N., & Aviram, M. 2005. Pomegranate juice inhibits oxidized LDL uptake and cholesterol biosynthesis in macrophages. *Journal of Nutritional Biochemistry*, *16*, 570–576. 10.1016/j.jnutbio.2005.02.009

Gamboa, R. A. 2006. Physiopathology of essential hypertension. *Medizinische Klinik*, *65*(17), 815–818.

Gimenez-Bastida, J. A., Avila-Galvez, M. A., Espín, J. C., & Gonzalez-Sarrías, A. 2021. Evidence for health properties of pomegranate juices and extracts beyond nutrition: A critical systematic review of human studies. *Trends in Food Science & Technology*, *114*, 410–423.

González-Muniesa, P., Mártinez-González, M. A., Hu, F. B., Després, J. P., Matsuzawa, Y., Loos, R. J. F., . . . Martinez, J. A. 2017. Obesity. *Nature Reviews Disease Primers*, *3*. https://doi.org/10.1038/nrdp.2017.34

Grabež, M., Škrbić, R., Stojiljković, M. P., Rudić-Grujić, V., Paunović, M., Arsić, A., . . . Vasiljević, N. 2020. Beneficial effects of pomegranate peel extract on plasma lipid profile, fatty acids levels and blood pressure in patients with diabetes mellitus type-2: A randomized, double-blind, placebo-controlled study. *Journal of Functional Foods*, *64*(August 2019). https://doi.org/10.1016/j.jff.2019.103692

Haghighian, M. K., Rafraf, M., Moghaddam, A., Hemmati, S., Jafarabadi, M. A., & Gargari, B. P. 2016. Pomegranate (Punica granatum L.) peel hydro alcoholic extract ameliorates cardiovascular risk factors in obese women with dyslipidemia: A double blind, randomized, placebo controlled pilot study. *European Journal of Integrative Medicine*, *8*(5), 676–682. https://doi.org/10.1016/j.eujim.2016.06.010

Hajipour, S., Sarkaki, A., Mohammad, S., Mansouri, T., Pilevarian, A., RafieiRad, M. 2014. Motor and cognitive deficits due to permanent cerebral hypoperfusion/ischemia improve by pomegranate seed extract in rats. *Pakistan Journal of Biological Sciences*, *17*, 991–998.

Hariri, M., & Reza, G. 2016. Cinnamon and chronic diseases in Drug discovery from mother nature, ed. S. C. Gupta, S. P. Bharat, & B. Aggarwal, 1–24, Springer.

Jordão, J. B. R., Porto, H. K. P., Lopes, F. M., Batista, A. C., & Rocha, M. L. 2017. Protective effects of ellagic acid on cardiovascular injuries caused by hypertension in rats. *Planta Medica*, *83*(10), 830–836. https://doi.org/10.1055/s-0043-103281

Kanda, H., Tateya, S., Tamori, Y., Kotani, K., Hiasa, K. I., Kitazawa, R., . . . Kasuga, M. 2006. MCP-1 contributes to macrophage infiltration into adipose tissue, insulin resistance, and hepatic steatosis in obesity. *Journal of Clinical Investigation*, *116*(6), 1494–1505. https://doi.org/10.1172/JCI26498

Kelishadi, R., Mortazavi, S., Hossein, T. R., & Poursafa, P. 2010. Association of cardiometabolic risk factors and dental caries in a population-based sample of youths. *Diabetology & Metabolic Syndrome*. www.dmsjournal.com/content/2/1/22

Liu, X., Cao, K., Lv, W., Feng, Z., Liu, J., Gao, J., Li, H., Zangh, W., & Liu, J. 2019. Punicalagin attenuates endothelial dysfunction by activating FoxOl, a pivotal regulating switch of mitochondrial biogenesis. *Free Radical Biology and Medicine*, *135*, 251–260. https://doi.org/10.1016/j.freeradbiomed.2019.03.0l1

López De Fez, C. M., Gaztelu, M. T., Rubio, T., & Castaño, A. 2004. Mecanismos de hipertensión en obesidad. *Anales Del Sistema Sanitario de Navarra*, *27*(2), 211–219. https://doi.org/10.4321/s1137-66272004000300006

Ludwig, D. S., & Ebbeling, C. B. 2018. The carbohydrate-insulin model of obesity: Beyond "calories in, calories out." *JAMA Internal Medicine*, *178*(8), 1098–1103. https://doi.org/10.1001/jamainternmed.2018.2933

Lynn, A., Hamadeh, H., Leung, W. C., Russell, J. M., & Barker, M. E. 2012. Effects of pomegranate juice supplementation on pulse wave velocity and blood pressure in healthy young and middle-aged men and women. *Plant Foods for Human Nutrition*, *67*, 309–314. doi: 10.1007/s11130–012–0295-z

MacRae, K., Connolly, K., Vella, R., & Fenning, A. 2019. Epicatechin's cardiovascular protective effects are mediated via opioid receptors and nitric oxide. *European Journal of Nutrition*, *58*, 515–527. https://doi.org/10.1007/s00394-018-1650-0

Manzur, F., Alvear, C., & Alayón, A. N. 2010. Adipocytes, visceral obesity, inflammation and cardiovascular disease. *Revista Colombiana de Cardiologia*, *17*(5), 207–213. https://doi.org/10.1016/S0120-5633(10)70243-6

Mohan, M., Waghulde, H., & Kasture, S. 2010. Effect of pomegranate juice on angiotensin II-induced hypertension in diabetic Wistar rats. *Phytotherapy Research*, *24*(Suppl 2), S196–S203. doi: 10.1002/ptr.3090

Qidwai, W., Yeoh, P. N., Inem, V., Nanji, K., & Ashfaq, T. 2013. Role of complementary and alternative medicine in cardiovascular diseases. *Evidence-Based Complementary and Alternative Medicine.* 2013; 2013:142898. doi: 10.1155/2013/14289

Redinger, R. N. 2007. The pathophysiology of obesity and its clinical manifestations. *Gastroenterology and Hepatology, 3*(11), 856–863.

Reyes, J. M. 2010. Inflammatory characteristics of obesity. *37,* 498–504.

Ruivo, J. 2016. *Complementary Therapy with Zingiber Officinalis Clinical Cases,* Thesis in Master Science. Instituto de Ciencias Biomedicas Abel Salazar, Universidade Du Porto.

San-Cristobal, R., Navas-Carretero, S., Martínez-González, M. Á., Ordovas, J. M., & Martínez, J. A. 2020. Contribution of macronutrients to obesity: Implications for precision nutrition. *Nature Reviews Endocrinology, 16,* 305–320. https://doi.org/10.1038/s41574-020-0346-8

Simpson, R. J., Hammacher, A., Smith, D. K., Matthews, J. M., & Ward, L. D. 1997. Interleukin-6: Structure-function relationships. https://doi.org/10.1002/pro.5560060501

Sohrab, G., Nasrollahzadeh, J., Tohidi, M., Zand, H., & Nikpayam, O. 2018. Pomegranate juice increases sirtuin1 protein in peripheral blood mononuclear cell from patients with type 2 diabetes: A randomized placebo controlled clinical trial. *Metabolic Syndrome and Related Disorders,* 446–451. https://doi.org/10.1089/met.2017.0146

Steiner, M., & Li, W. 2001. Aged garlic extract, a modulator of cardiovascular risk factors: A dose-finding study on the effects of AGE on platelet functions. *The Journal of Nutrition.*

Stockton, A., Farhat, G., McDougall, G. J., & Al-Dujaili, E. A. S. 2017. Effect of pomegranate extract on blood pressure and anthropometry in adults: A double-blind placebo-controlled randomised clinical trial. *Journal of Nutritional Science, 11,* 4–11. https://doi.org/10.1017/jns.2017.36

Sun, W. Y., Yan, C. H., Frost, B., Wang, X., Hou, C., Zeng, M. Q., Gao, H. L., Kang, Y. M., & Liu, J. K. 2016. Pomegranate extract decreases oxidative stress and alleviates mitochondrial impairment by activating AMPK-Nrf2 in hypothalamic paraventricular nucleus of spontaneously hypertensive rats. *Scientific Reports, 6,* 34246.

Tanaka, T., Narazaki, M., & Kishimoto, T. 2014. Il-6 in inflammation, immunity, and disease. *Cold Spring Harbor Perspectives in Biology, 6*(10). https://doi.org/10.1101/cshperspect.a016295

Tzanavari, T., Giannogonas, P., & Karalis, K. P. 2010. TNF-αlpha and obesity. *Current Directions in Autoimmunity, 11,* 145–156. https://doi.org/10.1159/000289203

Van Meijer, M., & Pannekoek, H. 1995. Structure of plasminogen activator inhibitor 1 (PAI-1) and its function in fibrinolysis: An update. *Fibrinolysis and Proteolysis, 9*(5), 263–276. https://doi.org/10.1016/S0268-9499(95)80015-8

Virdis, A., & Schiffrin, E. L. 2003. Vascular inflammation: A role in vascular disease in hypertension? *Current Opinion in Nephrology and Hypertension, 12*(2), 181–187. https://doi.org/10.1097/00041552-200303000-00009

Wang, D., Özen, C., Abu-Reidah, I. M., Chigurupati, S., Patra, J. K., Horbanczuk, J. O., . . . Atanasov, A. G. 2018. Vasculoprotective effects of pomegranate (Punica granatum L.). *Frontiers in Pharmacology, 9*(May), 1–15. https://doi.org/10.3389/fphar.2018.00544

Wongcharoen, W., & Phrommintikul, A. 2009. The protective role of curcumin in cardiovascular diseases. *International Journal of Cardiology, 133*(2), 145–151. doi: 10.1016/j.ijcard.2009.01.073

World Health Organization. www.who.int/health-topics/cardiovascular-diseases#tab=tab_1. Access date: January 20th, 2022.

Wu, D., Ma, X., & Tian, W. 2013. Pomegranate husk extract, punicalagin and ellagic acid inhibit fatty acid synthase and adipogenesis of 3T3-L1 adipocyte. *Journal of Functional Foods, 5*(2), 633–641. https://doi.org/10.1016/j.jff.2013.01.005

Yadav, A., Saini, V., & Arora, S. 2010. MCP-1: Chemoattractant with a role beyond immunity: A review. *Clinica Chimica Acta, 411*(21–22), 1570–1579. https://doi.org/10.1016/j.cca.2010.07.006

20 Review on Phytochemistry and Pharmacological Properties of *Momordica dioica* Roxb.
Special Emphasis on Cardioprotective Activity

Seema Mehdi, Tamsheel Fatima Roohi, Suman P., M. S. Srikanth and K. L. Krishna

CONTENTS

20.1	Introduction	314
20.2	Background	315
20.3	Description of MD	315
20.4	Habitat of MD	315
20.5	Botanical Description of MD	315
20.6	Nutritive Value	316
20.7	Phytochemical Composition of MD	316
20.8	Composition and Nutrient Value of MD	317
20.9	Cucurbitacin Triterpenoids	318
	20.9.1 Occurrence	318
	20.9.2 Structural Properties	318
	20.9.3 Chemical Properties	319
20.10	Ethnopharmacological Properties of MD	319
20.11	Pharmacological Activities of MD	320
20.12	Cardioprotective Biomolecular Activity Mechanism and Targets	322
	20.12.1 Hypertension	322
	20.12.2 Atherosclerosis	322
	20.12.3 Inflammation and Endothelial Function	323
20.13	Evidences That Support Cardioprotective Effects of MD	323
20.14	Conclusion	324
20.15	Other Foods, Herbs, Spices and Botanicals Used in Cardiovascular Health and Disease	324
20.16	Toxicity and Cautionary Notes	325
20.17	Acknowledgement	325
20.18	Summary Points	326
References		326

DOI: 10.1201/9781003220329-22

LIST OF ABBREVIATIONS

ADME	Absorption, Distribution, Metabolism and Excretion
CAD	Coronary Artery Disease
CCl_4	Carbon Tetrachloride
CKMB	Creatine Kinase Myocardial Band
CLA	Conjugated Linoleic Acid
CNS	Central Nervous System
COX-2	Cyclooxygenase-2
CTGF	Connective Tissue Growth Factor
CVDs	Cardiovascular Disease
DPPH	2,2-diphenyl-1-picrylhydrazyl
GSH	Glutathione
HDL	High-Density Lipoproteins
IL-10	Interleukin-10
LDH	Lactic Acid Dehydrogenase
LDL	Low-Density Lipoproteins
LPC	1-linolenoyl-lysophosphatidylcholine
LPS	Lipopolysaccharide
MAPK	Mitogen Activated Protein Kinase
MD	*Momordica diocia*
NFkB	Nuclear Factor Kappa B
PGE2	Prostaglandin E2
PPARs	Peroxisome Proliferator Activated Receptors
ROS	Reactive Oxygen Species
SARS-CoV-2	Severe Acute Respiratory Syndrome Coronavirus 2
SGOT	Serum Glutamic-Oxaloacetic Transaminase
SOD	Superoxide Dismutase
TG	Triglycerides
TGF-β	Tumour Growth Factor Beta
TLC	Thin Layer Chromatography
TNF-α	Tumour Necrosis Factor-Alpha

20.1 INTRODUCTION

This climbing creeper *Momordica dioica* (MD) Roxb. is an annual member of the Cucurbitaceae family and is commonly known as the spiny gourd or spine gourd, teasle gourd, ban karola or small bitter gourd (Nehra et al. 2021). In spite of its medicinal values, this plant is also used as vegetable which has significant nutritive values. Cardiovascular diseases (CVDs) are the leading reason for death on a global scale. CVD deaths account for more than three-quarters of all deaths in low- and middle-income nations. Conferring to the World Health Organization (WHO), around 75% of premature CVD is mostly avoidable and also by improving its associated risk factors can benefit to diminish the intensifying CVD load on patients affected role and healthcare staff. Currently, flavonoids are considered as an essential component in a number of therapeutic preparations and nutraceuticals due to their possible health benefits and medicinal relevance. Furthermore, these flavonoids have been shown to help reduce cardiovascular diseases (CVDs), possibly because of their potent antioxidant, anti-thrombotic and anti-atherogenic properties (Sebastian et al. 2019). The cardioprotective activity of dietary flavonoids is supported by many observational and interventional studies which also include *in vitro/in vivo* evidence for their antioxidant activities. Furthermore, consistent consumption of foods comprising flavonoids inhibits LDL oxidation and platelet aggregation as per the earlier studies. With all this evidence we can clearly correlate the cardioprotective mechanism which MD may possess.

20.2 BACKGROUND

Over thousands of years, MD has been utilised not only as a preventative and healing agent for abundant ailments, but also as an herb with high nutritional content. Often found budding wild and in hedges, teasel gourds are grown for their fruits, which are used in nutritional preparations. Teasel gourds are cucurbitaceous and are popular during the summer months. MD is rich in both primary and secondary metabolites in various areas. MD generates sugars, proteins and chlorophyll as main metabolites, with alkaloids, flavonoids and tannins as secondary metabolites. The fruit is rich in nutrition and valuable bioactive compounds which have potential for the preparation of products. Despite having various pharmacological properties such as hypoglycaemic, hypolipidaemic, anti-inflammatory, and antioxidant activity, MD's cardioprotective potential has yet to be proved at the molecular level. MD extracts can be used for an extensive assortment of ailments and indications because of their diverse biological qualities (Tungmunnithum et al. 2018). MD's phytotherapeutic and pharmacological potential includes a significant number of phytoconstituents, antioxidants and vitamins, which may aid in the treatment of diabetes, cancer and neurological illnesses. The widespread identification of MD and its bioactive compounds indicate it has many medicinal properties against many diseases. This chapter highlights MD's biological source, ethnopharmacology, plant characteristics, nutrient composition, different pharmacological uses with more emphasis on cardioprotective activities, along with its cellular and molecular activities.

20.3 DESCRIPTION OF MD

MD is a dioecious perennial climber which belongs to the *Cucurbitaceae* family. Spine gourd is its most common name. There have been comprehensive assessments of this multipurpose fruit's distribution, nutritional qualities, phytochemical composition, and medicinal capabilities due to its multiple uses in nutritious diet, traditional medicine and functional food ingredient (Jha et al. 2017; Jha et al. 2019).

20.4 HABITAT OF MD

- At present 80 species of MD have been identified (Bharathi et al. 2011).
- The origin of genus *Momordica* is from the Asian region (India and Bangladesh); it is also found in Southeast Asia, China and Sri Lanka (Haimed et al. 2019).
- In Assam, MD can be grown up to a height of 1500 meters.

20.5 BOTANICAL DESCRIPTION OF MD

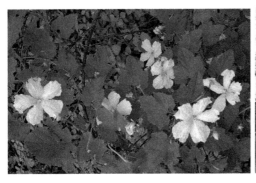
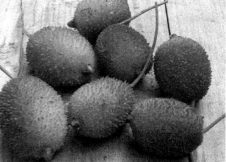

FIGURE 20.1 Plant and fruit of *Momordica dioica* Roxb.

- **Plant:** perennial, dioicous climbing creeper, grows up to height of 1500 metres.
- **Stem:** branched, slim with furrows and shining, tendrils are striate and elongated.
- **Leaves:** broadly ovate, membranous, cordate base, simple, entire but sometimes denticulate, varied length from 3.5 to 8 cm, lobed around three triangles and petiolated around 4 cm.
- **Texture of leaf:** pubescent and also glandular.
- **Flower:** solitary.
- **Male flower:** yellow coloured around 3 cm long. Petals are oblong, calyx five lobed, corolla five stamen in three.
- **Female flower:** yellow coloured, small bract below peduncle, calyx and corolla same as male flower, ovary covered with long soft papillae and has many ovules which are ellipsoid.
- **Fruit:** obtuse shape with red inner kernel, with short beak, echinate with smooth spines, greenish to yellow during matured stage.
- **Seed:** ellipsoid to rounded, compressed little, irregular enclosed with red pulp (Figure 20.1).

CONSUMPTION: The following are the ways to use it as a vegetable.

- Tender leaves and flowers are used as salad or sometimes cooked.
- Unripened fruits are cooked and consumed.

20.6 NUTRITIVE VALUE

- Fruit is rich in carotene when compared to all *Cucurbitaceae* members (162 mg/100 gm).

The MD leaves are of great medicinal value; it is indicated in worm infestation, to subside three humours of the body (i.e., *Vata*, *Pitta* and *Kapha*). It's also useful in anorexia, dyspnoea, fever, azoospermia, tuberculosis, cough and haemorrhoids.

TAXONOMY (ITIS-Report: *Momordica dioica* 2022)

Kingdom	Plantae
Subkingdom	Tracheobionata
Super	division Spermatophyta
Division	Magnoliphyta
Class	Magnoliopsida
Subclass	Dilleniidae
Order	Violales
Family	Cucurbitaceae
Genus	Momordica

PROPAGATION: The seeds or tubers are commonly used for the propagation of MD.

- It can be grown in both in tropical and subtropical regions. In India two main states cultivate this commercially (i.e., Karnataka and West Bengal). The average yield of this variety is 10, 15, 20 quintals/ha in the 1st, 2nd, 3rd year respectively (Rai et al. 2012).

20.7 PHYTOCHEMICAL COMPOSITION OF MD

The fruit is rich in various amino acids, β-sitosterol, saponins, glycosides, alkaloids, flavonoids and traceable amounts of manganese (Venkateshwarlu et al. 2017; Das et al. 2016). It also contains various vitamins like thiamine, riboflavin, carotene and niacin in smaller quantities (Vutukuri and Male 2020). Other important phytoconstituents present in the fruit include gypsogenin, oleanoic acid, alphaspiranosterol hederagenin, stearic acid and momordicaursenol. Various phytochemical studies have shown that the root of the Momordica plant contains three triterpenes: alphaspinasterol octadecanonate,

Properties of *Momordica dioica* Roxb. 317

alphaspinasterol-3-O-beta-D-glucopyranoside and 3-O-beta-D-glucuronopyranosyl gypsogenin. The root contains steroidal compounds, namely 3-O-beta-D-glucopyranosyl gypsogenin and 3-O-beta-D-glucopyranosyl hederagenin. 6-Methyl tritriacont-500n-*28*-Hydroxy-*6-methyl*-5-tritriacontanone and 8-methyl hentracont-3-ene along with the known pleuchiol was isolated from the fruit of MD. From MD seed Momordicaursenol, an unknown pentacyclic triterpene, was isolated and has been identified as urs-12, 18(19)-diene-3 beta-3 beta-ol on. Three triterpenes and two steroidal compounds were isolated from the MD dry root, spinasterol octadecanonate (I), alpha-spinasterol-3-O-beta-D-glucopyranoside (II), 3-O-beta-D-glucuronopyranosyl gypsogenin (III), 3-O-beta-D-glucopyranosyl gypsogenin (IV) and 3-O-beta-D-glucopyranosyl hederagenin (V) (Hitinayake et al. 2017).

20.8 COMPOSITION AND NUTRIENT VALUE OF MD

The fruit of MD contains 9.1% ash, 5.44% crude protein, 3.25% crude fat, 22.9% crude fibre and 59.31% carbohydrate. Its dry weight has a high energy value of 288.25 kcal/100 g. Potassium (4.63), sodium (1.62), calcium (7.37), iron (5.04) and zinc (5.04) are the mineral ranges (mg/100 g dry weight) (3.83). 84.1% moisture, 7.7 g carbohydrate, 3.1 g protein, 3.1 g fat, 3.0 g fibre and 1.1 g minerals were identified in the average nutritional value per 100 g edible fruit (Bawara et al. 2010). People with high blood pressure should drink fresh spine gourd fruit juice. Due to its high antioxidant activity, it promotes blood circulation and helps to prevent atherosclerosis. It has anti-lipid peroxidative properties, which means it protects and heals artery walls. It contains lectins, sitosterol, saponin glycosides, ursolic acid triterpenes, hederagenin, oleanolic acid, stearic acid, gypsogenin, momodicaursenol, and three new compounds named 3-o-benzoyl-11-oxo-ursolic acid, 3-o-benzoyl-6-oxo-ursolic acid and 3-o-β-D-glucuronopyranosyl gypsogenin (Hsu et al. 2012) (Table 20.1).

TABLE 20.1
Chemical Composition of MD Fruit

Active Ingredients/Phytochemicals	g/100 g	%
Moisture	–	84.1
Ash	–	6.7
Lipids	–	4.7
Fibre	–	21.3
Carbohydrate	–	42.98
Protein	–	19.38
Vitamin A	2.5	–
Vitamin B1 (Thiamine)	1.8	–
Vitamin B2 (Riboflavin)	3.5	–
Vitamin B3 (Niacin)	1.9	–
Vitamin B5 (Pantothenic Acid)	18	–
Vitamin B6 (Pyridoxine)	4.3	–
Vitamin B9 (Folic Acid)	3.6	–
Vitamin B12 (Cyanocobalamin)	4	–
Vitamin D2 and 3 (Cholecalciferol)	3	–
Vitamin H (Biotin) g/100g	6.5	–
Vitamin K (Phytonadione)	15	
Myristic Acid	–	3.589
Palmitic Acid	–	12.157
Stearic Acid	–	3.547
Oleic Acid	–	56.253
Linoleic Acid	–	22.511
Alpha-Linolenic Acid	–	1.943

20.9 CUCURBITACIN TRITERPENOIDS

Cucurbitacins are a type of triterpenoids found in many cucurbitaceous plants. They are known for their high toxicity and bitterness, so they are widely researched for their cytotoxic and anti-cancer activities. But they were not able to become a primary anti-cancer drug because of their non-specific cytotoxic activities; nowadays they are found to be used in anti-cancer therapy rarely under strict medical control. Beside their cytotoxic activity they hold many other *in vitro* and *in vivo* activities.

20.9.1 Occurrence

As it is mentioned, they are found mainly in cucurbitaceous plants like *Bryonia*, *Cucumis*, *Cucurbita*, *Luffa*, *Echinocystis*, *Lagenaria* and *Citrullus*. And also, in some other plant families like Brassicaceae, Scrophulariaceae, Begoniaceae, Elaeocarpaceae, Datiscaceae, Desfontainiaceae, Polemoniaceae, Primulaceae, Rubiaceae, Sterculiaceae, Rosaceae and Thymelaeaceae. In recent days, cucurbitacins are being isolated from different mushrooms including *Russula* and *Hebeloma* and even shell-less marine molluscs (*dorid nudibranchs*).

20.9.2 Structural Properties

They are characterised by a tetracyclic cucurbitane nucleus skeleton, which is 19-(10*9b)-abeo-10 alanosta-5-ene (9b-methyl-19-nor lanosta-5ene), which on modification by oxygen groups and double bonds gives rise to several Cucurbitacins with distinctive features. The majority of Cucurbitacins are crystallised and present as needles at room temperature, except Cucurbitacin H, which is an amorphous solid. The majority of Cucurbitacins is soluble in petroleum ether, chloroform, benzene, ethyl acetate, methanol, and ethanol, but are not so soluble in methanol. They are only slightly soluble in water. Cucurbitacins usually have absorption maxima for ultraviolet light between 228–234 nm (Zeng Y et al. 2021) (Figure 20.2).

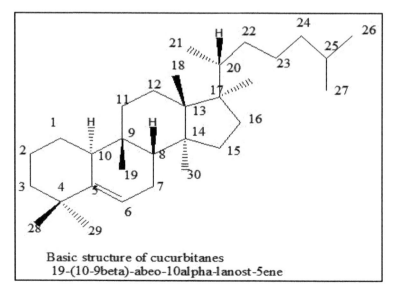

FIGURE 20.2 Basic skeletal structure of cucurbitacins.

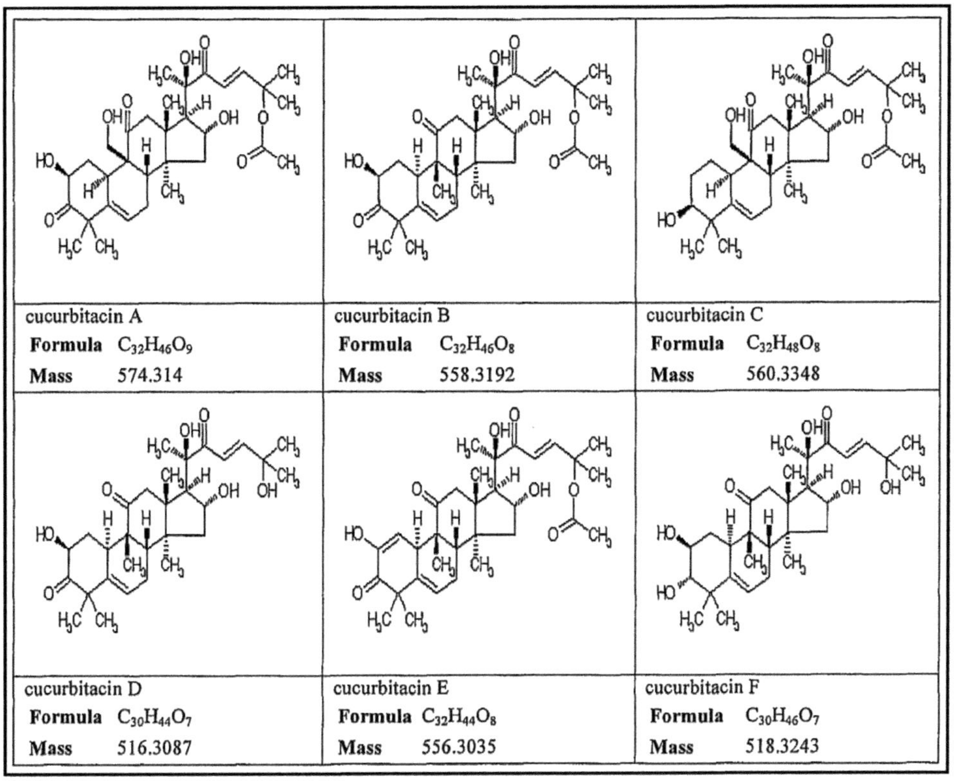

Properties of *Momordica dioica* Roxb.

FIGURE 20.3   Molecular formula and molecular mass of different cucurbitacins.

20.9.3 CHEMICAL PROPERTIES

Cucurbitacins are fairly polar in nature and have been isolated many times using methanol as a solvent. Most Cucurbitacins have aglycones that are soluble in moderately polar solvents like chloroform. Cucurbitacins extracted from methanol are partitioned between water and chloroform, which is typically used for *Cucurbitacin* purification. Chromatographic techniques such as open-column chromatography on silica gel, alumina or florosil, or thin layer chromatography (TLC) have been used to purify Cucurbitacins from plant extracts (Shyaula et al. 2021). The fruit of MD is high in Vitamin C and contains lectins, proteins, triterpenes and vitamins. Various amino acids, -sitosterol, many saponins, a lot of glycosides, similarly alkaloids and flavonoids are abundant in the fruit. Manganese is also present in trace concentrations. Gypsogenin, Oleanolic acid, alpha-spiranosterol hederagenin, stearic acid and momordicaursenol are some of the other phytoconstituents that are important. The alkaloid present in the seeds of the fruit is momordicin and the alkaloid present in the roots is called Momordica foetid (Samaddar et al. 2020). The root contains various steroidal compounds such as 3-O-beta-D-glucopyranosyl gypsogenin and 3-O-beta-D-glucopyranoside hederagenin (Garg et al. 2018) (Figure 20.3).

20.10 ETHNOPHARMACOLOGICAL PROPERTIES OF MD

Plants, animals and minerals have been used for centuries to treat disease. Pharmacognostical, phytochemical and pharmacological studies of traditional medicinal plants have been gaining attention.

TABLE 20.2
Ethnopharmacological Uses of MD Plant and Its Parts

Parts of MD Plant	Ethnopharmacological Uses
Fruit of MD	• Anti-inflammatory
	• Antioxidant
	• Anti-diabetic
	• Hepatoprotective
	• Analgesic
	• Anti-feedant
	• Anti-cancer
Leaves of MD	• Aphrodisiac
	• Anthelminthic
	• Respiratory disorders: bronchitis and asthma
	• Urinary infections
	• Jaundice
Seeds of MD	• Antiallergic
Root of MD	• Anti-cancer
	• Antimicrobial
	• Antioxidant

Currently, most of the natural sources whose compounds are used for medical purposes are actually used in ethnomedicine. MD plants from the Cucurbitaceae family have different parts – roots, stem, fruits, leaves – which can provide multiple bioactive functional ingredients, with a wide range of therapeutic applications. The metabolites obtained have anti-diabetic, anti-inflammatory, cytotoxic and immunosuppressive qualities as well as hepatoprotective, antimicrobial effects (Mukherjee et al. 2022) (Table 20.2).

20.11 PHARMACOLOGICAL ACTIVITIES OF MD

Antibacterial activity: A methanolic extract of its roots has been shown to possess antibacterial properties against both Gram-positive and Gram-negative bacteria. Both male and female plants were known to be antibacterial. *In vitro* studies carried out using Muller Hinton agar plate method suggest that the female plants have shown a higher inhibition zone compared to the male plants. The plant has shown its antibacterial activity against several microorganisms like *S. aureus*, *E coli* and *B. subtilis*. The leaves and the pericarp of the fruit are also known to be antibacterial. However, they show weakly active inhibition against various Gram-positive and Gram-negative bacteria like *S. aureus*, *S. typhi* and *Shigella* (Pingle et al. 2018).

Anti-diabetic activity: Methanolic fruit extracts of Momordica show excellent anti-diabetic activity against type I diabetes. The anti-diabetic activity was tested *in vivo* using rat model. Streptozotocin was used for induction of diabetes. After oral administration of the extract at dose 500 mg/kg for 30 days, rats showed recovery of body weight, reduction in fasting serum glucose, increase in serum insulin and hypolipidaemic effect. Various biochemical parameters like LDL, HDL, TG, glycolate haemoglobin were estimated to have proven the anti-diabetic properties of the fruit extract. Hence, MD is useful in betterment of the lipid profile and Diabetes mellitus mediated cardiovascular complications (Ahmad et al. 2016; Sravani et al 2013).

Anti-cancer activity: Active constituents like curcuminoids, phenolic acids, coumarin, lignans etc., are responsible for the overall antimitotic activity of the fruit. Aqueous extract of the fruit has been tested for its antimitotic activity using *Allium cepa* roots. Developed roots of *Allium cepa* were dipped in the aqueous extract. The tip parts of the roots were cut and fixed using fixing solution

Properties of *Momordica dioica* Roxb. 321

(45% v/v acetic acid and 95% v/v ethanol in 1:3 v/v ratio) (Ahirrao RA 2019; Revathy et al. 2014; Madesh et al. 2020).

Hepatoprotective activity: Fresh fruit extracts of MD prepared in ethanol showed good hepatoprotective activity. Hepatotoxicity was induced in Wistar albino rats using CCl_4. Oral administration of the fruit extract for 14 days, at dose 200 mg/kg containing phytoconstituents like triterpenoids, steroids, glycosides, saponins and tannins showed considerable hepatoprotective activity. The activity was confirmed by estimation of various biochemical parameters like total bilirubin, total protein, serum alanine transaminase, alkaline phosphatase and aspartate transaminase (Shankar et al. 2011; Jain et al. 2008).

Antioxidant property: The antioxidant effects of MD have been determined by radical scavenging activity. The extent of the antioxidant activity is proportional to the decreased absorbance of DPPH. The antioxidant activity of the methanolic extracts of the fruit and root of the plant was evaluated by scavenging stable DPPH radical (Anjamma and Lakshmi 2018).

Antiviral property: Recent in silico studies suggest that the biomolecules present in the MD plant like flavonoids and triterpenes possess notable antiviral properties. Flavonoids and triterpenes like quercetin, oleanolic acid, catechin and hederagenin are determined to be responsible for the antiviral properties of the plant. Activity against SARS-CoV-2 main protease, RNA dependent RNA polymerase, spike protein, etc., was evaluated by molecular docking studies and in silico ADME predicting methods (Sakshi et al. 2020).

Antiallergic and analgesic activity: Aqueous, ethanolic and methanolic extracts of MD seeds (200 mg/kg i.p.) were evaluated for potential analgesic and antiallergic activity. Amongst the various extracts, methanolic extract showed significant effects when tested *in vivo* using mice models. The models included milk-induced leucocytosis milk-induced eosinophilia and differential leukocytes count in mice. Analgesic activity was evaluated using hot plate activity and writhing test (Choudhary D et al. 2017).

Neuroprotective activity: Methanolic and aqueous extracts of MD fruit have been evaluated for potential CNS depressant activity. Locomotor activity and motor coordination activity were employed to evaluate the activity using Swiss albino mice. The extracts of the fruit produced significant effect on the locomotor activity and motor coordination concluded by Rotarod paradigm. Hence, it can be concluded that MD has significant analgesic and antipsychotic activity due to which it can be used to treat various CNS disorders (Rakh et al. 2010).

Antifertility activity: Ethanolic extract of MD fruit (dried) was tested for antifertility activity in both male and female rats *in vivo*. Thirty days continuous oral administration of the extract produced significant sperm abnormality and decreased sperm count and motility in male rats. In female rats, the extract produced significant reduction in oestrogen and progesterone levels. This activity of MD can be employed to produce herbal contraceptives with lower side effects (Pusuloori et al. 2017).

Antimalarial activity: *In vivo* and *in vitro* tests using alcoholic extracts of MD have been carried out widely. The extract has shown significant schizonticidal activity against NK 65 strain of *Plasmodium bergheli, Aegle marmelos,* etc. (Mishra et al. 1989).

Antiulcer activity: *In vivo* tests on male Sprague-Dawley rats have been conducted to evaluate antiulcer activity. Oral administration of hydroalcoholic extract of MD fruits at dose 200 mg/kg for 16 days produced significant protective effects against Pylorus ligation-induced ulcers. Ulcer scores and gastric content analysis were utilised to evaluate the activity. The extract produced significant decrease in H^+K^+ATPase, gastric juice volume and acid output. It also showed substantial increase in gastric mucus and pH (Rakh MS et al. 2021; Vijayakumar et al. 2011).

Nephroprotective activity: Ethanolic extract of MD containing phytoconstituents like flavonoids, glycosides, alkaloids and steroids was tested against Gentamicin-induced renal damage in rats. Oral administration of the extract at dose 200 mg/kg produced significant nephroprotective effects. The activity showed a significant decrease in elevated blood urea and serum creatinine levels. The nephroprotective activity was also confirmed in histopathological studies (Jain et al. 2010).

Cardioprotective activity: Hydroalcoholic and aqueous extracts of MD fruits were tested *in vivo* for their cardioprotective activity against stress and clozapine-induced cardiotoxicity. The extracts contain various phytochemicals like carbohydrates, steroids, alkaloids, flavonoids, tannins, anthraquinone glycosides and cardiac glycosides. Oral administration of the extract at 200 mg/kg dose showed significant decrease in QT and ST intervals during ECG recording. CKMB, SGOT and LDH levels were decreased in extract treated animals. The cardioprotective activity may result from antioxidant properties of the extract (Mehdi et al. 2020; Ramya et al. 2013; Chinmaya et al. 2020).

20.12 CARDIOPROTECTIVE BIOMOLECULAR ACTIVITY MECHANISM AND TARGETS

Numerous studies have shown that flavonoids are biologically active. Flavonoids are metabolised to phenolic acids, some of which remain radical scavenging compounds (Panche et al. 2016). Phytochemicals, in combination with minerals present in fruits and vegetables, may aid postponement of ageing progression and subordinate the hazard of abundant illnesses, according to research. These chemicals are known to be physiologically active, which means they might be to blame for their therapeutic effects and could be used to develop synthetically enhanced therapeutic medicines (Zhang et al. 2020). As antioxidants scavenge free radicals and reduce lipid peroxidation, they are able to provide resistance to oxidative stress (Figure 20.4).

20.12.1 Hypertension

For hypertension and diabetes, fresh fruit juice and cooked fruit with a modest quantity of oil are recommended. Despite its high potassium content and low Na+/K+ ratio, the crop is useful in treating hypertension and other cardiovascular disorders (Singh et al. 2008).

20.12.2 Atherosclerosis

Current studies have revealed that bitter gourd extracts may help to reduce obesity and hyperlipidaemia in animal models triggered by high fat diet (Sunshine et al. 2017). The majority of these investigations have simply used fruit pulps. This plant is known for activating the PPAR gene, which controls lipid metabolism; its active components, such as conjugated linoleic acid (CLA), override PPAR, enabling fatty acids to be oxidised within cells and preserving their metabolic consistency (Alam et al. 2015). More study is needed to determine whether the considerable drop in body weight of mice given 10% wild bitter gourd has deleterious physiological consequences (Gervois and Roxane 2012).

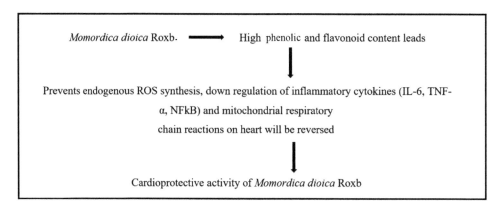

FIGURE 20.4 Possible mechanism showing cardioprotective activity of MD.

Properties of *Momordica dioica* Roxb.

20.12.3 Inflammation and Endothelial Function

The objective of anti-inflammatory medications is to ease the discomfort produced by inflammation by reducing the generation of inflammatory mediators (Abdulkhaleq et al. 2018). MD decreases the generation of pro-inflammatory cytokines and other compounds. The anti-inflammatory cytokine IL-10 rises dramatically as well, resulting in anti-inflammatory benefits. According to the existing research, a butanol-soluble fraction of its placenta extract substantially suppresses LPS-induced TNF production in RAW264.7 cells. 1-linolenoyl-lysophosphatidylcholine (LPC), 2-linolenoyl-LPC, 1-lynoleoyl-LPC and 2-linoleoyl-LPC were found as anti-inflammatory components (Ciou et al. 2014).

20.13 EVIDENCES THAT SUPPORT CARDIOPROTECTIVE EFFECTS OF MD

Another study reported that its fruits are a high-nutrient source of protein, carbohydrate, fat, calcium, crude fibre, iron and phosphorus. Many studies have demonstrated scientific evidence in support of MD for possessing anti-diabetic qualities which was discovered primarily via the investigation of organic and aqueous extracts from fruit and leaves. As it was mentioned earlier, natural-source compounds possess potent activity against free radicals; similarly various studies were performed using different extracts of MD to examine its free radical scavenging activity. It was proved to be potent with significant antioxidant activity, as one of the study reported that with 4000 g/ml ascorbic acid, the alcoholic extract of MD reduced the free radical generation in *in vitro* as per the reports (Shreedhara et al. 2006). In another study, the tuberous root's ability to scavenge free radicals was investigated using various *in vitro* methods, which included potent antioxidant activity using DPPH radical scavenging assay. Its fruit was identified as a powerful antioxidant due to the presence of flavonoids among those phytochemicals (Shrinivas et al. 2009).

According to autopsy findings, the evolution of CVDs in future years is unpredictable, hence care is essential. It has been proven that the protective advantages of eating nutritious fruits rich in flavonoids with potent antioxidant activity, eating vegetables and exercising regularly could help in preventing cardiovascular diseases. Cucurbitacin I has been reported to have cardioprotective activity by protecting the heart against cardiac hypertrophy via inhibition of CTGF/MAPK, and TGF-β/Smad facilitated events (Jeong MH et al. 2015). At low concentration (1 μM), cucurbitacin I inhibited the hypertrophic response *in vitro*, where phenylephrine-stimulated, cultured rat neonatal cardiomyocytes were used. There has been an increase in scientific interest in consumption of flavonoids to avoid CVDs and promote the health of our vascular system during the last decade.

Flavonoid-rich foods have been extensively researched and are widely regarded as powerful bioactive substances with a variety of biological functions, including involvement in a number of key signalling pathways linked to chronic disease (Khoo et al. 2017). Whereas stress caused by oxidative species is also a noteworthy factor to the pathophysiology involved in many diseases, a wide range of clinical diseases, including cardiovascular dysfunctions, atherosclerosis and diabetes. In the recent study conducted in diabetic rats, an extract of protein obtained from the fruit pulp of MD demonstrated a strong beneficial and protective outcome by maintaining glucose and lipid homeostasis, as well as reducing oxidative stress (Poovitha et al. 2017).

Another study reported that herbal supplements that are high in flavonoids have been reported to improve and manage the disorders caused by metabolic dysfunction such as CVDs and diabetes mellitus (Kumar et al. 2011). Myocardial infarction is caused mainly by the oxidative stress which is involved in the development of CVDs such as ischemic heart disease, which can result in deadly consequences such as cardiomyopathy and heart attack. MD has been evaluated for its cardioprotective activity against stress and clozapine-induced cardiotoxicity in both normal and diabetic rats. So, the reports of previous studies, though there are not many, still provide evidence that this plant has cardioprotective activity and that is mainly because of its constituents and their ability to protect tissue by free radical scavenging activity (Shamala and Krishna 2013).

There is another study which revealed that this plant's extracts have shown anti-diabetic and anti-hyperlipidaemic properties and hence it can also have cardioprotective properties. Both the ethanolic and aqueous extracts have shown antioxidant activity to scavenge free radicals. This activity might be once again connected to the presence of flavonoids in the extracts, which have been proven for their protective effects (Safia et al. 2013). As the studies revealed a high content of phenolic acids and flavonoids in MD, it acts as cardioprotective, perhaps by reducing reactive oxygen species (ROS) by a variety of mechanisms including direct neutralisation of various types of free radicals, metal chelation, increased creation of endogenous antioxidant enzymes such as catalase, glutathione (GSH) and superoxide dismutase (SOD) and also inhibition of cellular enzymes that are involved in generating ROS. Inflammation raised levels of ROS and amplified oxidative stress in response to harmful stimuli, as well as several complex signalling pathways (Akhlaghi M et al. 2009).

Plants and fruits that are rich with flavonoids supplementation have been shown in epidemiological studies to reduce inflammation in the biological system by lowering the values of inflammation-causing agents like pro-inflammatory cytokines and agents that could damage the tissue and thereby it helps in promoting the survival of cells and retaining their functionality (Sugamura et al. 2011). Studies have reported that there will be an imbalance in the metabolism of GSH in the body due to increased free radicals, which results in impairment of availability of antioxidants and their enzymes, which would result in increase in oxidative stress. It is characterised by decreased HDL, hypertriglyceridemia levels and increased LDL. According to the survey, it is reported that almost 80% of the patients who are diagnosed with type 2 diabetes are known to have hyperlipidaemia and reduced activity of lipoprotein lipase enzyme. The enzyme helps in conversion of triglycerides into free fatty acids, causes hyper-triglyceridemia which is considered as a risk to patients with diabetes to suffer with cardiovascular abnormalities. Hence having possible control over the aforementioned would help with metabolic disorders like diabetes. This all should be part of diabetes care, which further results in protecting the cardiovascular system (Alfaddagh et al. 2020; Fernandes et al. 2007). As per the recent study, which evaluated the activity of MD using its various extracts, it clearly states that natural compounds like MD do possess potent antioxidant activity and they are capable of reducing the levels of bad cholesterol, controlling hyperlipidaemia and diabetes, protecting the kidneys, liver and heart. MD has offered experimental support for its wide practice in supervision of diabetes-related complications. It can help in preventing cardiovascular dysfunction and hence, it can be a cardioprotective agent in future detailed investigations.

20.14 CONCLUSION

The ethnomedicinal, phytochemical, pharmacological and general study of MD has been reported in this review. Due to its active phyto ingredients, this medicinal plant has a twofold significance: first, as a possible future food source (as nutritive supplement), and second, as a source of future novel therapeutic remedies for many diseases and ailments, particularly novel cardioprotective phyto remedies. These findings from the literature study may serve as a starting point for academics and practitioners interested in phytochemistry, pharmacology, pharmacognosy and general research on this plant. As a result, effective extraction and application of this therapeutic plant should be prioritised.

20.15 OTHER FOODS, HERBS, SPICES AND BOTANICALS USED IN CARDIOVASCULAR HEALTH AND DISEASE

Hypertension, dyslipidaemia, endothelial dysfunction, vascular dysfunction, cardiomyopathy and peripheral vascular disease are caused by various risk factors such as smoking, unhealthy diet and lifestyle, no physical activity, diabetes mellitus, elevated levels of LDL and low levels of

Properties of *Momordica dioica* Roxb.

HDL. The herbal therapies for cardiovascular disorders exert protective and ameliorating effects on the pathogenesis exacerbated by these risk factors. The herbal extracts manifest high ameliorating effects against endothelial disorder, vascular smooth muscle cells alterations by acting as vasodilators, free radical scavengers, inflammatory inhibitors, and as an anti-proliferative. All of these changes may reduce mitochondrial activity, leading to malfunction that in turn boosts the availability of nitric oxide and the formation of new blood vessels. The predictable measures which were used for the supervision of cardiovascular disorder exhibited so many unpleasant side effects and accompanying complications, herbal therapies are needed to be researched. They are less toxic towards the human body and showed better efficacious results towards the diseases and ailments (Reiner Z et al. 2019). *Allium sativum* (garlic) is a well-known example of an herb used to treat CVDs. It is well known for its multiple characteristics. It inhibits cardiovascular related disorders such as high blood pressure, imbalances between oxidation and free radicles generation, inflammation and hyperlipidaemia (Sun M et al. 2018). Garlic can be used to treat atherosclerosis and hyperlipidaemia by lowering total cholesterol and LDL levels, decreasing lipid content in arterial cells, and suppressing VSMC growth. *Astragaloside IV*, the plant's principal bioactive ingredient, is globally used as an antioxidant and for protection against ischemic-related CVDs (Zhou J et al. 2000). *Ginseng* has hypotensive properties because it improves vascular function. Ginsenosides have been shown to help in vasorelaxation in rat aortas, murine coronary arteries and monkey cerebral arteries (Lee H et al. 2016). *Ginsenoside Rg3* activates eNOS gene expression and induces nitric oxide generation. Bioactive compounds in *Ganoderma lucidum* have modulatory effects on the immune system, inhibit oxidative properties, and have hepatoprotective, anti-cancer properties (Wachtel-Galor S et al. 2011).

20.16 TOXICITY AND CAUTIONARY NOTES

The toxicity profile of MD is not reported in any Ayurvedic text and is found to be a most safe plant. Fruits of MD are being consumed as vegetables in many parts of India and have many health benefits because of their bitter properties. Ayurvedic classical references quote no toxicity profiles of MD and point out its safety and health benefits. Only a few publications in scientific literature are available regarding the toxicity of MD and its parts. Jha DK et al. (2019) studied the toxicity of saponin from the methanolic extraction of the fruits of MD. The saponin was tested for acute, sub-acute and chronic toxicity testing with a dose of 250, 500, 1000 and 5000 mg/kg/b.w. No death ratio was found in toxicity testing as well as no recorded behavioural changes were observed. The saponin methanolic extract of MD was not toxic and did not produce any signs or symptoms on histopathology and biochemical alteration. Khan MF et al. (2019) determined the LD_{50} values in seed extract of *M. charantia* in which 50 μg/ml was injected to embryos of Zebrafishes. Different irregularities were observed at sub-lethal concentration in Zebrafish embryos. The fruit extract showed much better results and did not produce any lethality. There is a report of acute oral toxicity effects of *M. Charantia* in SD rats, and they found no lethality at different doses, 300 and 2000 mg/kg/bw. After administration of test drug, the animals showed dizziness and depression during the first 30 minutes of study. The body weight, food intake, water intake and weight gain of animals did not show any significant reduction. The blood parameters, lipid profile did not show any sign and symptoms and no significant differences (Husna RN et al. 2013).

20.17 ACKNOWLEDGEMENT

The authors thanks Principal, JSS College of Pharmacy, JSS AHER, Mysuru for encouraging and supporting writing of this review. Also, thanks, JSS Academy of Higher Education and Research for providing the necessary infrastructure to carry out the review process.

20.18 SUMMARY POINTS

- This chapter focusses on ethnopharmacological and pharmacological activities of different parts of *Momordica Dioica* Roxb (MD).
- The origin of genus *Momordica* is from Asian region (India and Bangladesh), it is also found in Southeast Asia, China and Sri Lanka.
- MD fruit is consumed as a vegetable, and known for its nutritive and medicinal values for many years.
- MD extract effects on metabolic disorders like diabetes and hypercholesteremia are very well documented.
- Many pieces of literature are in support of the beneficial role of MD fruit for cardiovascular ailments; this chapter discusses this in detail.
- MD can be exploited as a source for many bioactive phytopharmaceuticals for various diseases and ailments.

REFERENCES

Abdulkhaleq, L.A., Assi, M.A., Abdullah, R., Zamri-Saad, M., Taufiq-Yap, Y.H. and Hezmee, M.N.M. 2018. The crucial roles of inflammatory mediators in inflammation: A review. *Veterinary World*, 11(5):627–635.

Ahirrao, R.A. 2019. Anticancer activity of Fruits of Momordica Dioica by using MTT assay. *Madridge Journal of Immunology*, 3(2):89–92.

Ahmad, N., Noorul, H., Zeeshan, A., Mohd, Z. and Seikh, Z. 2016. Momordica charantia: For traditional uses and pharmacological actions. *Journal of Drug Delivery and Therapeutics*, 6(2):40–44.

Akhlaghi, M. and Brian, B. 2009. Mechanisms of flavonoid protection against myocardial ischemia-reperfusion injury. *Journal of Molecular and Cellular Cardiology*, 46(3):309–317.

Alam, M.A., Uddin, R., Subhan, N., Rahman, M.M., Jain, P. and Reza, H.M. 2015. Beneficial role of bitter melon supplementation in obesity and related complications in metabolic syndrome. *Journal of Lipids*, 2015:1–18.

Alfaddagh, A., Seth, S.M., Thorsten, M.L., Erin, D.M., Michael, J., Blaha, Charles, J.L., Steven, R.J. and Peter, P. 2020. Toth. Inflammation and cardiovascular disease: From mechanisms to therapeutics. *American Journal of Preventive Cardiology*, 4, 100130:1–19.

Anjamma, M., and Lakshmi N.B. 2018. Comparative antibacterial and antioxidant activity from root and fruit extracts of Momordica charantia L. and Momordica dioica Roxb. *International Journal of Scientific Research in Science and Technology*, 4(5):1710–1716.

Bawara, B., Mukesh, D., Chauhan, N.S., Dixit, V.K. and Saraf, D.K. 2010. Phyto-pharmacology of Momordica dioica Roxb. ex. Willd: A review. *International Journal of Phytomedicine*, 2(1):1–9.

Bharathi, L.K., Munshi, A.D., Shanti, C., Behera, T.K., Das, A.B. and Joseph John, K. 2011. Cytotaxonomical analysis of Momordica L. (Cucurbitaceae) species of Indian occurrence. *Journal of Genetics*, 90(1):21–30.

Chinmaya, N.K., Chandan, H.M., Krishna, K.L., Seema, M., Nandini, H.S., Abhinav, R.G. and Bhooshitha, A.N. 2020. Pre-treatment with cucurbitacin triterpenoids rich biofraction of Momordica dioica Roxb. fruit protected the cardiotoxicity induced by isoproterenol and stress in rats. *International Research Journal of Pharmacy*, 11(3):5–13.

Choudhary, D., Bhattacharyya, S. and Bose, S. 2017. Efficacy and safety of ashwagandha (Withania somnifera (L.) Dunal) root extract in improving memory and cognitive functions. *Journal of Dietary Supplements*, 14(6):599–612.

Ciou, S.Y., Cheng-Chin, H., Yueh-Hsiung, K. and Che-Yi, C. 2014. Effect of wild bitter gourd treatment on inflammatory responses in BALB/c mice with sepsis. *BioMedicine*, 4(3):1–7.

Das, D.R., Anupam, K.S., Mohd, S. and Mohd, I. 2016. Phyto-pharmacology of momordca dioica: A review. *Asian Journal of Pharmaceutical Research and Development*, 4(1):1–6.

Fernandes, Nafisa P.C., Lagishetty, C.V., Vandana, S.P. and Naik, S.R. 2007. An experimental evaluation of the antidiabetic and antilipidemic properties of a standardized Momordica charantia fruit extract. *BMC Complementary and Alternative Medicine*, 7(1):1–8.

Garg, S., Sunil, C.K., and Renu, W. 2018. Cucurbitacin B and cancer intervention: Chemistry, biology and mechanisms. *International Journal of Oncology*, 52(1):19–37.

Properties of *Momordica dioica* Roxb.

Gervois, P. and Roxane, M.M. 2012. PPARα as a therapeutic target in inflammation-associated diseases. *Expert Opinion on Therapeutic Targets*, 16(11):1113–1125.

Haimed, Y.A.S., Suman, S.A.M.D. and Deepak, K.J. 2019. An investigation on antidiabetic activity of phytochemical (s) isolated from Momordica dioica in type I diabetes mellitus. *International Journal of Research and Analytical Reviews*, 6(1):786–798.

Hitinayake, H.M.C., Sumanarathne, J.P., Abesekara, W.A.D.S., Madushika, K.G.N., Danushka, W.M. and Sawarnalatha, K.G. 2017. Yield improvement of spine gourd through. *Annals of Sri Lanka Department of Agriculture*, 19(2):71–78.

Hsu, C.H., Tsung-Hsien, T., You-Yi, L., Wen-Huey, W., Ching-Jang, H. and Po-Jung, T. 2012. Wild bitter melon (Momordica charantia Linn. var. abbreviata Ser.) extract and its bioactive components suppress Propionibacterium acnes-induced inflammation. *Food Chemistry*, 135(3):976–984.

Husna, R.N., Noriham, A., Nooraain, H., Azizah, A.H., Amna, O.F. 2013. Acute oral toxicity effects of Momordica charantia in Sprague dawley rats. *International Journal of Bioscience, Biochemistry and Bioinformatics*, 3(4):408.

ITIS Report: Momordica Dioica. 2022. Accessed March 7. www.itis.gov/servlet/SingleRpt/SingleRpt?search_topic=TSN&search_value=505903#null.

Jain, A., Manish, S., Lokesh, D., Anurekha, J., Rout, S.P., Gupta, V.B. and Krishna, K.L. 2008. Antioxidant and hepatoprotective activity of ethanolic and aqueous extracts of Momordica dioica Roxb. leaves. *Journal of Ethnopharmacology*, 115(1):61–66.

Jain, A. and Singhai, A.K. 2010. Effect of Momordica dioica Roxb on gentamicin model of acute renal failure. *Natural Product Research*, 24(15):1379–1389.

Jeong, M.H., Shang-Jin, K., Hara, K., Kye, W.P., Woo, J.P., Seung Yul, Y. and Dong Kwon, Y. 2015. Cucurbitacin, I attenuates cardiomyocyte hypertrophy via inhibition of connective tissue growth factor (CCN2) and TGF-β/Smads signaling. *PLoS One*, 10(8):e0136236.

Jha, D.K., Koneri, R., Samaddar, S. 2019. Toxicity studies of a saponin isolated from the fruits of *Momordica dioica* in rats. *International Journal of Pharmaceutical Sciences and Research*, 10(10):4462–4476.

Jha, D.K., Raju K. and Suman, S. 2017. Potential bio-resources of momordica dioica roxb: A review. *International Journal of Pharmaceutical Sciences Review and Research*, 45(2):203–209.

Jha, D.K., Raju, K. and Suman, S. 2019. Antidiabetic activity of Phyto saponin in STZ-Induced type I diabetes in rats. *Research Journal of Pharmacy and Technology*, 12(8):3919–3926.

Khan, M.F., Abutaha, N., Nasr, F.A., Alqahtani, A.S., Noman, O.M., Wadaan, M.A. 2019. Bitter gourd (Momordica charantia) possesses developmental toxicity as revealed by screening the seeds and fruit extracts in zebrafish embryos. *BMC Complementary and Alternative Medicine*, 19(1):1–3.

Khoo, H.E., Azrina, A., Sou Teng, T. and See Meng, L. 2017. Anthocyanidins and anthocyanins: Coloured pigments as food, pharmaceutical ingredients, and the potential health benefits. *Food & Nutrition Research*, 61(1):1361779.

Kumar, C., Hari, A., Ramesh, J.N., Kumar, S. and Mohammed Ishaq, B. 2011. A review on hepatoprotective activity of medicinal plants. *International Journal of Pharmaceutical Sciences and Research*, 2(3):501.

Lee, H., Choi, J., Shin, S.S. and Yoon, M. 2016. Effects of Korean red ginseng (Panax ginseng) on obesity and adipose inflammation in ovariectomized mice. *Journal of Ethnopharmacology*, 178, 229–237.

Madesh, T., Abhinav, R.G., Krishna, K.L., Seema, M., Nandini, H.S., Chandan, H.M. and Bhooshitha, A.N. 2020. Anti-tumor potential of cucurbitacin triterpenoids of Momordica dioica Roxb. fruit by EAC induced ascites tumor model. *International Journal of Research in Pharmacy and Science*, 11(2):1793–1797.

Mehdi, S., Das, A., Krishna, K.L., Vengal Rao, P., Nandini, H.S. 2020. Cardioprotective effect of Momordica dioica roxb. fruit upon stress and clozapine induced cardiotoxicity in rat model. *Journal of Global Trends in Pharmaceutical Sciences*, 11(1):7318–7326.

Mishra, P., Pal, N.L., Guru, P.Y., Katiyar, J.C. and Tandon, J.S. 1989. Antimalarial activity of traditional plants against erythrocytic stages of plasmodium bergheli. *International Journal of Pharmacognosy*, 29(1):19–23.

Mukherjee, P.K., Singha, S., Kar, A., Chanda, J., Banerjee, S., Dasgupta, B., Haldar, P.K. and Sharma, N. 2022. Therapeutic importance of Cucurbitaceae: A medicinally important family. *Journal of Ethnopharmacology*, 282, 114599.

Nehra, M. 2021. An ethnomedicinal, phytochemistry of Momordica dioica roxb. *Journal of Phytological Research*, 34(2):93–102.

Panche, A.N., Diwan, A.D. and Chandra, S.R. 2016. Flavonoids: An overview. *Journal of Nutritional Science*, 5(e47):1–15.

Pingle, M.T., Snehal, S.G., Snehal, K.B. and Surana, S.J. 2018. Antibacterial activity of Momordica dioica Roxb. fruit pericarp and leaves in bacterial species. *Journal of Pharmaceutical and BioSciences*, 6(2):41.

Poovitha, S., Muddineni Siva, S. and Madasamy, P. 2017. Protein extract from the fruit pulp of Momordica dioica shows anti-diabetic, anti-lipidemic and antioxidant activity in diabetic rats. *Journal of Functional Foods*, 33:181–187.

Pusuloori, R., Pusuloori, R. and Yakaiah, V. 2017. Evaluation of effect of momordica dioica extract on reproductive system of male and female rats. *Biomedical and Pharmacology Journal*, 10(3):1419–1425.

Rai, G.K., Major, S., Neha, P.R., Bhardwaj, D.R. and Sanjeev, K. 2012. In vitro propagation of spine gourd (Momordica dioica Roxb.) and assessment of genetic fidelity of micropropagated plants using RAPD analysis. *Physiology and Molecular Biology of Plants*, 18(3):273–280.

Rakh, M.S. and Banurekha, J. 2021. Comparative review of momordica charantia and momordica dioica: An update. *International Journal of Pharmaceutical Sciences and Research*, 12(8):4101–4114.

Rakh, M.S. and Sanjay, R.C. 2010. Evaluation of CNS depressant activity of Momordica dioica Roxb willd fruit pulp. *International Journal of Pharmaceutical and Sciences*, 2(4):124–126.

Ramya, S.B. and Krishna, K.L. 2013. Cardioprotective activity of triterpenoid rich bio fraction of momordica diocia roxb. *Indian Journal of Pharmacology*, 45(1):B S160–E S160.

Reiner, Z., Laufs, U., Cosentino, F. and Landmesser, U. 2019. The year in cardiology 2018: Prevention. *European Heart Journal*, 40(4):336–344.

Revathy, S., Bhavana, V., Krishna, K.L., Mahalakshmi, A.M., Ramprasad, K.L., Tekuri, M.K. 2014. Anti-tumor activity of fruit extracts of Momordica dioica Roxb. *World Journal of Pharmaceutical Research*, 4(1):1–13.

Safia, A. and Krishna, K.L. 2013. Evaluation of hypolipidemic and anti-obesity activities of Momordica dioica Roxb. fruit extracts on atherogenic diet induced hyperlipidemic rats. *Pharmacophore*, 4(6):215–221.

Sakshi, C., Harikrishnan, A., Selvakumar, J., Ahana Roy, C. and Veena, V. 2020. Predictive medicinal metabolites from Momordica dioica against comorbidity related proteins of SARS-CoV-2 infections. *Journal of Biomolecular Structure and Dynamics*, 1–14.

Samaddar, S., Deepak, K.J. and Raju, K. 2020. Optimization of pancreatic islet isolation from rat and evaluation of islet protective potential of a saponin isolated from fruits of Momordica dioica. *Journal of Applied Pharmaceutical Science*, 10(7):089–099.

Sebastian, S., Katie, F., Matthias, O., Sanela, K., Marin, K., Maria Teresa Bayo, J., Ksenija, M.V., Johanna, H., Swenja K.S., Thomas, M. and Andreas, D. 2019. Vascular inflammation and oxidative stress: Major triggers for cardiovascular disease. *Oxidative Medicine and Cellular Longevity*, 709215:1–26.

Shamala, S. and Krishna, K.L. 2013. Cardioprotective activity of fruit extracts of momordica dioca roxb. on doxorubicin induced toxicity on rats. *Science International*, 1(12):392–400.

Shankar, P., Prasanna Kumar, B.R. and Mohammed, K. 2011. Hepatoprotective activity of momordica diocia roxb fruits in CCl4-induced hepatotoxicity in rats. *Iranian Journal of Pharmaceutical Sciences*, 7(4):279–282.

Shreedhara, C.S. and Vaidya, V.P. 2006. Screening of momordica dioica for hepatoprotective, antioxidant, and antiinflammatory activities. *Natural Product Sciences*, 12(3):157–161.

Shrinivas, B., Samleti, A., Melisa, P. and Manisha, S. 2009. Evaluation of antimicrobial and antioxidant properties of Momordica dioica Roxb. (Ex Willd). *Journal of Pharmaceutical Research*, 2(6):1075–1078.

Shyaula, Sajan L. and Manandhar, M.D. 2021. Secondary metabolites of cucurbitaceae, occurrence, structure and role in human diet. *Comprehensive Insights in Vegetables of Nepal*, 235–245.

Singh, D., Bahadur, V., Singh, D.B. and Ghosh, G. 2008. Spine gourd (*Momordica dioica*): An underutilized vegetable with high nutritional and medicinal values: International symposium on the socio-economic impact of modern vegetable production technology in Tropical Asia. *Acta Hortic*, 809:241–249.

Sravani, C.H., Sindhura, J., Krishna, K.L. 2013. Evaluation of nephroprotective activity of momordica dioica roxb fruit. Indian Journal of Pharmacology, 45(1):B S218–E S219.

Sugamura, K. and Keaney Jr, J.F. 2011. Reactive oxygen species in cardiovascular disease. *Free Radical Biology and Medicine*, 51(5):978–992.

Sun, M., Chai, L., Lu, F., Zhao, Y., Li, Q., Cui, B., Gao, R. and Liu, Y. 2018. Efficacy and safety of Ginkgo Biloba pills for coronary heart disease with impaired glucose regulation: Study protocol for a series of N-of-1 randomized, double-blind, placebo-controlled trials. *Evidence-Based Complementary and Alternative Medicine*:7571629;8.

Sunshine, H., and Luisa Iruela-Arispe, M. 2017. Membrane lipids and cell signaling. *Current Opinion in Lipidology*, 28(5):408–413.

Tungmunnithum, D., Areeya, T., Apinan, P. and Yangsabai, A. 2018. Flavonoids and other phenolic compounds from medicinal plants for pharmaceutical and medical aspects: An overview. *Medicines*, 5(93):1–16.

Venkateshwarlu, M., Nagaraju, M., Odelu, G., Srilatha, T., and Ugandhar, T. 2017. Studies on phytochemical analysis and biological activities in Momordica dioica Roxb through Fruit. *The Pharma Innovation Journal*, 6(12):437–440.

Vijayakumar, M., Bavani Eswaran, M., Ojha, S.K., Rao, C.V. and Rawat, A. K. S. 2011. Antiulcer activity of hydroalcoholic extract of Momordica dioica roxb. fruit. *Indian Journal of Pharmaceutical Sciences*, 73(5):572–577.

Vutukuri, S. and Male, A. 2020. A review on Momordica dioica fruits. *Journal of Advancements in Plant Science*, 3(1):1–5.

Wachtel-Galor, S., Yuen, J., Buswell, J.A. and Benzie, I.F. 2011. Ganoderma lucidum (Lingzhi or Reishi). *Herbal Medicine: Biomolecular and Clinical Aspects*. 2nd edition. CRC Press/Taylor & Francis.

Zeng, Y., Jin, W., Qinwan, H., Yuanyuan, R., Tingna, L., Xiaorui, Z., Renchuan, Y. and Jilin, S. 2021. Cucurbitacin IIa: A review of phytochemistry and pharmacology. *Phytotherapy Research*, 35(8):4155–4170.

Zhang, Y.J., Ren-You, G., Sha, L., Yue, Z., An-Na Li, Dong-Ping X. and Hua-Bin Li. 2020. Antioxidant phytochemicals for the prevention and treatment of chronic diseases. *Molecules*, 20(12):21138–21156.

Zhou, J., Fan, Y., Kong, J., Wu, D. and Hu, Z. 2000. Effects of components isolated from Astragalus membranaceus Bunge on cardiac function injured by myocardial ischemia reperfusion in rats. *Zhongguo Zhong Yao Za Zhi*, 25(5):300–302.

21 Saptrees (Genus *Garcinia*) and Cardioprotection
Molecular, Cellular, and Metabolic Aspects

Elvine Pami Nguelefack-Mbuyo and Télesphore Benoît Nguelefack

CONTENTS

21.1 Introduction 332
21.2 Background 332
21.3 Anti-Inflammatory Effects of Saptrees 333
21.4 Anti-Apoptotic Effects of Saptrees 335
21.5 Mitophagic Effects of Saptrees 336
21.6 Antioxidant Effects of Saptrees 336
21.7 Anti-Atherogenic Effects of Saptrees 338
     21.7.1 Preclinical Studies 338
     21.7.2 Clinical Studies 339
21.8 Effects of Saptrees against Cardiac Remodeling 339
21.9 Effects of Saptrees against Vascular Remodeling 340
21.10 Other Foods, Herbs, Spices, and Botanicals Used in Cardiovascular
     Health and Disease 341
21.11 Toxicity and Cautionary Notes 341
21.12 Summary Points 342
References 342

LIST OF ABBREVIATIONS

ACLY   ATP-citrate lyase
Bcl-2   B-cell lymphoma 2
BNP   brain natriuretic peptide
CAT   catalase
CVDs   cardiovascular diseases
ERK   extracellular signal-regulated kinase
FAS   fatty acid synthase
GA   gambogic acid
GPx   glutathione peroxidase
GSH   reduced glutathione
HDL   high-density lipoprotein
IL   interleukin
iNOS   inducible nitric oxide synthase
I/R   ischemia/reperfusion

DOI: 10.1201/9781003220329-23

JNK	c-Jun N-terminal kinase
LDL	low-density lipoprotein
MAPK	mitogen-activated protein kinase
MDA	malondialdehyde
MI	myocardial infarction
NF-κB	nuclear factor kappa B
PI3K	phosphatidylinositol-3-kinase
PPARα	peroxisome proliferators-activated receptor alpha
ROS	reactive oxygen species
SOD	superoxide dismutase
SREBP-1c	sterol regulatory element-binding protein-1c
STAT	signal transducer and activator of transcription
TC	total cholesterol
TG	triglycerides
TNF-α	tumor necrosis factor-alpha

21.1 INTRODUCTION

Cardiovascular diseases (CVDs) refer to diseases of the heart and blood vessels. They are a severe public health issue that has devastating socioeconomic effects worldwide. CVDs are the world's largest cause of death (WHO, 2021) with an estimated 17.9 million deaths in 2019, representing 32% of all global deaths (WHO, 2021). Heart diseases represent an important part of CVDs, and include coronary artery disease, cardiac arrhythmias, heart failure, heart valve disease, pericardial disease, dilated cardiomyopathy, myocardial infarction (MI), hypertrophic cardiomyopathy, and congenital heart disease. Among these, MI is the most violent and the deadliest (Jayaraj et al., 2018). It is commonly known as heart attack and represents a true emergency condition.

MI, defined as cardiomyocyte necrosis, is a result of prolonged myocardial ischemia caused by an imbalance between coronary blood supply and myocardial demand (Boarescu et al., 2019). Clinically, the management of MI consists of an urgent recovery of blood flow to the heart known as reperfusion (Herrera-Zelada et al., 2021). However, reperfusion itself is associated with a second episode of cardiomyocyte death that can culminate in cardiac arrhythmias and ventricular function collapse (van der Weg et al., 2019). Given the vital importance of the heart, novel and effective therapeutic strategies are needed to protect the cardiac muscle from injuries. The term "cardioprotection" is used to describe "all measures and interventions to prevent, attenuate, and repair myocardial injury" (Herrera-Zelada et al., 2021). In the search for new cardioprotective agents, medicinal plants appear as a valuable asset.

Since the dawn of time, humankind has always drawn from nature everything needed for survival. As such, the use of plants as a remedy by humans dates back from time immemorial and they have significantly contributed to establishing good health and well-being through their therapeutic properties. Medicinal plants have played a key role in the development of pharmaceutical industries. In fact, 39% of the 520 new drugs approved between 1983 and 1994 were natural compounds or derived from natural compounds (Shaito et al., 2020). To contribute to the drug discovery using plants, a number of pharmacological studies have been carried out using saptrees. This review focuses on the molecular, cellular, and metabolic mechanisms underlying the cardioprotective effect of saptrees (genus *Garcinia*).

21.2 BACKGROUND

The genus *Garcinia* comprises about 250 species and is part of the family Clusiaceae (Baruah et al., 2021). The plants in this genus are commonly called saptrees, kokum, mangosteens, garciniasor, or monkey fruit (Hemshekhar et al., 2011). The genus is native to tropical Asia, Africa, New Caledonia, Polynesia, and Brazil (Espirito Santo et al., 2020) and can be divided into Asian and African groups though some species were introduced in South America (Maňourová et al., 2019). *Garcinia* species are evergreen polygamous trees or shrubs, usually with a yellow resin having simple, opposite, or nearly opposite, leathery leaves in whorls of three often with glandular and resinous cells (Angami et al., 2021).

Almost all parts of the plant (root, bark, stem, seed, rind, pericarp, fruits, flowers, and leaves) of the genus *Garcinia* are used for multiple purposes. In Asian countries, *Garcinia* is used for culinary purposes as a condiment and flavoring agent in place of tamarind or lemon (Chuah et al., 2013). Many species of *Garcinia* bear edible fruits that are eaten locally and among all, *Garcinia mangostana* is regarded as the queen of fruits for its beautiful purple-blue pericarp and delicious flavor (Angami et al., 2021). Young leaves of *G. anomala*, *G. pedunculata*, and *G. paniculata* are eaten cooked by some tribes in the northeast region of India (Baruah et al., 2021). In Cameroon, *G. kola* and *G. lucida* are the most commonly used species and their stem bark served as an additive in palm wine processing (Guedje et al., 2017; Maňourová et al., 2019). The leaves of *G. lucida* are thought to fight against evil spirits or to chase away ghosts (Guedje et al., 2017).

Plants of the genus *Garcinia* are also reputed for their medicinal potential. They are traditionally used in the treatment of various diseases and conditions including microbial infections, cancer, and obesity (Hemshekhar et al., 2011). In Indian folk medicine, *G. cambogia*, also known as Malabar tamarind, is used as a purgative in the treatment of intestinal worms and other parasites, and as a cardiotonic (Chuah et al., 2013). In addition, it is used to treat ulcers, rheumatism, hemorrhoids, diarrhea, dysentery, and cancers (Chuah et al., 2013; Espirito Santo et al., 2020). In Cameroon folk medicine, *G. kola* also called "bitter kola" because of its typical bitter taste, and *G. lucida*, known as "essok," are among the most important medicinal plants. Both species, mostly the seeds and the bark, are used to treat digestive tract disorders, gynecological pains and infections, sexually transmittable diseases, generalized pain, cancers, and mostly, as an antidote (Guedje et al., 2017; Maňourová et al., 2019). *G. kola* seeds are chewed by men for their claimed aphrodisiac effects. *G. kola* and *G. lucida* are used by some Cameroonian traditional healers for the management of cardiovascular ailments (Sonfack et al., 2021).

A broad range of bioactive secondary metabolites has been identified and/or isolated from *Garcinia* species. These metabolites include xanthones, flavonoids (especially biflavonoids), benzophenones (mostly derivates of polyisoprenylated benzophenones), lactones, and phenolic acid (Espirito Santo et al., 2020; Angami et al., 2021) and they have gained considerable attention from a pharmacological point of view. In fact, natural products from saptrees have demonstrated anti-inflammatory, anti-apoptotic, mitophagic, antioxidant, anti-atherogenic, and remodeling activities. The following parts will give more insights into these pharmacological properties.

21.3 ANTI-INFLAMMATORY EFFECTS OF SAPTREES

Inflammation is a complex process comprising molecular and cellular patterns that are essential in the host's defense mechanism. However, persistent inflammation is associated with deleterious effects and has been recognized as a hallmark of myocardial infarction (MI) and reperfusion injury, and plays a critical role in myocardial hypertrophy. Inflammation is typically characterized by the infiltration of inflammatory cells (neutrophils, monocytes, macrophages, lymphocytes, and fibroblasts) and the release of pro-inflammatory cytokines/chemokines.

Among the molecular mechanisms that activate inflammatory response, nuclear factor kappa B (NF-κB), a transcription factor, is the best known (Fiordelisi et al., 2019). The NF-κB family consists of five members, of which the p50/p65 heterodimer is the most abundant and is responsible for the majority of NF-κB canonical transcriptional activity (Kumar et al., 2013; Fiordelisi et al., 2019). In the inactive state, NF-κB is bound to an inhibitory kappa B (IκB) protein in the cytoplasm (Kumar et al., 2013; Fiordelisi et al., 2019). It has been shown that extracts and compounds from *Garcinia* species exhibit anti-inflammatory properties.

Gambogic acid (GA) is the main active ingredient isolated from *G. hanburyi* (Liu et al., 2013) and *G. maingayi* (Na et al., 2018). In a model of hypoxia-induced right ventricular hypertrophy, Zhao et al. (2013) showed that treatment with GA at the dose of 0.75 mg/kg inhibited the proteasome activity and increased IκBα accumulation in cardiac tissues resulting in the blockade of NF-κB translocation from the cytoplasm to the nucleus, thus decreasing NF-κB DNA-binding activity and reducing interleukin (IL)-2 levels. Similar results were observed by Liu et al. (2013) who found that GA (1.5 mg/kg), administered every other day for 2 weeks suppressed pressure overload-induced left ventricular hypertrophy via the inhibition of the proteasome and NF-κB pathway.

Intraperitoneal administration of 1 mg/kg GA inhibited MI-induced cardiac damage by altering multiple inflammatory pathways, including decreased activity of pro-inflammatory cytokines such as tumor necrosis factor-alpha (TNF-α) and interleukin-6 (IL-6) while increasing the activity of IL-10, an anti-inflammatory cytokine (Na et al., 2018). Inducible nitric oxide synthase (iNOS) production was likewise lowered by GA associated with the blockade of NF-κB/p65, and p38/mitogen-activated protein kinase (MAPK) pathway (Na et al., 2018).

Jiang et al. (2020) in their study showed that α-mangostin, a major constituent extracted from the hull of *G. mangostana* (Fang et al., 2018) achieves its cardioprotective effect by inhibiting the protein expression of NF-κB and cyclooxygenase-2 (COX-2) in an experimental model of ischemia/reperfusion. In the same line, Soetikno et al. (2020) showed that treatment with α-mangostin inhibited the infiltration of immune cells in hypertrophic cardiomyocytes of diabetic rats coupled to a reduction in monocyte chemoattractant protein-1 expression. In addition, α-mangostin also diminished TNF-α mRNA and cardiac protein expression of inflammatory cytokines such as TNF-α, IL-6, and IL-1β.

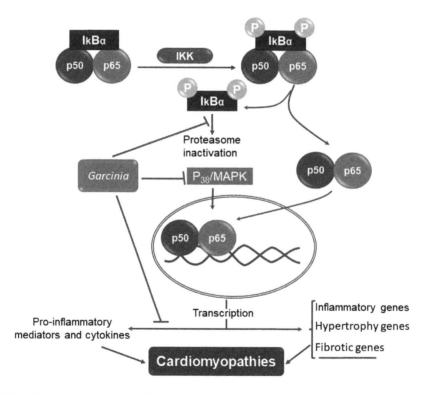

FIGURE 21.1 Molecular pathway underlying the anti-inflammatory-mediated cardioprotective effect of *Garcinia* species.

Note: Garcinia inactivates the proteasome activity leading to IκBα accumulation. The accumulation of IκBα inhibits the translocation of the heterodimer p50 and p65 of NF-κB leading to the inhibition of downstream genes and pro-inflammatory factors. *Garcinia* inhibits the expression of p38/MAPK protein resulting in the negative regulation of NF-κB transcriptional activity. IκBα: inhibitory kappa B alpha; IKK: I kappa B kinase.

The cardioprotective effect of Kolaviron, a biflavonoid complex isolated from the seed extract of *G. kola* against cyclophosphamide-induced cardiac toxicity was explored by Omole et al. (2018). Kolaviron, which is composed of Garcinia biflavonoids – GB1, GB2, and kolaflavanone (Oyagbemi et al., 2017; Oyagbemi et al., 2018) – mitigates cyclophosphamide-induced cardiac injury by preventing myeloperoxidase activity. Concordantly, *G. lucida* was found to inhibit the infiltration of inflammatory cells in cardiac tissue of rats chronically administered with adenine (Sonfack et al., 2021). The anti-inflammatory mechanisms of saptrees are summarized in Figure 21.1.

21.4 ANTI-APOPTOTIC EFFECTS OF SAPTREES

Apoptosis is a form of programmed cell death that plays an essential role in tissue homeostasis. However, excessive apoptosis is harmful to the tissue and has been involved in the pathophysiology of cardiac diseases. Apoptosis has been implicated in cardiomyocyte death during MI and ischemia/reperfusion (I/R) with caspases playing a key role in this process. Many authors have demonstrated that *Garcinia* species exert their cardioprotective effect by suppressing pro-apoptotic or enhancing anti-apoptotic pathways. Treatment with *G. kola* or kolaviron improved left ventricle function and coronary flow during I/R by down-regulating the protein expression of p38 MAPK, caspase-3, cleaved caspase-3 (Asp 175), cleaved poly adenosine diphosphate ribose polymerase, c-Jun N-terminal kinase (JNK) 1 and 2, and phosphorylated JNK1 (Tyr 185) and 2 (Thr 183) pro-apoptotic pathways (Oyagbemi et al., 2017; Oyagbemi et al., 2018). Moreover, the expression of anti-apoptotic factors like signal transducer and activator of transcription 3 (STAT3) and STAT5, phosphorylated STAT3 (Tyr 705), heat shock protein 27 (Hsp27), and phosphorylated Hsp27 (Ser 82) was increased following *G. kola* or kolaviron exposure (Oyagbemi et al., 2018) (Figure 21.2).

Another mechanism by which *G. kola* and kolaviron abrogated apoptosis is the activation of the so-called "reperfusion injury salvage kinase (RISK)" pathway. The RISK pathway is composed of

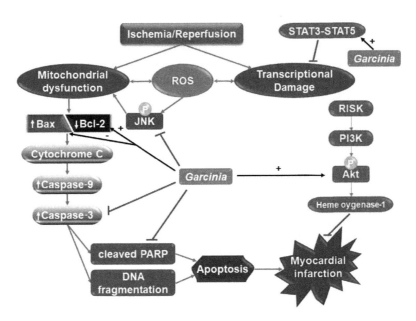

FIGURE 21.2 Caspase inhibition and activation of PI3K/Akt pathways contribute to the cardioprotective effects of *Garcinia* plant species in myocardial infarction.

Note: Bcl-2: B-cell lymphoma 2; Bax: Bcl-2-associated X protein; JNK: c-Jun N-terminal kinase; PARP: poly adenosine diphosphate ribose polymerase; STAT: signal transducer and activator of transcription; PI3K: phosphatidylinositol-3-kinase.

two parallel cascades: phosphatidylinositol-3-kinase/Akt (PI3K/Akt) and mitogen-activated protein kinase 1/extracellular signal-regulated protein kinase 1/2 (MEK1/ERK1/2) (Rossello and Yellon, 2018). The administration of *G. kola* or kolaviron enhanced the total Akt and phosphorylated Akt (Oyagbemi et al., 2018) (Figure 21.2).

Fang et al. (2018) have evaluated the anti-apoptotic effect of α-mangostin, in an experimental model of CoCl2-induced hypoxia in H9C2 cardiac cells. The results show that α-mangostin prevents apoptosis of H9C2 cells through up-regulation of the gene and protein expression of B-cell lymphoma 2 (Bcl-2), an anti-apoptotic factor. These authors further demonstrated that α-mangostin down-regulated mRNA of Bax, caspase-9, and caspase-3 as well as that of the corresponding proteins. In another study, it was demonstrated that α-mangostin reduced the expression of the pro-apoptotic protein Bcl2 interacting protein 3 (Jiang et al., 2020).

Garcinol, a polyisoprenylated benzophenone found in the fruit of *G. indica*, similar to α-mangostin effectively prevented apoptosis in rats with isoproterenol-induced heart failure and in H9C2 cardiac cells by increasing mRNA and protein expression of Bcl-2. In addition, garcinol reduced the mRNA and protein levels of caspase-3, cleaved caspase-3, and Bax (Li et al., 2020) (Figure 21.2). ATP depletion has been reported to initiate mitochondrial dysfunction that can further lead to the so-called intrinsic pathway-induced apoptosis (Dong et al., 2019; Jiang et al., 2020). It was demonstrated by Jiang et al. (2020) that one of the mechanisms by which α-mangostin protects rat cardiac tissues from I/R is the inhibition of ATP depletion.

21.5 MITOPHAGIC EFFECTS OF SAPTREES

Mitochondria are cell organelles responsible for the production of energy in the organism and they are often injured during reperfusion following an ischemic episode (Xiang et al., 2020). Damaged mitochondria are cytotoxic and need to be cleared. This is achieved by a process known as mitophagy (Xiang et al., 2020) whereby damaged mitochondria trigger their own destruction. Adequate mitophagy is thought to be cardioprotective during I/R (Killackey et al., 2020).

Gerontoxanthone I and macluraxanthone were isolated from the leaves of *G. bracteata* by Xiang et al. (2020) and their ability to induce mitophagy was tested using H9C2, YFP-Parkin HeLa, and SH-SY5Y cells. The results showed that gerontoxanthone I and macluraxanthone attenuated I/R injury in H9C2, increased the accumulation of PTEN-induced kinase 1 (PINK1), promoted Parkin puncta accumulation, and reduced the protein levels of translocase of outer membrane 20 (Tom20) and translocase of inner membrane 23 (Tim23) with no effect on the mRNA levels of Tim23 and Tom20. These latter results suggest that gerontoxanthone and macluraxanthone favor the post-transcriptional degradation of Tim23 and Tom20. These same authors also found that treatment with gerontoxanthone and macluraxanthone up-regulated the expression of autophagy receptors, namely nuclear dot protein 52 kDa (NDP52) and microtubule-associated protein 1A/1B-light chain 3 (LC3) II, as well as the phosphorylation and ubiquitination of Parkin. Taken together, the results show that gerontoxanthone and macluraxanthone induce *in vitro* cardioprotective effects by activating mitophagy through the PINK1-Parkin pathway. The mechanism of gerontoxanthone and macluraxanthone-induced mitophagy is summarized in Figure 21.3.

21.6 ANTIOXIDANT EFFECTS OF SAPTREES

Oxidative stress is defined as an imbalance between oxidants also known as reactive oxygen species (ROS) and antioxidants in favor of the oxidants. Increased ROS production can cause damage to DNA, protein, cell membranes, and other macromolecules (D'Oria et al., 2020). Oxidative stress mediates various physiopathological mechanisms involved in cardiac injury like inflammation, cardiac and vascular remodeling, and plaque formation (Donia and Khamis, 2021). As such it has become an attractive target to achieve cardioprotection (Donia and Khamis, 2021).

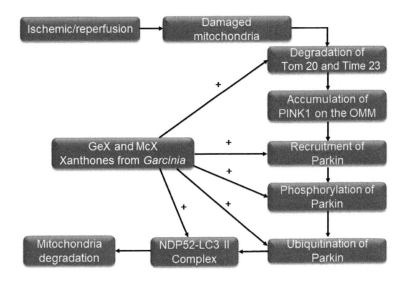

FIGURE 21.3 Mitophagy activation contributes to the cardioprotective effects of xanthone secondary metabolites from saptrees.

Note: The degradation of Tom 20 and Tim 23 by gerontoxanthone I and macluraxanthone causes the accumulation of PINK1 on the outer membrane of the damaged mitochondria with subsequent recruitment of Parkin. PINK then phosphorylates and ubiquitinates Parkin which in turn ubiquitinates mitochondrial proteins. The activation of the NDP52-LC3 II complex recognized the ubiquitinated mitochondria and triggers its degradation. Tom: translocase of outer membrane 20; Tim 23: translocase of inner membrane 23; PINK1: PTEN-induced kinase 1; OMM: outer mitochondrial membrane; NDP52: nuclear dot protein 52 kDa; LC3 II: microtubule-associated protein 1A/1B-light chain 3 two.

Panda et al. (2014) used a model of isoproterenol-induced cardiac necrosis in rats to demonstrate the antioxidant efficacy of a hydroethanolic extract of *G. indica* fruit rind. Treatment with *G. indica* at dosages of 400 mg/kg and 800 mg/kg prevented lipid peroxidation, as shown by lower cardiac malondialdehyde (MDA) levels in this study. *G. indica* also restored catalase (CAT), superoxide dismutase (SOD), glutathione peroxidase (GPx), and glutathione reductase activities, which had been decreased by isoproterenol treatment.

Adaramoye and Lawal (2015) show that kolaviron at doses of 100 or 200 mg/kg improved the redox status in isoproterenol-treated rats' cardiac tissue by limiting the rate of formation of MDA, a lipid peroxidation marker, and preventing the depletion of non-enzymic and enzymic antioxidants, such as reduced glutathione (GSH), GST, GPx, SOD, and CAT. When normal rats were given kolaviron, however, there was no change in the levels of oxidative stress markers (Adaramoye and Lawal, 2015). Apart from the aforementioned antioxidant properties of kolaviron, Oyagbemi et al. (2017) discovered that this biflavonoids complex was also capable of lowering the amount of oxidized glutathione (GSSH) and increasing the GSH/GSSH ratio under I/R conditions.

The incubation of H9C2 cardiac cells with α-mangostin at concentrations of 0.06 or 0.3 mM 24 h prior to $CoCl_2$ addition has been shown to suppress ROS and MDA production and enhance SOD activity (Fang et al., 2018). This *in vitro* antioxidant activity of α-mangostin was further confirmed *in vivo* in a model of I/R by Jiang et al. (2020). It was observed during this study that the administration of α-mangostin abrogated ROS production, decreased levels of lipid peroxides, and increased the activity of cellular antioxidant defense mechanisms such as SOD, reduced glutathione (GSH), glutathione peroxidase (GPx), and glutathione S-transferase (GST). This antioxidant activity of α-mangostin was mediated by the activation of the nuclear factor erythroid 2-related factor 2 (Nrf-2)/heme oxygenase-1 (HO-1) signaling pathway (Jiang et al., 2020). Importantly α-mangostin did not affect the redox status of healthy male Sprague Dawley rats (Jiang et al., 2020). Recently, Labban et al. (2021) show that when the aqueous extract of *G. mangostana* (from which α-mangostin was extracted) was administered to normal Wistar rats, no change in their redox status was noticed, supporting the finding that *G. mangostana* and its derivative compound α-mangostin exert their antioxidant effect by preventing an imbalance between oxidative and antioxidant mechanism and not by up-regulating the level of antioxidant defense mechanism. It was shown in the study of Sari et al. (2021) that α-mangostin reduces ROS in primary neonatal rat fibroblasts by down-regulating the expression of NADPH oxidase 4 mRNA, a key player in the generation of oxidative stress in the heart.

21.7 ANTI-ATHEROGENIC EFFECTS OF SAPTREES

Atherosclerosis is a disease characterized by the formation of a plaque (also called atheroma) made up of fatty deposits in the vascular wall of small or large arteries. The protrusion or the rupture of the plaque can lead to partial or complete obstruction of blood flow to the heart when built on a coronary vessel resulting in MI. Atherosclerosis is triggered by hypercholesterolemia with low-density lipoprotein (LDL) oxidation as the starting point. Also, platelet aggregation at the site of plaque rupture may cause arterial thrombus formation leading to MI. Using LDL and platelets isolated from the blood of healthy volunteers, Saputri and Jantan (2012) demonstrated that *G. hombroniana* and specifically 3,5,3′,5′-tetrahydroxy-4-methoxybenzophenone and 1,7-dihydroxyxanthone strongly inhibit LDL oxidation and platelet aggregation.

Tabares-Guevara et al. (2017) used *in vitro* and *in vivo* approaches to study the anti-atherogenic properties of biflavonoids (morelloflavone, volkensiflavone, fukugiside) and the biflavonoid fraction (85% morelloflavone, 10% volkensiflavone, and 5% amentoflavone) isolated from G. *madruno.* Morelloflavone, fukugiside, and biflavonoid fractions inhibit LDL oxidation triggered by Cu^{2+} and prevent enhanced electronegativity of the LDL's apolipoprotein component (ApoB-100). The biflavonoids used in this study also inhibited the surface expression of the proatherogenic receptor CD36 and its subsequent transformation into foam cells, as well as limiting oxidized LDL uptake and cholesterol accumulation. G. *kola* biflavonoid fractions were reported to reduce serum total cholesterol (TC), triglycerides (TG), LDL, and increased HDL levels (Adejor et al., 2017).

G. cambogia and its main active ingredient, (–)-Hydroxycitric acid have been intensively studied for their hypocholesterolemic effects in both preclinical and clinical studies.

21.7.1 PRECLINICAL STUDIES

The administration of flavonoids from *G. cambogia* to normal and hypercholesterolemic rats resulted in a reduction of serum and tissue lipids, probably related to the decrease in liver β-hydroxy β-methyl glutaryl coenzyme A (HMG-CoA) reductase activity (Koshy et al., 2001). In addition, the activity of plasma lecithin cholesterol acyltransferase, an enzyme responsible for the maturation of HDL cholesterol was also boosted while the activity of glucose-6-phosphate dehydrogenase and isocitrate dehydrogenase was highly reduced. These results show that flavonoids from *G. cambogia* display a hypolipidemic effect through the inhibition of lipogenesis and the stimulation of lipolysis (Koshy et al., 2001).

The study conducted by Han et al. (2016) explores the effect of a diet supplemented with (–)-Hydroxycitric acid (the active ingredient extracted from the rind of *G. cambogia* fruit) on lipid metabolism with a particular focus on genes involved in fatty acids synthesis or degradation in broiler chickens. They found that (–)-Hydroxycitric acid induced low serum TG and LDL levels. Besides, liver TG was decreased, while non-esterified fatty acids and hepatic lipase activity were enhanced. The sterol regulatory element-binding protein-1c (SREBP-1c), ATP-citrate lyase (ACLY) and fatty acid synthase (FAS) mRNA levels were markedly decreased, while AMP-activated protein kinase β2 (AMPKβ2) and peroxisome proliferators-activated receptor alpha (PPARα) mRNA expression was up-regulated. SREBP-1c is a transcription factor involved in the activation of genes responsible for the synthesis of fatty acids like ACLY, FAS, and acetyl CoA carboxylase (ACC) (Han et al., 2016; Chen et al., 2021). The phosphorylation of SREBP-1c by AMPK inhibits its nuclear translocation resulting in the down-regulation of its target genes (Chen et al., 2021). PPARα has been reported to promote fatty acid β-oxidation (Han et al., 2016). These results clearly show that (−)-Hydroxycitric acid inhibited lipogenesis by down-regulating the gene expression of ACLY, SREBP-1c, and FAS in the one hand, and accelerated lipolysis through enhancing hepatic lipase activity and PPARα expression on the other hand.

21.7.2 CLINICAL STUDIES

Some clinical trials investigated the effect of *G. cambogia* on lipid metabolism and results are conflicting. In a double-blind placebo-controlled clinical trial performed by Hayamizu et al. (2003) on obese patients, the authors observed that *G. cambogia* extract containing 60% (−)-Hydroxycitric acid, has no significant effect on TC, TG, free fatty acids, HDL, and LDL despite a reduction in abdominal fat accumulation after 16 weeks of treatment. On the opposite, Al-Kuraishy and Al-Gareeb (2016) conducted a 3-month randomized, population-based controlled study during which obese patients were treated with either *G. cambogia*, orlistat, or the combination of both. They observed that *G. cambogia* significantly improved lipid parameters as evidenced by low TC, TG, and LDL levels. Moreover, the atherogenic index (log (TG/HDL)) and the cardiac risk ratios were also reduced. One possible reason that could explain the discrepancy between these studies could be the source of *G. cambogia* used.

21.8 EFFECTS OF SAPTREES AGAINST CARDIAC REMODELING

Cardiac remodeling is a series of cellular and molecular alterations that result in a change in the shape, size, and function of the heart. It may occur in response to hemodynamic stress, cardiac injury, inflammation, and neurohormonal activation as adaptive or maladaptive mechanisms (Figure 21.4). Alpha-skeletal actin (α-SK-actin) and brain natriuretic peptide (BNP) genes are abundantly expressed in fetal hearts and down-regulated in adults under normal physiological conditions. However, in some pathological circumstances, such as heart hypertrophy, the reactivation of these fetal genes may occur (Zhao et al., 2013; Liu et al., 2013). One of the mechanisms underpinning the protective effect of GA against right ventricular hypertrophy in rats exposed to chronic hypoxia (Zhao et al., 2013) or left ventricular hypertrophy induced by abdominal aorta constriction is the suppression of α-SK-actin and BNP reactivation (Liu et al., 2013). In addition, GA prevents ventricular remodeling by reducing the protein expression of matrix metalloproteinase 2 (MMP-2), MMP-9, and intercellular adhesion molecule-1 (Na et al., 2018).

The efficacy of α-mangostin against phenylephrine-induced hypertrophy of primary neonatal rat cardiomyocytes was recently investigated by Sari et al. (2021). They discovered that α-mangostin abolished cardiomyocyte enlargement via lowering the levels of the mRNAs for atrial natriuretic factor (ANF) and BNP. They further investigated the role of signaling pathways linked with cardiomyocyte hypertrophy, particularly the Akt-ERK-p38 pathway and found that α-mangostin strongly reduced phenylephrine-induced Akt activation, but not ERK or p38 phosphorylation. Sari et al. (2021) also observed that α-mangostin inhibits collagen synthesis by blocking L-proline incorporation and down-regulating periostin (a collagen synthesis mediator) mRNA. In cultured cardiac fibroblasts, treatment with α-mangostin inhibited the differentiation of fibroblasts into myofibroblasts as evidenced by the decrease in the protein and gene expression of alpha smooth muscle actin (α-SMA), a marker of activated myofibroblasts. Boonprom et al. (2017) demonstrated that the aqueous extract from *G. mangostana* pericarp protects against cardiac remodeling in Nω-nitro-L-arginine methyl ester (L-NAME) hypertensive rats by preventing oxidative stress and enhancing NO bioavailability through the suppression of the NADPH oxidase subunit p47phox expression. Another mechanism

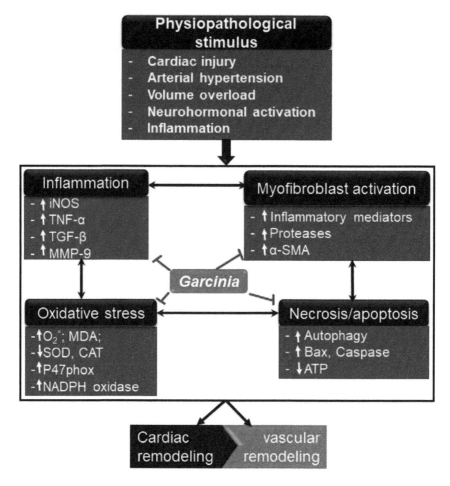

FIGURE 21.4 Protective effects of *Garcinia* species against cardiovascular remodeling.

Note: Garcinia species prevent cardiac and vascular remodeling by inhibiting inflammatory, oxidative, and necrotic/apoptotic pathways.

by which *G. mangostana* extract prevented cardiac remodeling was the decrease in plasma TNF-α and suppression of iNOS protein expression (Figure 21.4).

21.9 EFFECTS OF SAPTREES AGAINST VASCULAR REMODELING

Vascular remodeling is a complex process contributing to the phenotypic change of blood vessels that promote neointima formation. This process involves cellular mechanisms such as cell growth, cell death, cell migration, and the production or degradation of the extracellular matrix. During atherosclerosis, vascular remodeling is associated with plaque instability (Wihastuti et al., 2014). *In vitro* and *in vivo* experiments were conducted by Pinkaew et al. (2009) to assess the ability of morelloflavone, an active principle isolated from *G. dulcis* to prevent restenosis. They found that morelloflavone inhibited vascular smooth muscle migration and invasion in the scratch wound test, inhibited the formation of lamellipodia, and reduced injury-induced neointima formation in ApoE-/- mice. These effects were found to be mediated by the de-activation of some key migration molecules such as RhoA, Cdc42, focal adhesion kinase, and ERK (Pinkaew et al., 2009).

Wihastuti et al. (2014) have examined the anti-angiogenic effect of the ethanolic extract from *G. mangostana* pericarp in Wistar rats given a hypercholesterolemic diet. The results showed that treatment

Saptrees (Genus *Garcinia*) and Cardioprotection 341

with *G. mangostana* significantly lowered the number of vasa vasorum formed. This effect was accompanied by a decrease in vascular endothelial growth factor receptor-1 (VEGFR1), hypoxia-inducible factor-1 alpha (HIF-1α), NF-κB, and iNOS in aortic tissues. VEGF is a proangiogenic factor whose expression is stimulated by HIF-1α under hypoxic conditions (Wihastuti et al., 2014; Li et al., 2020) and binds to tyrosine kinase receptors VEGFR-1. NF-κB and iNOS, apart from their role in inflammation, have been reported to play an important role in the angiogenic process (Wihastuti et al., 2014). Thus, a decrease in VEGFR-1, HIF-1α, NF-κB, and iNOS is associated with an anti-angiogenic response. In a later study, Wihastuti et al. (2019) demonstrated that *G. mangostana* pericarp inhibits vascular cell adhesion molecule-1 expression and decreases the intima-media thickness in the aorta of rats fed a high-fat diet.

21.10 OTHER FOODS, HERBS, SPICES, AND BOTANICALS USED IN CARDIOVASCULAR HEALTH AND DISEASE

Aframomum pruinosum (Zingiberaceae) and *Crinum zeylanicum* (Amaryllidaceae) are medicinal plants used in Cameroon for the management of cardiovascular disorders including cardiac palpitations and arterial hypertension. The aqueous and ethanolic seed extract from *A. pruinosum* were evaluated for their cardioprotective effects against isoproterenol-induced MI. The results showed that both extracts reduced cardiomyocyte necrosis and fibrosis through anti-inflammatory (reduced nitric oxide and myeloperoxidase levels) and antioxidant mechanisms (reduced MDA levels and increased SOD and CAT activity) (Nguelefack-Mbuyo et al., 2022). In addition, these extracts were shown to exhibit vasorelaxant activity that was partially mediated by nitric oxide production. This latter mechanism was thought to contribute to the cardioprotective effect of *A. pruinosum* by decreasing cardiac workload (Nguelefack-Mbuyo et al., 2022). Ndjenda et al. (2021a) show that *C. zeylanicum* methanol leaf extract completely reversed L-NAME-induced hypertension. Later on, they show that this same extract was able to reduce the beating rate and the beating amplitude of cardiomyocytes, suggesting its negative chronotropic and inotropic effects (Ndjenda et al., 2021b).

Draginic et al. (2021) reported that *Melissa officinalis* (Lamiaceae) also known as honey balm exhibits antiarrhythmic effects as evidenced by a slower heart electrical conduction through partial PR and QTc prolongation in the electrocardiogram. This antiarrhythmic effect was shown to be mediated by the stimulation of muscarinic receptors (Draginic et al., 2021). *M. officinalis* also protects against MI and I/R injury by down-regulating the expression of NF-κB, TNF-α, and COX-2 on the one hand, and by decreasing the expression of proapoptotic factors, Bax and caspase-3, on the other hand. The improvement of the redox status (decreased MDA levels and increased SOD) also contributes to the cardioprotective effects of *M. officinalis* (Draginic et al., 2021).

21.11 TOXICITY AND CAUTIONARY NOTES

Despite the huge number of experimental studies evidencing the cardioprotective effect of *Garcinia* species, the translation of these findings into clinical settings is still needed. Until now, just a few clinical trials have been conducted on the hypolipidemic effects of *G. cambogia* and the results are conflicting. Although no clear toxicity has been evidenced with use of saptrees, caution should be taken concerning the use of some *Garcinia* species. *G. cambogia* or its active ingredient, hydroxycitric acid, is widely used as a dietary supplement for weight loss, and its consumption has been associated with adverse effects in rare cases. For instance, two cases of hepatic failure requiring transplantation were reported in a 34-year-old Hispanic male and in a 26-year-old obese woman following *G. cambogia* intake for 5 and 7 months, respectively (Lunsford et al., 2016; Ferreira et al., 2020). Additional studies are needed to assess the long-term toxicity of saptrees natural products in humans.

21.12 SUMMARY POINTS

- This chapter highlights the molecular, cellular, and metabolic mechanisms that support the cardioprotective effect of saptrees (genus *Garcinia*).
- Saptrees are native to tropical Asia, Africa, New Caledonia, Polynesia, and Brazil.
- All parts of the plants are used for medicinal purposes, including cardiac protection.
- Saptrees exert their cardioprotective effect through anti-inflammatory, anti-apoptotic, antioxidant, anti-atherogenic, and antiremodeling mechanisms.
- The NF-κB/p65, PI3K/Akt, extracellular signal-regulated protein kinase 1/2 (ERK1/2) and p38/mitogen-activated protein kinase (MAPK) pathways seem to play a pivotal role in the cardioprotective effect of saptrees.
- Xanthones and biflavonoids account for the majority of the cardioprotective effect of saptrees.
- No considerable side effect of saptrees was observed. Nevertheless, hepatotoxicity has been mentioned as the common side effect of *G. cambogia* used as a dietary supplement.

REFERENCES

Adaramoye, O.A., and S.O. Lawal. 2015. Kolaviron, a biflavonoid fraction from *Garcinia kola*, protects against isoproterenol-induced injury by mitigating cardiac dysfunction and oxidative stress in rats. *Journal of Basic and Clinical Physiology and Pharmacology* 26, no. 1 (January 1). www.degruyter.com/document/doi/10.1515/jbcpp-2013-0139/html.

Adejor, E.B., D.A. Ameh, D.B. James, O.A. Owolabi, and U.S. Ndidi. 2017. Effects of *Garcinia kola* biflavonoid fractions on serum lipid profile and kidney function parameters in hyperlipidemic rats. *Clinical Phytoscience* 2: 19.

Al-Kuraishy, H., and A. Al-Gareeb. 2016. Effect of orlistat alone or in combination with *Garcinia Cambogia* on visceral adiposity index in obese patients. *Journal of Intercultural Ethnopharmacology* 5: 408.

Angami, T., L. Wangchu, P. Debnath, P. Sarma, B. Singh, A.K. Singh, S. Singh, et al. 2021. *Garcinia* L.: A gold mine of future therapeutics. *Genetic Resources and Crop Evolution* 68: 11–24.

Baruah, S., P. Barman, S. Basumatary, and B. Bhuyan. 2021. Diversity and ethnobotany of genus *Garcinia* L. (clusiaceae) in Assam, Eastern Himalaya. *Ethnobotany Research and Applications* 21, no. 1 (June 29). http://ethnobotanyjournal.org/index.php/era/article/view/2571.

Boarescu, P.-M., I. Chirilă, A.E. Bulboacă, I.C. Bocşan, R.M. Pop, D. Gheban, and S.D. Bolboacă. 2019. Effects of curcumin nanoparticles in isoproterenol-induced myocardial infarction. *Oxidative Medicine and Cellular Longevity* 2019: 1–13.

Boonprom, P., O. Boonla, K. Chayaburakul, J.U. Welbat, P. Pannangpetch, U. Ukongviriyapan, V. Kukongviriyapan, P. Pakdeechote, and P. Prachaney. 2017. *Garcinia Mangostana* pericarp extract protects against oxidative stress and cardiovascular remodeling via suppression of P47 Phox and iNOS in nitric oxide deficient rats. *Annals of Anatomy – Anatomischer Anzeiger* 212: 27–36.

Chen, Y.-C., R.-J. Chen, S.-Y. Peng, W.C.Y. Yu, and V.H.-S. Chang. 2021. Therapeutic targeting of nonalcoholic fatty liver disease by downregulating SREBP-1C expression via AMPK-KLF10 axis. *Frontiers in Molecular Biosciences* 8: 751938.

Chuah, L.O., W.Y. Ho, B.K. Beh, and S.K. Yeap. 2013. Updates on antiobesity effect of *Garcinia* Origin (–)-HCA. *Evidence-Based Complementary and Alternative Medicine* 2013: 1–17.

Dong, Y., H. Chen, J. Gao, Y. Liu, J. Li, and J. Wang. 2019. Molecular machinery and interplay of apoptosis and autophagy in coronary heart disease. *Journal of Molecular and Cellular Cardiology* 136: 27–41.

Donia, T., and A. Khamis. 2021. Management of oxidative stress and inflammation in cardiovascular diseases: Mechanisms and challenges. *Environmental Science and Pollution Research* 28: 34121–353.

D'Oria, R., R. Schipani, A. Leonardini, A. Natalicchio, S. Perrini, A. Cignarelli, L. Laviola, and F. Giorgino. 2020. The role of oxidative stress in cardiac disease: From physiological response to injury factor. *Oxidative Medicine and Cellular Longevity* 2020: 1–29.

Draginic, N., V. Jakovljevic, M. Andjic, J. Jeremic, I. Srejovic, M. Rankovic, M. Tomovic, et al. 2021. *Melissa Officinalis* L. as a nutritional strategy for cardioprotection. *Frontiers in Physiology* 12: 661778.

Espirito Santo, B.L.S. do, L.F. Santana, W.H. Kato Junior, F. de O. de Araújo, D. Bogo, K. de C. Freitas, R. de C.A. Guimarães, et al. 2020. Medicinal potential of *Garcinia* species and their compounds. *Molecules* 25: 4513.

Fang, Z., W. Luo, and Y. Luo. 2018. Protective effect of α-mangostin against CoCl$_2$-induced apoptosis by suppressing oxidative stress in H9C2 rat cardiomyoblasts. *Molecular Medicine Reports* (March 6). www.spandidos-publications.com/10.3892/mmr.2018.8680.

Ferreira, V., A. Mathieu, G. Soucy, J.-M. Giard, and D. Erard-Poinsot. 2020. Acute severe liver injury related to long-term *Garcinia cambogia* intake. *ACG Case Reports Journal* 7: e00429.

Fiordelisi, A., G. Iaccarino, C. Morisco, E. Coscioni, and D. Sorriento. 2019. NFkappaB is a key player in the crosstalk between inflammation and cardiovascular diseases. *International Journal of Molecular Sciences* 20: 1599.

Guedje, N.M., F. Tadjouteu, J.M. Onana, E. NnaNga Nga, and O. Ndoye. 2017. *Garcinia lucida* Vesque (Clusiaceae): From traditional uses to pharmacopeic monograph for an emerging local plant-based drug development. *Journal of Applied Biosciences* 109: 10594.

Han, J., L. Li, D. Wang, and H. Ma. 2016. (–)-Hydroxycitric acid reduced fat deposition via regulating lipid metabolism-related gene expression in broiler chickens. *Lipids in Health and Disease* 15: 37.

Hayamizu, K., Y. Ishii, I. Kaneko, M. Shen, Y. Okuhara, N. Shigematsu, H. Tomi, M. Furuse, G. Yoshino, and H. Shimasaki. 2003. Effects of *Garcinia cambogia* (Hydroxycitric acid) on visceral fat accumulation: A double-blind, randomized, placebo-controlled trial. *Current Therapeutic Research* 64: 551–567.

Hemshekhar, M., K. Sunitha, M.S. Santhosh, S. Devaraja, K. Kemparaju, B.S. Vishwanath, S.R. Niranjana, and K.S. Girish. 2011. An overview on genus *Garcinia:* Phytochemical and therapeutical aspects. *Phytochemistry Reviews* 10: 325–351.

Herrera-Zelada, N., U. Zuñiga-Cuevas, A. Ramirez-Reyes, S. Lavandero, and J.A. Riquelme. 2021. Targeting the endothelium to achieve cardioprotection. *Frontiers in Pharmacology* 12: 636134.

Jayaraj, C., J.K. Davatyan, S.S. Subramanian, and J. Priya. 2018. Epidemiology of myocardial infarction. In *Myocardial Infarction*, ed. B. Pamukçu. IntechOpen. www.intechopen.com/books/myocardial-infarction/epidemiology-of-myocardial-infarction.

Jiang, H., W. Guo, D. Zhu, W. Zhang, J. Yu, M. Feng, X. Wang, et al. 2020. α-Mangostin protects against myocardial ischemia reperfusion injury by suppressing the activation of HIF-1α. *Tropical Journal of Pharmaceutical Research* 19: 25–31.

Killackey, S.A., D.J. Philpott, and S.E. Girardin. 2020. Mitophagy pathways in health and disease. *Journal of Cell Biology* 219: e202004029.

Koshy, A.S., L. Anila, and N.R. Vijayalakshmi. 2001. Flavonoids from *Garcinia cambogia* lower lipid levels in hypercholesterolemic rats. *Food Chemistry* 72: 289–294.

Kumar, R., Q.C. Yong, and C.M. Thomas. 2013. Do multiple nuclear factor kappa B activation mechanisms explain its varied effects in the heart? *The Ochsner Journal* 13: 157–165.

Labban, R.S.M., H.A. Alfawaz, A.T. Almnaizel, M.N. Al-Muammar, R.S. Bhat, and A. El-Ansary. 2021. *Garcinia Mangostana* extract and curcumin ameliorate oxidative stress, dyslipidemia, and hyperglycemia in high fat diet-induced obese wistar albino rats. *Scientific Reports* 11: 7278.

Li, M., X. Li, and L. Yang. 2020. Cardioprotective effects of garcinol following myocardial infarction in rats with isoproterenol-induced heart failure. *AMB Express* 10: 137.

Liu, J., H. Wang, and J. Li. 2016. Inflammation and inflammatory cells in myocardial infarction and reperfusion injury: A double-edged sword. *Clinical Medicine Insights: Cardiology* 10: CMC.S33164.

Liu, S., C. Zhao, C. Yang, X. Li, H. Huang, N. Liu, S. Li, X. Wang, and J. Liu. 2013. Gambogic acid suppresses pressure overload cardiac hypertrophy in rats. *American Journal of Cardiovascular Disease* 3: 227–238.

Lunsford, K.E., A.S. Bodzin, D.C. Reino, H.L. Wang, and R.W. Busuttil. 2016. Dangerous dietary supplements: *Garcinia cambogia*-associated hepatic failure requiring transplantation. *World Journal of Gastroenterology* 22: 10071.

Maňourová, A., O. Leuner, Z. Tchoundjeu, P. Van Damme, V. Verner, O. Přibyl, and B. Lojka. 2019. Medicinal potential, utilization and domestication status of bitter kola (*Garcinia kola* Heckel) in West and Central Africa. *Forests* 10: 124.

Na, D., H. Aijie, L. Bo, M. Zhilin, and Y. Long. 2018. Gambogic acid exerts cardioprotective effects in a rat model of acute myocardial infarction through inhibition of inflammation, iNOS and NF-κB/p38 pathway. *Experimental and Therapeutic Medicine* (December 5). www.spandidos-publications.com/10.3892/etm.2017.5599.

Ndjenda II, M.K., E.P. Nguelefack-Mbuyo, A.D. Atsamo, C.K. Fofie, C. Fodem, F. Nguemo, and T.B. Nguelefack. 2021a. Antihypertensive effects of the methanol extract and the ethyl acetate fraction from *Crinum zeylanicum* (Amaryllidaceae) leaves in L-NAME-treated rat. *Evidence-Based Complementary and Alternative Medicine* 2021: 2656249.

Ndjenda II, M.K., E.P. Nguelefack-Mbuyo, J. Hescheler, T.B. Nguelefack, and F. Nguemo. 2021b. Assessment of the *in vitro* cytotoxicity effects of the leaf methanol extract of *Crinum zeylanicum* on mouse induced pluripotent stem cells and their cardiomyocytes derivatives. *Pharmaceuticals* 14: 1208.

Nguelefack-Mbuyo, E.P., F. Nokam, N.L. Tchinda, A.F. Goumtsa, N. Tsabang, and T.B. Nguelefack. 2022. Vasorelaxant and antioxidant effects of *Aframomum pruinosum* Gagnep. (Zingiberaceae) seed extracts may mediate their cardioprotective activity against isoproterenol-induced myocardial infarction. *Evidence-Based Complementary and Alternative Medicine* 2022: 7257448.

Omole, J.G., O.A. Ayoka, Q.K. Alabi, M.A. Adefisayo, M.A. Asafa, B.O. Olubunmi, and B.A. Fadeyi. 2018. Protective effect of kolaviron on cyclophosphamide-induced cardiac toxicity in rats. *Journal of Evidence-Based Integrative Medicine* 23: 215658721875764.

Oyagbemi, A.A., D. Bester, J. Esterhuyse, and E. Farombi. 2017. Kolaviron, a biflavonoid of *Garcinia kola* seed mitigates ischaemic/reperfusion injury by modulation of pro-survival and apoptotic signaling pathways. *Journal of Intercultural Ethnopharmacology* 6: 42.

Oyagbemi, A.A., D. Bester, J. Esterhuyse, and E. Farombi. 2018. Kolaviron and *Garcinia kola* seed extract protect against ischaemia/reperfusion injury on isolated rat heart. *Drug Research* 68: 286–295.

Panda, V., S. Kamble, Y. Desai, and S. Sudhamani. 2014. Antioxidant and cardioprotective effects of *Garcinia indica* (Kokoberry), an Indian super fruit in isoproterenol induced myocardial necrosis in rats. *Journal of Berry Research* 4: 159–174.

Pinkaew, D., S.G. Cho, D.Y. Hui, J.E. Wiktorowicz, N. Hutadilok-Towatana, W. Mahabusarakam, M. Tonganunt, et al. 2009. Morelloflavone blocks injury-induced neointimal formation by inhibiting vascular smooth muscle cell migration. *Biochimica et Biophysica Acta (BBA) – General Subjects* 1790: 31–39.

Rossello, X., and D.M. Yellon. 2018. The RISK pathway and beyond. *Basic Research in Cardiology* 113: 2.

Saputri, F.C., and I. Jantan. 2012. Inhibitory activities of compounds from the twigs of *Garcinia Hombroniana* Pierre on human low-density lipoprotein (LDL) Oxidation and Platelet Aggregation. *Phytotherapy Research* 26: 1845–1850.

Sari, N., Y. Katanasaka, Y. Sugiyama, Y. Miyazaki, Y. Sunagawa, M. Funamoto, K. Shimizu, S. Shimizu, K. Hasegawa, and T. Morimoto. 2021. Alpha mangostin derived from *Garcinia Magostana* Linn ameliorates cardiomyocyte hypertrophy and fibroblast phenotypes *in vitro*. *Biological and Pharmaceutical Bulletin* 44: 1465–1472.

Shaito, A., D.T.B. Thuan, H.T. Phu, T.H.D. Nguyen, H. Hasan, S. Halabi, S. Abdelhady, G.K. Nasrallah, A.H. Eid, and G. Pintus. 2020. Herbal medicine for cardiovascular diseases: Efficacy, mechanisms, and safety. *Frontiers in Pharmacology* 11: 422.

Soetikno, V., A. Murwantara, P. Andini, F. Charlie, G. Lazarus, M. Louisa, and W. Arozal. 2020. Alpha-Mangostin improves cardiac hypertrophy and fibrosis and associated biochemical parameters in high-fat/high-glucose diet and low-dose streptozotocin injection-induced type 2 diabetic rats. *Journal of Experimental Pharmacology* 12: 27–38.

Sonfack, C.S., E.P. Nguelefack-Mbuyo, J.J. Kojom, E.L. Lappa, F.P. Peyembouo, C.K. Fofié, T. Nolé, T.B. Nguelefack, and A.B. Dongmo. 2021. The aqueous extract from the stem bark of *Garcinia lucida* Vesque (Clusiaceae) exhibits cardioprotective and nephroprotective effects in adenine-induced chronic kidney disease in rats. Ed. Priscila Souza. *Evidence-Based Complementary and Alternative Medicine* 2021: 1–11.

Tabares-Guevara, J.H., O.J. Lara-Guzmán, J.A. Londoño-Londoño, J.A. Sierra, Y.M. León-Varela, R.M. Álvarez-Quintero, E.J. Osorio, and J.R. Ramirez-Pineda. 2017. Natural biflavonoids modulate macrophage-oxidized ldl interaction in vitro and promote atheroprotection in vivo. *Frontiers in Immunology* 8: 923.

van der Weg, K., F.W. Prinzen, and A.P. Gorgels. 2019. Editor's choice-reperfusion cardiac arrhythmias and their relation to reperfusion-induced cell death. *European Heart Journal: Acute Cardiovascular Care* 8: 142–152.

WHO. 2021. Cardiovascular diseases. www.who.int/en/news-room/fact-sheets/detail/cardiovascular-diseases-(cvds).

Wihastuti, T.A., F.N. Aini, C.T. Tjahjono, and T. Heriansyah. 2019. Dietary ethanolic extract of mangosteen pericarp reduces VCAM-1, perivascular adipose tissue and aortic intimal medial thickness in hypercholesterolemic rat model. *Open Access Macedonian Journal of Medical Sciences* 7: 3158–3163.

Wihastuti, T.A., A. Tjokroprawiro, S. Soeharto, M.A. Widodo, D. Sargowo, and N. Permatasari. 2014. *Vasa Vasorum* anti-angiogenesis through H_2O_2, HIF-1α, NF-κB, and iNOS Inhibition by mangosteen pericarp ethanolic extract (*Garcinia Mangostana* Linn) in hypercholesterol-diet-given *Rattus norvegicus* Wistar strain. *Vascular Health and Risk Management* 10: 523–531.

Xiang, Q., M. Wu, L. Zhang, W. Fu, J. Yang, B. Zhang, Z. Zheng, H. Zhang, Y. Lao, and H. Xu. 2020. Gerontoxanthone I and Macluraxanthone induce mitophagy and attenuate ischemia/reperfusion injury. *Frontiers in Pharmacology* 11: 452.

Zhao, C., S. Liu, C. Yang, X. Li, H. Huang, N. Liu, S. Li, X. Wang, and J. Liu. 2013. Gambogic acid moderates cardiac responses to chronic hypoxia likely by acting on the proteasome and NF-κB pathway. *American Journal of Cardiovascular Disease* 3: 135–145.

22 Watermelon (*Citrullus lanatus*) and Cardiovascular Protection
A Focus on the Effects of Citrulline

Bilgehan Ozcan, Christophe Moinard and Elise Belaïdi

CONTENTS

22.1 Introduction 346
    22.1.1 Watermelon: Background 346
    22.1.2 Antioxidant Properties of Watermelon 346
    22.1.3 Watermelon and Cardiovascular Health 346
22.2 Citrulline 348
    22.2.1 Discovery 348
    22.2.2 Generalities 348
    22.2.3 Citrulline-Arginine Metabolism: A Dual Role in Nitrogen
             Homeostasis and Cardiovascular Regulation 348
    22.2.4 Citrulline-Arginine Cooperation in Endothelial Cells 350
22.3 Citrulline and Cardiovascular Health 351
    22.3.1 Citrulline and Vessels 351
    22.3.2 Citrullin and Heart..352
22.4 Other Citrulline Resources Than Watermelon 353
22.5 Toxicity and Cautionary Notes 353
22.6 Summary Points 353
References..354

LIST OF ABBREVIATIONS

ADMA   Asymmetric dimethylarginine
ASL   Argininosuccinate lyase
ASS   Argininosuccinate synthase
cGMP   Cyclic guanosine monophosphate
eNOS   Endothelial nitric oxide synthase
NO   Nitric oxide
OTC   Ornithine transcarbamylase
PDE   Phosphodiesterase
PKG   Protein kinase G
ROS   Reactive oxygen species
sGC   Soluble guanylyl cyclase
VCAM1   Vascular cell adhesion protein 1

DOI: 10.1201/9781003220329-24

22.1 INTRODUCTION

Citrullus lanatus, better known as watermelon, belongs to the family of Cucurbitaceae. Mostly, the fruit's flesh is consumed raw, but is possible to find recipes with cooked rind and seeds in different cultures.

22.1.1 WATERMELON: BACKGROUND

The wild watermelon originates from the deserts of Africa and was cultivated by multiple civilizations since prehistoric times. A fun fact is that the wild watermelon had a yellow and bitter interior. Selective breeding since the 3rd century developed the sweet red domesticated watermelons known and loved today – the gene that gives the red color is paired with the gene that makes the watermelon sweet (Strauss 2015). Tracking the watermelon's medicinal properties is challenging because watermelon's name changed a lot during history, but now the scientific community is agreeing to call it by its modern name "*Citrullus lanatus*".

In the past, watermelon was used for different properties in several civilizations. In ancient Egypt, it was commonly used as a water source (Strauss 2015). Marwat et al. 2008 report that watermelon was used for its diuretic properties in the old Islamic communities between years 613–687 (Marwat et al. 2008). In ancient Greece, it was used as diuretic and the rind was applied on the top of the heads of children suffering from heat stroke. In Nigeria, seeds of watermelon were used as a vermifuge and roots were recognized for their purgative and emetic properties (Ed 2020).

22.1.2 ANTIOXIDANT PROPERTIES OF WATERMELON

Actually, watermelon flesh, seeds and rind contain carotenoids, vitamins and amino acids which all have antioxidant properties (Sorokina et al. 2021; Sol Zamuz et al. 2021).

Carotenoids are pigments of the flesh with highly antioxidant properties. The red-fleshed watermelons contain mostly lycopens and β-carotens, while yellow flesh contains mostly neoxhantin. Ten percent of the lycopens in red-fleshed watermelon is cis-lycopens, which is the isoform found in human serum and tissues, and watermelon is the only source that readily has the cis-lycopens. Due to their antioxidant role, lycopens are shown to be effective against cancer, gastritis, atherosclerosis, cardiovascular diseases (Story et al. 2010).

β-carotene is the second most abundant pigment in watermelon. It is the precursor of vitamin A that exerts critical roles for development, eyesight and immune system homeostasis. Vitamin A is also involved in skin photoprotection due to its antioxidant properties (Grune et al. 2010).

Other than these two carotens, watermelon has phytoene and phytofluene which are known to be the precursors of other carotenoids. Both have been demonstrated to have antioxidant and anti-inflammatory effects (Meléndez-Martínez et al. 2018).

The phenolic compounds found in the cell vacuoles and walls of watermelon also have antioxidant effects.

Watermelon seeds are rich in linoleic acid (61% of watermelon seed's fatty acid), a polyunsaturated fatty acid known for its role in prevention of cardiovascular diseases.

22.1.3 WATERMELON AND CARDIOVASCULAR HEALTH

As the antioxidant capacity of watermelon extract has been really highlighted and suggested as a natural antioxidant (Asghar et al. 2013), it is interesting to discuss its supplementation against different pathologies. This chapter focuses on metabolism risk and associated cardiovascular pathologies. In obese and diabetic rats, supplementation of watermelon juice for 4 weeks has been shown to improve systemic metabolic parameters (i.e. fat accumulation, plasmatic glucose, plasmatic arginine concentration, free fatty acid), to decrease plasmatic cardiovascular risk factors (i.e. homocysteine, dimethyl-arginines) and to improve vascular dysfunction characterized by an increase in acetylcholine-induced

Watermelon (*Citrullus lanatus*) and Cardiovascular Protection 347

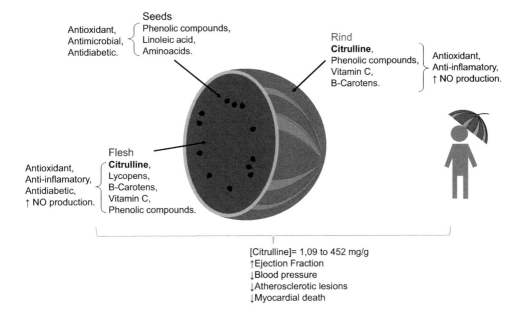

FIGURE 22.1 Watermelon's cardioprotective components.

Note: Watermelon seeds are a main source of antioxidant, antidiabetic and antimicrobial phenolic compounds as well as linoleic acid and different amino acids. Watermelon flesh shows strong antioxidant, anti-inflammatory and antidiabetic properties, thanks to carotens like lycopens and β-carotens, phenolic compounds and the vitamin C that it contains. Watermelon rind also holds vitamin C, phenolic compounds and β-carotens showing antioxidant and anti-inflammatory properties. Watermelon flesh as well as its rind contains citrulline known to have antioxidant and anti-inflammatory properties and to increase plasma nitric oxide (NO) concentration. Citrulline concentration in watermelons varies between 1.09 to 4.52 mg/g and citrulline supplementation increases ejection fraction and decreases blood pressure, atherosclerotic lesions and myocardial death.

vasorelaxation (Wu et al. 2007). In line, watermelon extract supplemented in atherosclerosis-prone mice exhibited reduced fat mass, plasma cholesterol and atherosclerosis. Indeed, some clinical trials also demonstrated the beneficial effects of watermelon in the context of atherosclerosis. In postmenopausal overweight and obese women, watermelon extract consumption decreased atherosclerosis risk characterized by a decrease in vascular cell adhesion protein 1 (VCAM). VCAM is a protein that mediates immune cells adhesion in the vascular wall, corresponding to an early step of the atherosclerosis process (Shanely et al. 2020). Currently, watermelon has also been described to reduce blood pressure. Indeed, aortic systolic blood pressure was reduced after watermelon juice supplementation (Figueroa et al. 2011). Watermelon extract given to middle-aged patients diagnosed with prehypertension also reduced arterial systolic blood pressure (Figueroa et al. 2013). Moreover, in these studies, watermelon has been evidenced to improve systemic vascular hemodynamics characterized by an improvement in aortic and bronchial pulse and blood pressure.

In 2021, Michael and collaborators reported a work based on lead poisoning. Lead poisoning induces many deaths every year and is associated with hypertension and right cardiac hypertrophy. Lead positioning also induces hyperuricemia that contributes to a reduction in nitric oxide (NO) bioavailability and endothelial dysfunction, suggesting that watermelon extract could reverse the toxic effects of lead. In a rat model of lead poisoning, watermelon rind extracts increased NO serum levels and this is accompanied with an increase in antioxidant defenses and a reestablishment of arterial blood pressure as well as a decrease in right ventricular heart weight (Michael et al. 2021).

Finally, and importantly, the studies demonstrating cardiovascular improvements after watermelon supplementation also observed an increase in plasma citrulline concentration (nearly twofold in Poduri et al. (2013).

Indeed, watermelon is the natural source of citrulline, a non-essential amino acid which is the precursor of arginine and usually considered as an intermediate molecule in the urea cycle. In a fresh watermelon, the flesh contains more citrulline than the rind; however, in dried watermelon, there are more citrulline in the rind than in the flesh (Rimando and Perkins-Veazie 2005). Besides watermelon's antioxidant properties, a large part of its cardioprotective effects are attributed to the citrulline, very well-recognized for its involvement in NO metabolism (Allerton et al. 2018) and possibly for its antioxidant properties.

22.2 CITRULLINE

22.2.1 Discovery

Though it is a C3 type of plant, watermelon is the only green plant in the desert that can resist severe drought and hot conditions (Kawasaki et al. 2000). Under these circumstances, an increase in the content of a one particular free amino acid is detected: L-citrulline.

L-citrulline was first isolated by Koga and Ohtake from *Citrullis vulgaris* in 1914 then characterized and named by Wage in 1930 (Fragkos and Forbes 2011). This amino acid is a very efficient hydoxyl radical scavenger that accumulates under drought conditions in the plant. It is thought that citrulline is increased in watermelon in order to protect the plant from oxidative injuries and from hydric stress (Yokota 2002).

Same as watermelon, the name of this molecule is also hard to track in historical documents because from 1882 to 1920 the term "citrulline" was used for a resinoide substance extracted from the pulp of *Citrullis Colocynthis*, also known as colocynth or bitter apple. This explains some confusion in the effects of citrulline sometimes described as a purgative and a laxative in old resources (Ed 2020; Michael et al. 2021). However the actual L-citrulline extracted from watermelon has been chemically defined in 1914 and has been specifically described for at least three important physiological processes: citrulline has been described to be involved in the urea cycle (1932); citrulline has been demonstrated to be transformed into arginine in the kidneys (1943) and citrulline is recycled thanks to the transformation of arginine into NO in endothelial cells (1988). Finally, after several years, citrulline emerged as a major factor in the control of nitrogen homeostasis in humans (for review see Breuillard et al. 2015).

22.2.2 Generalities

The most important fact to know about citrulline is probably that citrulline is the precursor of arginine, a non-essential proteinogenic amino acid playing a key role in immunity, cardiovascular and nitrogen homeostasis, and in many other metabolism processes. Though not essential, the production of endogenous arginine can be insufficient in some contexts (during growth and pathologies like trauma, infection, etc.) which requires an exogeneous supplementation.

As arginine, citrulline is also a non-essential amino acid produced endogenously by most of the mammalians. Most of the citrulline comes from glutamine, arginine and proline conversion to ornithine in the enterocytes (Figure 22.2A). The transformation of ornithine into citrulline is realized by the ornithine transcarbamylase (OTC) in the mitochondria of enterocytes, as in the mitochondria of hepatocytes (Figure 22.2B) (Couchet et al. 2021). Therefore, citrulline plasmatic level is now accepted as a reliable biomarker of the gut function as demonstrated by the pioneering papers from Crenn and collaborators (Crenn et al. 2000, 2003).

22.2.3 Citrulline-Arginine Metabolism: A Dual Role in Nitrogen Homeostasis and Cardiovascular Regulation

The control of nitrogen homeostasis is ensured through close cooperation between the liver and the intestine. Indeed, nitrogen flows must be regulated because many amino acids have neurotoxic

Watermelon (*Citrullus lanatus*) and Cardiovascular Protection

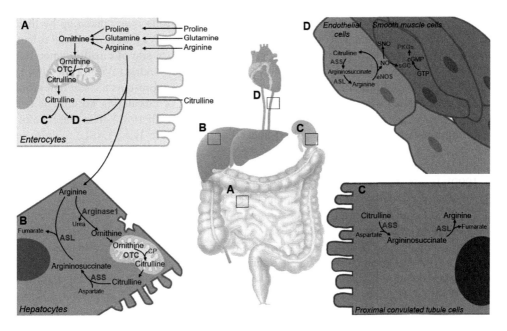

FIGURE 22.2 Citrulline production and systemic circulation.

Note: (A) Citrulline may be absorbed from nutriments in the small intestines. Otherwise, proline, glutamine and arginine from nutriments are absorbed in the intestines, and following different pathways, are transformed to ornithine. Ornithine enters in the mitochondria in order to meet ornithine transcarbamylase (OTC). OTC uses carbamoyl phosphate (CP) and ornithine to produce citrulline. Citrulline exits the mitochondria and is released into the systemic circulation. Most of it is captured by kidneys (C) while some stays in plasma which may be internalized by endothelial cells (D).

(B) Most of the arginine absorbed from nutriments, once in the systemic circulation, is captured by the liver which activates the urea cycle. Arginine is transformed to ornithine by arginase 1 while creating urea. Ornithine enters in the mitochondria and by OTC activity, it is transformed to citrulline, then exits the mitochondria. Citrulline produced in hepatocytes is not released into the circulation as in enterocytes. Instead, the urea cycle continues by citrulline's transformation to argininosuccinate by argininosuccinate synthase (ASS) and to arginine once again by argininosuccinate lyase (ASL).

(C) Some of citrulline released by intestines is captured by proximal convoluted tubule cells in kidneys. This citrulline is taken by ASS and ASL in order to produce arginine which is released into the blood circulation.

(D) The citrulline released from the intestines but not captured by the kidneys circulates in the vascular system. Endothelial cells may capture this citrulline and transform it to arginine by an incomplete urea cycle. This arginine is the substrate of endothelial nitric oxide synthase (eNOS) to produce nitric oxide (NO). This gas molecule either directly S-nitrosylate proteins (SNO) or diffuses into the smooth muscle cells in order to activate soluble guanylyl cyclase (sGC) which transforms guanosine triphosphate (GTP) into cyclic guanosine monophosphate (GMP) which activates protein kinase G (PKG) to stimulate further pathways.

properties when present in excess in the systemic circulation. Contrary to what is observed for many nutrients (such as calcium), the intestinal absorption of amino acids is not limiting: it is 95 to 99% regardless of the protein intake. The control site is the liver, which physiologically purifies about 50% of the nitrogen provided by the diet. The rate of clearance is partly regulated by the portal flow of arginine. This amino acid is an activator of N-acetylglutamate synthetase (NAGS), an enzyme allowing the transformation of glutamate into N-acetyl-glutamate (NAG), an allosteric activator of carbamoylphosphate synthase I (CPS I: 1st step of the urea cycle) (Cynober et al. 1995).

However, the portal flux of arginine (the regulatory element of ureogenesis) is itself controlled by the gut. Indeed, there is an intestinal expression of arginase and OTC (Figure 22.2A), allowing the intestine to release citrulline. It is important to note that the expression of these enzymes is dependent on the level of protein intake, thus limiting ureagenesis to a level proportional to the protein intake (Ventura et al. 2011). Citrulline is not taken up by the liver but it is taken up by the kidneys (Figure 22.2C). Hence, the kidneys play an essential role in the metabolism of arginine and citrulline. Indeed, they are the main site of citrulline metabolism. Thus, Dhanakoti and collaborators have shown that the kidneys extract 35% of the circulating citrulline and the quantity of citrulline captured by the kidneys represents 83% of that produced by the intestine (Dhanakoti et al. 1990). Furthermore, 75% of circulating arginine is derived from renal neosynthesis from citrulline (Windmueller and Spaeth 1981). The presence of significant argininosuccinate synthase (ASS) and argininosuccinate lyase (ASL) activity in the kidney makes this organ the primary site of endogenous arginine production. Indeed, about 60% of arginine synthesis in adult mammals originates from the kidneys (Yu et al. 1995; Dhanakoti et al. 1990). In general, renal arginine synthesis is independent of dietary arginine intake, which suggests that the control point is intestinal metabolism. Furthermore, it has been shown (Morris et al. 1989) that renal expression of ASS and ASL mRNA is elevated at low protein intake. This can be considered as an adaptive mechanism to maintain arginine homeostasis at different levels of protein intake. In humans, the work of Castillo and collaborators (Castillo et al. 1993) has shown that *de novo* arginine synthesis is not modified by a diet lacking this amino acid. These observations indicate that renal arginine synthesis is not related to the status of this amino acid and that the main regulatory element of arginine metabolism is at the level of its catabolism (O'Sullivan et al. 2000; Castillo et al. 1993). In fact, the capacity of the kidneys to synthesize arginine from citrulline is much greater than the capacity of the intestine to produce it. Thus, all the data in the literature strongly suggest that intestinal production of citrulline is the crucial element of renal arginine synthesis.

In conclusion, this tight equilibrium allows control of nitrogen homeostasis and ensures arginine availability at the whole body level.

22.2.4 CITRULLINE-ARGININE COOPERATION IN ENDOTHELIAL CELLS

In 1988 the scientific world already knew the existence of NO as an endothelium-dependent relaxing factor, but Richard and collaborators have reported that the same enzyme that produces NO from arginine produces also citrulline in endothelial cells. Nitric oxide synthase (NOS) uses arginine and O_2 as a substrate to produce NO and citrulline. There are three known isomers of NOS called NOS 1, 2, 3 or neuronal (n); inducible (i) and endothelial (e) NOS, respectively. It is largely accepted that there are mainly eNOS and nNOS in the heart and the vessels during physiological conditions.

NO is a gas molecule known to have protective effects on tissues. First, when produced in the endothelial cells by eNOS, NO diffuses to vascular smooth muscle cells to activate cytosolic soluble guanylyl cyclase (sGC) which transforms guanosine triphosphate (GTP) to cyclic guanosine 3',5'-monophosphate (cGMP). cGMP activates cGMP-dependent protein kinases (PKGs) that lead to the activation of several signaling pathways notably involved in smooth muscle relaxation, cardiac protection, endothelial permeability, gene transcription (Keravis and Lugnier 2012) (Figure 22.2D). An important amount of cGMP is able to activate phosphodiesterases (PDEs), that in turn modulate cGMP content and associated processes. Particularly, the involvement of PKG and PDE signaling have been well explored in vascular smooth muscles. PKG mediates vasodilation and the balance between PKG and PDE has been deeply studied to understand mechanisms involved in heart hypertrophy and contractility (Tsai and Kass 2009).

Second, NO uses another way to protect against stress. Indeed, NO can be added to cysteine thiol residues on proteins leading to their S-Nitrosylation (SNO) that modulates their activity. This process is mostly recognized to protect against tissue injury (Farah and Reboul 2015).

Citrulline produced by enterocytes and released to the blood circulation can be transported into these endothelial cells (i.e. pulmonary arterial cells) by a Na^+-dependent neutral amino acid transporter, SNATs (particularly SNAT1) (Fike et al. 2012). This suggests that citrulline that is not captured by the kidneys (nearly 27%) is essential for other tissues. This is other proof of the fact that citrulline's

Watermelon (*Citrullus lanatus*) and Cardiovascular Protection

functions, apart from being a mask for arginine, need to be explored. This also suggests that citrulline extracted from watermelon could represent an interesting therapeutic strategy in various diseases.

As a proof of fact, in 2001, Flam and collaborators demonstrated that exogenous citrulline levels stimulate NO production even though there were saturating levels of arginine in and outside of cells (Flam et al. 2001). This finding supports the fact that endothelial cells need *de novo* synthetized arginine from citrulline for NO production. In histological experiments, eNOS in caveolar membrane colocalizes with ASS and ASL and only uses the arginine that comes from this activity (Figure 22.2D) (Simon et al. 2003).

The homeostasis of NO by arginine and citrulline is under fine regulation. Any perturbation (eNOS uncoupling observed under some pathologies) or intervention (citrulline or arginine supplementations) of this balance results in the "arginine paradox". The hypothesis is that there are two intracellular arginine pools in human endothelial cells. The first one is a non-stable arginine pool that can freely exchange arginine with outside of the cell. However, the second pool is the one that eNOS uses. This second pool is composed of *de novo* synthesized arginine from citrulline as well as the arginine that comes from proteolysis (Simon et al. 2003).

Hence, in some pathological conditions, asymmetrically dimethylated arginine (ADMA) that comes from proteolyze of methylated proteins, accumulates in cells and competes with arginine for eNOS. Once fixed to eNOS, ADMA uncouples eNOS, impairing its activity and leading to a decreases in NO production and an increase in ROS production. Therefore, ADMA is a well-known cardiovascular risk marker. However, arginine that comes from citrulline can not be methylated. Thus, citrulline supplementation may show benefits against ADMA by accumulating non-methylated arginines to compete with ADMA (McCarty 2016). Even so, citrulline's effect on ADMA concentrations is yet to be investigated.

22.3 CITRULLINE AND CARDIOVASCULAR HEALTH

Lots of pre-clinical studies support a beneficial effect of citrulline in terms of cardiovascular health. However, there are a small number of studies that investigate specifically the mechanisms involved in citrulline protection. These following paragraphs will summarize the literature and this will lead to opening new avenues in studying citrulline supplementation impact.

22.3.1 CITRULLINE AND VESSELS

Pre-clinical studies support the hypothesis that endothelial function and vessel dilatation may be enhanced by the capability of citrulline supplementation to increase arginine levels and NO biosynthesis (indirectly) (Wijnands et al. 2015). In spontaneous hypertensive rats, where NO availability is impaired, citrulline restored NO levels and increased L-arginine/ADMA ratio (Chien et al. 2014).

Though there are arguments in favor of an improvement in vasodilation function that can be assessed using brachial artery flow mediated dilatation, studies demonstrated opposite effects depending of the context (young/old participants; the presence of another pathologies; treatment duration and citrulline dose) (Allerton et al. 2018). Often, citrulline supplementation is beneficial in complex models such as pre-clinical models that present a metabolic risk. For example, in rabbits submitted to a high cholesterol diet, citrulline preserves endothelial function by increasing endothelium-dependent vasorelaxation and decreasing atherosclerotic lesions. It seems that this effect was not conferred only to an alteration in eNOS function but also to antioxidative properties of citrulline characterized, for example, by a decrease in superoxide anion production (Hayashi et al. 2005). This is a very interesting point allowing one to think that citrulline-induced beneficial effects are not conferred only to the increase in NO bioavailability. This also explains why citrulline supplementation does not exert the same protective effects in all the studies performed in humans. Antioxidant properties of citrulline can be attributed to eNOS activity increase, which in turn, reduces reactive oxygen species (ROS) formation but also to the citrulline itself. Indeed, citrulline has been described to be a ROS scavenger and this is associated with an increase in vascular function (Coles 2007).

Taken together, citrulline plays a protective role at different levels of vessels remodeling, atherosclerosis processes including endothelial damages and vascular function impairment. However, the specific contexts and mechanisms by which citrulline is vasoprotective depends on several contexts and they remain to be elucidated.

Taking into account that citrulline activates cGMP signaling in order to induce vasodilatation, several studies investigated its ability to decrease arterial blood pressure. Interestingly, in clinical studies, the same team demonstrated that watermelon juice supplementation increases mean arterial blood pressure (Bailey et al. 2016), whereas citrulline diet decreases mean arterial blood pressure (Bailey et al. 2015). This impact of citrulline is associated with an improvement of exercise performance in healthy adults probably due to an increase in muscle perfusion after moderate exercise (Bailey et al. 2016) and these studies highlight a specific action of citrulline on arterial blood pressure. Otherwise, on postmenopausal and obese women, a reduction in aortic systolic and diastolic blood pressure and an improvement in systemic aortic circulation characterized by an enhanced wave reflection amplitude in aorta and radial artery is reported (Figueroa et al. 2013). In a pre-clinical model, citrulline supplementation has been demonstrated to decrease blood pressure in spontaneously hypertensive rats and this was associated with an increase in L-arginine/ADMA ratio (Chien et al. 2014).

22.3.2 Citrullin and Heart

Myocardial infarction and subsequent heart failure is one of the major causes of death worldwide. Limiting myocardial infarction risk factors such as obesity, denutrition, hypertension is the first way to limit its occurrence and to control its deleterious consequences such as the progression of heart failure. Then, because heart failure is mostly induced by myocardial infarction and is a consequence of myocardial infarction-induced cardiomyocyte death, researchers aim at deciphering the mechanisms involved in myocardial infarction-generated infarct size in order to limit cardiomyocyte death. Though the number of studies investigating the impact of citrulline supplementation is weak, the following paragraph reports how citrulline is currently studied in the context of cardiac pathologies.

First, it is very interesting to note that NO bioavailability is primordial to maintain vessels and heart homeostasis since it is primordial to maintain perfusion. Very interestingly, using metabolomic, two recent studies measured citrulline as a marker of NO bioavailability and thus, as a marker of cardiovascular health. The first one reported that empaglifozin (a sodium glucose transporter 2 inhibitor which is now largely studied for its beneficial effects against heart failure) suppresses endothelial apoptosis and improves systolic dysfunction via eNOS/NO pathway. These effects of empaglifozin are associated with an increase in citrulline levels (Nakao et al. 2021). The second one was performed in participants of the Framinghalm Heart study and demonstrates that citrulline increase is associated with an improvement of cardiometabolic profile elicited with acute exercise (Nayor et al. 2020). In rats, citrulline increase was associated with a delay in mitochondrial permeability transition pore opening which is a clear determinant of cardiomyocyte death induced by myocardial infarction (Akopova et al. 2016).

Second, blood pressure control and sympathovagal balance maintenance avoid myocardial decompensation because they limit myocardial over-supply and thus, preserve its function. Promising effects of citrulline supplementation have been reported in humans: citrulline improves sympathovagal balance (measured by heart rate variability study) and decreases blood pressure (Wong et al. 2016; Alsop and Hauton 2016). In patients with chronic systolic heart failure, daily supplementation of citrulline increased left and right ventricular ejection fraction, endothelial function as well as the heart failure functional class (Balderas-Munoz et al. 2012). Very interestingly, heart failure with preserved ejection fraction also seems to be improved by citrulline supplementation with a decreased pulmonary arterial hypertension (Orozco-Gutiérrez et al. 2010).

Watermelon (*Citrullus lanatus*) and Cardiovascular Protection

The final aspect is citrulline's anti-inflammatory and antioxidant capacity. Zhou and collaborators indicate that sepsis may induce myocardial injury causing cardiac dysfunction in sepsis patients. However, in rat models of sepsis induced by cecal ligation and puncture, citrulline increased the survival rate after operation and controlled the inflammatory response by reducing leucocytes and neutrophils in blood. Citrulline also reduced inflammatory cell infiltration between the myocardial cells and eased myocardial injury. Additionally, as expected, citrulline improved antioxidant ability of septic rats heart and reduced lipid peroxidation-induced damage. Interestingly, as during sepsis, iNOS produces excessive amount of NO, causing accumulation of reactive nitrogen species that damages the organism; citrulline reduced serum NO concentration in early sepsis (Zhou et al. 2018).

22.4 OTHER CITRULLINE RESOURCES THAN WATERMELON

Even though through this whole chapter the red-fleshed watermelon is discussed, yellow-fleshed watermelon is actually reported to have more citrulline (Sol Zamuz 2021).

Citrulline was a well-conserved amino acid during evolution. It is present in animals, plants, bacteria and fungi. Even though watermelon is accepted as "the" source of citrulline, buffalo gourd, cantaloupe, pumpkin and cucumber also present this amino acid. Even almonds, cocoa, chickpeas, garlic, onions, walnuts, peanuts, prune juice, mushrooms, salmon, soy sauce and wine have citrulline; however it is really scarce compared to the watermelon (Joshi and Fernie 2017). Of course, consuming these foods will provide citrulline; however, watermelon has the richest nutrition in terms of citrulline (1.09 to 4.52 mg/g) (Davis et al. 2011). The minimum effective dose of citrulline to increase plasmatic arginine is 3 g/day and the maximum is 10 g/day. Which means, in the best case, a person should eat 663.71 g of watermelon/day to increase plasmatic arginine. Knowing that, eating other resources which have less citrulline than watermelon may not show any effects. Plus, as mentioned in de Souza et al. 2021, citrulline stability in other resources is not guaranteed. Anyway, isolated citrulline supplementation seems like a more reasonable choice to protect our cardiovascular system.

22.5 TOXICITY AND CAUTIONARY NOTES

Pre-clinical and clinical trials studying citrulline supplementation showed no harmful effect caused by citrulline. This is because citrulline, contrary to arginine, is not captured by the liver, so liver damage is out of the question. Moinard and collaborators tested different doses of oral citrulline supplementation in healthy men (2, 5, 10 and 15 g) with tolerance and safety tests. These doses were well tolerated by subjects and did not cause any gastrointestinal disorders even for the subjects who received high dose of citrulline (Moinard et al. 2008). The biggest concern with amino acid supplementations is calcium loss with increased urination. However, citrulline supplementation, even in high doses, did not interfere with calcium homeostasis. Citrulline supplementation did also not modify plasmatic concentration of other amino acids apart from ornithine and arginine. The same authors tested 10 g of oral citrulline supplementation and 9.94 g of oral arginine supplementation in elderly men Moinard et al. 2016. The results confirmed the previous results as citrulline is very well tolerated even in elderly subjects. These results suggest together that citrulline, even in high doses, does not show toxicity.

22.6 SUMMARY POINTS

- *Citrullus lanatus*, the watermelon, is reported to have cardioprotective properties.
- These observations are mostly attributed to its antioxidant capacity but also to its anti-inflammatory, citrulline content.
- *Citrillus lanatus* is rich in citrulline content, an amino acid, the precursor of arginine.
- Citrulline is essential for nitrogen homeostasis and arginine bioavailability.

- Citrulline supplementation may decrease blood pressure and improve heart functions.
- The increase in NO bioavailability and citrulline's antioxidant properties seems to be the key players of cardiometabolic risk control.

REFERENCES

Akopova, O., A. Kotsiuruba, Y. Korkach, L. Kolchinskaya, V. Nosar, B. Gavenauskas, Z. Serebrovska, I. Mankovska, and V. Sagach. 2016. "The effect of NO donor on calcium uptake and reactive nitrogen species production in mitochondria." *Cell Physiol Biochem* 39 (1):193–204. doi: 10.1159/000445616.

Allerton, Timothy, David Proctor, Jacqueline Stephens, Tammy Dugas, Guillaume Spielmann, and Brian Irving. 2018. "l-citrulline supplementation: Impact on cardiometabolic health." *Nutrients* 10 (7):921. doi: 10.3390/nu10070921.

Alsop, Paige, and David Hauton. 2016. "Oral nitrate and citrulline decrease blood pressure and increase vascular conductance in young adults: A potential therapy for heart failure." *European Journal of Applied Physiology* 116 (9):1651–1661. doi: 10.1007/s00421-016-3418-7.

Asghar, Muhammad Nadeem, Muhammad Tahir Shahzad, Iram Nadeem, and Chaudhry Muhammad Ashraf. 2013. "Phytochemical and in vitro total antioxidant capacity analyses of peel extracts of different cultivars of cucumis melo and citrullus lanatus." *Pharmaceutical Biology* 51 (2):226–232. doi: 10.3109/13880209.2012.717228.

Bailey, S. J., J. R. Blackwell, E. Williams, A. Vanhatalo, L. J. Wylie, P. G. Winyard, and A. M. Jones. 2016. "Two weeks of watermelon juice supplementation improves nitric oxide bioavailability but not endurance exercise performance in humans." *Nitric Oxide* 59:10–20. doi: 10.1016/j.niox.2016.06.008.

Bailey, Stephen J, Jamie R Blackwell, Terrence Lord, Anni Vanhatalo, Paul G Winyard, and Andrew M Jones. 2015. "l-Citrulline supplementation improves O2 uptake kinetics and high-intensity exercise performance in humans." *Journal of Applied Physiology*.

Balderas-Munoz, Karla, Lilia Castillo-Martínez, Arturo Orea-Tejeda, Oscar Infante-Vázquez, Marcelo Utrera-Lagunas, Raúl Martínez-Memije, Candace Keirns-Davis, Bryan Becerra-Luna, and Gabriela Sánchez-Vidal. 2012. "Improvement of ventricular function in systolic heart failure patients with oral L-citrulline supplementation." *Cardiology Journal* 19 (6):612–617. doi: 10.5603/cj.2012.0113.

Breuillard, C., L. Cynober, and C. Moinard. 2015. "Citrulline and nitrogen homeostasis: An overview." *Amino Acids* 47 (4):685–691. doi: 10.1007/s00726-015-1932-2.

Castillo, L., T. E. Chapman, M. Sanchez, Y. M. Yu, J. F. Burke, A. M. Ajami, J. Vogt, and V. R. Young. 1993. "Plasma arginine and citrulline kinetics in adults given adequate and arginine-free diets." *Proceedings of the National Academy of Sciences of the United States of America* 90 (16):7749–7753. doi: 10.1073/pnas.90.16.7749.

Chien, S. J., K. M. Lin, H. C. Kuo, C. F. Huang, Y. J. Lin, L. T. Huang, and Y. L. Tain. 2014. "Two different approaches to restore renal nitric oxide and prevent hypertension in young spontaneously hypertensive rats: L-citrulline and nitrate." *Transl Res* 163 (1):43–52. doi: 10.1016/j.trsl.2013.09.008.

Coles, Kirsten Elizabeth. 2007. "An investigation into the antioxidant capacity of l-arginine and l-citrulline in relation to their vascular protective properties." Doctor degree, Cardiology, Cardiff University (U584160).

Couchet, M., C. Breuillard, C. Corne, J. Rendu, B. Morio, U. Schlattner, and C. Moinard. 2021. "Ornithine transcarbamylase – from structure to metabolism: An update." *Front Physiol* 12:748249. doi: 10.3389/fphys.2021.748249.

Crenn, P., C. Coudray-Lucas, F. Thuillier, L. Cynober, and B. Messing. 2000. "Postabsorptive plasma citrulline concentration is a marker of absorptive enterocyte mass and intestinal failure in humans." *Gastroenterology* 119 (6):1496–505. doi: 10.1053/gast.2000.20227.

Crenn, P., K. Vahedi, A. Lavergne-Slove, L. Cynober, C. Matuchansky, and B. Messing. 2003. "Plasma citrulline: A marker of enterocyte mass in villous atrophy-associated small bowel disease." *Gastroenterology* 124 (5):1210–9. doi: 10.1016/s0016-5085(03)00170–7.

Cynober, Luc, Jacques Le Boucher, and Marie-Paule Vasson. 1995. "Arginine metabolism in mammals." *The Journal of Nutritional Biochemistry* 6 (8):402–413. doi: https://doi.org/10.1016/0955-2863(95)00066-9.

Davis, Angela, Charles Webber, Wayne Fish, Todd Wehner, Stephen King, and Penelope Perkins. 2011. "L-citrulline levels in watermelon cultigens tested in two environments." *HortScience* 46:1572–1575. doi: 10.21273/HORTSCI.46.12.1572.

de Souza, Mônica Volino Gonçalves, Vivian dos Santos Pinheiro, Gustavo Vieira de Oliveira, Carlos Adam Conte Junior, and Thiago da Silveira Alvares. 2021. "Storage stability of L-citrulline in cucumber

(Cucumis sativus) and watermelon (Citrullus lanatus) juices." *Brazilian Journal of Development* 7 (3):26849–26859.

Dhanakoti, S. N., J. T. Brosnan, G. R. Herzberg, and M. E. Brosnan. 1990. "Renal arginine synthesis: Studies in vitro and in vivo." *Am J Physiol* 259 (3 Pt 1):E437–42. doi: 10.1152/ajpendo.1990.259.3.E437.

Ed, Hassan Abdullahi Dachia B.Sc. 2020. "Medicinal values of watermelon (Citrullus Lanatus)." *International Journal of Scientific and Management Research* 3 (2):78–84.

Farah, Charlotte, and Cyril Reboul. 2015. "NO better way to protect the heart during Ischemia – reperfusion: To be in the right place at the right time." *Frontiers in Pediatrics* 3. doi: 10.3389/fped.2015.00006.

Figueroa, A., M. A. Sanchez-Gonzalez, P. M. Perkins-Veazie, and B. H. Arjmandi. 2011. "Effects of watermelon supplementation on aortic blood pressure and wave reflection in individuals with prehypertension: A pilot study." *American Journal of Hypertension* 24 (1):40–44. doi: 10.1038/ajh.2010.142.

Figueroa, A., A. Wong, S. Hooshmand, and M. A. Sanchez-Gonzalez. 2013. "Effects of watermelon supplementation on arterial stiffness and wave reflection amplitude in postmenopausal women." *Menopause* 20 (5):573–7. doi: 10.1097/GME.0b013e3182733794.

Fike, Candice D., Marta Sidoryk-Wegrzynowicz, Michael Aschner, Marshall Summar, Lawrence S. Prince, Gary Cunningham, Mark Kaplowitz, Yongmei Zhang, and Judy L. Aschner. 2012. "Prolonged hypoxia augments l-citrulline transport by System A in the newborn piglet pulmonary circulation." *Cardiovascular Research* 95 (3):375–384. doi: 10.1093/cvr/cvs186.

Flam, B. R., P. J. Hartmann, M. Harrell-Booth, L. P. Solomonson, and D. C. Eichler. 2001. "Caveolar localization of arginine regeneration enzymes, argininosuccinate synthase, and lyase, with endothelial nitric oxide synthase." *Nitric Oxide* 5 (2):187–97. doi: 10.1006/niox.2001.0340.

Fragkos, K. C., and A. Forbes. 2011. "Was citrulline first a laxative substance? The truth about modern citrulline and its isolation." *Nihon Ishigaku Zasshi* 57 (3):275–92.

Grune, Tilman, Georg Lietz, Andreu Palou, A. Catharine Ross, Wilhelm Stahl, Guangweng Tang, David Thurnham, Shi-An Yin, and Hans K. Biesalski. 2010. "β-carotene is an important vitamin A source for humans." *The Journal of Nutrition* 140 (12):2268S–2285S. doi: 10.3945/jn.109.119024.

Hayashi, Toshio, Packiasamy A. R. Juliet, Hisako Matsui-Hirai, Asaka Miyazaki, Akiko Fukatsu, Jun Funami, Akihisa Iguchi, and Louis Joseph Ignarro. 2005. "l-Citrulline and l-arginine supplementation retards the progression of high-cholesterol-diet-induced atherosclerosis in rabbits." *Proceedings of the National Academy of Sciences of the United States of America* 102 38:13681–13686.

Joshi, Vijay, and Alisdair R. Fernie. 2017. "Citrulline metabolism in plants." *Amino Acids* 49 (9):1543–1559. doi: 10.1007/s00726-017-2468-4.

Kawasaki, Shinji, Chikahiro Miyake, Takayuki Kohchi, Shinichiro Fujii, Masato Uchida, and Akiho Yokota. 2000. "Responses of wild watermelon to drought stress: Accumulation of an ArgE homologue and citrulline in leaves during water deficits." *Plant and Cell Physiology* 41 (7):864–873. doi: 10.1093/pcp/pcd005.

Keravis, Thérèse, and Claire Lugnier. 2012. "Cyclic nucleotide phosphodiesterase (PDE) isozymes as targets of the intracellular signalling network: Benefits of PDE inhibitors in various diseases and perspectives for future therapeutic developments." *British Journal of Pharmacology* 165 (5):1288–1305. doi: 10.1111/j.1476–5381.2011.01729.x.

Marwat, Sarfaraz Khan, Muhammad Aslam Khan, and Fazal-ur-Rehman. 2008. "Ethnomedicinal study of vegetables mentioned in the Holy Qura'n and Ahadith." *Ethnobotanical Leaflets* 2008:170.

McCarty, Mark. 2016. "Asymmetric dimethylarginine is a well established mediating risk factor for cardiovascular morbidity and mortality – should patients with elevated levels be supplemented with citrulline?" *Healthcare* 4 (3):40. doi: 10.3390/healthcare4030040.

Meléndez-Martínez, Antonio J., Paula Mapelli-Brahm, and Carla M. Stinco. 2018. "The colourless carotenoids phytoene and phytofluene: From dietary sources to their usefulness for the functional foods and nutricosmetics industries." *Journal of Food Composition and Analysis* 67:91–103. doi: https://doi.org/10.1016/j.jfca.2018.01.002.

Michael, O. S., O. Bamidele, P. Ogheneovo, T. A. Ariyo, L. D. Adedayo, O. I. Oluranti, E. O. Soladoye, C. O. Adetunji, and F. O. Awobajo. 2021. "Watermelon rind ethanol extract exhibits hepato-renal protection against lead induced-impaired antioxidant defenses in male Wistar rats." *Curr Res Physiol* 4:252–259. doi: 10.1016/j.crphys.2021.11.002.

Moinard, C., J. Maccario, S. Walrand, V. Lasserre, J. Marc, Y. Boirie, and L. Cynober. 2016. "Arginine behaviour after arginine or citrulline administration in older subjects." *British Journal of Nutrition* 115 (3):399–404. doi: 10.1017/s0007114515004638.

Moinard, C., I. Nicolis, N. Neveux, S. Darquy, S. Bénazeth, and L. Cynober. 2008. "Dose-ranging effects of citrulline administration on plasma amino acids and hormonal patterns in healthy subjects: The Citrudose pharmacokinetic study." *British Journal of Nutrition* 99 (4):855–862. doi: 10.1017/s0007114507841110.

Morris, Sidney M., Carole L. Moncman, Jennifer S. Holub, and Yaacov Hod. 1989. "Nutritional and hormonal regulation of mRNA abundance for arginine biosynthetic enzymes in kidney." *Archives of Biochemistry and Biophysics* 273 (1):230–237. doi: https://doi.org/10.1016/0003-9861(89)90183-5.

Nakao, Masaaki, Ippei Shimizu, Goro Katsuumi, Yohko Yoshida, Masayoshi Suda, Yuka Hayashi, Ryutaro Ikegami, Yung Ting Hsiao, Shujiro Okuda, Tomoyoshi Soga, and Tohru Minamino. 2021. "Empagliflozin maintains capillarization and improves cardiac function in a murine model of left ventricular pressure overload." *Scientific Reports* 11 (1). doi: 10.1038/s41598-021-97787-2.

Nayor, Matthew, Ravi V. Shah, Patricia E. Miller, Jasmine B. Blodgett, Melissa Tanguay, Alexander R. Pico, Venkatesh L. Murthy, Rajeev Malhotra, Nicholas E. Houstis, Amy Deik, Kerry A. Pierce, Kevin Bullock, Lucas Dailey, Raghava S. Velagaleti, Stephanie A. Moore, Jennifer E. Ho, Aaron L. Baggish, Clary B. Clish, Martin G. Larson, Ramachandran S. Vasan, and Gregory D. Lewis. 2020. "Metabolic Architecture of Acute Exercise Response in Middle-Aged Adults in the Community." *Circulation* 142 (20):1905–1924. doi: 10.1161/circulationaha.120.050281.

O'Sullivan, D., J. T. Brosnan, and M. E. Brosnan. 2000. "Catabolism of arginine and ornithine in the perfused rat liver: Effect of dietary protein and of glucagon." *Am J Physiol Endocrinol Metab* 278 (3):E516–E521. doi: 10.1152/ajpendo.2000.278.3.E516.

Orozco-Gutiérrez, J. J., L. Castillo-Martínez, A. Orea-Tejeda, O. Vázquez-Díaz, A. Valdespino-Trejo, R. Narváez-David, C. Keirns-Davis, O. Carrasco-Ortiz, A. Navarro-Navarro, and R. Sánchez-Santillán. 2010. "Effect of L-arginine or L-citrulline oral supplementation on blood pressure and right ventricular function in heart failure patients with preserved ejection fraction." *Cardiol J* 17 (6):612–618.

Poduri, Aruna, Debra L. Rateri, Shubin K. Saha, Sibu Saha, and Alan Daugherty. 2013. "Citrullus lanatus 'sentinel' (watermelon) extract reduces atherosclerosis in LDL receptor-deficient mice." *The Journal of Nutritional Biochemistry* 24 (5):882–886. doi: 10.1016/j.jnutbio.2012.05.011.

Rimando, Agnes M., and Penelope M. Perkins-Veazie. 2005. "Determination of citrulline in watermelon rind." *Journal of Chromatography. A* 1078 1–2:196–200.

Shanely, R., Jennifer Zwetsloot, Thomas Jurrissen, Lauren Hannan, Kevin Zwetsloot, Alan Needle, Anna Bishop, Guoyao Wu, and Penelope Perkins. 2020. "Daily watermelon consumption decreases plasma sVCAM-1 levels in overweight and obese postmenopausal women." *Nutrition Research* 76. doi: 10.1016/j.nutres.2020.02.005.

Simon, Alexandra, Lars Plies, Alice Habermeier, Ursula Martiné, Marco Reining, and Ellen I. Closs. 2003. "Role of neutral amino acid transport and protein breakdown for substrate supply of nitric oxide synthase in human endothelial cells." *Circulation Research* 93 (9):813–820. doi: 10.1161/01.res.0000097761.19223.0d.

Sol Zamuz, Paulo E.S. Munekata, Beatriz Gullón, Gabriele Rocchetti, Domenico Montesano, José M. Lorenzo. 2021. "Citrullus lanatus as source of bioactive components: An up-to-date review." *Trends in Food Science & Technology* 111:208–222. doi: https://doi.org/10.1016/j.tifs.2021.03.002.

Sorokina, Maria, Kira S. McCaffrey, Erin E. Deaton, Guoying Ma, José M. Ordovás, Penelope M. Perkins-Veazie, Christoph Steinbeck, Amnon Levi, and Laurence D. Parnell. 2021. "A catalog of natural products occurring in watermelon – citrullus lanatus." *Frontiers in Nutrition* 8. doi: 10.3389/fnut.2021.729822.

Story, Erica N., Rachel E. Kopec, Steven J. Schwartz, and G. Keith Harris. 2010. "An update on the health effects of tomato lycopene." *Annual Review of Food Science and Technology* 1 (1):189–210. doi: 10.1146/annurev.food.102308.124120.

Strauss, Mark. 2015. "The 5,000-year secret history of the watermelon." *National Geographic*, 21 August 2015.

Tsai, Emily J., and David A. Kass. 2009. "Cyclic GMP signaling in cardiovascular pathophysiology and therapeutics." *Pharmacology & Therapeutics* 122 (3):216–238. doi: 10.1016/j.pharmthera.2009.02.009.

Ventura, G., C. Moinard, F. Sinico, V. Carrière, V. Lasserre, L. Cynober, and J. P. De Bandt. 2011. "Evidence for a role of the ileum in the control of nitrogen homeostasis via the regulation of arginine metabolism." *British Journal of Nutrition* 106 (2):227–236. doi: 10.1017/s0007114511000079.

Wijnands, Karolina, Tessy Castermans, Merel Hommen, Dennis Meesters, and Martijn Poeze. 2015. "Arginine and citrulline and the immune response in sepsis." *Nutrients* 7 (3):1426–1463. doi: 10.3390/nu7031426.

Windmueller, H. G., and A. E. Spaeth. 1981. "Source and fate of circulating citrulline." *Am J Physiol* 241 (6):E473–E480. doi: 10.1152/ajpendo.1981.241.6.E473.

Wong, A., O. Chernykh, and A. Figueroa. 2016. "Chronic l-citrulline supplementation improves cardiac sympathovagal balance in obese postmenopausal women: A preliminary report." *Auton Neurosci* 198:50–53. doi: 10.1016/j.autneu.2016.06.005.

Wu, Guoyao, Julie K. Collins, Penelope Perkins-Veazie, Muhammad Siddiq, Kirk D. Dolan, Katherine A. Kelly, Cristine L. Heaps, and Cynthia J. Meininger. 2007. "Dietary supplementation with watermelon pomace juice enhances arginine availability and ameliorates the metabolic syndrome in Zucker diabetic fatty rats." *The Journal of Nutrition* 137 (12):2680–2685. doi: 10.1093/jn/137.12.2680.

Yokota, A. 2002. "Citrulline and DRIP-1 protein (ArgE Homologue) in drought tolerance of wild watermelon." *Annals of Botany* 89 (7):825–832. doi: 10.1093/aob/mcf074.

Yu, Y. M., C. M. Ryan, J. F. Burke, R. G. Tompkins, and V. R. Young. 1995. "Relations among arginine, citrulline, ornithine, and leucine kinetics in adult burn patients." *Am J Clin Nutr* 62 (5):960–968. doi: 10.1093/ajcn/62.5.960.

Zhou, Ji-Qiu, Xiong Xu, Wei-Wei Zhen, Yu-Long Luo, Bin Cai, and Sen Zhang. 2018. "Protective effect of citrulline on the hearts of rats with sepsis induced by cecal ligation and puncture." *BioMed Research International* 2018:1–10. doi: 10.1155/2018/2574501.

Section III

Resources

23 Recommended Resources on Cardiovascular Health and Disease in Relation to Foods, Plants, Herbs and Spices in Human Health

Rajkumar Rajendram, Daniel Gyamfi,
Vinood B. Patel and Victor R. Preedy

CONTENTS

23.1 Introduction 361
23.2 Resources 362
23.3 Other Resources 368
23.4 Summary Points 368
23.5 Acknowledgements (in Alphabetical Order) 368
References 369

23.1 INTRODUCTION

Dietary modification and medications are standard treatments to control risk factors related to cardiovascular disease and therapeutic options also include percutaneous coronary interventions, and open cardiac surgery. These approaches have considerably improved the morbidity and mortality associated with cardiovascular disease. However, cardiovascular disease is still the leading cause of mortality worldwide (World Health Organization, 2021). Thus, finding more efficacious alternatives is required.

Many cultures use traditional remedies derived from medicinal plants to treat cardiovascular diseases including angina, heart failure and arrhythmias (Rastogi et al., 2016, 2017; Naveed et al., 2020). Ancient remedies derived from plants have also been used to treat the risk factors for cardiovascular disease such as diabetes and hypertension (Naveed et al., 2020; Deutschländer et al., 2009; Li et al., 2004). The amount of text-based material related to the treatment of cardiovascular-related conditions is considerable.

We have previously presented resources to assist experienced researchers and clinicians to navigate such information. Those embarking on research into foods, plant-based remedies and cardiovascular disease can also be guided on where to begin their exploration by the tables containing resources recommended by active researchers and practitioners.

The list of acknowledgements to follow includes all the experts who helped to compile these valuable resources.

DOI: 10.1201/9781003220329-26

23.2 RESOURCES

Tables 23.1–5 list the most up-to-date information on the regulatory bodies (Table 23.1), professional societies (Table 23.2), books (Table 23.3), emerging technologies, platforms (Table 23.4) and other resources of interest (Table 23.5) that are relevant to an evidence-based approach to foods, plants, herbs, spices and cardiovascular disease in human health. Some organisations are listed in more than one table as they occasional fulfil multiple roles.

TABLE 23.1

Websites, Regulatory Bodies or Organisations Dealing with the Study of Foods, Plants, Herbs, Spices and Cardiovascular Disease or Related Fields and Areas

Regulatory Body or Organisation	Web Address
Academy of Nutrition and Dietetics	www.eatrightpro.org/
American Congress of Rehabilitation Medicine	https://acrm.org/
Botanical Safety Consortium	https://botanicalsafetyconsortium.org/
British Heart Foundation	www.bhf.org.uk/
Centers for Disease Control and Prevention	www.cdc.gov/
Diabetes Canada	www.diabetes.ca/
European Commission	https://ec.europa.eu/
European Food Safety Authority (EFSA)	www.efsa.europa.eu/en
European Heart Network	www.ehnheart.org/
European Medicines Agency	www.ema.europa.eu/en
Food and Agriculture Organization of the United Nations (FAO)	www.fao.org/
Food and Drug Administration Center for Food Safety and Applied Nutrition	www.fda.gov/food/
Food with Health Claims, Food for Special Dietary Uses, and Nutrition Labelling, Japan	www.mhlw.go.jp/english/topics/foodsafety/fhc/
Healthline Media	www.healthline.com/
Heart and Stroke Foundation of Canada	www.heartandstroke.ca/
International Olive Council (IOC)	www.internationaloliveoil.org/?lang=es
Linus Pauling Institute: Oregon State University	https://lpi.oregonstate.edu
Micronutrient Forum	https://micronutrientforum.org/
Ministry of Health, Labour and Welfare, Japan	www.mhlw.go.jp/english/
National Academy of Medicine	https://nam.edu/
National Agency for Food and Drug Administration and Control	www.nafdac.gov.ng/
National Center for Complementary and Integrative Health (NCCIH)	www.nccih.nih.gov/
National Health and Medical Research Council (NHMRC)	www.nhmrc.gov.au/
National Health Service (NHS)	www.nhs.uk/
National Health Service (NHS) England	www.england.nhs.uk/
National Institute of Cardiology, Mexico	www.cardiologia.org.mx/
National Institute on Aging	www.nia.nih.gov/
National Institutes of Health	www.nih.gov/
National Pharmaceutical Regulatory Agency	https://npra.gov.my/index.php/en/
Nutrition.gov: U.S. Department of Agriculture	www.nutrition.gov/
Office of Dietary Supplements: National Institutes of Health	https://ods.od.nih.gov/
Physicians Committee for Responsible Medicine	www.pcrm.org/
PublicHealth	www.publichealth.org/
Swedish Nutrition Foundation	https://snf.ideon.se/
U.S. Department of Agriculture (USDA)	www.usda.gov/
U.S. Food and Drug Administration	www.fda.gov/

Recommended Resources on Cardiovascular Health and Disease

Table 23.1 *(Continued)*
Websites, Regulatory Bodies or Organisations Dealing with the Study of Foods, Plants, Herbs, Spices and Cardiovascular Disease or Related Fields and Areas

Regulatory Body or Organisation	Web Address
World Food safety Organisation (WFSO)	https://worldfoodsafety.org/
World Health Federation	https://world-heart-federation.org/
World Health Organization (WHO)	www.who.int/

Note: This table lists the regulatory bodies and organisations involved with the study of foods, plants, herbs, spices and cardiovascular disease. Some of the links have indirect references to this topic. The links were accurate at the time of going to press but may move or alter. Some societies and organisations have a preference for shortened terms, such as acronyms and abbreviations. See also Table 23.2.

TABLE 23.2
Professional Societies Associated with the Study of Foods, Plants, Herbs, Spices and Cardiovascular Disease or Related Fields and Areas

Society Name	Web Address
American Heart Association	www.heart.org/
American Nutrition Association	https://theana.org/
American Society for Nutrition	https://nutrition.org/
American Society for Parenteral and Enteral Nutrition	www.nutritioncare.org/
American Society for Preventive Cardiology	www.aspconline.org/
American Society of Hypertension (ASH US)	www.ash-us.org/
Canadian Nutrition Society	www.cns-scn.ca/
Chinese Nutrition Society	www.cnsoc.org/
Czech Society for Nutrition	www.vyzivaspol.cz/
Danish Nutrition Society	www.sfe.dk/dansk1
European Society for Clinical Nutrition and Metabolism	www.espen.org/
European Society of Cardiology	www.escardio.org/
Federation of African Nutrition Societies	http://fanus.org/
Federation of European Nutrition Societies	https://fensnutrition.org/
German Society for Nutritional Medicine	www.dgem.de/
Hong Kong Nutrition Association	www.hkna.org.hk/
Inter-American Society of Cardiology	www.siacardio.com/
International American Association of Clinical Nutritionists	www.iaacn.org
International Confederation of Dietetic Associations (ICDA)	www.internationaldietetics.org/
International Society for Ethnopharmacology	https://ethnopharmacology.org/
International Union of Nutritional Sciences (IUNS)	https://iuns.org/
Japan Atherosclerosis Society	www.j-athero.org/jp/english/
Malaysian Natural Products Society	www.mymnps.org/
Mexican Society of Cardiology	www.smcardiologia.org.mx/
National Association of Nutrition Professionals	https://nanp.org/
Nutrition Society	www.nutritionsociety.org
Royal Pharmaceutical Society	www.rpharms.com/
Royal Society of Chemistry	www.rsc.org/
Society for Medicinal Plant and Natural Product Research (GA)	https://ga-online.org/
Society for Nutrition Education and Behavior	www.sneb.org/
Society of Japanese Food Studies	https://washoku-bunka.jp/greeting.html

(Continued)

364 Ancient and Traditional Foods, Plants, Herbs and Spices

TABLE 23.2 *(Continued)*
Professional Societies Associated with the Study of Foods, Plants, Herbs, Spices and Cardiovascular Disease or Related Fields and Areas

Society Name	Web Address
Swiss Society for Nutrition	www.sfkn.se/
United Nations System Standing Committee on Nutrition	www.unscn.org/
Universal Society of Food and Nutrition	www.usfn.net/

Note: This table lists the professional societies involved with foods, plants, herbs, spices and cardiovascular disease in human health. Some of the links have indirect references to this topic. The links were accurate at the time of going to press but may move or alter. In these cases, the use of the "Search" tabs should be explored at the parent address or site. Some societies and organisations have a preference for shortened terms, such as acronyms and abbreviations. See also Table 23.1.

TABLE 23.3
Books on Foods, Plants, Herbs, Spices and Cardiovascular Disease or Related Fields and Areas

Book Title	Authors or Editors	Publisher	Year of Publication
Aromatic Herbs in Food	Galanakis CM	Academic Press	2021
Bioactive Food as Dietary Interventions for Cardiovascular Disease: Bioactive Foods in Chronic Disease States	Watson RR, Preedy VR	Academic Press	2013
Biologie Et Pathologie Du Cœur Et Des Vaisseaux	SFC-GRRC	John Libbey Eurotext	2019
Botanical Medicine and Clinical Practice	Watson RR, Preedy VR	CABI Publishing	2008
Evidence-Based Nutrition and Clinical Evidence of Bioactive Foods in Human Health and Disease	Duttaroy AK	Academic Press	2021
Evidence-Based Validation of Herbal Medicine: Translational Research on Botanicals	Mukherjee PK	Elsevier	2022
Food Bioactives and Health	Galanakis CM	Springer Nature	2021
Functional Foods	Gibson GR, Williams CM	Woodhead Publishing Limited	2000
Functional Foods, Cardiovascular Disease and Diabetes	Arnoldi A	CRC	2004
Functional Foods, Nutraceuticals, and Degenerative Disease Prevention	Paliyath G, Bakovic M, Shetty K	Wiley Blackwell	2011
Handbook of Herbs and Spices	Collin H	Woodhead Publishing	2006
Handbook of Medicinal Herbs	Duke JA	CRC Press	2002
Heart Physiology: From Cell to Circulation. 4th edition	Opie LH	Lippincott Williams & Wilkins	2003
Herbal and Traditional Medicine: Molecular Aspects of Health	Packe L, Ong C, Halliwell B	Marcel Dekker, New York	2004
Herbal Medicine: Biomolecular and Clinical Aspects. 2nd edition	Benzie IFF, Wachtel-Galor S	CRC Press	2011
Herbs and Molecular Basis of Cardiovascular Protection	Joshi S, Paliwal VM, Priya VV, Sahu BD	CRC Press	2022
Herbs and Natural Supplements, Volume 2: An Evidence-Based Guide. 4th edition	Braun L, Cohen M	Churchill Livingstone	2015

Recommended Resources on Cardiovascular Health and Disease

TABLE 23.3 *(Continued)*

Books on Foods, Plants, Herbs, Spices and Cardiovascular Disease or Related Fields and Areas

Book Title	Authors or Editors	Publisher	Year of Publication
Herbs and Spices	Ahmad RS	IntechOpen	2021
Herbs of Malaysia: An Introduction to the Medicinal, Culinary, Aromatic and Cosmetic Use of Herbs	Wong KM	Marshall Cavendish Editions	2009
Indian Materia Medica	Nadkarni KM	Bombay Popular Prakashan Private Limited	1976
Indian Medicinal Plants	Sala AV	Orient Longman Private Limited	1995
Indian Medicinal Plants	Basu BD	International Book Distributors	1999
Malaysian Herbal Monograph 2015	Malaysian Herbal Monograph Committee	Institute of Medical Research, Malaysia	2016
Malaysian Medicinal Plants for the Treatment of Cardiovascular Diseases	Goh SH	Pelanduk Publications	1995
Medicinal Herbs in Primary Care: An Evidence-Guided Reference for Healthcare Providers	Bokelmann JM	Elsevier	2021
Nature's Medicine: A Collection of Medicinal Plants from Malaysia's Rainforest	Hussain AG, Hussin K, Noor MN	Landskap Malaysia	2018
Obesity: Oxidative Stress and Dietary Antioxidants	Marti A, Aguilera CM	Academic Press	2018
Olive Oil and Health	Quiles JL, Ramirez-Tortosa MC and Yaqoob P	CABI Publishing	2006
Recent Development in Plant Research	Capasso A	Research Signpost	2007
Traditional Malay Medicinal Plants	Zakaria M	Oxford Fajar Sdn. Bhd.	2010
Tratado de Nutrición	Gil A	Editorial Médica Panamericana	2017

Note: This table lists books relevant to the study of foods, plants, herbs and spices and cardiovascular disease.

TABLE 23.4

Emerging Techniques, Instruments and Analytical Platforms or Devices for Investigating Foods, Plants, Herbs, Spices and Cardiovascular Disease or Related Fields and Areas

Organisation or Company Name	Web Address
AD Instruments	www.adinstruments.com/
Artificial Intelligence in Cardiology	www.dicardiology.com/videos/video-acc-efforts-advance-evidence-based-implementation-ai-cardiovascular-care
Diagnostic and Interventional Cardiology (DAIC): 8 Cardiovascular Technologies to Watch in 2020	www.dicardiology.com/content/blogs/8-cardiovascular-technologies-watch-2020
Emka Technologies	www.emkatech.com/
Gordon Center for Medical Imaging	https://gordon.mgh.harvard.edu/gc/research/quantitative-petspect/
Heart Research Institute: Cardiovascular Medical Devices	www.hri.org.au/our-research/cardiovascular-medical-devices

(Continued)

366 Ancient and Traditional Foods, Plants, Herbs and Spices

TABLE 23.4 *(Continued)*

Emerging Techniques, Instruments and Analytical Platforms or Devices for Investigating Foods, Plants, Herbs, Spices and Cardiovascular Disease or Related Fields and Areas

Organisation or Company Name	Web Address
IDTechEx	www.idtechex.com/en/reports/photonics/116
IITC Life Science	www.iitcinc.com/
Measuring Development Engineering	www.mdegmbh.eu/en/
MedTechIntelligence	www.medtechintelligence.com/feature_article/emerging-trends-in-cardiovascular-devices/
Nestle Health Science	www.nestlehealthscience.com/
Panlab	www.panlab.com/en/
PlantNet	https://identify.plantnet.org/the-plant-list/species/Momordica%20dioica%20Roxb.%20ex%20Willd./data
Ugo Basile	www.ugobasile.com/
Useful Tropical Plants Databases	https://tropical.theferns.info/viewtropical.php?id=Momordica+dioica
ZOE: In-Depth Nutrition	https://joinzoe.com/

Note: This table lists technologies or platforms relevant to foods, plants, herbs, spices and cardiovascular disease in human health. Please note, occasionally the location of the websites or web address changes.

TABLE 23.5

Other Resources of Interest or Relevance for Health Care Professionals or Patients Related to the Study of Foods, Plants, Herbs, Spices and Cardiovascular Disease or Related Fields and Areas

Name of Resource or Organisation	Web Address
Australian Regulatory Guidelines for Listed Medicines and Registered Complementary Medicines	www.tga.gov.au/publication/australian-regulatory-guidelines-listed-medicines-and-registered-complementary-medicines
Better Health Channel: Department of Health, State Government of Victoria, Australia	www.betterhealth.vic.gov.au/health/conditionsandtreatments/heart-disease-and-food
Biodiversity for Food and Nutrition	www.b4fn.org/resources/species-database/detail/momordica-dioica/
Centre for Advanced Functional Foods Research and Entrepreneurship: Ohio State University	https://u.osu.edu/caffre/
Cleveland HeartLab: Top Herbs for Your Heart	www.clevelandheartlab.com/blog/top-herbs-for-your-heart/
Diversity of WASHOKU: Ministry of Agriculture, Forestry and Fisheries (MAFF)	www.maff.go.jp/e/policies/market/divers.html
European Commission: Cardiovascular Diseases	https://ec.europa.eu/info/research-and-innovation/research-area/health-research-and-innovation/cardiovascular-dieases_en
European Commission's Food Safety	https://ec.europa.eu/food/overview_en/
European Federation of Pharmaceutical Industries and Associations: Working with Patient Groups	www.efpia.eu/relationships-code/patient-organisations/
European Food Safety Authority: Material on Botanicals	www.efsa.europa.eu/en/topics/topic/botanicals
European Medicines Agency: Cardiovascular Diseases	www.ema.europa.eu/en/news-events/therapeutic-areas-latest-updates/cardiovascular-diseases
Global Biodiversity Information Facility	www.gbif.org/
Global Information Hub on Integrated Medicine (GlobinMed)	www.globinmed.com/

TABLE 23.5 *(Continued)*

Other Resources of Interest or Relevance for Health Care Professionals or Patients Related to the Study of Foods, Plants, Herbs, Spices and Cardiovascular Disease or Related Fields and Areas

Name of Resource or Organisation	Web Address
Global Plants Database	https://plants.jstor.org/
Health: Ministry of Health, Labour and Welfare, Japan	www.mhlw.go.jp/english/policy/health-medical/health/index.html
Healthy Eating: Diabetes Canada	www.diabetes.ca/nutrition – fitness/healthy-eating
Heart and Stroke Foundation of Canada: Healthy Eating	www.heartandstroke.ca/healthy-living/healthy-eating
Herbs and Supplements for Heart Disease: Healthline Media	www.healthline.com/health/heart-disease/herbs-supplements
Integrated Taxonomic Information System (ITIS) Report	www.itis.gov/servlet/SingleRpt/SingleRpt?search_topic=TSN& search_value=505903#null
International Association for Plant Taxonomy (IAPT)	www.iaptglobal.org/
International Plant Name Index	www.ipni.org/
International Regulatory Cooperation for Herbal Medicines (IRCH)	www.who.int/initiatives/international-regulatory-cooperation-for-herbal-medicines#:~:text=International%20Regulatory%20 Cooperation%20for%20Herbal%20Medicines%20(IRCH)%20is%20 a%20global,improved%20regulation%20for%20herbal%20 medicines.
Japanese Food Culture National Council	https://washokujapan.jp/
Micronutrient Information Centre: Oregon State University	https://lpi.oregonstate.edu/mic
Mushrooms Canada	www.mushrooms.ca/
National Cancer Institute: Complementary and Alternative Medicine	www.cancer.gov/about-cancer/treatment/cam
National Center for Natural Products Research: The University of Mississippi	https://pharmacy.olemiss.edu/ncnpr/research-programs/medicinal-plant-research/
National Centre for Complementary and Integrative Health: Resources for Health Care Providers	www.nccih.nih.gov/health/providers
National Centre for Complementary and Integrative Health: Clinical Practice Guidelines	www.nccih.nih.gov/health/providers/clinicalpractice
National Institute of Neurological Disorders and Stroke: Patient Organisations	www.ninds.nih.gov/Disorders/Support-Resources/ Patient-Organizations
Natural and Non-Prescription Health Products Directorate: Government of Canada	www.canada.ca/en/health-canada/corporate/about-health-canada/ branches-agencies/health-products-food-branch/natural-non-prescription-health-products-directorate.html
Natural Health Products Regulations: Government of Canada	https://laws-lois.justice.gc.ca/eng/regulations/SOR-2003-196/page-1. html
Nestle Nutrition Institute	https://nnia.nestlenutrition-institute.org/
Nutrition and Healthy Eating: Government of Canada	www.canada.ca/en/health-canada/services/food-nutrition/healthy-zating.html
Plant Identification: University of Massachusetts	https://extension.umass.edu/plant-identification/common/all
PublicHealth: Heart Disease Resources	www.publichealth.org/resources/heart-disease/
Regulatory Frameworks for Nutraceuticals: Australia, Canada, Japan, and the United States	https://pubmed.ncbi.nlm.nih.gov/34345505/

(Continued)

TABLE 23.5 *(Continued)*

Other Resources of Interest or Relevance for Health Care Professionals or Patients Related to the Study of Foods, Plants, Herbs, Spices and Cardiovascular Disease or Related Fields and Areas

Name of Resource or Organisation	Web Address
Regulatory Frameworks for Nutraceuticals: Different Countries of the World	https://pubmed.ncbi.nlm.nih.gov/32427089/
Tang Centre for Herbal Medicine Research: University of Chicago	www.uchicago.edu/education-and-research/center/tang_center_for_herbal_medicine_research/
The Patients Association	www.patients-association.org.uk/
The Plant List	www.theplantlist.org/
UMass Amherst Plant Identification	https://extension.umass.edu/plant-identification/
UniProt Taxonomy	www.uniprot.org/taxonomy/
WHO Global Report on Traditional and Complementary Medicine 2019	www.who.int/traditional-complementary-integrative-medicine/WhoGlobalReportOnTraditionalAndComplementaryMedicine2019
World Flora Online	www.worldfloraonline.org/
World Health Organization: Nutrition	www.who.int/health-topics/nutrition

Note: This table lists other resources of interest or relevance to the study of foods, plants, herbs, spices and cardiovascular disease in human health. Please note, occasionally the location of the websites or web address changes.

23.3 OTHER RESOURCES

The Wellcome Collection (https://wellcomecollection.org/collections) and the British Library (www.bl.uk/) also hold material on topics related to foods and plant-based approaches to the study of cardiovascular disease.

Other chapters on resources relevant to nutrition and cardiovascular disease (recommended by authors and practitioners) have been published previously (Alzaid et al., 2015; Rajendram et al., 2013a, 2013b; Rajendram et al., 2014, 2015, 2016, 2019a, 2019b, 2020, 2022a, 2022b).

This list of material in these tables is included to provide general information only. It does not constitute any recommendation or endorsement of the activities of these sites, facilities, or other resources listed in this chapter, by the authors or editors of this book.

23.4 SUMMARY POINTS

- The use of traditional remedies for the treatment of cardiovascular disease is widespread in many cultures.
- Cardiovascular disease is one of the most common causes of morbidity and mortality worldwide.
- Natural remedies have gained tremendous importance as sources of drugs for the treatment of cardiovascular disease and other communicable and non-communicable diseases.
- This chapter lists resources relevant to foods, plants, herbs, spices and cardiovascular disease.

23.5 ACKNOWLEDGEMENTS (IN ALPHABETICAL ORDER)

We thank the following authors for their contributions to the development of this resource. We apologise if some of the suggested material was not included in this chapter or has been moved to different sections.

Asgharzadeh, Fereshteh
Belaidi, Elise

Borradaile, Nica M.
Jaramillo Flores, María Eugenia
Fong, Lai Yen
Mesa García, María Dolores
Moinard, Christophe
Nguelefack, Télesphore Benoît
Nguelefack-Mbuyo, Elvine Pami
Ozcan, Bilgehan
Tomlinson, Brian
Wilson, Rachel B.
Yong, Yoke Keong

REFERENCES

Alzaid, F., Rajendram, R., Patel, V.B., Preedy, V.R. (2015). Expanding the knowledge base in diet, nutrition and critical care: Electronic and published resources. In Rajendram, R., Preedy, V.R., Patel, V.B. (Editors). Diet and Nutrition in Critical Care. Springer, Germany.

Deutschländer, M., Lall, N., Van De Venter, M. (2009). Plant species used in the treatment of cardiovascular disease by South African traditional healers: An inventory. Pharm. Biol., 47, 348–365.

Guo, X., Li, H., Xu, H., Woo, S., Dong, H., Lu, F., Lange, A.J., Wu, C. (2012). Glycolysis in the control of blood glucose homeostasis. Acta Pharm. Sinica B, 2, 358–367.

Hossain, M.S., Urbi, Z., Evamoni, F.Z., Zohora, F.T., Rahman, K.M.H. (2016). A secondary research on medicinal plants mentioned in the Holy Qur'an. J. Med. Plants, 3 (59), 81–97.

Li, W., Zheng, H., Bukuru, J., De Kimpe, N. (2004). Natural medicines used in the traditional Chinese medical system for therapy of cardiovascular disease mellitus. J. Ethnopharmacol., 92, 1–21.

Naveed, M., Majeed, F., Taleb, A., Zubair, H.M., Shumzaid, M., Farooq, M.A., Baig, M., Abbas, M., Saeed, M., Changxing, L. (2020). A review of medicinal plants in cardiovascular disorders: Benefits and risks. The American Journal of Chinese Medicine, 48(2), 259–286.

Rajendram, R., Gyamfi, D., Patel, V.B., Preedy, V.R. (2022a). Recommended resources for biomarkers of nutrition. In Preedy, V.R. and Patel, V.B. (Editors). Biomarkers of Nutrition. Elsevier, USA (in press).

Rajendram, R., Gyamfi, D., Patel, V.B., Preedy, V.R. (2022b). Recommended resources for biomarkers in diabetes: Methods, discoveries, and applications. In Patel, V.B., Preedy, V.R. (Editors). Biomarkers in Diabetes. Biomarkers in Disease: Methods, Discoveries and Applications. Springer, Cham. https://doi.org/10.1007/978-3-030-81303-1_58-2

Rajendram, R., Patel, V.B., Preedy, V.R. (2014). Web based resources and suggested reading. In Rajendram, R., Patel, V.B., Preedy, V.R. (Editors). Glutamine in Health and Disease (pp. 527–532). Springer, USA.

Rajendram, R., Patel, V.B., Preedy, V.R. (2015). Web based resources and suggested reading. In Rajendram, R., Patel, V.B., Preedy, V.R. (Editors). Branched Chain Amino Acids in Health and Disease. Springer, USA.

Rajendram, R., Patel, V.B., Preedy, V.R. (2016). Recommended resources on biomarkers in cardiovascular disease. In Patel, V., Preedy, V. (Editors). Biomarkers in Cardiovascular Disease. Springer, Dordrecht. https://doi.org/10.1007/978-94-007-7741-5_52-1

Rajendram, R., Patel, V.B., Preedy, V.R. (2017). Recommended resources on maternal nutrition. In Rajendram, R., Patel, V.B., Preedy, V.R. (Editors). Nutrition and Diet in Maternal Diabetes (pp. 495–500). Springer, USA.

Rajendram, R., Patel, V.B., Preedy, V.R. (2019a). Resources in famine, starvation, and nutrient deprivation. In Patel, V.B., Preedy, V.R. (Editors). Famine, Starvation, and Nutrient Deprivation (pp. 2399–2406). Springer, USA.

Rajendram, R., Patel, V.B., Preedy, V.R. (2019b). Resources in diet, nutrition and epigenetics. In Patel, V.B., Preedy, V.R. (Editors). Nutrition and Epigenetics (pp. 2309–2314). Springer, USA.

Rajendram, R., Patel, V.B., Preedy, V.R. (2020). Recommended resources for nutrition, oxidative stress, and dietary antioxidants. In Martin, C.R., Preedy, V.R. (Editors). Nutrition, Oxidative Stress, and Dietary Antioxidants (pp. 393–397). Elsevier, USA.

Rajendram, R., Rajendram, R., Patel, V.B., Preedy, V.R. (2013a). Interlinking diet, nutrition, the menopause and recommended resources. In Hollins-Martin, C.J., Watson, R.R., Preedy, V.R. (Editors). Nutrition and Diet in Menopause. Springer, Germany.

Rajendram, R., Rajendram, R., Patel, V.B., Preedy, V.R. (2013b). Diet quality: What more is there to know? In Preedy, V.R., Hunter, L.-A., Patel, V.B. (Editors). Diet Quality: An Evidence-Based Approach (pp. 397–401). Springer, Germany.

Rastogi, S., Pandey, M.M., Rawat, A.K. (2016). Traditional herbs: A remedy for cardiovascular disorders. Phytomedicine: International Journal of Phytotherapy and Phytopharmacology, 23(11), 1082–1089.

Rastogi, S., Pandey, M.M., Rawat, A. (2017). Spices: Therapeutic potential in cardiovascular health. Current Pharmaceutical Design, 23(7), 989–998.

World Health Organization. Fact Sheet. (2021, 16 June). Available online: www.who.int/news-room/fact-sheets/detail/cardiovascular-diseases-(cvds) (accessed on 10 October 2022).

Index

Note: **Boldface** page references indicate tables. *Italic* references indicate figures.

A

adiponectin, 274, *275*
Aframomum pruinosum (Zingiberaceae), 341
African plants and cardiovascular health, 237, 241–242
alginate, 71
allergy management, 148, 242, 321
Allium sativum (garlic), 13, 55–56, 59, 308, 325
Aloe forex mill, 242
Aloysia Paláu genus
antibacterial activity of, 220
chemical constituents, 220, **221–223**, *224*, **224**, **225**
description of, 215–216, *216*
flavonoids in, *225*
general usage, 218
health promotion of, 218
leaf infusion, 218
leaves of, 217–218, *217*
pharmacobotany, 216–219
pharmacological investigations, 219–220
safety evaluations, 220
species, 116
stems of, *217*
toxicity/cautions, 220
traditional usage of, 216–219
amaranth, slender/green (*Amaranthus viridis*), 56–57
Amaryllidaceae (*Crinum zeylanicum*), 341
American Heart Association, 5
analgesic activity of *Momordica dioica*, 321
Andrographis paniculata, see kalmegh
angiotensin-converting enzyme (ACE), 51, 56, 151, 184, 249–250, 308
anthocyanins, 52, 299
antibacterial activity of *Aloysia Paláu/Momordica dioica*, 220, 320
antifertility activity of *Momordica dioica*, 321
antimalarial activity of *Momordica dioica*, 321
antioxidants, *see also* phytochemicals; *specific type*
in balloon vine, 138
in black cumin, 12
cardiovascular diseases and, 8, *9*
in date palm tree/fruit, 163
flavonoids and, 138
in *Ganoderma lucidum*, 248–249
hypertension and decreased levels of, 6
in kalmegh, 205
in mango, 12–13
in *Momordica dioica*, 321
natural, in hypertension management, 8–13, *9*, *13*
plants with properties of, 12–13
in saptrees, 336–338
in watermelon, 346
antiseizure activity of black cumin, 148
antiulcer activity of *Momordica dioica*, 321
antiviral property of *Momordica dioica*, 321
apigenin, 54, 137–138, 140, 180
Apium graveolens L. (celery), 12

apolipoprotein/apolipoprotein B, 305, 338
apoptosis, 118–119, 151–152, 170, 204, 335–336, 352
arginine, 348–351, *349*
argininosuccinate lyase (ASL), 350
argininosuccinate synthase (ASS), 350
arjuna ghee, 104
Artemisia genus
in cancer management, 179, **179–180**
chemical structure of, 179, *179*
description of, 177–178
distribution of, 178, *178*
general usage of, 178
historical perspective of, 177–178
in hypertension management, 184, *184*, **185–186**, 186–187
pharmacological activities of, main, 179, *179*, **179–180**
phytochemicals in, 180, **181–183**
toxicity/cautions, 187
Artemisia herba-alba, 241–242
ascorbic acid (AA), 9–10
asiatic acid, 86
asiaticoside, 85
asiatic pennywort, *see Centella asiatica*
Aspalathus linearis, 242
atherosclerosis (AS)
baicalein in inhibiting, 115, *116*
cardiovascular disease associated with, 168
Centella asiatica in inhibiting, 84–85
Momoridica dioica in inhibiting, 322
mushrooms and, 285–286, 288–290
pomegranate in inhibiting, 305–307
saffron and, 55
saptrees in inhibiting, 338–339
vitamin C and, 10
autophagy, 152
Ayurvedic medicine, 79, 95–96, 128, 196–197
azhal thamaraga noi, 133

B

baicalein
absorption of, 113–114
in apoptosis modulation, 118–119
in atherosclerosis inhibition, 115, *116*
cardiovascular health and, 114–117, 120
chemical structure of, 113, *113*
excretion of, 113–114
extraction of, 112–113
in heart failure management, 116–117
in hypertension management, 115–116, *116*
in inflammation mitigation, 118
in ischemia/reperfusion injury, 117–119, *119*
metabolism of, 113–114
oxidative stress inhibition and, 117–118
purification of, 113
source of, 113–114
toxicity/cautions, 120
vascular action and, 119, *119*

371

Index

balloon vine (*Cardiospermum halicacabum* L.)
aerial parts of, 129–130
antioxidants in, 138
in Ayurvedic medicine, 128
cardio-cerebral disease and, 133–135
cardiovascular health and, 113, 132–133
cell membrane properties and, modification of, 137
description of, 127–129
enzymatic activity and, inhibition of, 138–139
financial significance of, 132
flavonoids in, 131, 134–135, *134*
general usage of, 129
ion channels and, modulation of, 137
leaves of, 130
metabolites and, *139*, 140
nitric oxide synthase and, 137
phytochemicals in, 134–135
phytoconstituents of, 131
receptors and, 138
risks associated with, 131–132
roots of, 130–131
seed of, 130
species of, 128
synonyms for, 128, **128**
toxicity/cautions, 131, 140
traditional usage of, 129–131
transporter mechanism and, 138
vernacular names of, 128, **128–129**
Bax, 170–171
Berberis aristata DC, 53–54
B-carotene, 346
betel vine (*Piper betel*), 13
BF, *see Bridelia ferruginea* Benth
bioactive compounds
in black cumin, 146–147, **147**
in *Ganoderma lucidum*, 248, 325
in Mexican orchid, 263, **264–271**
in pomegranate, 298–305, **298**
in virgin olive oils, 37–38, **38**
bioavailability of phenolic compounds, 42, 305, *305*
biodiversity, Brazilian, 224, 226–227
black cumin (*Nigella sativa* L.)
anti-apoptotic effects of, 151–152
anti-fibrotic effects of, 152–154, *153*
antioxidants in, 12
antioxidative effects of, 149–151, *150*
antiseizure activity of, 148
bioactive compounds in, 146–147, **147**
cardiovascular health and, 148–154
chemical composition, 146–147, **147**
in diabetes management, 148
in inflammation management, 148–149, *149*
plant morphology, 146, *147*
reactive oxygen species and, 149–151
therapeutic potential of, 148, **148**
toxicity/cautions, 154
blood glucose, 283, 286–287, 289, *see also* diabetes
blood pressure, 4–5, **5**, 11, 71, 352, *see also* hypertension
blueberry extract, 12
Brazilian plants, 224, 226–227
Bridelia ferruginea Benth (BF)
cardiovascular health and, 236–237
chemical structure of, 232, **234–235**
description of, 232

distribution of, 232, *233*
extracts, 232–233
flavonoids in, 236
future of, 241
general usage of, 232, *233*
metabolites in leaves of, 236
quercetin in, 236
safety concerns with, 241
squalene in, 236
toxicity/cautions, 241–242
vitamin E in, 237
British Herbal Pharmacopoeia, 79

C

cancer management/protection, 13, 66–68, 71, 148, 162,
        165–166, 179, 219–220, 318, 320–321, 333
cardiac fibrosis, 116, 152–154, *153*
cardiac hypertrophy, 82, **84**, 98–100, 204
cardiac remodeling, 339–340, *340*
Cardiospermum halicacabum L., *see* balloon vine
cardiovascular diseases (CVDs), *see also* cardiac health;
        specific type
antioxidants and, 8, *9*
atherosclerosis-associated, 168
definition of, 4, 146, 332
dietary oils and, 36
epidemiology on, global, 237, *238*
evolution in future years, 323
fasting plasma glucose and, impaired, 303
glucose tolerance and, impaired, 303
health ailments linked to, 4, 50, 168, 237
herbs/spices in treating, 154
incidence of, 237, *238*
mortality rate, 36, 50, 114, 146, 168, 237, 298, 332
obesity and, 276
oxidative stress and, 4
prevention of, 36
risk factors, 168
seaweed and risk of, 68, 71
in Siddha system, 133
treatments of, typical, 114
cardiovascular health
African plants, 237, 241–242
baicalein, 114–117, 120
balloon vine, 113, 132–133
black cumin, 148–154
Brazilian plants, 224, 226–227
Bridelia ferruginea, 236–237
Centella asiatica and, 57, *58*, 80, *81*
citrulline, 351–352
date palm tree/fruit, 164, 168–171, *170*
dietary oils, 43
flavonoids, 134–140, *134*, 171
fruits, **307**
herbs/spices, 51–58, *58*, *59*, 71, 86–87, **87**, 104–105,
        135, **135–136**, 154, 171, 208, **209**, 224, 226–227,
        307–308, 324–325, 341
Japanese diet, 22, 71
kalmegh and, 197, *198–201*, **202–203**, 204–208, *208*
Malaysian plants, 208, **209**
Mexican orchid, 263, 276
Momordica dioica, 322–324, *322*
mushrooms, 283–286

Index

373

oleic acid, 40–41
olive oil, 40–42, *40*
phenolic compounds, 41–42
pomegranate, 298–305, **298**, **307**
Terminalia arjuna, 94–95
triterpenes, 42
watermelon, 346–348, *347*
cardiovascular regulation, 348–349, *349*
carotenoids, 12, 165, 171, 346
caspase-3, 118, 170–171
catechins, 11
celery (*Apium graveolens* L.), 12
cell membrane properties, modification of, 137
Centella asiatica
in atherosclerosis inhibition, 84–85
cardiac hypertrophy inhibition and, 82, **84**
cardiovascular health and, 57, *58*, 80, *81*
chemical structure of, 79, *80*
description of, 78, *79*
diabetes management and, 83, **84**
endothelial function improvement and, 86, **87**
extraction of, 78
general usage of, 79–80
health promotion of, 79
historical perspective of, 79
in hyperlipidaemia management, 82–83, **84**
in hypertension management, 85
in myocardial infarction protection, 80–82
in obesity management, 82–83, **84**
toxicity/cautions, 87–88
in venous insufficiency improvement, 85–86
CH, *see* balloon vine (*Cardiospermum halicacabum*)
China Health and Nutrition Survey, 28
Chinese herbal medicine (CHM), 112, *112*
Chinese scholar tree, *see* Japanese pagoda tree
cholesterol
date palm tree/fruit, and 168–169
dyslipidaemia, 250, *251*, 299–300
function of, 299
high-density cholesterol and, 41, 299–300
hyperlipodaemia and, 82–83, **84**, 209, 283, 299
lipid metabolism and, 100–101
low-density lipoprotein and, 10, 41, 51, 54, 56, 71, 164, 236, 299–300, 306
triglyceride levels and, 306
triglycerides and, 23, 29, 52–53, 55–56, 71, 82, 250, 283–290, 299–300, 306, 324
very-low density lipoprotein and, 51, 56, 306
cinnamon, 307–308
cinnamon bark (*Tinospora cordifolia*), 57–58, *59*, 105
Circulatory Risk in Communities Study (CIRCS), 68
citrulline
arginine metabolism and, 348–349, *349*
cardiovascular health and, 351–352
cardiovascular regulation and, 348–349, *349*
cooperation with arginine in endothelial cells, *349*, 350–351
discovery of, 348
in endothelial function improvement, *349*, 350–351
general properties of, 348
heart and, 352–353
in inflammation management, 353
nitrogen homeostasis and, 348–349, *349*
sources of, 353
toxicity/cautions, 353

vessels and, 351–352
Citrullus lanatus, *see* watermelon
cocoa products, 13
coconut oil, 43
coenzyme 10 (CoQ), 10–11
collagen, 41, 99, 104, 116, *117*, 152–153, 197, 204, 339
Crataegus spp. (hawthorn), 51
C-reactive protein (CRP), 40, 56–57, 82, 103, 115, *116*, 133, 249, 263
Crinum zeylanicum (Amaryllidaceae), 341
crocin, 55
Crocus sativus L. (saffron), 55
cucurbitacin triterpenoids, 318–319, *318*, *319*
curcumin, 307
cyanidin glucoside, 306
cytokines, 52, 54, 57, 99, 102, 115, 118, 153, 165–166, 170, 206, 276, 300, 304–305, 323, 334

D

DASH-JUMP diet, 24
date palm tree/fruit (*Phoenix dactylifera*)
antioxidants in, 163
cardiovascular health and, 164, 168–171, *170*
cholesterol and, 168–169
description of, 162
edible parts of, **164**, 165–166, **167**, 168
experimental research on edible parts, 165–166, **167**, 168
flavonoids in, 164–165, **164**
general use of, 162–163
health promotion of, 163–165, *166*
lipid metabolism and, 168–169
magnesium in, 165
minerals in, 165
non-edible parts of, 162
parts of, 162
phenolic compounds in, 163–164, **164**
therapeutic properties of, 165, *166*
toxicity/cautions, 171
vitamins in, 165
diabetes
black cumin in managing, 148
cardiovascular system and, 273
Centella asiatica in managing, 83, **84**
Ganoderma lucidum in managing, 250–253
Mexican orchid in managing, 272–273, *272*
Momordica dioica in managing, 320, 324
pomegranate in managing, 302–303
diabetic cardiomyopathy, 273, 303, 306
diastolic blood pressure, 4–5
diazinon, 55
Dietary Approaches to Stop Hypertension (DASH) diet, 24–25
dietary fats/oils, *see also* olive oil
cardiovascular diseases and, 36
cardiovascular health and, 43
health promotion of, 36
monounsaturated fatty acids, 36, 40–41
polyunsaturated fatty acids, 36, 43
saturated fatty acids, 36–38
toxicity/cautions, 43
dietary fiber, 286–289
DNA/RNA oxidation, 7–8
doxorubicin (DOX), 96–97
dyslipidaemia, 250, *251*, 299–300

374 Index

E

ellagic acid, 302, 308
endothelial function improvement
  Centella asiatica and, 86, **87**
  citrulline and, *349*, 350–351
  kalmegh and, 206
  Momordica dioica and, 323
  olive oil and, 42
enzymatic activity, inhibition of, 138–139
epicatechin, 307
epigallocatechin, 138
ergothioneine (EGT), 289–290
E-selectin, 306
eugenol, 13
eupatilin, 180
EUROLIVE (Effect of Olive Oil Consumption on
  Oxidative Damage in European
  Populations), 41
European Food Safety Authority (EFSA), 36
extra virgin olive oil (EVOO), 36–37, 41

F

fasting plasma glucose (FPG), impaired, 303
fatty acid synthase (FAS), 305
fish oil, 43
5-Adenosine monophosphate-activated protein kinase
  (AMPK), 55
flavonoids
  in *Aloysia Paláu*, 225
  antioxidants in, 138
  in balloon vine, 131, 134–135, *134*
  in *Bridelai ferruginea*, 236
  cardiovascular health and, 134–140, *134*, 171
  cell membrane properties and, modification
    of, 137
  chemical structure of, 135
  in date palm tree/fruit, 164–165, **164**
  definition of, 112
  enzymatic activity and, inhibition of, 138–139
  in hypertension management, 11
  in inflammation management, 324
  ion channels and, modulation of, 137
  in kalmegh, 56
  metabolites and, *139*, 140
  in *Momordica dioica*, 314
  receptor perspective and, 138
  research on foods rich in, 323
  transporter mechanism and, 138
Food and Agriculture Organization of the
    United Nations Statistics Divsion
    database (FAOSTAT), 29
free radicals, 12–13, 97–98, 117–118, 138, 149, 205, 248,
    323–324
fruits, 171, **307**, *see also specific type*
fucoidan, 71

G

gambogic acid (GA), 333–335
Ganoderma lucidum
  antioxidants in, 248–249
  bioactive compounds in, 248, 325

chemical structure of, 250, *251*
clinical studies of, 252–253
description of, 248
in diabetes management, 250–253
in dyslipidaemia management, 250, *251*
general usage of, 248
in hypertension management, 249–250
in hypoglycaemia management, 250–252
in inflammation management, 249
names of, 248
peptidoglycans in, 248
polysaccharides in, 248
toxicity/cautions, 253
triterpenes in, 248
Garcinia genus, *see* saptrees
garcinol, 336
garlic (*Allium sativum*), 13, 55–56, 59, 308, 325
gerontoxanthone I, 336
ginger, 307
ginseng (*Panax ginseng*), 12, 325
Global Burden of Disease (GBD) database, 20
glucose tolerance, impaired, 303, *see also* diabetes
glut transporter (GLUT)-4 proteins, 138
Glycyrrhiza glabra (licorice), 13
green chiretta, *see* kalmegh
Guduchi, 57–58, *59*

H

hawthorn (*Crataegus* spp.), 51
Healthy Diet Indicator (HDI), 25
Healthy Eating Index (HEI) diet, 24–25
healthy life expectancy (HALE), 30, *31*
heart failure, 4, 7–8, 96, 100–101, 116–117, *117*, 152, 197,
    273, 275, 352
heart fibrosis, 152–154, *153*
heptoprotective activity of *Momordica dioica*, 321
herbal ghee, 104
herbal supplements, 323
herbs/spices, *see also specific type*
  in cardiovascular disease management/treatment, 135,
    135–136, 154
  cardiovascular health and, 51–58, *58*, *59*, 71, 86–87,
    87, 104–105, 154, 171, 208, **209**, 224, 226–227,
    307–308, 324–325, 341
  general usage of, 50
  health promotion of, 50–51
  as phytomedicine, 50
  toxicity/cautions, 58–59
high blood pressure, *see* hypertension
high-density lipoprotein (HDL), 41, 299–300
hijiki, 66
homocysteine, 133
honey balm (*Melissa officinalis*), 341
hydroxytyrosol, 41
hyperglycaemia, 283, *see* diabetes
hyperglyceridemia, 29
hyperlipodaemia, 82–83, **84**, 209, 283, 299
hypertension
  antioxidants and, decreased levels of, 6
  Artemisia genus in managing, 184, *184*, **185–186**,
    186–187
  baicalein in managing, 115–116, *116*
  Centella asiatica in managing, 85

Index 375

circle of, vicious, 301, *301*
coenzyme Q10 in managing, 10–11
definition of, 4–5, 301
DNA/RNA acid oxidation and, 7–8
essential, 302
flavonoids in managing, 11
Ganoderma lucidum in managing, 249–250
lipid peroxidation and, 7
metabolic disorders and, 5
Momordica dioica in managing, 322
mortality rate, 5
natural antioxidants in managing, 8–13, *9, 13*
nucleic acid oxidation and, 7–8
oxidative stress and, 6–7
phytochemicals in managing, 12–13
pomegranate in managing, 300–302
protein oxidation and, 7
reactive oxygen species and, 5–6, *6, 8*
Renin Angiotensin Aldosterone System and, 5–6, *5*
sirtuins in managing, 11
vitamin A in managing, 8
vitamin C in managing, 9–10
vitamin E in managing, 10
hypertriglycemia, 29, 289, 324
hypoglycaemia, 250–252, *251, 252,* 272–273, *272, see also*
        diabetes

I

inflammation
baicalein in mitigating, 118
black cumin in managing, 148–149, *149*
citrulline in managing, 353
cytokines and, 52, 54, 57, 99, 102, 115, 118, 153, 165–166,
        170, 206, 276, 300, 304–305, 323, 334
flavonoids in managing, 324
Ganoderma lucidum in managing, 249
heart fibrosis and, 153
kalmegh in managing, 205–206
lemon balm and, 54
Mexican orchid in managing, 273–274, *273*
Momordica dioica in managing, 323
myocarditis and, 198, 204
phenolic compounds in managing, 41
pomegranate in managing, 305–307
production of, 170
reactive oxygen species and, 115, 304
saptrees in managing, 333–335, *334*
Terminalia arjuna in managing, 101–104, *102*
vascular, 301
inflammation cytokines and, 52
insulin resistance, 272, *see also* diabetes
interleukin-6 receptor (IL-6), 304
interleukin-10 receptor (IL-10), 305
interleukin-18 receptor α (IL-18Rα), 101–102, *102*
ion channels, 137, 204–205
ischemia/reperfusion (I/R) injury, 117–119, *119*
ischemic heart disease (HID)
incidence of, 20, *20, 21,* 237, *238*
Japanese diet and, 20–22, *20, 21,* 28–29, *30*
mitochondrial dysfunction in, 238, *239*
seaweed and, 65–68, *69–70,* 70
isoproterenol (ISO), 98–100
iyya thamaraga noi, 133

J

Japan Collaborative Cohort Study for the Evaluation of
        Cancer Risk (JACC) Study, 67–68
Japanese diet
cardiovascular health and, 22, 71
description of, 19
dishes in, 21, *22*
Food Guide Spinning Top, 26–27, *26*
future of, 29–31
healthy life expectancy and, 30, *31*
intervention trial, 27–28
ischemic heart disease and, 20–22, *20, 21,* 28–29, *30*
obesity and, 29–30, *29*
score compared to other diets, 24–25
studies on usefulness of, 22–24
traditional score, 30
unique score of, 25–27, *29*
Japanese Diet Index (JDI), 24
Japanese pagoda tree (*Styphnolobium japonicum*
        L./*Sophora japonica*), 51–52
Japan Multi-Institutional Collaborative
        Cohort Study, 23
Japan National Health and Nutrition Survey
        (NHNS), 22
Japan Public Health Center-based prospective (JPHC)
        study, 21, 25, 66–67

K

kalmegh (*Andrographis paniculata*)
antioxidants in, 205
Ayurvedic formulations of, 196–197
cardiovascular health and, 197, *198–201,* **202–203,**
        204–208, *208*
description of, 194–196
direct cardioprotective mechanism of action, 197–198,
        198, 199, 201, **202–203,** 204–205
endothelial function improvement and, 206
flavonoids in, 56
general usage of, 196–197
health promotion of, 56
high fat diet-induced cardiac hypertrophy and, 204
indirect cardioprotective mechanism of action, 205–208, *208*
in inflammation management, 205–206
ion channels and, 204–205
in myocardial infarction protection, 204
in myocarditis protection and, 198, 204
phytochemicals in, 197, *198–201*
plant morphology of, *195,* 196
platelets and, 207
reactive oxygen species and, 205
taxonomic hierarchy of, 196, **196**
toxicity/cautions, 210
vascular muscle tone and, 206–208
King of Bitter, *see* kalmegh
kombu, 66
Korea National Health and Nutrition Examination
        Survey, 29

L

left ventricular end diastolic pressure (LVEDP), 99–101
left ventricular pressure (LVP), 99

lemon balm (*Melissa officinalis* L.), 54
Leonurus cardiaca L. (motherwort), 53
licorice (*Glycyrrhiza glabra*), 13
lingonberry (*Vaccinium vitis-idaea* L.), 52–53
Lingzhi, *see Ganoderma lucidum*
lipid metabolism, 100–101, 168–169
lipid oxidation (LPO), 7
lipid peroxidation, 7
liver glucose metabolism, 285, 288–289
liver lipid metabolism, 283–285, 287–289, *287*
Longevity Sciences-Longitudinal Study of Aging, 24
long pepper (*Piper longum* L.), 54–55
low-density lipoprotein (LDL), 10, 41, 51, 54, 56, 71, 163, 236, 299–300, 306
luteolin, 135, 138, 140, *140*, 180
lycopene, 12

M

macluraxanthone, 336
magnesium, 165
Malaysian plants and cardiovascular health, 208, **209**
manganese superoxide dismutase (MnSOD), 118
mango (*Mangifera indica*), 12–13
medicinal plants, 332, *see also specific type*
Mediterranean (MED) diet, 24–25, 36–37, 40
Melissa officinalis (honey balm), 341
Melissa officinalis extract (MOE), 54
Melissa officinalis L. (lemon balm), 54
metabolic disorders, 5, *see also specific type*
metabolites, *139*, 140, 154, 236, 333
Mexican orchid (*Prosthechea karwinskii*)
adiponectin levels and, 274, *275*
bioactive compounds in, 263, **264–271**
cardiovascular health and, 263, 276
cardiovascular risk and, decreasing, 276
chemical structure of, 263, **264–271**
description of, 260, *260*, 261
in diabetes management, 272–273, *272*
extraction, 261, *261*
general usage of, 261–262, *262*
historical perspective of, 261, *262*
in hypocglycaemia management, 272–273, *272*
in inflammation management, 273–274, *273*
knowledge of, medicinal, 260–261, *261*, *262*, **262**
pericardial fat and, 263, *272*
reactive oxygen species and, 275–276, **275**
toxicity/cautions, 276
weight loss and, 263, *272*
mitochondrial DNA (mtDNA), 7–8, 149–150
mitochondrial dysfunction, 238, *239*
mitophagy activation, 336, *337*
Moldenke, *see Aloysia Paláu* genus
Momordica dioica Roxb.
in allergy management, 321
analgesic activity of, 321
antibacterial activity of, 320
antifertility activity of, 321
antimalarial activity of, 321
antioxidants in, 321
antiulcer activity of, 321
antiviral property of, 321
in atherosclerosis inhibition, 322
in cancer management, 320–321

cardiovascular health and, 322–324, *322*
chemical composition of, 317, **317**
chemical structure of, 318, *318*
cucurbitacin triterpenoids in, 318–319, *318, 319*
description of, 314–316, *315*
in diabetes management, 320, 324
in endothelial function improvement, 323
ethnopharmacological properties of, 319–320, **320**
flavonoids in, 314
general usage, 315
habitat of, 315, *315*
hepatoprotective activity of, 321
historical perspective of, 315
in hypertension management, 322
in inflammation management, 323
in myocardial infarction inhibition, 324
nephroprotective activity of, 321
neuroprotective activity of, 321
nutritive value of, 316–317, **317**
parts of, 316
pharmacological activities of, 320–322
phytochemicals in, 316–317
toxicity/cautions, 325
Mondei white, 242
monocyte chemoattractant protein 1 (MCP-1), 304
monounsaturated fatty acids (MUFAs), 36, 40–41
motherwort (*Leonurus cardiaca* L.), 53
mukkutra thamaraga noi, 133
Multi-Ethnic Cohort study of Chinese, Malay, and Indian population, 29
mushrooms
atherosclerosis and, 285–286, 288–290
cardiovascular health and, 283–286
consumption of, 282
dietary fiber in, 286–289
ergothioneine in, 289–290
general usage of, 282–283
health promotion of, 282–283, *284*
in hyperglycaemia management, 283
in hyperlipidaemia, 283
liver glucose metabolism and, 285, 288–289
liver lipid metabolism and, 283–285, 287–289, *287*
mortality rate and, reduced, 282
overview, 282
polysaccharides in, 286–289, *287*
toxicity/cautions, 290
myocardial infarction (MI)
Bridelia ferruginea in protection from, 240–241
cell survival/death in, 239
Centella asiatica in protection from, 80–82
cross-talk between liver and heart during, 240
definition of, 238–239, 332
in heart mitochondria, 238, *239*
kalmegh in protection from, 204
Momordica dioica in inhibiting, 323
mortality rate, 352
oxidative stress and, 323
pathophysiology of, 237–238, *239*
permeability transition pore in, 240
saptrees in inhibiting, 335, *335*
Terminalia arjuna in protection from, 104
myocardial I/R injury, 117–119, *119*
myocarditis, 198, 204
myricetin, 11

Index

377

N

natural antioxidants, 8–13, *9*, *13*, *see also* phytochemicals
nephroprotective activity of *Momordica dioica*, 321
neuronal NOS, 137
neuroprotective activity of *Momordica dioica*, 321
Nigella sativa L., *see* black cumin
nitric oxide synthase, 137
nitrogen homeostasis, 348–349, *349*
non-alcoholic fatty liver disease (NAFLD), 283
nori, 66
NS, *see* black cumin
nucleic acid oxidation, 7–8
NUTRAOLEUM study, 42
Nutrient-Rich Food Index (NRF), 24

O

obesity
cardiovascular diseases and, 276
Centella asiatic in managing, 82–83, **84**
etiology, 304
fatty acid synthase and, 305
Japanese diet and, 29–30, *29*
pomegranate in managing, 303–305, *305*
Ohsaki National Health Insurance Cohort study, 23
Olea europaea, 36
oleic acid, 37, 40–41
oleuropein, 41
olive oil
cardiovascular health and, 40–42, *40*
chemical structure of, 38, *39*
composition of, 36–37
in endothelial function improvement, 42
extra virgin, 36–37, 41
Mediterranean diet in, 36, 43
oleic acid from, 40–41
phenolic compounds in, 41–42
toxicity/cautions, 43
triterpenes from, 42
types of, 37, *37*
virgin, 36–38, **38**, *39*, 40
oxidative stress
baicalein in inhibiting, 117–118
balloon vine and, 138
cardiovascular diseases and, 4
definition of, 5, 96, 138, 336
hyperglycemia-induced cardiac injury and, 303
hypertension and, 6–7
manganese superoxide dismutase in managing, 118
myocardial infarction and, 323
reactive oxygen species and, 6–7, *8*, 96

P

pakkavatham (stroke), 133–135
Panax ginseng (ginseng), 12, 325
peptides, 71
peptidoglycans, 248
pericardial fat, 263, *272*, 276
phenolic compounds
bioavailability of, 42, 305, *305*
cardiovascular health and, 41–42

in date palm tree/fruit, 163–164, **164**
in inflammation management, 41
in olive oil, 41–42
Phonenix dactylifera, *see* date palm tree/fruit
phytochemicals, *see also specific type*
in *Artemisia* genus, 180, **181–183**
in balloon vine, 134–135
in hypertension management, 12–13
in kalmegh, 197, *198–201*
in *Momoridica dioica*, 316–317
in part plants, different, **95**
toxicity/cautions, 13–14
phytomedicine, 50, *see also* herbs/spices
Piper betel (betel vine), 13
Piper longum L. (long pepper), 54–55
plasma lipids, 283, 286–287, 289
plasminogen activator inhibitor 1 (PAI-1), 304
platelet-derived growth factor (PDGF), 208
platelets aggregation, 41, 54–57, 101, 103, 115, 197, 207, 263, 272, 299, 338
polyphenols, 12–13, 165, 171
polysaccharides, 248, 286–289, *287*
polyunsaturated fatty acids (PUFAs), 36, 43
pomegranate (*Punica granatum*)
in atherosclerosis inhibition, 305–307
bioactive compounds in, 298–305, **298**
cardiovascular health and, 298–305, **298**, **307**
cyanidin glucoside in, 306
in diabetes management, 302–303
in dyslipideaemia management, 300
ellagic acid in, 302
E-selectin in, 306
ethanolic extract of peel of, 302
in hyperlipidaemia management, 299
in hypertension management, 300–302
in inflammation management, 305–307
in obesity management, 303–305, *305*
punicalagin in, 303
toxicity/cautions, 308
Prevention with Mediterranean Diet (PREDIMED) study, 40
Prosthechea karwinskii, *see* Mexican orchid
protein oxidation (PO), 7
Punica granatum, *see* pomegranate
punicalagin, 303

Q

quercetin, 11, 13, 54, 56, 131, 135, 137–138, 164, 180, 232, 236

R

reactive oxygen species (ROS), 96–98, *97*, 115
black cumin and, 149–151
electrons and, unpaired, 248
hypertension and, 5–6, *6*, *8*
inflammation and, 115, 304
kalmegh and, 205
Mexican orchid and, 275–276, **275**
oxidative stress and, 6–7, *8*, 96
protein oxidation and, 7
Terminalia arjuna and, 96–98, *97*
receptor perspective, 138

378   Index

red wine, 12
Renin Angiotensin Aldosterone System, 5–6, *5*
resources
books, 362, **364–365**
function of, 361
for health care professionals/patients, 362, **366–368**
investigative techniques, 362, **365–366**
other, 368
professional societies, 362, **363–364**
regulatory bodies, 362, **362–363**
Resveratrol, 12–13
retinoids, 8
rutin, 56, 135, 138, 164

S

saffron (*Crocus sativus* L.), 55
salt intake, 21–24, 71
saptrees (*Garcinia* genus)
antioxidants in, 336–338
apoptosis and, 335–336, *335*
in atherosclerosis inhibition, 338–339
cardiac remodeling and, 339–340, *340*
description of, 332–333
gambogic acid in, 333–335
garcinol in, 336
general usage of, 333
gerontoxanthone I in, 336
in inflammation management, 333–335, *334*
macluraxanthone in, 336
medicinal potential of, 333
metabolites in, 333
mitophagy activation and, 336, *337*
in myocardial infarction inhibition, 335, *335*
species, 332
toxicity/cautions, 341
vascular remodeling and, 340–341
saturated fatty acids (SFAs), 36–38
seaweed
cancer and, 67–68
cardiovascular disease risk and, 68, 71
CIRCS Study, 68
consumption, 65–66
ischemic heart disease and, 65–68, *69–70*, 70
JACC Study, 67–68
JPHC Study, 66–67
meta-analysis of evidence, 68, *69–70*, 70
nutrients in, 65
toxicity/cautions, 71–72
types of, 66
seizure management, 148
selenium, 162
sirtuins, 11
Sophora japonica (Japanese pagoda tree), 51–52
spices, *see* herbs/spices; *specific type*
squalene, 236
stroke, 133–135
Styphnolobium japonicum L. (Japanese pagoda tree), 51–52
sunflower oil, 36, 43
systolic blood pressure, 4–5, **5**, 11

T

Takayama Cohort study, 27
Terminalia arjuna (Roxb.)

in Ayurvedic medicine, 95–96
bark extracts, 96, 100, 105
cardiotonic behavior of, in clinical trials, 101
cardiovascular health and, 94–95
cellular aspects of, 104
description of, 94–95
general usage of, 95–96
in inflammation management, 101–104, *102*
lipid metabolism and, 100–101
in myocardial infarction protection, 104
physiological aspects of, 96
reactive oxygen species and, 96–98, *97*
toxicity/cautions, 105
Terminalia arjuna aqueous extract (TAAE), 96–102, *97,*
        102, 104
thrombin, 207
thymol, 151
thymoquinone, 13–14
Tinospora cordifolia (cinnamon bark), 57–58, *59*, 105
tomato/tomato extract, 12
toxicity/cautions
Aloysia Paláu genus, 220
Artemisia genus, 187
baicalein, 120
balloon cine, 131, 140
black cumin, 154
Bridelia ferruginea, 241–242
Centella asiatica, 87–88
citrulline, 353
date palm tree/fruit, 171
dietary oils, 43
Ganoderma lucidum, 253
herbs/spices, 58–59
kalmegh, 210
Mexican orchid, 276
Momordica dioica, 325
mushrooms, 290
olive oil, 43
phenolic compounds, 42–43
phytochemicals, 13–14
pomegranate, 308
saptrees, 341
seaweed, 71–72
Termninalia arjuna, 105
watermelon, 353
Traditional Chinese Medicine (TCM), 112, *112*, 197, 248
traditional medicine, 232, 261
trans fatty acids, 36
transporter mechanism, 138
triglycerides, 23, 29, 52–53, 55–56, 71, 82, 250, 283–290,
    299–300, 306, 324
triterpenes, 42, 57, 83, 85–86, 248, 316–319, *318, 319*,
    321

U

ulcer protection, 321
Unani system of medicine, 79

V

Vaccinium vitis-idaea L. (lingonberry), 52–53
vali thamaraga noi, 133
vascular action/muscle tone, 119, *119*, 206–208
vascular remodeling, 340–341

Index

vegetables, 171, *see also specific type*
venous insufficiency improvement, 85–86
very-low-density lipoprotein (VLDL), 51, 56, 306
virgin olive oil (VOO), 36–38, **38**, *40*, 43
virus protection, 321
vitamin A, 8
vitamin C, 9–10
vitamin E, 10, 237
vitamins, 165, *see also specific type*

W

wakame, 66
watermelon (*Citrullus lanatus*), *see also* citrulline
antioxidants in, 346
cardiovascular health and, 346–348, *347*

description of, 346
general usage of, 346
health promotion of, 13
historical perspective of, 346
toxicity/cautions, 353
Wellcome Collection, 368
WHO-Coordinated Cardiovascular Diseases and Alimentary Comparison study, 22
Wight and Arn, *see Terminalia arjuna* (Roxb.)
Withania somnifera stem, 105
World Health Organization (WHO), 22, 25, 50, 114, 154, 314

Z

Zingiberaceae (*Aframomum pruinosum*), 341

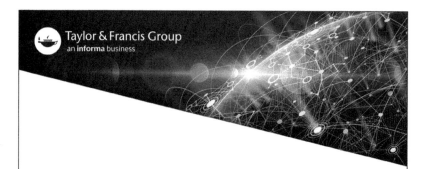

9781032115344